e Art and Scienc
⁺al Health Nursing

f Principles and Practice

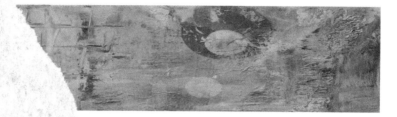

Second Edition

The Art and Science of Mental Health Nursing

A Textbook of Principles and Practice

Second Edition

Edited by Ian Norman and Iain Ryrie

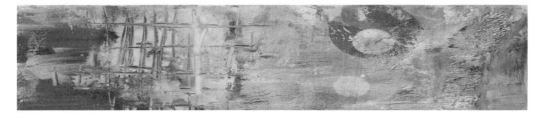

McGraw Hill

Open University Press

Open University Press
McGraw-Hill Education
McGraw-Hill House
Shoppenhangers Road
Maidenhead
Berkshire
England
SL6 2QL

email: enquiries@openup.co.uk
world wide web: www.openup.co.uk

and Two Penn Plaza, New York, NY 10121—2289, USA

First published 2009

A catalogue record of this book is available from the British Library

ISBN-10: 0-335-22293-5
ISBN-13: 978-0335-22293-3

Library of Congress Cataloguing-in-Publication Data
CIP data applied for

Typeset by Kerrypress Ltd, Luton, Bedfordshire
Printed in the UK by Bell and Bain Ltd, Glasgow

Fictitious names of companies, products, people, characters and/or data that may be used herein (in case studies or in examples) are not intended to represent any real individual, company, product or event.

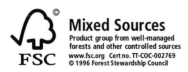

Mixed Sources
Product group from well-managed
forests and other controlled sources
www.fsc.org   Cert no. TT-COC-002769
© 1996 Forest Stewardship Council
FSC

The **McGraw·Hill** Companies

To our fathers: Ken and Tom

Contents

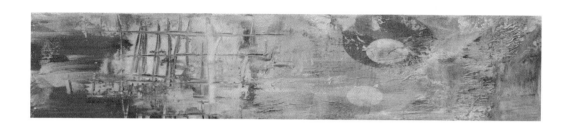

PART 5 Core procedures · 619

PART 6 Future directions · 747

Contributors

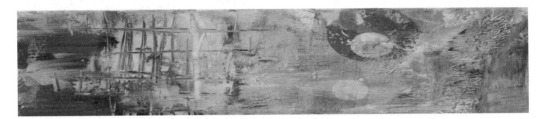

Anne Aiyegbusi, West London Mental Health NHS Trust, St Bernard's Hospital, Middlesex, UK.

Robin Basu, Child Psychiatrist, Surrey Oaklands NHS Trust, Epsom, Surrey, UK.

Geoff Brennan, Nurse Consultant Psychosocial Interventions, Berkshire Healthcare NHS Trust, Prospect Park Hospital, Berkshire, UK.

Daniel Bressington, Senior Lecturer in Mental Health, The Department of Social Work, Community and Mental Health, Faculty of Health and Social Care, Canterbury Christ Church University, Canterbury, Kent, UK.

Heather Castillo, Chief Executive, The Haven Project, Colchester, Essex, UK.

Howard Chadwick, Senior Lecturer in Mental Health, Faculty of Health and Social Care Sciences, Kingston University and St George's London University, Honorary Tutor and Researcher at the Institute of Psychiatry, King's College London, UK.

Philip Confue, Head of Mental Health, Tribal Consulting, Plymouth, UK.

Jacqueline Curthoys, Publisher and manic depressive, London, UK.

Graham Durcan, Research and Development Manager, Criminal Justice Programme, the Sainsbury Centre for Mental Health, London, UK.

Alison Faulkner, Independent Service User Consultant, London, UK.

Philip Fennell, Professor, Cardiff University Law School, UK.

Richard Ford, Director, National Institute for Mental Health in England, South-East Development Centre, Basingstoke, UK.

Lynne Friedli, Mental Health Promotion Specialist, London, UK.

Catherine Gamble, Consultant Nurse, South West London and St George's Mental Health NHS Trust, UK.

Judith Gellatly, Department of Health Research Fellow, School of Nursing, Midwifery and Social Work, University of Manchester, UK.

Lina Gega, Lecturer in Health Psychology, School of Medicine, University of East Anglia, UK.

Richard Gray, Professor, School of Nursing, University of East Anglia, UK.

Sue Gurney, Head of Nurse Education, Surrey and Borders Partnership NHS Trust, Epsom, Surrey, UK.

Kevin Hope, Senior Lecturer, University of Manchester, UK.

John Keady, Professor, School of Nursing, Midwifery and Social Work, University of Manchester, UK.

Stephan Kirby, Senior Lecturer in Forensic Mental Health, School of Health and Social Care, University of Teesside, UK.

Cheryl Kipping, Nurse Consultant, Alcohol and Addiction Service, Maudsley Hospital, London, UK.

Karina Lovell, Professor, School of Nursing, Midwifery and Social Work, University of Manchester, UK.

Andrew McCulloch, Chief Executive, Mental Health Foundation, London, UK.

Steve Morgan, Practice Development Consultant for Mental Health, Blackheath, London, UK.

Ian Noonan, Lecturer, Mental Health Section, Florence Nightingale School of Nursing and Midwifery, King's College London, UK.

Ian Norman, Professor, Florence Nightingale School of Nursing and Midwifery, King's College London, UK.

Kingsley Norton, Consultant Psychiatrist in Psychotherapy, Head of Psychotherapy, St Bernard's Hospital, Middlesex, UK.

Steve Onyett, Senior Development Consultant, Care Service Improvement Partnership SW (incorporating NIMHE), Bristol, UK.

Jane Padmore, Lead Clinician, Lambeth CAMHS, South London and Maudsley NHS Foundation Trust, UK.

Sean Page, Clinical Nurse Specialist, Manchester Mental Health and Social Care Trust, and Teaching Fellow, School of Nursing, Midwifery and Social Work, University of Manchester, UK.

Jean Penny, Professor, NHS Institute for Innovation and Improvement, University of Warwick, UK.

Rachel Perkins, Clinical Director of Quality Assurance and User/Carer Experience, South West London and St George's Mental Health NHS Trust, London, UK.

Karen Pilkington, Senior Research Fellow, School of Integrated Health, University of Westminster, London, UK.

Chris Prestwood, Acting Children's Service Manager and Clinical Co-ordinator, Eating Disorders Service, Truro Health Office, Truro, UK.

Hagen Rampes, Consultant Psychiatrist and Honorary Clinical Senior Lecturer, North East CMHT, Middlesex, UK.

Debbie Robson, Programme Leader and Research Nurse in Medication Management, Section of Mental Health Nursing, Health Services and Population Research, Institute of Psychiatry, King's College London, UK.

Julie Repper, Professor, Faculty of Health and Wellbeing, Sheffield Hallam University, UK.

Iain Ryrie, Consultant, Tribal Consulting Limited, London, UK.

Susan Sookoo, Head of Mental Health Care Department, Florence Niightingale School of Nursing and Midwifery, King's College London, UK.

Marc Thurgood, Specialist Practitioner in Community Mental Health Nursing, South London and Maudsley NHS Trust, UK.

Andrew Wetherell, Co-director, ARW Mental Health Training and Consultancy, Essex, UK.

Toby Williamson, Associate Head of Service Improvement and Workforce Development, Mental Health Foundation, London, UK.

Victoria Yeates, Senior Lecturer in Law, University of Glamorgan Law School, UK.

Preface

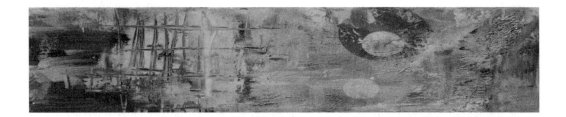

The first edition of this book, published in 2004, quickly became a best-seller and is now an established core text for mental health nurses who are trained and in training. This second edition has been extended and revised substantially to incorporate changes to the policy context of mental health nursing, the legal framework of mental health care within the UK, advances in treatment and changes in the philosophy and principles of mental health care.

Our aim, as for the first edition, has been to produce a comprehensive textbook for mental health nurses and students in training, which takes account of the diversity of mental health nursing as a practice discipline and the contemporary context in which nursing is practised. In so doing we have sought to avoid the tendency of debates within academic nursing, and some other textbooks, to present a restrictive concept of mental health nursing as a uni-dimensional activity – typically as an 'art' concerned with nurses' therapeutic relationships with 'people' in distress, or as a 'science', concerned with evidence-based interventions that can be applied to good effect by nurses, often working in what might be seen as extended roles, to 'patients' with defined mental illness. The polarized views expressed by both artists and scientists within mental health nursing are becoming less relevant today than previously as the focus of mental health care changes towards an emphasis on promoting social inclusion and recovery, reducing social stigma and supporting principles such as choice. Thus, evidence-based practice and interventions are now framed within a recovery-oriented approach which emphasizes the central place of the person with mental health problems and the impact of services upon his/her life journey, rather than the place of the patient within mental health services. In reality, practising nurses must be artists and scientists simultaneously and they need to find ways of integrating these elements while meeting policy directives for mental health services and service users' demands. This book seeks to be a resource to practising nurses to help them meet this remit.

It seems to us that any contemporary account of mental health nursing as a practice discipline needs to establish its case within three broad parameters:

- professional diversity;
- national policy; and
- service users' expectations.

Professional diversity

We avoid aligning the discipline of mental health nursing to any one theoretical perspective but, rather, acknowledge the breadth and complexity of the perspectives upon which mental health nurses draw in their work. The title of this book reflects our aim, therefore, which is to provide an integrative account of the discipline that accommodates its many origins, influences and practices. To assist this process we introduce a schema in Chapters 1 and 2 which integrates explanatory models of mental health and illness, and which demonstrates each one's crucial, though partial, contribution to our understanding of the human condition. We contend that all mental health nursing, whatever its origin or theoretical basis, can be mapped onto this schema. Further, no one part of the schema is, itself, adequate to deal with people's changing needs in relation to mental health and mental illness.

National policy

The UK National Health Service (NHS) and social care provision have long been subject to government policy. As a consequence professionals who work in these organizations must be expected to adjust their practice to meet contemporary demands. This second edition of this book, as with the first, is anchored in the National Service Framework (NSF) for Mental Health (DH 1999), and subsequent policy documents which together provide a blueprint for the development of mental health services in the United Kingdom (UK) into the future. The first edition of this book pre-empted the findings of the Chief Nursing Officer for England's (2006) review of mental health nursing in its call for mental health nurses to incorporate the principles of recovery into their work with service users and focus on improving their health outcomes. In looking to the future this new edition reflects moves internationally to widen the focus of mental health services from a concern with individuals suffering from mental disorder and their families to improve the mental health of communities and populations as a whole. We do not advocate substituting individual care with population and public health perspectives but we do argue the need for mental health nurses to incorporate these perspectives into their work. Chapter 6 deals with mental health policy specifically, and the content of subsequent chapters is shaped by the policy context within which mental health nurses operate. While most examples reflect practice in the UK context we have tried to produce a text that is not too parochial and which can cross geographical boundaries.

Service-user perspectives

An important tenet that underpins this textbook is our belief that mental health nursing is concerned primarily with helping people find meaning and purpose in their lives, and assisting them in the process of recovery. Nurses cannot do this adequately unless they (we) are prepared to hear service users' accounts of their difficulties and appreciate their own preferences for a meaningful life. This fact is so central to understanding how mental health nurses can help that we have sought to make it explicit throughout the book, rather than confine it to a single chapter. Thus, each contributor incorporates user perspectives into their chapter. The terminology used to describe recipients of mental health services does however vary between contributors. There are chapters that use the term 'patient' and others that refer to 'service user' or to 'clients'; these terms tell us something about the perspective that the contributor brings to bear on their work. Following the introduction of the schema in Chapters 1 and 2, which is used to integrate explanatory models of mental health and illness, it follows that all perspectives are valid though each is partial. We have, therefore, chosen not to standardize these terms (into service user, for example), but have allowed contributors to speak for themselves.

Content and organization

The book is divided into six parts. Part 1, Foundations, deals with the historical origins and contemporary basis of mental health nursing. Chapter 1 introduces a schema that provides an integrative account of the many and varied factors that influence our sense of mental health and well-being. In Chapter 2 the schema is used to explore a range of aetiological theories for understanding mental illness, and Chapter 3 provides a detailed account of mental health promotion and public mental health. Chapter 4 examines the origins and traditions of mental health nursing, and Chapter 5 deals with recovery and social inclusion as a fundamental orientation for contemporary care.

Part 2, Contexts, considers the policy context (Chapter 6) and the legislative and ethical frameworks (Chapter 7) within which mental health nurses practise. The other two chapters in this part of the book consider the organization of mental health services through a consideration of functional teams and whole systems (Chapter 8) and also how these services can be continually improved and developed (Chapter 9).

Part 3, Interventions, incorporates eight chapters that represent the main therapeutic approaches available to nurses in their work. Two chapters are devoted to assessment (Chapters 10 and 11), and one chapter examines the concept of therapeutic milieus in the context of contemporary inpatient care settings (Chapter 12). The other chapters in this part of the book deal with lifestyle interventions (Chapter 13), psychosocial interventions (Chapter 14), psychopharmacological and complementary therapies (Chapters 16 and 17), and physical health care of people suffering from mental disorder (Chapter 15).

Part 4, Client groups, examines the major challenges confronting those who use mental health services and outlines evidence-based interventions available to the mental health nurse. Each of the nine chapters in this section is oriented to a particular type or group of disorders that a person can experience (Chapters 18–26).

Part 5, Core procedures, covers the fundamental processes of mental health nursing care. The chapters here have a very practical orientation. They are concerned with the 'know-how' of mental health nursing, with the skills needed by nurses working in partnership with clients in any care setting. Chapters 27 and 28 discuss how to engage clients in treatment and work with them to identify and solve their problems. Chapter 29 focuses on the contribution of self-help and how nurses can work with clients to foster self-care. Chapters 30, 31 and 32 are concerned with the practical application of behavioural and cognitive techniques with clients and the management of their medication; these chapters demonstrate application of some of the interventions previously discussed in Part 2. Chapters 33 and 34 are concerned with the therapeutic management of psychiatric emergencies; of aggression and violence and attempted suicide and self-harm.

Part 6, Future directions, is devoted to anticipated future developments for mental health nursing (Chapter 35).

Each chapter is preceded by an overview which outlines its scope and content and concludes with a set of bullet points to summarize the main points, questions for reflection and discussion, and an annotated bibliography which points the reader towards more detailed reading. Case studies are used within some chapters to illustrate the practical application of the material. This new edition is supported by a website, which can be accessed at www.openup.co.uk/normanryrie. Though written primarily for mental health nurses and nursing students the book aims also to provide a useful reference for other health care professionals, lay carers and for people with mental health problems.

We owe the success of the first edition of this book to our excellent contributors, a number of whom have also contributed to this second edition in which they have been joined by 20 new authors. The book's contributors have been chosen to reflect the many diverse professional perspectives within mental health care. All are experts in their field and in writing their chapter each was asked to draw upon their specialist knowledge and practice rather than try to relate their subject to a narrow definition of mental health nursing.

Without the commitment and patience of each author, this book would not have been written. We are grateful to each of them for taking time out of their busy lives to produce their chapters. This book will have been successful if it goes some small way to helping mental health nurses become skilful, well-informed and sensitive practitioners who work confidently in the context of mental health services to promote mental health and in partnership with service users to help them regain control over their lives.

Ian Norman and Iain Ryrie
London, UK

References

Department of Health (1999) The National Service Framework for Mental Health. London: DH.
Chief Nursing Officer (England) (2006) Review of Mental Health Nursing: from values to action. London: DH.

Foreword

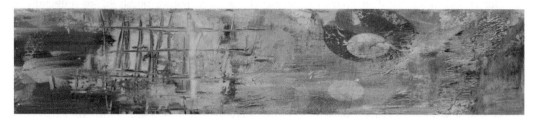

A good textbook functions as a mirror. Superficially it only reflects appearances, such as established policy, procedures and interventions. But a good observer can also detect changes over time, such as the introduction of new concepts and their popularity and, with some caution, can anticipate future directions. This book on mental health nursing offers plenty of the core content of a textbook for mental health nursing, but also sends a strong signal about the scope and priorities of mental health care in general. Changes from the previous edition are highly significant.

An important change, and no doubt a powerful signal of intent, is the placing of the chapter on Mental health at the beginning of this book. The term 'mental health' is increasingly ambiguous, since too often it is used as a euphemism for mental illness, but not so here. It is only very recent that the scope of mental health care has been broadened to cover concepts such as mental health promotion and prevention at population level within books designed for practitioners. This reflects the challenge for governments to address the burden of disease posed by mental disorders, the largest cause of disability in Western countries, and the importance to develop comprehensive services, including promotion and prevention. It is not a coincidence that intergovernmental agencies, such as the World Health Organization and the European Community, give growing attention to the exploration of activities that strengthen well-being and resilience of the population. A key question is who should be responsible for delivering such interventions. Are nurses primarily focusing on people with mental disorders, or is an essential part of their responsibility the prevention of mental health problems? This book suggests a strong shift in the latter direction, although rightly at the heart of the book remain the parts dealing with interventions, client groups and core procedures.

However, the titles and content of the chapters in these parts also show that mental health care in general, and nursing specifically, have liberated themselves from their traditional care and support roles to embrace treatment and patient centred models of care, having discovered that clients are active and essential participants in their recovery. The chapters on self-help, lifestyle options and psychosocial interventions reinforce this message. In past books on psychiatric nursing it was surprising how many pages could be covered with information about a limited range of supportive care in hospital settings. In this modern book it is astonishing how much diverse and complex material is covered in its 34 chapters, each deserving a book in its own right. Nurses have moved on in a very short time to become experts in a wide range of topics and working in a large number of settings.

Faced with so many potential skills and roles as presented in this book, all requiring education and training, it is obviously impossible for any person to achieve expertise in all. This poses a question about mental health nursing as a generic profession or as an assortment of specialist practitioners. Probably the decision point has already been passed, if not yet formalized, with the proliferation of higher degree courses and specialist treatment settings, varying from primary care to forensic hospitals. It can be predicted that mental health nursing will soon be used as a collective term that branches off into growing levels of sub-specialization. The role of a book such as this is to provide a compendium of knowledge, a point of reference for what is held in common.

The growing specialization is common across the workforce, and this raises a question at a higher level, which is the differentiation between groups active in mental health care. Originally staff groups had their origin in different roles in hospital settings, such as doctors, occupational therapists, psychologists and social workers. This resulted in considerable tensions in multi-disciplinary teams when settings and challenges changed, since nurses were no longer content to fill the gap between psychologists offering assessments and therapies and social workers addressing financial, employment and family issues. Nurses considered themselves sharing many of the objectives and competencies. It is telling that most of these are covered in this book. Is this book therefore marking boundaries around the core competencies of nursing, or could this book be of equal value to other staff groups, aiming to address shared areas of importance to mental health care in general? For me, it has achieved to find a compromise, interpreting common themes of importance from a nursing perspective, thus defining nursing as a unique area of practice with its own set of values, while scrutinizing all available evidence in a very open-minded fashion.

A final question of interest to me is whether this wide-ranging book has value beyond the UK. It is no doubt very much ahead of its time in countries that still heavily rely on asylums and traditional staff divisions, but it might be read even there as a vision of the future, of what can be achieved. In some European countries much of the book is of immediate relevance, and some of its content has the potential to assist the development of policies and new ways of working internationally. I would be happy to carry around copies on my travels, and hand them out to leaders of the profession.

I have no doubt that this very well-considered and innovative book has the potential to challenge and inform, and therefore to change practice, nationally and internationally, and that it will be strongly welcomed.

Matt Muijen
Regional Advisor for Mental Health World Health Organization (WHO) Europe

Technology to enhance learning and teaching

Vist **www.openupco.uk/normanryrie** *today*

Online Learning Centre (OLC)

After completing each chapter, log on to the supporting Online Learning Centre website. Take advantage of the study tools offered to reinforce the material you have read in the text, and to develop your knowledge of psychology in a fun and effective way.

Resources for students include:

- *Additional material on law and ethics*
- *Reflections from the authors on the end-of-chapter learning activities*
- *Links to useful websites*
- *Links to annotated bibliography*

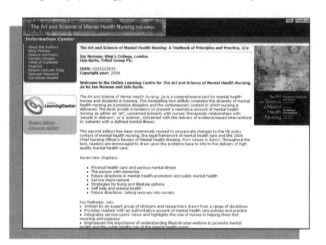

Foundations

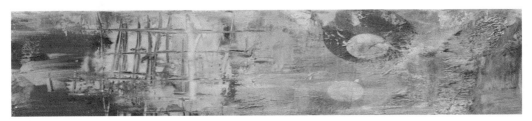

Chapter contents

CHAPTER 1

Mental health

Iain Ryrie and Ian Norman

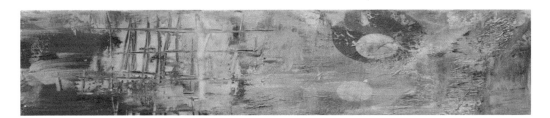

Chapter overview

    " There is no health without mental health.

(World Health Organization 2007) **"**

Whether you begin this book as a student nurse or an experienced practitioner the World Health Organization's (WHO) assertion sets a significant challenge for mental health nursing. It certainly implies that physical health counts for little if people do not also enjoy mental health. Cardiovascular fitness or an immune system that provides protection from the common cold may be of little value to a person who is in the depths of depression or experiencing an acute episode of schizophrenia. But the WHO's assertion is, in fact, more profound. Whatever people experience is dependent on their mental faculties since all of life is realized through mental awareness. In its most rudimentary form, mental health is the culmination of everything that comes into human awareness, and if mental health is 'everything', then safeguarding and promoting mental health is perhaps the ultimate nursing challenge.

Paradoxically, in most practice contexts mental health has usually meant mental illness. Mental health nurses in the UK work in a national health service that deals with illness, apply the Mental Health Act where there is evidence of illness, and care for people with mental health problems which, in many cases, are severe and debilitating illnesses. This is not an indictment of the profession but rather a sign of the times through which it has developed. One hundred years ago most people, by and large, would have had their life course set from birth. Individual opportunity was subservient to family and community expectations. Nowadays people are much more likely to believe that 'the world is their oyster' and to value individual opportunity more highly than family or community ties. While this attitude of mind may be regarded as a good thing, loss of a sense of community has, in our view, highlighted its importance to our sense of mental health. Similarly, 100 years ago people could not have known what planet earth looked like from space, nor understand the fragility of its biosphere and the dynamic systems that maintain life. Now this is understood, there is in many people an unsettling awareness, a degree of angst not previously experienced as they have come to understand the importance of the environment to their mental health. As so often in life, it is only when something is lost or depleted that its true quality and worth becomes apparent. This is true of mental health, which in recent decades as a word and as a concept has emerged in the collective consciousness, freed from illness and born independently as a concept in its own right.

In this opening chapter we introduce a simple framework which may be used to map everything that is possibly within human experience. The framework is used as a starting point for understanding mental health and some contemporary definitions of mental health are presented and mapped onto the framework. The chapter then demonstrates how mental health arises from the integration of all that we experience and fluctuates as all things relative to it change. The emergence of mental health as a complex, integral phenomenon is clarified and its implications for the work of mental health nurses are explored. The reader is also signposted to subsequent chapters in which these themes are developed further. In summary this chapter covers:

- A framework for everything;
- The nature of mental health;
- Definitions of mental health;
- Integral mental health;
- Implications for nursing.

A framework for everything

It may seem a little ambitious if foolhardy to present a framework for everything that is within human experience. However, there have been important developments in this respect over the last 30 years. The experience and reflections of all major human civilizations from pre-modern to post-modern times are now open to study and there has been an extensive search by evolutionary psychologists for a comprehensive map of human potentials (Beck and Cowan 1996; Wilber 2001, 2007). Some deceptively simple and elegant patterns have emerged from this search.

To begin with there are just two key dimensions that capture everything that is within human experience. The first of these is quite easy to discern; me and you, I and we, mine and theirs. This dimension simply differentiates between what is you and what is everything else, what is 'self' and what is 'other'. Within the context of this chapter 'community' is substituted for 'other' so that the first dimension runs from 'self' to 'community'.

The second dimension is a little more subtle but equally encompassing. Human beings have an interior, subjective sense of themselves but also an exterior objective-self. The former includes thoughts and feelings and the latter the physical body, which includes its organs, chemical and physical structures. The subjective-self can be described, even written down but remains wholly within a person's own experience and is not directly accessible to others. The objective-self can be quantified and measured, and in this sense is accessible to the direct experience of others who may be doing the measuring. It also follows that communities have interior (subjective) and exterior (objective) characteristics. The second dimension therefore runs from 'subjective' to 'objective' and when crossed with the first dimension from 'self' to 'community' formulates a four quadrant schema or framework (Figure 1.1).

Figure 1.1 contains reference to the physical and psychosocial elements that arise within each quadrant. Thus, from the subjective-self quadrant a person formulates their personal intentions while it is from the subjective-community quadrant that a collective sense of culture is forged. From the objective-self arises behaviours that can be observed and

	Subjective	Objective
Self	Interior individual Intentional (upper-left)	Exterior individual Behavioural (upper-right)
Community	Interior collective Cultural (lower-left)	Exterior collective Social (lower-right)

Figure 1.1: Framework of Human Experience I (After Wilber, 2001)

measured while in the objective-community reside social systems and structures. Thus, the framework incorporates everything that is within human awareness and provides an important starting point for understanding the nature of mental health.

The nature of mental health

This section describes the quadrants and provides some examples of the contribution each makes to people's sense of mental health. To a certain extent this is an artificial exercise since no quadrant acts in isolation or can be completely responsible on its own for an individual's experience of mental health. There is some inevitable overlap of information therefore as each of the quadrants is discussed. This is a useful starting point however and a more integral account is provided further on in the chapter.

Objective-self

In the upper right or objective-self quadrant reside the physical attributes of an individual. This includes a person's anatomical form and biochemical functioning as well as their physical behaviours. It also includes a person's genes.

Genes

Genetic determinism is a highly contested area though the current weight of opinion is against the idea that genes alone are responsible for most complex traits (Strohman 2003). Interactions between DNA and signals from other genes as well as from the environment influence the development of a trait. Within such a context it is hard to follow a deterministic line. Dobbs (2007) reports conclusions drawn by the Nobel Prize winning neuroscientist Eric Kandel, who states that genes are not simply the determinants of behaviour but are also the servants of the environment. Genes have an integral role to play in the human condition as Figure 1.1 suggests, rather than a starring role as many neuroscientists had originally thought. In essence this means that much can be done by people to promote and maintain good mental health regardless of any genetic load they may have inherited.

Anatomical form

Anatomical form and in particular the different regions and aspects of the brain are key factors that influence a person's sense of mental health. Of particular importance are the reptilian brain stem, the limbic system or mammalian brain and the cerebrum, each of which represents a seismic leap in the evolution of the human being. The reptilian brain stem drives many of our basic instincts such as the need for food and water. It also stimulates sensorimotor actions essential for self-preservation including reflexes and fight or flight impulses. It is focused in a rather limited way on self, on the preservation of 'me'.

The mammalian brain or limbic system evolved millions of years after the reptilian brain and provides more sophisticated functions including the generation of feelings, desires, emotions, sexual impulses and interpersonal needs. Common to all mammals is their tendency to protect and nurture their young, and to a lesser extent, to experience and communicate empathy. This aspect of the brain introduced a collective sense of 'us' rather than just the limited 'me' of the reptilian brain. It is these qualities that allow humans to forge meaningful relationships with other mammals such as horses, dogs and dolphins. There is now a wealth of evidence that demonstrates pet ownership and pet therapy can engender emotional bonds that support mental health (e.g. Servan-Schreiber 2004).

The cerebrum is the rational, analytical brain that evolved only 200,000 years ago. It governs visual processing, sound, speech, calculation and pattern matching. It integrates several functions such as thinking, analysing, conceptualizing and planning. It has allowed humans to develop the written language and to generate ideas and concepts (Plant and Stephenson 2008). It is now recognized that different aspects of a person's brain are associated with different experiences of mental health (or illness). In particular the older reptilian and mammalian brains generate feelings and emotions, the cerebrum registers those feelings and enables people to express them and to a certain extent control them.

The mammalian brain is also responsible for the physiological functioning of the body's organs. The autonomic nervous system begins in the mammalian brain and spreads throughout the body via two distinct branches; the sympathetic and the parasympathetic nervous systems. The former releases the hormones adrenaline and noradrenaline, which focus a person's attention on threats, increases their heart rate and determines a fight or flight response. The latter releases acetylcholine, which induces relaxation, slows the heart rate and generates calm. This is why humans literally feel their emotions. The sympathetic nervous system creates some of the most unpleasant physical symptoms associated with anxiety and depression including rapid or irregular heartbeats, dry mouth and cold sweats (Plant and Stephenson 2008).

Being able to feel emotions for what they are and to understand and respond to them appropriately is important to mental health (see subjective-self). Achieving a balance between the emotional (mammalian) brain and cognitive (cerebrum) brain is therefore necessary but so is a balance between the sympathetic and parasympathetic nervous systems. Dominant sympathetic activity leads to feelings of acute anxiety, edginess and ultimately emotional and physical exhaustion. Too much parasympathetic activity leads to understimulation, disengagement and blunted feelings.

The cognitive brain can respond well to talking therapies, which assist people to better control feelings and their impact. However, the emotional brain does not respond only to language and may be better cared for by other means; these are considered in detail later.

Biochemical functioning

The biochemical functioning of the human brain and autonomic nervous system is too vast a subject to cover in any detail here. However, there are a number of key functions that mental health nurses should be aware of, particularly the role of neurotransmitters, which control the electrical circuits of the brain and nervous system by allowing messages to transfer between the nerve cells or neurons. If levels of key neurotransmitters become depleted or unbalanced then the electrical circuits will not function properly and mental health is threatened.

Plant and Stephenson (2008) provide a useful account of the role of neurotransmitters. Table 1.1 presents an overview of what are considered to be some of the most important neurotransmitters for mental health. Reference is also made to these chemicals in Chapter 13.

Neurotransmitter	Type of effect
Glutamate	Excitory, agitating
Gamma-aminobutyric acid (GABA)	Inhibitory, calming
Dopamine	Physical arousal
Noradrenaline	Attention
Adrenaline	Fight or flight
Serotonin	Optimism
Endorphins	Pleasure
Acetylcholine	Relaxation

Table 1.1 Neurotransmitters and their general effects

Behaviour

There are a number of individual behaviours that support mental health through their direct effect on different parts of the brain and on its chemical messengers. The Mental Health Foundation has produced a series of valuable reports in these respects, two of which are 'Up and Running' (MHF 2005a) and 'Feeding Minds' (MHF 2005b). The former makes the case for exercise and the latter for a healthy diet.

It is possible for example to staunch the flow of anxiety and agitation from the emotional brain by gentle but consistent exercise through which natural endorphins are released. It is also possible to calm the mind by eating a diet rich in the precursors of specific neurotransmitters. Each of these is addressed in more detail in Chapter 13. There is also evidence for the benefits of behaviours that induce relaxation such as mindfulness exercises, meditation and yoga. These promote balance and coherence between the sympathetic and parasympathetic nervous systems, regulating heartbeat and calming the emotional brain (see Chapter 17). Servan-Schreiber (2004) and Plant and Stephenson (2008) deal in considerable detail with these matters. Both emphasize the role of diet, exercise and relaxation methods among a range of approaches that can promote a person's sense of mental health and well-being.

There are other individual behaviours that can severely threaten a person's mental health not least of which is the use of alcohol and drugs. Although there is evidence linking light drinking with improved emotional, mental and physical health there is an emerging picture of alcohol use as a way of masking problems and helping people deal with emotions they would otherwise find too difficult to manage. A problem with this approach is that regular alcohol consumption changes the chemistry of the brain, particularly levels of the neurotransmitter serotonin, which become depleted (MHF 2006a). This chemical is implicated in the development of depression and a cyclical process can be established. A person may drink to relieve their low mood or sense of depression, become more depressed as levels of serotonin are depleted and therefore drink more alcohol to medicate the depression. It is now estimated that up to 12 million adults in the UK drink alcohol to help them relax or overcome feelings of depression (MHF 2006a).

Subjective-self

In the upper left or subjective-self quadrant reside immediate thoughts, feelings, emotions and sensations all described in first person terms. This represents a person's interior, subjective world made up of emotions and cognitive processes. A form of intelligence that people use to understand and regulate their emotions is known as emotional intelligence (Mayer *et al.* 2000). In objective-self terms it reflects biochemical cooperation between the emotional and cognitive brains. Its subjective-self qualities are characterized by a person's ability to:

- accurately identify their emotional state;
- grasp the natural course of their emotions, what generates them and how they ebb and flow;
- reason about their emotions, being aware of the consequences of different courses of action they could take;
- regulate their emotions, taking charge appropriately (Mayer *et al.* 2000).

It is not unusual for people to misinterpret emotions, particularly in an age that is characterized by constant demand on their time and resources. One of the most frequent misinterpretations is between stress or fatigue and hunger. In a society where food is abundantly available and stress very common overeating has become quite ordinary. Naish (2008) draws attention to an emerging phenomenon in society of the 'Eat All You Can' buffet style restaurant. Not eat all you 'like' or 'need' but eat all you 'can'! Humans possess instincts within their reptilian and mammalian brains to eat whatever food appears in front of them. In earlier times when food was scarce this was a necessary mechanism for preservation of self and the species. Marketing of the 'Eat All You Can' variety taps into these basic instincts and seeks to bypass cognitions and emotional intelligence. Gradually it is being recognized that poor mastery of emotions, fuelled by crude marketing, is one reason for the growing incidence of obesity in society (Servan-Schreiber 2004).

A range of individual concepts have also been formulated to express mental health in subjective-self terms. Some are indicated in Table 1.1, such as feeling agitated, calm or optimistic. One of the most recent to garner attention is happiness which is explored in more detail in Chapters 3 and 35. Following Tudor (1996) others include:

- coping;
- tension and stress management;
- self-concept and identity;
- self-esteem;
- self-development;
- autonomy and self-determination;
- self-efficacy;
- hope.

An expression of the subjective-self that has received less attention is the role of spirituality in contributing to a person's sense of mental health. The Mental Health Foundation has published a literature review on this subject that reports anecdotal, quantitative and qualitative evidence to support a positive, though often modest, relationship between spirituality and mental health (MHF 2006b). This may be explained by a number of emotions that are encouraged in many spiritual traditions including hope, contentment, love and forgiveness. Other explanations rest on the premise that spiritual beliefs may allow a person to reframe or reinterpret uncontrollable events in such a way as to make them seem less stressful or more meaningful. It is true also that spiritual support from others can be a valuable source of self-esteem, information, companionship and practical help that enables people to cope more effectively with stress and negative life events. The last explanation rests on a person's relationship with others, which moves this discussion to the community quadrants of the framework.

Subjective-community

In the lower left or subjective-community quadrant reside collective thoughts, feelings and world views often referred to as culture. A person's sense of belonging to a friendship, family, community or nation is a key factor that influences mental health, and belonging is also mediated by emotional intelligence. Mayer *et al.*'s (2000) original work applied to others as well as to the individual. Thus, emotional intelligence is also characterized by a person's ability to accurately identify, grasp, reason and regulate the emotions of others. This capacity for relating to others makes a significant contribution to mental health and in children is predictive of success in adulthood (Servan-Schreiber 2004).

If people do not belong they feel excluded and social exclusion is a significant threat to mental health. It should be of concern to the mental health nursing profession that mental health is not yet part of mainstream discourse. Its exclusion avoids the need to think about it, which is detrimental to public mental health. A 2006 policy paper produced by the Sainsbury Centre for Mental Health (SCMH) states that: 'A more tolerant and understanding society ... would bring about the biggest improvement in the lives of people with mental health problems' (2006: 12).

Stigma refers to the way a society views individuals and represents a negative feeling or world view about the group or individuals in question. It is pernicious and damaging not least because of the internalization of those collective messages by the individuals to whom they are aimed. This leads to lower self-esteem and a seemingly self-imposed reluctance to engage in mainstream life and to do the things that a person might really want to do. Furthermore it stops people seeking help for treatment or sharing their difficulties with others.

Stigma is not a tangible commodity therefore but a subjective quality that is harboured in the lower left quadrant of the framework and which threatens the mental health of those who experience it. In the mental health field it has been recognized in different forms for more than 100 years. Emile Durkheim's classic theory of suicide proposed in 1897 attributes some suicides to weakened ties and connections between the suicidal individual and others (cf. Chapter 35). Today there are dedicated programmes to tackle the stigma and discrimination surrounding mental health in England (Shift)[1] and Scotland (See Me).[2]

The marginalization and exclusion in society of people with mental health problems and the mental health discourse itself are forms of social deprivation. It is only in recent decades that this concept has been fully articulated, distinct from an earlier preoccupation with material deprivation. Another recent concept used to describe the opposite of social deprivation is social capital. This is the invisible glue that binds communities together, giving them a shared sense of identity, enabling them to work together for mutual benefit (Kawachi *et al.* 1997). Research into social capital suggests that indicators of community cohesion and efficacy, including levels of trust, tolerance, reciprocity and participation, are important influences on mental health (Friedli 2000). In a sense tolerance and inclusion or intolerance and exclusion are in some way structural, aided or otherwise by mental health services and legislation.

Objective-community

In the lower right or objective-community quadrant reside the physical attributes of a community, its legislature, policy, services and environment.

Legislation

Legislation has a key role to play, particularly that which promotes tolerance and inclusion. Listed below are three key Government Acts and Regulations that support the mental health of the public:

- **The Disability Discrimination Act (DDA) 2005**: The DDA requires public bodies to promote equality of opportunity for disabled people. The 2005 Act amended and extended existing provisions of the DDA 1995. This includes extended protection to cover people who experience mental health problems.
- **Employment Equality (Religion or Belief) and Employment Equality (Sexual Orientation) Regulations 2003:** These regulations outlaw discrimination in employment on the grounds of religion or belief or sexual orientation and came into effect from 2 December 2003. Age related regulations came into force some three years later in October 2006.
- **The Civil Partnership Act 2004**: This Act came into operation on 5 December 2005 and enables a same-sex couple to register as civil partners of each other. Register offices or

---

[1]   http://www.shift.org.uk/
[2]   http://www.seemescotland.org.uk/

other approved premises in England and Wales can be used for this purpose providing a venue and formal procedure for same-sex couples to make a public declaration of their commitment and for families and loved ones to support them in their commitment.

It is worth considering the employment and relationship stability that members of society would experience if these Acts and Regulations had not come into force and how this might impact on their mental health.

Legislative developments are often underpinned by related initiatives that provide more tangible support. One example is that of the Shaw Trust[3] which offers an online resource to equip line managers with the information necessary to support employees who may be dealing with mental health conditions. It aims to help employees stay in work and encourages employers to be more open to recruiting employees who disclose that they manage a mental health condition.

Other types of support that stem from legislation include mental health policy and service structures (cf. Chapter 6). Mental health promotion and public mental health have become important policy strands and drivers for service developments (Bywaters 2005). The contribution of mental health nursing to public mental health is in its infancy but there is reason to be optimistic about its future. The principles of recovery and social inclusion, discussed by Perkins and Repper in Chapter 5, are now prominent in mental health nursing practice. These provide an egalitarian discourse and a social approach to the delivery of care, freed from the strictures of traditional psychiatry, which can be applied to communities and the public as well as to individuals. This premise is discussed in more detail in Chapters 3 and 35.

Environment

Chapters 3 and 35 also discuss the close association between poor mental health and aspects of the environment including unemployment, low income and low material standards of living. This represents material deprivation, which is a corollary to the social deprivation discussed under the subjective-community quadrant. Other elements of the environment are also implicated in mental health including the built environment and the natural environment. In a systematic review of the built environment conducted in the UK Clark *et al.* (2006) identified the following relationships:

■ Urban birth is associated with schizophrenia.
■ Rural residence in adulthood is associated with suicide among males.
■ Neighbourhood violence is associated with poorer mental health.
■ Perceived neighbourhood disorder is associated with poorer mental health.
■ Housing and neighbourhood regeneration is associated with improved mental health.
■ Chronic noise exposure is associated with poorer mental health.

Another review from Australia examined relationships between the natural environment, in terms of green space, and mental health (Maller *et al.* 2002). Among other findings the authors were able to conclude that access to green space results in:

■ improved self-awareness, self-esteem and mood;
■ reductions in negative feelings such as anger, anxiety and fear;

---

[3]   http://www.tacklementalhealth.org.uk/

- improved psychological health, especially emotional and cognitive function;
- restored capacity for attention and concentration.

The Association of Public Health Laboratories has produced a report containing more than 70 indicators of public mental health including their rationale (Wilkinson *et al.* 2007). These echo many of the points raised in discussions of the four quadrants including employment, alcohol and drug use, physical activity, healthy eating, social capital, spirituality, social networks, neighbourliness, violence and safety. Mental health nurses need to acquaint themselves with this type of knowledge to better understand the contributions they can make to community and public mental health.

There is another contemporary indicator that deserves inclusion and which stems from the objective-community quadrant. It concerns a growing preoccupation with the consumption of material goods. A report in the *American Journal of Psychiatry* (Koran *et al.* 2006) found that more than one in 20 individuals meet criteria for compulsive buying. This is characterized by people buying things they do not need, do not use or cannot afford resulting in debt and interpersonal problems, particularly with spouses.

When there is no longer room to store unwanted goods in homes people buy storage space to maintain their hoarding. In 2005 the UK self-storage industry made £310 million and is reported to be growing by 40 per cent each year (Naish 2008). In America, self-storage space occupies three times the area of Manhattan Island and makes more money per annum than America's movie business or its music business (Naish 2008). This 'grab and stash' phenomenon is fuelled by dissatisfaction with self, greed and envy of others. These are the subjective-self and community correlates of behaviours in the objective-community quadrant that result in the unnecessary purchase of material goods. Behaviours that are perpetuated by intense marketing that tap into the emotional brain, which millions of years ago did indeed need to grab and stash whatever was available to ensure survival. From the time of Karl Marx many have argued convincingly that the survival of capitalism as an economic system requires people to be dissatisfied with what they have in order that they will desire the next product on the market. How far such an economic system is sustainable in the long term is open to debate. But for the maintenance of their mental health it might be that the public need support and encouragement to understand their behaviours and identify more mature responses to their needs.

Definitions of mental health

Having provided an overview of each quadrant we consider here the different ways that mental health has been defined. In this respect there are likely to be as many different definitions of mental health as there are readers of this book; with reference to the framework presented in Figure 1.1 it is possible to identify any number of factors in each of the quadrants that an individual might feel has some bearing on their mental health. While differences between individuals, cultures, social classes and genders impede achieving a consensus definition of mental health, it is also true that a common understanding between people and communities is essential if we are to understand how mental health can be improved and/or protected. In this section some historical and contemporary definitions of mental health are presented and appraised for their value with recourse to the framework (Figure 1.1).

Making it Happen was published by the Department of Health (England) in 2001 to support implementation of Standard 1 of the National Service Framework for Mental Health (DH 1999), which requires health and social services to promote mental health and reduce the discrimination and social exclusion associated with mental health problems. Within the context of promotion *Making it Happen* (DH 2001) defined mental health as 'thinking, feeling and physical health and well-being'. This definition appears limited given the framework approach since it appears to refer only to the upper quadrants of Figure 1.1. In fairness the report's authors acknowledge that communities and organizations (lower quadrants) also think and feel but this was not explicit in their diagrammatic representation of mental health promotion.

The World Health Organization (WHO) provides several definitions of (mental) health. For example, their constitution states that 'health is a state of complete physical, mental and social well-being and not merely the absence of disease or infirmity' and more recently 'mental health is more than the absence of mental disorders' (WHO 2001). These definitions are of little value. In the latter case mental health is not defined positively at all but rather in terms of what it is not, i.e. not just the absence of mental disorders. We would also challenge a key assumption underlying both definitions, that health and illness are mutually exclusive complete states. In our experience it is quite possible for a person with a diagnosed mental illness, say schizophrenia, to also experience a degree of mental health such as meaningful employment. In the same way it is possible for a person with a physical illness, say macular degeneration, to also experience a degree of physical health such as cardiovascular fitness. Health and illness frequently co-exist and are mutually exclusive only if health is defined in a restrictive way as the absence of disease (Sartorius 1990).

A more recent definition by the WHO (2007) holds more promise:

66   Mental health can be conceptualized as a state of well-being in which the
      individual realizes his or her own abilities, can cope with the normal stresses
      of life, can work productively and fruitfully, and is able to make a
      contribution to his or her community. In this positive sense, mental health is
      the foundation for well-being and effective functioning for an individual and
      for a community.   99

This definition provides a much more integrative account of mental health and draws from both the 'self' and 'community' quadrants of Figure 1.1. It recognizes that mental health resides within individuals and within communities and establishes the case for public mental health interventions, which are addressed in some detail in Chapter 3. The definition is quite complex however and a simpler approach to definition has been proposed by a number of authors including Keyes (2002) and Huppert (2005). These authors distinguish two dimensions that encompass positive mental health and well-being:

■ hedonic: positive feelings and positive affect, which reflect subjective well-being;
■ eudaimonic: positive functioning, which includes engagement, fulfilment and social well-being.

These dimensions of mental health together offer an integrative account of the concept that incorporates the upper (self) and lower (community) quadrants of Figure 1.1. However, it lacks the breadth contained in Figure 1.1. For example it tends to focus on the left hand quadrants (both self and community/social) but draws little from the right hand quadrants. It nevertheless offers a useful delineation of some individual and collective factors and is elaborated further in Chapters 3 and 35.

In sum, defining mental health has proved a difficult task. While some definitions offered above can be of utility for those charged with promoting mental health we would recommend adopting a more open stance that recognizes the interplay of the four quadrants in Figure 1.1. There is still much to be learned about that interplay and pinning mental health down to a single definition tends to limit those opportunities. Recognizing that mental health arises from a state of balance that includes the self and community in both their subjective and objective forms will, we believe, help individuals, professionals and communities better understand how to promote and protect it.

Integral mental health

This chapter has hitherto presented the four quadrants and dealt with each in turn to provide a sense of their individual content and impact on mental health. Our purpose in this section, is to put these jigsaw pieces back together and so provide an integral understanding of mental health. A basic premise that underpins this approach is the fact that mental health (and mental illness) has at least four dimensions (the quadrants). It may be tempting to ask which is the right or best quadrant for interventions to support mental health, but an integral approach would assert that all are right, each is vital but also representative of a partial explanation of the phenomenon, because there are three other contributing quadrants. In more abstract terms this implies that every single moment of awareness contains elements from all four quadrants. This is illustrated by Figure 1.2 which shows the framework introduced previously but now containing the pronouns that major languages use to describe different aspects of human experience. Thus, a person can witness an event from the point of view of 'I' in terms of what I see and feel about the event; or from the point of view of 'we' in terms of how others or 'we' collectively feel about the event; and then again it can be viewed as an 'it' or 'its' in terms of the objective facts of the event (Wilber 2007). All events or phenomena in the manifest world can be interpreted from each of these four dimensions (I, it, we and its) each of which are vital though partial accounts of the event or phenomenon.

This can be demonstrated with reference to the thought 'I'll go to the shops'. As Wilber (2001) points out the thought evokes images, concepts and memories (subjective-self), while at the same time there are chemical processes going on in the brain (objective-self). The language used is a cultural phenomenon that only has meaning in relation to a specific cultural background (subjective-community), and there are also socioeconomic factors through the existence of shops (objective-community). An even simpler thought such as Descartes' proof of his own existence 'I think therefore I am' contains all four quadrants; the thought, chemical activity, the meaning of the language and the structure of the language in terms of its written words and sentence structure. The four quadrants are all pervasive, all of the time, in any moment of human awareness.

We turn now to the empirical evidence which demonstrates the integral nature of the human condition. An orthodox or conventional medical practitioner (upper right quadrant) might prescribe anxiolytic medication to calm the limbic and sympathetic nervous systems, both of which are involved in the development of anxiety and depression. However, the

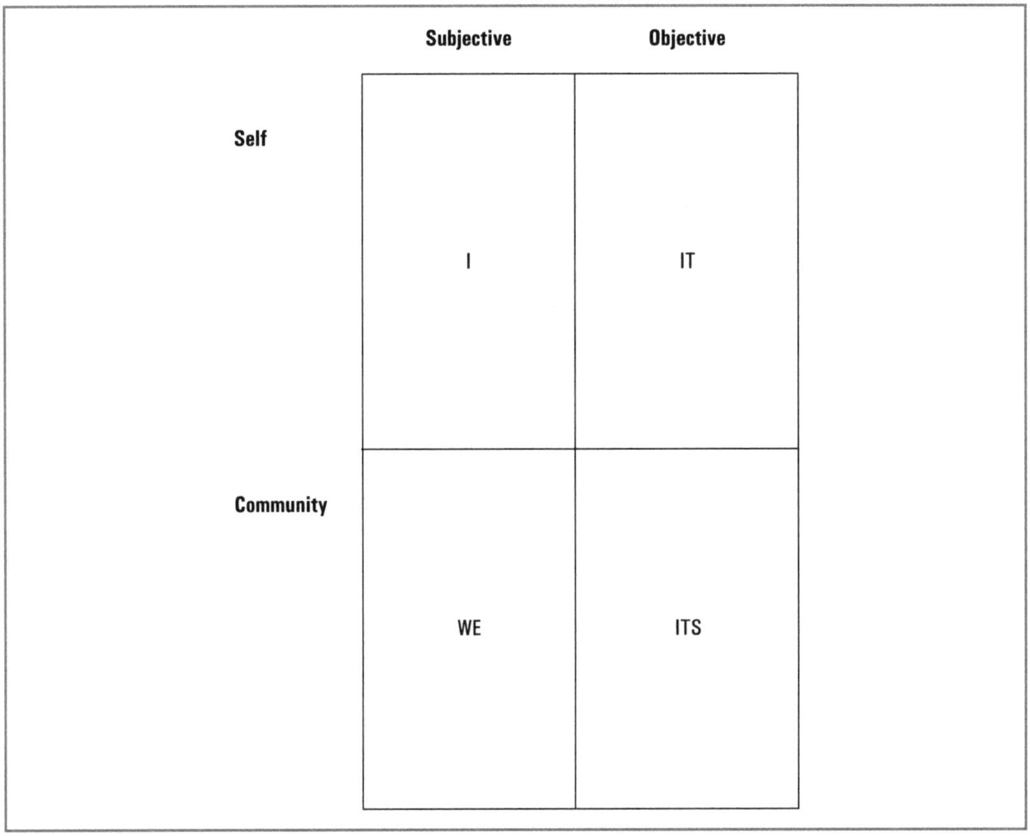

	Subjective	Objective
Self	I	IT
Community	WE	ITS

Figure 1.2 Framework of Human Experience II (After Wilber, 2001)

integral approach suggests there are other dimensions to the physical phenomena of excited limbic and sympathetic nervous systems, one of which is expressed through a person's thoughts and feelings (upper left quadrant). It should therefore be possible to calm these physiological functions by non-physiological approaches as the integral framework suggests. Research into the mechanisms by which talking therapies, including cognitive behavioural therapy (CBT), have a therapeutic affect would appear to confirm this.

Brain scans of individuals who receive CBT for depressive symptoms indicate that the therapy may help the prefrontal cortex (cognitive brain) take better control of the emotional brain. As the person with depressive symptoms struggles between their feelings and the corrective guidance of CBT there are high levels of prefrontal activity in their brain. Once they achieve some success or correction of their thoughts the prefrontal lobes relax and brain scans demonstrate significantly reduced activity (Plant and Stephenson 2008). Thus, there would appear to be an integrated system in human beings through which brain chemistry can alter our emotions and equally, our emotions can alter our brain chemistry. This highlights the importance of identifying the wider issues that impact on brain function, in this instance the subjective, integral correlates of an over-stimulated limbic and sympathetic nervous systems.

The integral nature of the human condition is also evident in the literature that explores relationships and social networks. In human beings and other mammals, physiological balance (upper right quadrant) is dependent on the love we receive from others (lower left quadrant). This was strikingly demonstrated in a study conducted in the 1960s which was published in the *British Medical Journal* (Parkes *et al.* 1969). The team of researchers studied two groups of elderly men of the same age. One group had been widowed while the wives of the other group were still alive. The average survival time of the widowers was significantly less than the married group. Servan-Schreiber (2004) has used this study and others, which demonstrate clear links between emotionally supportive relationships, social networks, and health to argue that the physiology of social mammals is not separate from the rest of their being, particularly their mental health. Humans are integral beings and optimum mental and physical functioning depends on relationships with others, especially those that offer close emotional ties. It is of little surprise therefore that when mental health service users are asked about the strategies they find 'most helpful', relationships with others is top of their list (Faulkner and Layzell 2000).

Psychiatrists at the University of San Francisco refer to this phenomenon as 'limbic regulation' and argue that a relationship is a physiological process as much as it is a social process, as real and as potent as any pill or surgical procedure (Lewis *et al.* 2000). People can die from broken hearts and Servan-Schreiber (2004) argues that love is quite literally a biological need.

We conclude this section by drawing on other chapters in this volume, and work carried out by the Mental Health Foundation (McCulloch and Ryrie 2006) and NHS Health Scotland (Friedli *et al.* 2007) to populate the framework with variables that provide a contemporary, integral account of mental health (Figure 1.3). From this perspective, mental health is a complex phenomenon that arises from the integration of everything that is within human experience and fluctuates as all things relative to that experience change. While this is undoubtedly complex the framework allows understanding of its meaning and suggests implications for mental health nursing practice, which we now explore.

Implications for nursing

Figure 1.3 represents the art and science of mental health nursing. It contains its subjective and objective orientations, its interpersonal and evidence-based traditions, between which there has been growing consensus and cross-fertilization over the past five years since the first edition of this book was published (cf. Chapter 4). Those traditions, which developed principally around the care of people with mental illness, can now be understood in relation to mental health.

From this understanding there are, in our view, two overarching themes that have implications for the practice of mental health nursing. The first concerns the delivery of care to promote the mental health of people who experience mental disorders. This is additional to the profession's established tradition of delivering interventions designed to manage the mental disorder itself. The second concerns extension of the profession's role to support the mental health and well-being of communities and the public. A number of chapters in this book address these matters (cf. Chapters 3, 5, 6, 13, 17, 29, 35).

Mental health of the individual

While the care and management of mental disorders remains a primary focus for mental health nursing, a complementary focus on mental health provides nurses with opportunities

Subjective	Objective
Self	
Thought	Brain function
Feelings	Autonomic nervous
Self-acceptance	system function
Cognitive style	Physiological balance
Emotional intelligence	Exercise
Spirituality	Diet
Creativity	Alcohol and drug use
Talking	Rest
I	**IT**
WE	**ITS**
Community	
Relationships	Legislation
Belonging	Policy
Inclusion	Services
Social support	Employment
Social capital	Material wealth
Community	Built environment
participation	Nature
Tolerance	Public health indicators

Figure 1.3 Integral Mental Health
After Wilber (2001)

to strengthen their clients' resilience to the debilitating consequences of their condition and to help them forge a meaningful quality of life irrespective of that condition.

Nursing work focused on promoting mental health is best undertaken in the context of innovative services which integrate some aspects of practice discussed in this chapter into mainstream service provision. One such example (cited in the Mental Health Foundation's report *Feeding Minds* (MHF 2005b) is of an early intervention team in Yorkshire for people who experience a first episode of psychosis, which includes nutritional and physical activity assessments as part of routine care. Nutritional deficiencies in the diet are initially increased by supplements with the aim of achieving optimum nutrition from a balanced diet as care progresses. Physical activity programmes are also developed to suit individual users with the support of community sports staff who exercise together with the service users.

Another example is the use of exercise referral schemes of which there are now more than 1000 across the UK (MHF 2005a). The schemes operate in a variety of forms, often involving a partnership between primary care trusts and local leisure services. Health professionals can refer people who might benefit and an increasing number offer a dedicated service for people with mental health problems. Once referred, people are seen by a qualified exercise professional who makes a detailed assessment of their fitness and develops an individual activity plan. Throughout the programme the service user can draw on the exercise professional for support and follow-up and assessments are scheduled at key points during the programme. Exercise referral schemes of this type may be of particular value as their impact spans all quadrants of the framework presented in this chapter. Mechanisms by which they are believed to have a beneficial effect include:

■ increased release of endorphins that promote feelings of well-being
■ building new social networks and relationships that promote inclusion and help prevent feelings of anxiety and depression
■ boosting self-esteem and worth as service users master new skills and achieve goals
■ distraction from preoccupations with negative thoughts by providing an alternative focus for attention (MHF 2005b).

Mental health of the public

In 2004 the national clinical director for mental health for England reviewed progress towards the standards contained in the National Service Framework for Mental Health (DH 1999) and stated:

   66   We are entering a new phase in which the emphasis will move on from specialist mental health care, crucial though that will remain, to the mental health and well-being of the community as a whole

      (DH 2004: 71). 99

Mental health nurses as a professional group may feel cautious moving from a dedicated focus on the needs and care of the individual to incorporate one that is oriented toward the public. However, the integral nature of mental health demonstrates that interventions at the public or community level also have an effect on the experience of individuals. In Chapters 3 and 35 this premise is further explored with reference to the work of Huppert (2005).

Government public consultations on contemporary health policy have found a considerable demand for more support to promote mental health and emotional well-being (Wilkinson *et al.* 2007). The work of the Mental Health Foundation has been important in these respects providing a series of reports on different aspects of mental health and sharing this information with the public through standard media channels. An example of this work is provided in Chapter 35.

Conclusion

In summary this chapter has outlined an integral understanding of the human condition and has used this to map those elements that have a bearing on the mental health of individuals and communities. This stands in contrast to more familiar professional terrain that is predicated on mental disorders, which are the subject of the next chapter. This understanding has the potential to extend mental health nurses' role among those to whom it already provides services and among the wider public. The potential contribution of mental health nurses to positive health and well-being in the twenty-first century is considerable and the chapters that follow are testament to this claim.

In summary the main points are:

■ In recent decades, 'mental' health as a concept has emerged in the collective consciousness, freed from illness and born independently as a concept in its own right.

■ Mental health is an integral phenomenon that can be understood using a four quadrant framework to recognize its objective and subjective elements as well as those that relate to the individual and their communities.

■ The physiological basis of mental health is a vital if partial piece of the jigsaw that needs to be understood by the profession and the public.

■ Equally important are the subjective and community correlates of mental health, which can themselves affect physiological functioning.

■ The integral nature of mental health provides opportunity to work at the level of the individual or the community to enhance mental health for all.

■ Mental health nurses as a professional group have the potential to incorporate this knowledge into their evidence base and make significant contributions to the mental health and well-being of people who experience mental health problems and to the public at large.

Questions for reflection and discussion

1   Using the four quadrant framework make in inventory of those factors in each of the quadrants that have an impact on your own mental health.
2   Think about your community or nation and reflect on any subjective tendencies or objective markers that might be damaging to its mental health.
3   Think of a service user you have cared for or a service in which you have practised and consider how their care or the service could be enhanced with reference to the material contained in this chapter.
4   What contributions do you consider the mental health nursing profession can make to develop communities and environments that support mental health and well-being.

Annotated bibliography

■ Servan-Schreiber, D. (2004) *Healing without Freud or Prozac*. London: Rodale International Ltd. This textbook demonstrates how it is possible to support mental health without recourse to traditional or orthodox treatments. It provides an overview of seven highly effective interventions that work through the body to tap into the emotional brain's self-healing process. It combines cutting edge science with alternative medicine and points the way to mental health practice of the future.

■ Plant, J. and Stephenson, J. (2008) *Beating Stress, Anxiety and Depression*. London: Piatkus Books. Jane Plant and Janet Stephenson provide a contemporary account of the ways in which we can all support our own mental health and prevent the onset of mental health problems. It provides a rigorous analysis of the physiological correlates of mental health and offers ten lifestyle and nutritional factors that can decrease the chances of mental illness and dramatically improve mental well-being.

■ Mental Health Foundation (2005) *Up and Running: Exercise therapy and the treatment of mild or moderate depression in primary care* (2005); *Feeding Minds: The impact of food on mental health* (2005); *The Impact of Spirituality on Mental Health* (2006); *Cheers? Understanding the relationship between alcohol and mental health* (2006). London: MHF.

These are just four of many publications produced for public consumption by the Mental Health Foundation. They explore a range of factors that contribute to mental health, case study innovative interventions and provide individual guidance to those who wish to care more effectively for their mental health.

References

Beck, D. and Cowan, C. (1996) *Spiral Dynamics: Mastering Values, Leadership and Change.* Oxford: Blackwell Publishing.

Bywaters, J. (2005) Public Mental Health in England since 1997: past present and future. *Journal of Public Mental Health* **4**: 13–16.

Clark, C., Candy, B. and Stansfield, S. (2006) *A Systematic Review on the Effect of the built and physical Environment on Mental Health.* London: MHF.

Department of Health (1999) *A National Service Framework for Mental Health.* London: The Stationery Office.

Department of Health (2001) *Making it Happen: A guide to delivering mental health promotion.* London: DH.

Department of Health (2004) *The National Service Framework for Mental Health – Five Years On.* London: DH.

Dobbs, D. (2007) Eric Kandel: From mind and brain and back again. *Scientific American* Mind **33**: 33–7.

Faulkner, A. and Layzell, S. (2000) *Strategies for Living: A Report of user-led research into people's strategies for living with mental distress.* London: Mental Health Foundation.

Friedli, L. (2000) *Mental Health Improvement 'concepts and definitions': Briefing paper for the National Advisory Group.* Edinburgh: Scottish Executive.

Friedli, L., Oliver, C., Tidyman, M. and Ward, G. (2007) *Mental Health Improvement: Evidence based messages to promote mental wellbeing.* Edinburgh: NHS Health Scotland.

Huppert, F. (2005) Positive mental health in individuals and populations, in: F. Huppert, N. Bayliss and B. Keverne (eds) *The Science of Well-Being.* Oxford: Oxford University Press.

Kawachi, I., Kennedy, B. and Lochner, K. (1997) Health and social cohesion: why care about income inequality? *British Medical Journal* **314**: 1037–40.

Keyes, C. (2002) The mental health continuum: from languishing to flourishing in life. *Journal of Health and Social Research* **43**: 207–22.

Koran, L., Faber, R., Aboujaoude, E., Large, M. and Serpe, R. (2006) Estimated prevalence of compulsive buying behavior in the United States. *American Journal of Psychiatry* **163**: 1806–12.

Lewis, T., Amini, F. and Lannon, R. (2000) *A General Theory of Love.* New York: Random House.

Maller, C., Townsend, M., Brown, P. and St. Leger, L. (2002) Healthy Parks, Healthy People: the health benefits of contact with nature in a park context: a literature review. Victoria, Australia: Deakin University.

Mayer, J., Salovey, A. and Capuso, A. (2000) Models of emotional intelligence, in: R. Steinberg (ed.) *Handbook of Intelligence.* Cambridge: Cambridge University Press.

McCulloch, A. and Ryrie, I. (2006) The impact of diet on mental health. *The Mental Health Review* **11**: 19–22.

Mental Health Foundation (MHF) (2005a) *Up and Running: Exercise therapy and the treatment of mild or moderate depression in primary care.* London: Mental Health Foundation.

Mental Health Foundation (2005b) *Feeding Minds: The impact of food on mental health.* London: MHF.

Mental Health Foundation (2006a) *Cheers? Understanding the relationship between alcohol and mental health.* London: MHF.

Mental Health Foundation (2006b) *The Impact of Spirituality on Mental Health.* London: MHF.

Naish, J. (2008) *Enough: Breaking free from the world of more.* London: Hodder and Stoughton.

Parkes, M., Benjamin, C. and Fitzgerald, R. (1969) Broken heart: a statistical study of increased mortality among widowers. *British Medical Journal* **646**: 740–3.

Plant, J. and Stephenson, J. (2008) *Beating Stress, Anxiety and Depression.* London: Piatkus Books.

Sainsbury Centre for Mental Health (2006) *The Future of Mental Health: A Vision for 2015.* London: SCMH.

Sartorius, N. (1990) Preface, in: Goldberg D. and Tantam, D. (eds) *The Public Health Impact of Mental Disorders.* Toronto: Hogrefe and Huber.

Servan-Schreiber, D. (2004) *Healing without Freud or Prozac.* London: Rodale International Ltd.

Strohman, R. (2003) Genetic determinism as a failing paradigm in biology and medicine. *Journal of Social Work Education* **39**: 169–91.

Tudor, K. (1996) *Mental Health Promotion: Paradigms and Practice.* London: Routledge.

Wilber, K. (2001) *A Theory of Everything.* Dublin: Gateway.

Wilber, K. (2007) *The Integral Vision.* Massachusetts: Shambhala Publications Inc.

Wilkinson, J., Bywaters, J., Chappel, D. and Glover, G. (2007) *Indicators of Public Health in the English Regions: Mental Health.* York: Association of Public Health Observatories.

World Health Organization (2001) *The World Health Report Mental Health: New Understanding, New Hope.* Geneva: WHO.

World Health Organization (2007) Mental Health: Strengthening mental health promotion. Fact Sheet No. 220. Available at: http://www.who.int/mediacentre/factsheets/fs220/en/

CHAPTER 2

Mental disorder

Iain Ryrie and Ian Norman

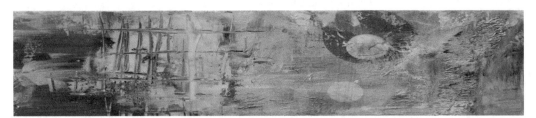

Chapter overview

Chapter 1 described mental health as a state of balance that includes the self and community in both their subjective and objective forms. This chapter uses the same framework to examine mental disorder. The point at which an individual's experience or behaviour might be considered disordered is a highly contested area since different schools of thought have their own explanatory models. Where the boundary is drawn or which shades of human experience constitute disorder is therefore open to debate. We do not draw conclusions in this respect but encourage the reader to consider an integrated explanation of human experience, and thus, of mental disorder. Different models or ways of understanding mental disorder are described both as singular explanations and as building blocks for a more integrated understanding. From this perspective, and as a corollary to mental health, mental disorder is presented as a state of imbalance that includes the self and community in both their subjective and objective forms. Systems that classify mental disorder are reviewed, and the prevalence and symptoms of key disorders are described.

In summary this chapter covers:

- Models of mental disorder;
- Integrating models of mental disorder;
- The classification of mental disorder;
- Key symptoms of mental disorder;
- Prevalence and incidence of mental disorders.

Models of mental disorder

This section describes the approaches taken by different schools of thought to explain the aetiology of mental disorder. It outlines also a number of treatment implications for each of the models.

The disease model

A disease is present if it harms the individual, reduces his or her capacity to reproduce and thereby places them at a biological disadvantage (Scadding 1967; Tyrer and Steinberg 2005).

This can be understood in terms of a physical disease, such as a cancer, a damaged heart valve, or a pathogen that can be transmitted between people. These conditions do place individuals at some sort of disadvantage. Disease theorists similarly attribute mental disorders, or psychiatric illnesses, to physiological and chemical changes in the individual, particularly in the brain but also in other parts of the body (Tyrer and Steinberg 2005).

Thus we can understand clearly the basis for disorders of perception and cognition among say, people with dementia or those who have suffered brain injuries. Observable physiological changes in brain structure have correlates in human behaviour. The disease model extends beyond these organic conditions to explain disorders such as depression, which can be attributed to changes in serotonin levels or to some other chemical fluctuation. Similarly, schizophrenia has been attributed to chemical abnormalities and also to physiological differences such as the size of the temporal lobe in the human brain (Gournay 1996).

The disease model, following traditional medicine, endeavours to identify through scientific objectivity the presence of a stable phenomenon that is called 'mental disorder'. Clinical syndromes become refined into diagnoses, which are essentially codes for heterogeneous, and often unstable collections of symptoms (Craig 2000). Objectivity in psychiatry is at best quite 'fuzzy', but remains a gold standard. Such a gold standard affords incredible power to its possessor. Clinical syndromes and diagnoses are codified languages, available only to those who have willingly immersed themselves in that particular paradigm. They can provide an efficient means to communicate complex phenomena, but only to those in the know.

Correspondingly, the treatment armoury of the disease theorist is elitist, being available only to the qualified practitioner. Medicines are prescribed to balance chemical imbalances, electroconvulsive therapy is administered to shunt neural pathways into shape, positron emission tomography may be requested to check those temporal lobes and, in the most extreme of cases, pieces of the brain may be removed.

A consistent criticism of the disease model is the possibility that people with mental disorders can become passive recipients of treatment and the nurse or doctor an authority on the person's experience. However, this is not a consequence of the disease model per se, but reflects something of the way in which practitioners apply their knowledge. Passive receipt of care can accompany any model if practitioners fail to speak to people as people, but instead believe they are dealing with symptoms, syndromes or a collection of behavioural problems. There is no reason why the disease model cannot take account of the person behind the symptoms or syndrome, and indeed in our experience this has largely been the case, though not always so.

There has been a recent resurgence of interest in the disease model particularly in terms of its diagnostic capabilities. Biochemical correlates of mental disorder in the form of organic compounds can be analysed in urine and blood samples to determine which neurotransmitters are too high or too low. Saliva samples can be analysed to determine levels of cortisol, which provide an indication of the degree of stress an individual is experiencing. Some commentators recommend that these procedures should be included in assessments for mental disorder, particularly before prescribing medications that act on specific neurotransmitters (Plant and Stephenson 2008).

The psychodynamic model

The psychodynamic model is more accurately described as a style of human interaction and understanding that draws on a broad philosophy, which includes clinical, biological and evolutionary theory as well as religion and the arts (Tyrer and Steinberg 2005). Psychodynamic practice may conjure an image of the psychoanalyst listening to their patient's stream of consciousness as the patient lies on a couch at their side. This may occur but the psychodynamic model has many branches including some forms of family therapy, group therapies and art therapy (Tyrer and Steinberg 2005).

Common to all psychodynamic approaches, which delineate them from other psychotherapeutic perspectives (for example, behaviour therapy), is their primary focus on the ideas and feelings behind the words and actions that constitute human behaviour. Psychiatric disorders are not viewed as illnesses with disease-based aetiologies but as conflicts between different levels of mental functioning. Of critical importance are the conscious and unconscious levels. Substantial amounts of mental activity that occur beyond human awareness are believed to determine much of our behaviour.

Human development is important in this respect since a person's early experiences can produce a particular *gestalt* or view of the person and their world, which they will take with them into adult life. This *gestalt* will include mental tricks and mechanisms to protect the person's sense of self. Problems may arise if a person's *gestalt*, that they necessarily cling to, is at odds with the real circumstances they find themselves in as adults.

A simple example is a man whose childhood was coloured by restraint, control, uncertainty and occasional pleasure. Then as an adult he works hard to please others, to demonstrate control and restraint in the expectation that doing for others will bring occasional pleasure. If this man was a priest then his *gestalt* may fit his real circumstances. But suppose this man spent his life struggling to forge a career in marketing or in the stock market to please his father? Though a simplistic example, conflict is likely to dominate this man's experience. Conflict between his personal aspirations and the expectations of others. Conflict between his working alliances and the impossibility of any harmony in such a work environment. Conflict between his relative failings as a merchant banker and his father's exacting standards. He may not be conscious of these specific conflicts but will nevertheless be affected by them as unconscious mental activity tries to reconcile the irreconcilable. Quite literally, the psychodynamic therapist views psychological distress as the upshoots of unconscious thought (Tyrer and Steinberg 2005). This simple principle is central to most if not all psychodynamic therapies.

Different theories have been put forward within the psychodynamic tradition to explain different human experiences, but the founding father of the psychodynamic school was Sigmund Freud (1856–1939). Freud was a biological thinker interested primarily in an organism's attraction to pleasure and repulsion from pain. Application of the pain/pleasure continuum to the human mind and its development led Freud to divide mental life into the *id*, *ego* and *superego*. The id represents basic primitive instincts, present at birth, which tend toward the pursuit of pleasure or gratification. As gratification is pursued people become aware also of an external reality separate from themselves and this realization necessitates the formulation of a self or ego. Others in their world have helped shape the external reality in terms of laws, rules and social expectations. This realization leads to the development of the superego, which is more easily understood as a person's conscience.

So people have needs (id), wishes (ego) and a conscience (superego) and, perhaps not surprisingly, psychological distress arises from the struggles that take place between them. Many of these struggles take place in the unconscious and Freudian analysts are concerned with healing the radical split between the conscious and unconscious, thereby creating a strong and healthy ego that is an accurate and acceptable self-image.

Freud's contemporaries and his followers have built subsequently upon his work to elaborate the psychodynamic school. Carl Jung (1875–1961) studied under Freud, who designated Jung his successor and crown prince. However, after less than ten years of collaboration they fell out over theoretical disagreements and never spoke to each other again! While Freud had dedicated his work to the ego level of personal functioning, Jung was more inclined to examine transpersonal levels of human awareness. For Jung there were aspects of a person that appeared to transcend or go beyond the person, and this premise was incomprehensible to Freud, whose work had been confined to the realms of the ego or self.

Jung had studied the great mythologies of the world, particularly their totems, ancient symbols, images and mythological motifs. What he discovered was that these images appeared with some regularity in the dreams and fantasies of modern Europeans, the majority of whom had never been exposed to these myths. His basic premise was that these primordial images, or *archetypes* as he called them, are common to all people. They do not belong to single individuals but are in fact transindividual or transcendent of the self.

Jung called this deep layer of the psyche, in which the archetypes reside, the 'collective unconscious'. Notice this is not individual consciousness but is something that resides deep within everyone. According to Jung these archetypes live on, whether people are aware of them or not, and continue to move individuals deeply in creative but also destructive ways. As an example, Jungian therapists are interested in people's key dreams and understanding the symbolism within them with recourse to ancient mythology. Knowing what mythological images have meant over time to the human race as a whole enables people to understand what the images may mean in their experience of the *collective unconscious*. It follows that through such conscious integration people are no longer forcibly moved by unconscious archetypes. Therefore, though related to Freud's ideas, Jung extended them beyond the organism to the cultural context within which the organism lives and used this context (or collective unconscious) to understand the psychic distress encountered by people.

Melanie Klein (1882–1960) is another key psychodynamic theorist whose work focused on the first two to three months of a child's life at a time when she believed the ego struggles to differentiate between itself and external reality. Unable to comprehend that good and bad can be present in the same object the infant assumes the *paranoid position* in which all things are either good or bad but never both. When able to comprehend that these qualities do exist in a single object (for example both the mother's love and her chastisement) the infant experiences this new discovery and moves to the *depressive position*. Therefore in Kleinian terms the experience and acceptance of depression is considered a maturational step necessary for personal growth (Tyrer and Steinberg 2005).

The influence of these early works on more contemporary psychodynamic therapies such as 'humanistic therapy', 'drama therapy', 'art therapy' and some forms of counselling is without doubt (Tyrer and Steinberg 2005). Equally, the psychodynamic tradition has influenced mental health nursing, particularly through the works of Hildegard Peplau and Annie Altschul (cf. Chapter 4; see also annotated bibliography).

The behavioural model

The behavioural model has a scientific basis in Learning Theory. Symptoms are considered to be learned habits arising from the interaction between external events or stressors and an individual's personality. Persistent, distressing symptoms are considered maladaptive responses rather than being markers for some underlying disease or illness. For the behaviour therapist the symptoms and their associated behaviours *are* the disorder (Tyrer and Steinberg 2005).

Learning theory posits that two forms of conditioning are responsible for the formation of symptoms; *classical* and *operant*. Classical conditioning refers to a neutral stimulus that becomes associated with an unrelated but established stimulus response sequence. Seminal experimental work in this area was conducted by the Russian physiologist Pavlov (1927) who conditioned dogs to salivate in response to a bell rather than to the established stimulus of food. Initially food was provided to the animals when a bell sounded. After several such trials the animals would salivate at the sound of the bell even when unaccompanied by food.

Operant conditioning results from behaviour rather than as the consequence of a stimulus. Skinner (1972) conducted seminal work in this field with a box in which one or more levers could be pressed. Rats would be placed in the box and through natural curiosity they would eventually press one or all of the levers. When the appropriate lever was pressed food would be deposited in the box. Gradually the rats would learn to continually press the appropriate lever until their appetites were satisfied. Thus it is not a neutral stimulus or the manipulation of an experimenter that conditioned the rats, but their own behaviour.

These theories provide a rationale for the development of some human behavioural problems. Take as a simple example a phobia or fear of spiders in a parent. When the parent encounters a spider their response may be at odds with the threat that a spider poses. They may appear to panic, perhaps scream and will certainly try to avoid the spider. It is possible that the children in this family will also develop a similar response since they have been subject to the classical conditioning of the parent. Thus they may learn to fear and avoid spiders, which can become self-perpetuating as their fear confirms the danger spiders pose, and their avoidance obviates any opportunity to realize that spiders pose no threat.

The behaviour therapist is interested in replacing maladaptive responses with adaptive behaviour patterns. This is usually done by gradually removing the fear response through such techniques as graded exposure and systematic desensitization. So the parent in our example may first be encouraged to imagine spiders, then view pictures of them in a book, followed by seeing them in a jar across the room, then holding the jar and finally holding the spider. Each of these stages will invoke a fear response but these will gradually subside if the person is encouraged to remain with the present situation through which they learn that spiders are actually quite harmless.

An important principle of behaviour therapy is a collaborative working partnership between client and therapist. A person's behaviour is part of their own responsibility and not something that can be handed over to a doctor to sort out (Tyrer and Steinberg 2005). The therapist does not view the person as being abnormal or ill, but regards them as an equal partner in an unlearning, or new learning process. Furthermore, behaviour therapists see this partnership as critical if the individual is to maintain and develop their new adaptive behaviours once therapy has finished.

This approach to managing human behaviour has had a major influence on mental health nursing, for example, through the work of Isaac Marks (Marks *et al.* 1978; Marks 1987) who, though not a nurse, has championed nurse behaviour therapists. Their contribution to health care has since been evaluated by Gournay *et al.* (2000).

The cognitive model

The cognitive model posits that people interpret their thoughts, which in turn are the main determinants of behaviour (Tyrer and Steinberg 2005). This stands in sharp contrast to the behavioural or disease models, which do not accommodate the cognitive mechanisms involved in behaviour and illness. For the cognitive therapist primacy is given to errors or biases in thinking and it is these dysfunctional thought patterns that create mental disorders.

An important framework used by many cognitive therapists is the ABC model first described by Ellis (1962). A stands for 'activating event', B stands for 'beliefs' about the 'activating event', and C stands for the emotional or behavioural 'consequence' that follows, B, given A. Thus, a person who comes across a spider (activating event) may think it harmless or dangerous (beliefs) and will either continue their usual activity or be unable to do so (consequence).

While the behavioural model focuses on the fear response, or consequence in the above example, the crux of the problem according to the cognitive model rests in the beliefs that people hold. Repetitive thoughts (ruminations) can lead to persistent actions (rituals), which can prevent normal functioning. Significant change in a person's mental health necessarily involves significant change in their cognitions (Tyrer and Steinberg 2005).

Though the reverse of the behavioural model, the two are rarely in major conflict. Open, collaborative working partnerships are established by respective therapists, and in the case of cognitive therapy, the client is encouraged to explore their thinking patterns and consider more appropriate and adaptive thoughts that fit the evidence. Furthermore, a growing discipline of cognitive behavioural therapy has emerged in recent decades (Grant *et al.* 2004; Kinsella and Garland 2008).

The cognitive model is the youngest of those described and it remains to be seen how it may develop and to what ends. Of contemporary interest, however, is the use of this model to manage distressing delusions, hallucinations and feelings of paranoia that people may experience in the course of a mental disorder (Morrison *et al.* 2003).

The social model

The social model is concerned with the influence of social forces as the causes or precipitants of mental disorder. While the psychodynamic model is principally concerned with the individual and their personal relations, the social model focuses on the person in the context of their society as a whole (Tyrer and Steinberg 2005).

Evidence that social forces are central to the aetiology of mental disorder can be traced to the work of Emile Durkheim (1897) who demonstrated that social factors, particularly isolation and the loss of social bonds, were predictive of suicide. We may be more familiar with associations between poor living circumstances in deprived geographical areas and the incidence of physical health problems (Whitehead 1992). However, this relationship holds also for mental disorders, perhaps because the associated deprivation is usually accompanied by unemployment, loss of social role and a subsequent sense of alienation from mainstream society (Pilgrim and Rogers 1999).

At the heart of this model is the premise that people are prone to mental disturbance when unpleasant events strike them without warning. This fact led Holmes and Rahe (1967) to develop the Social Readjustment Rating Scale, which attributes a severity score to 42 life events according to the degree of change or adaptation they produce in people. Perhaps not surprisingly, bereavement, divorce and starting a new job are high on the list.

There is an intuitive appeal to the social model since many people are likely to have experienced major upheavals in their lives that may have caused them to feel psychological distress. Anxiety and low mood, for example, may be experienced in the run up to a series of exams or in response to the frustrations associated typically with moving house. The social model provides also a rationale for the origin of other types of psychological distress in which delusions, hallucinations and an apparent loss of contact with reality occur. For example, it is known that unexpected life events are associated with the onset of schizophrenia (Brown and Birley 1968). Furthermore, the levels of critical 'expressed emotion' experienced by a person with schizophrenia from family members is predictive of the severity of the person's condition and, in particular, the likelihood of relapse (Falloon 1995).

Proponents of the social model do not have fixed ideas about what constitutes a psychiatric illness. Indeed, the model is concerned that labelling people with a psychiatric illness may create a disorder itself (Tyrer and Steinberg 2005). All symptoms and behaviour have to be understood in the context of the society from which they emanate. There are no independent, objective criteria for mental disorder according to the social model, only a boundary line between normal and abnormal that has been set by society.

Supporters of the social model aim to help people take up an acceptable role in society once more, rather than to correct a chemical imbalance or recondition specific behaviours (Tyrer and Steinberg 2005). This may involve social skills training, some systemic family therapies and more general family interventions involving education on the influence of critical 'expressed emotion' (Gamble and Brennan 2005).

The basic premise of the social model is reflected in Standard 1 of the National Service Framework (NSF) for Mental Health (DH 1999), which acknowledges that mental health problems can arise from the adverse effects of social exclusion. Subsequently, the Office of the Deputy Prime Minister published a major report on *Mental Health and Social Exclusion* (ODPM 2004). Though an important contribution to the field its impact has been disappointing partly due to the waning influence and eventual disappearance of the Office of the Deputy Prime Minister (cf. Chapter 6)

Integrating models of mental disorder

There are key features that differentiate each of the models according to the four quadrant framework introduced in Chapter 1. For example, the disease model is concerned with physical, biological and chemical markers of mental disorder. These markers can be observed and measured, and are therefore representative of an *objective* orientation. In contrast, the cognitive model deals with internal thought processes unique to individuals. This orientation is therefore primarily *subjective*.

There is a further difference to note. The behavioural model is concerned with *a person's* behaviour. Attention to this alone will suffice for the behaviour therapist. This model is clearly orientated to the *self*. In contrast, the social model is concerned not with *self* but with forces beyond a person's control in the society in which they live. This orientation is referred to as *community*.

These two dimensions, *subjective–objective* and *self–community*, are used to formulate the four-quadrant framework (Figure 2.1). Each of the models is positioned in their respective quadrants. Thus, the disease model, which is concerned with a person's biophysiological profile is upper right (*objective–self*). Similarly, the behavioural model, which deals with a person's observable behaviours is also upper right. The cognitive model however, is upper left (*subjective–self*) since its primary focus is on the internal thought processes of the individual.

	Subjective	Objective
Self	Cognitive	Disease
	Freudian Psychodynamics	Behavioural
Community	Jungian Psychodynamics	
	Social	Social

Figure 2.1 Framework for models of mental disorder

Freudian psychodynamics are certainly upper left (*subjective–self*) dealing as they do with our inner world and specifically our sense of self. However, Jungian psychodynamics are premised on a transcendent self, borne of intersubjective culture and mythology (community). For this reason we feel inclined to position Jung in the lower left quadrant (*subjective–community*). Finally, the social model is certainly community oriented but straddles both lower quadrants. Unemployment and poverty are quantifiable attributes, and each is associated with mental disorder. This interpretation of the social model reflects the lower right quadrant (*objective–community*). On the other hand, intersubjective experiences such as kinship and expressed emotion are also associated with mental disorder. This interpretation reflects the lower left quadrant (*subjective–community*).

Figure 2.1 illustrates the general orientation of different schools of thought in explaining the aetiology of mental disorder and points of comparison and contrast. But things are more complex than appear here, and there is certainly blurring across the quadrants. Cognitive behavioural therapy is a good example, since cognitive therapists might argue that although they deal initially with unique internal thought processes, they endeavour to alter these with recourse to external, observable evidence (*objective–self*). Nevertheless, it remains true that they are primarily concerned with, and rooted in, a person's subjective experience. All models have something to contribute to a contemporary understanding of mental disorder precisely because human experience is made up of a subjective and objective sense of self, and a subjective and objective sense of community.

We suggest, therefore, that the models of mental disorder considered here have many more points in common than difference because they each tap into a limited but, nevertheless, vital aspect of the human condition. Human experience arises from all four quadrants and mental health nurses need to draw on them all in their practice rather than discount some but not others on grounds of preference or prejudice.

The stress vulnerability model

An integrated, second-order model was developed by Zubin and Spring (1977) to specifically explain the aetiology of schizophrenia. Incorporating all other models, it has as its common denominator the relationship between stress and vulnerability. Stress is the variable that influences the manifestation of symptoms and a person's vulnerability represents their predisposition to such manifestations.

Two types of stress are at play here. The first is known as ambient stress and reflects the general concerns and pressures that people face in their everyday lives. Although such stressors are necessary to function and perform some people experience more ambient stress than others. The second type of stress arises from life events such as those included in Holmes and Rahe's (1967) Social Readjustment Rating Scale.

Similarly, there are two types of vulnerability. The first is inborn and will probably include genetic loading and the neurophysiology of the person. The second is acquired and will be specific to an individual's life experiences but may include perinatal complications, maladaptive learned behaviours or thought patterns, and adolescent peer interactions (Zubin and Spring 1977). Notice that these descriptions include features from the single models previously described and can, therefore, be mapped according to the four quadrants in Figure 2.1: for example, vulnerability can be upper left (thought patterns) or upper right (genetic loading) but also lower left (adolescent peer interactions).

Zubin and Spring's (1977) central hypothesis is that the interface between an individual's vulnerability and the stress they experience in the course of their lives is the basis for the development or otherwise of schizophrenic symptomatology. There will, of course, be a range of vulnerabilities in any population, with some people being extremely prone to illness even when experiencing relatively mild levels of stress, to those whose vulnerability is so low that they are able to tolerate high levels of stress for significant periods without any trace of psychiatric symptoms.

Since its publication in 1977 this model has had considerable impact in the field of mental health care. It offers hope to those who experience mental disorders because it suggests that coping mechanisms can be acquired to counter the effects of stress and thus reduce the risk of continued illness or relapse. The model is also of considerable value to mental health staff, since it provides a rationale for the use of psychosocial as well as medicinal interventions, and nursing has significantly developed its psychosocial skills base as a result.

The classification of mental disorder

Systems for classifying mental disorder or 'illness' stem from the medical model, which as Tyrer and Steinberg (2005) point out is not an aetiological model itself but an approach to diagnosing individual disorder. In a general sense all models apply this process, with exception perhaps of the social model, although the systems that are used for classification purposes vary between models. For example, the cognitive model uses Ellis's (1962) ABC framework for defining specific cognitive problems that arise between an activating event and the behavioural or cognitive consequence. Problem-oriented statements can be constructed from such an analysis, which represent one approach to classification. For example, 'When I make eye contact with strangers in public (Activating event), I believe they immediately think bad of me (Belief), and therefore I avoid social interaction (Consequence).' This statement classifies a cognitive or behavioural problem depending on your perspective.

Medical diagnosis is another classification system, which represents the dominant frame of reference for most mental health workers internationally. These diagnoses are described in two classification systems; the *International Classification of Disease* (ICD-10 World Health Organization (WHO) 1992); and the *Diagnostic and Statistical Manual for Mental Disorders* (DSM-IV American Psychiatric Association (APA) 1994). At the time of writing both systems are undergoing consultation and development. ICD-11 is scheduled for implementation in 2015 following draft publication in 2010. It will be designed in three different formats; for primary care, specialist services and research. DSM-V is scheduled for publication in 2012.

Ideally each diagnosis should be mutually exclusive and stand independently of other symptoms associated with other diagnoses. Rarely in practice is this achieved. More often than not a range of symptoms may indicate the relevance of two or more diagnoses. This point is particularly pertinent to the ICD-10 classification system, which uses a single axis on which to select diagnoses for a specific disorder. If more than one is selected they may appear to contradict each other (Tyrer and Steinberg 2005). However, psychiatric diagnoses are based on a hierarchical system so that each disorder can manifest symptoms present in disorders lower down the hierarchy, but not above it (Sturt 1981). For example, an individual who experiences persistent low mood may receive a diagnosis of *depression*. However, if the low mood is accompanied by delusional thought patterns, a diagnosis of *schizoaffective disorder* will take precedence over a diagnosis of depression.

In contrast to the single-axis approach of ICD-10 there is an increasing tendency to use multi-axial approaches in which clinical diagnosis is only one part. Thus, in DSM-IV the clinical diagnosis is axis 1, personality status is described in axis 2, and developmental delay, intellectual status, physical health, social functioning and reactions to stress are all separate axes. This approach allows several descriptors to be attributed to an individual's symptoms and their general condition.

Before examining ICD-10 diagnostic categories, which is the dominant frame of reference in the UK, it is important to stress that any system classifies syndromes and conditions, but not individuals. Anyone can suffer from one or more disorders of either a mental or physical nature at different times in their lives. It is meaningless, therefore, as well as stigmatizing, to use diagnostic labels to describe people. A person should never be equated with a disorder, physical or mental (WHO 2001).

ICD-10 diagnostic categories

Table 2.1 presents the main diagnostic groupings in ICD-10 together with their key features. The table presents an overview and readers are referred to subsequent chapters for more detailed accounts of many of these conditions. Equally, we recommend an examination of the WHO (1992) classification manual, particularly Chapter 5, which provides detailed information on all 100 categories of classification (though a proportion of these remain unused at present).

Psychoses and neuroses

The terms 'psychoses' and 'neuroses' are second-order classifications that group several of the conditions in Table 2.1. The psychoses are disorders in which '… people's capacity to recognize reality, their thinking processes, judgements and communications are seriously impaired, together with the presence of delusions and hallucinations' (Craig 2000: 54). In turn, these are divided into 'organic' and 'functional' psychoses. The former are represented by the group F00–F09 in Table 2.1 in which pathological processes affecting the brain result in psychotic symptoms. The functional psychoses are group F20–F29 and include schizophrenia and delusional disorders but also affective psychoses in which a primary disturbance of mood is accompanied by psychotic symptoms. In keeping with the hierarchical nature of diagnosis, any disorder in the F30–F39 group that incorporates psychotic symptoms will be elevated to a diagnosis within the F20–F29 group.

Individuals who experience neuroses are different from the general population only in the degree of the symptoms they experience. Thus, anxiety and low mood are common to people's experience of life. Indeed anxiety needs to be present to some degree before an important exam in order to enhance performance. However, if this anxiety becomes so great that it debilitates an individual, so that they cannot even attend the exam, then this may indicate a neurotic mental disorder. Therefore, in contrast to the psychoses, in which a person's grasp of reality is uncertain, the neuroses are characterized by the heightening of normal human experiences but to levels that interfere with a person's ability to function. The neuroses are represented by groups F30–F39 and F40–F48 in Table 2.1.

A group that falls outside of the psychoses/neuroses divide are the personality disorders represented by F60–F69. Personality is a familiar concept and one that people use to describe friends and colleagues. We may, for example, say that someone is always cheerful or shy. However, the personality disorders contained in F60–F69 are indicative of habitual behaviours that lead people into conflict with society. These deeply ingrained maladaptive behavioural patterns have been classified into different types of personality disorder including obsessive, avoidant, schizoid, paranoid, borderline, antisocial, dependent, schizotypal, histrionic and narcissistic (WHO 1992).

Diagnostic groupings	Key features
F00–F09 Organic mental disorders including dementias and delirium	Brain dysfunction resulting in disturbances of cognition, mood, perception and/or behaviour
F10–F19 Psychoactive substance use including intoxication, abuse, dependence and withdrawal states	Typically present when substance use interferes with a person's physical, mental or social functioning to the detriment of their well-being
F20–F29 Schizophrenia, schizotypal, delusional and schizoaffective disorders	Mental states characterized by distortions of thinking, perception and mood, but not due to an organic condition
F30–F39 Mood (affective) disorders including depression, manic disorder and bipolar disorders	The key symptom is a disturbance in mood though other features will also be present associated with this mood change for example social isolation accompanying depression
F40–F48 Neurotic, stress-related and somatoform disorders including phobias, obsessive compulsive disorder and stress reactions	A range of symptoms may be present including tension, anxiety, problems with concentration and ritualistic behaviours
F50–F59 Behavioural syndromes including eating disorders, sleep disorders and post-partum mental disorders	Symptoms vary according to the condition, for example weight loss with certain eating disorders. However, physiological and hormonal factors appear to play a part in these conditions
F60–F69 Disorders of adult personality and behaviour including personality disorders, gender identity disorders and impulse disorders	Disorders in which clinically significant behaviour patterns are persistent and reflect the person's lifestyle and way of interacting with others
F70–F79 Mental retardation of varying degrees from mild to profound	Usually manifest by the impairment of skills associated with intelligence
F80–F89 Disorders of psychological development including autism, speech disorders, disorders in scholastic skills and developmental disorders of motor functions	Originating in infancy or childhood these disorders delay the development of functions related to maturation of the central nervous system
F90–F98 Behavioural and emotional disorders of childhood including conduct disorders and hyperkinetic disorders	Only common features are an onset early in life and a fluctuating or unpredictable course

Table 2.1 ICD-10 classification of mental and behavioural disorders (*Adapted from WHO 1992; and Tyrer and Steinberg 2005*)

There has been considerable debate regarding how best to provide services for individuals with a diagnosis of personality disorder. Traditionally this diagnosis has often resulted in the neglect of the individual by psychiatric services. This is no longer acceptable and there has been a significant programme of service development and research in recent years, supported by England's Department of Health. The origins, processes and outputs of this programme are discussed in Chapter 26.

Serious mental illness and common mental health problems

A further distinction between different types of mental disorder is made with reference to 'serious mental illness' (SMI) and 'common mental health problems'. Current mental health policy and practice has been influenced significantly by the concept of SMI, the origins of which are many, though there have been two predominant influences from the past decade.

In 1990, White reported a tendency among community psychiatric nurses (CPNs) to provide primary care based liaison services through which they were more likely to encounter patients with neurotic rather than psychotic symptoms. Alongside this increasing awareness of CPN activity the British media reported a number of high-profile homicides committed by people with a mental illness, which they argued demonstrated the failure of community care. Public concern was countered by the Department of Health who began to target services towards people with SMI. Thus, the *Health of the Nation: Key Area Handbook* (DH 1994a) identified those with SMI to be the priority target group for services. The Mental Health Nursing Review Team report of the same year recommended that '... the essential focus for the work of mental health nurses lies in working with people with serious or enduring mental illness in secondary and tertiary care ...' (DH 1994b: 16).

These terms are still used today but with less frequency. A complementary classification approach has developed based on the severity or complexity of individual need. The Chief Nursing Officer's review of mental health nursing published in 2006 states that 'mental health nurses should ... focus on working directly with people with high levels of need and supporting other workers to meet less complex needs' (DH 2006: 2). This has not moved far from the original classification with SMI equating in general terms to complex need and common mental health problems to less complex need.

Key symptoms of mental disorder

The key symptoms of mental disorder are typically classified according to their impact on a person's mood, thought processes, perceptions and behaviour.

Mood

Anxiety

Anxiety is distinguished from general tension by its accompanying physical sensations (autonomic nervous system arousal), including palpitations, sweating and tremor. Anxiety may occur in response to phobic situations or specific thoughts but can also occur independently of any such trigger (free-floating anxiety), or be linked to a sense that something dreadful is about to occur (anxious foreboding) (Craig 2000). Anxiety may also occur abruptly for short periods during which the person experiences marked fearfulness and may feel they are losing control (panic attacks).

Depression

'Sad', 'gloomy' and 'low spirits' are synonymous with depressed mood. More severe forms of this experience encompass additional features including a reduced emotional response to the ups and downs of life (flattened or blunted affect). The individual may also experience disturbed sleep patterns, loss of appetite and a lack of interest in and engagement with life. More extreme forms of this experience can be accompanied by feelings of hopelessness, possibly leading to suicidal thoughts. Other terms associated with this experience include *self-deprecation* (loss of confidence in self and a developing sense of worthlessness) and *pathological guilt* (feeling responsible for actions that may be inconsequential to others).

Elation

Individuals who experience elation in the course of a mental health problem may feel euphoric and excited but also irritable and impatient (Craig 2000). Typically, concentration is impaired, there is over-talkativeness, a reduced need for sleep and reckless acts are not uncommon, for example excessive spending sprees. Common to these symptoms is an underlying self-esteem that is exaggerated, and grandiose beliefs, such as having special intelligence, are not uncommon.

Thought processes

Obsessional thoughts and compulsions

A person's thoughts are considered obsessional when they become intrusive, unwanted and no longer amenable to self-control (obsessional ruminations). *Obsessional incompleteness* refers to an overriding desire to ensure every aspect of a task has been correctly executed before the individual can consider it complete. Intrusive thoughts of this type may be accompanied by repetitive, *ritualistic behaviour*. An important feature that distinguishes these types of thought is the person's awareness that they are their own.

Delusions

A delusion is a false impression or belief that we can all be subject to from time to time. In the mental health field additional qualities associated with delusional thought distinguish it as a symptom of mental disorder. The belief is usually held with absolute and compelling conviction, is typically idiosyncratic and resistant to modification through experience or discussion (Craig 2000). Different types of delusion have been classified including *delusions of persecution* and *delusions of reference*. The latter often involves people feeling that news items on the TV, radio or in newspapers have a double meaning and make reference specifically to them.

Thought possession

Some people with mental health problems encounter the sensation that the innermost workings of their mind are amenable to outsiders (Craig 2000). Different sorts of experience have been described including *thought broadcasting* (a person believes that their thoughts are heard aloud by those around them), and *thought insertion* (a loss in the ownership of a person's own thoughts, usually accompanied by a delusional explanation for how thoughts are placed in their mind).

Perceptions

Perception among people who experience mental health problems can become diminished, heightened or distorted (Craig 2000). Hallucinations are a key symptom in this respect, which are defined as false perceptions in so far as there is no adequate external stimulus for the experience. Each of the five human senses can be affected by hallucinations. Thus, hallucinations are typically referred to as auditory, visual, olfactory, tactile and gustatory.

Behaviour

The behaviour and appearance of people with mental disorders may appear strange or unusual. A lack of self-care and accompanying self-neglect are not uncommon, but neither are they necessarily an indication of mental disorder. The specific patterns and qualities of a person's speech are more useful indicators of a mental disorder. Symptoms may include *pressure of speech* (a rush of words that is difficult to stop), *flight of ideas* (skipping from topic to topic with no logical association), and *poverty of speech* (speaking freely but in such a vague manner that no meaningful information is communicated).

The symptoms associated with the functional psychoses are sometimes also referred to as 'positive' and 'negative'. Brennan explores these terms in detail in Chapter 18.

Prevalence and incidence of mental disorders

Prevalence, expressed as a percentage, refers to the number of people with a particular disorder within a given population. Incidence, on the other hand, also expressed as a percentage, refers to the number of new cases that arise within a given population in a given time period. Actual estimates of prevalence and incidence of mental disorders vary from one epidemiological study to the next. Different samples will have been studied and there may be real differences between populations. Also different instruments might have been used, and the results from these might have been interpreted in different ways to define a 'case'.

The NSF for Mental Health (DH 1999) used a variety of sources to present prevalence data including World Health Organization figures, which generate European and other world region estimates, rather than country specific data (though the most recent report (WHO 2001) does provide estimates for Manchester as a marker for UK data). The NSF (DH 1999) also relied on a survey of psychiatric morbidity for adults conducted in the UK in 1994 (Meltzer *et al.* 1995). More recently this survey was repeated by Singleton *et al.* (2001) who sampled more than 15,000 private households in England, Wales and Scotland. Important work has also been conducted by the Mental Health Foundation (2005, 2007) to collate data on the prevalence of mental health problems from various sources, and by the Sainsbury Centre for Mental Health (SCMH 1998). Data from these sources indicate that:

■ One in four people will experience some kind of mental health problem in the course of a year. Between 10 and 25 per cent of the population present with mental health problems each year, usually in primary care. Within this figure, 2–4 per cent have a severe mental illness. Only 0.3–1.5 per cent of the population as a whole have severe and enduring mental health problems at any one time.

- Neuroses or common mental health problems are the most common form of mental health problem. The Office for National Statistics (ONS) survey in 2000 (Singleton *et al.* 2001) reported that 1 in 6 adults were assessed as having a neurotic disorder in the week before interview. Somewhere between 1 in 4 and 1 in 6 people will have serious depression at some stage in their lives. Clinical depression is second only to coronary heart disease in terms of international health burden. One in 10 people will have a disabling anxiety disorder at some stage in their lives. This may be a general anxiety mental health problem or a more specific phobia or obsessive compulsive disorder. Most neuroses last under one year, although there is a strong chance of recurrence. The ONS survey found that prevalence rates for all neurotic disorders, except for panic disorder, were higher among women than men. The highest prevalence rates were for people aged 40–54 and lowest for those over the age of 65. There were few differences between the 1993 and 2000 ONS surveys.

- Psychoses are less common. One in 100 people will suffer from bipolar illness and 1 in 100 from schizophrenia at some stage in their lives. Between a quarter and one half of people recover completely after a psychosis. Most people have multiple 'acute' episodes but only a minority of these have systematically reduced psychological function between episodes. An estimated 10–15 per cent of people with schizophrenia develop severe long-term disabilities. Again the ONS surveys of 1993 and 2000 show few changes over time in prevalence rates.

- Eating disorders are often not recognized or reported and studies may under-estimate prevalence. Anorexia nervosa affects 1 per cent of women aged 15–30. Half of these cases occur before the age of 20 and women outnumber men by 12 to 1. Bulimia nervosa affects 1–2 per cent of adult women.

- For the first time the 2000 ONS survey investigated the prevalence of personality disorder. Overall, 1 in 25 adults were assessed as having a disorder. The most common diagnosis was obsessive compulsive personality disorder with avoidant, schizoid, paranoid, borderline and anti-social disorders each having a prevalence of less than 1 per cent, although diagnosis of personality disorder is particularly controversial. Slightly more men than women were considered to have a personality disorder.

- Problems with drinking alcohol are common. The ONS 2000 survey revealed a prevalence of 38 per cent of men and 15 per cent of women as having a hazardous pattern of drinking during the year before interview. This prevalence decreased markedly with increasing age. Alcohol dependence was assessed as affecting 12 per cent of men and 3 per cent of women. Hazardous and harmful drinking was found to be affecting 32 per cent of men and 15 per cent of women in the 2004 national alcohol needs assessment (Drummond 2004). Alcohol abuse is associated with a range of mental disorders as well as alcohol disorders and is recognized as one possible and significant factor in the development of depression (WHO 2004).

- Overall, 13 per cent of men and 8 per cent of women reported using illegal drugs in the ONS 2000 survey. Cannabis was the most commonly used drug (10 per cent) with amphetamines, cocaine and ecstasy each used by 2 per cent of adults aged 16–74. As with alcohol use, prevalence of illegal drug use declines sharply with increasing age. The ONS 2000 survey assessed dependence using a low threshold and found 4 per cent of the population to be dependent on one or more illegal drugs (6 per cent for men, 2 per cent for women). This is double the figure reported in the 1993 survey.

■ Mental health problems in children and young people are also common. Studies have shown that 10 per cent of children and young people require specialist help and 1 in 5 have psychiatric symptoms at any one time. Anxiety, depression, hyperactivity and conduct disorder are the most common mental health problems. Estimates of prevalence vary widely because of different definitions and the high level of hidden morbidity.

■ Common mental health problems affect older people but may go unrecognized or untreated. Dementia affects 1 per cent of people aged 60–65, 5 per cent of those over 65 and perhaps as many as 20 per cent of those aged over 80. One in 1000 people under 65 have Alzheimer's disease (the most common form of dementia).

Mental health problems do not affect all groups of people equally. Many factors are associated with mental health problems. It must, however, be remembered that association is not the same as causality. For example social isolation may both lead to mental health problems and be a psychological and social response to mental health problems. Epidemiological studies have found the following:

■ **Isolation**: people with a neurosis and more markedly people with a psychosis are more likely than the general population to be separated or divorced and/or to live in a one-person family unit.

■ **Social class**: people with a probable psychosis are more likely to be defined as being in social classes IV or V.

■ **Unemployment**: 39 per cent of people with a neurosis and 70 per cent with a psychosis were found to be economically inactive compared to 28 per cent with no disorder.

■ **Social deprivation**: there are clear associations between social deprivation (e.g. poor housing/homelessness, employment and education) and mental illness. The Department of Health's psychiatric needs index shows a four-fold variation in need between the most affluent local authorities and the most deprived. Many authors argue that the variation in need is even greater for the most severe mental health problems. It is thought that the need for assertive outreach style services for people with the most severe difficulties varies from 12 to 200 people per 100,000 people aged 16 to 64 (Sainsbury Centre for Mental Health 1998).

■ **Physical ill health**: 57 per cent of people with a neurosis and 62 per cent with a psychosis reported having a physical complaint, compared to 38 per cent of those with no mental health problem.

■ **Black and minority ethnic communities**: Asian and African-Caribbean people are less likely to have mental health difficulties recognized by their GP. The prevalence of schizophrenia among Black African and African-Caribbean people is a much contested area of research. Whatever the underlying issues it is clear that Black people are considerably over-represented in secure settings and detentions under the Mental Health Act 1983. Many authors have argued that the cause is institutional racism, although this is seldom seen as the only factor and interventions coming too late in the development of problems is also a major issue. Mental health services are also seen as failing to meet the needs of these communities (Soni Raleigh 1995). More positive ways of responding have been proposed (Sainsbury Centre for Mental Health 2002) and there have been recent policy developments, but a lack of systematic implementation.

■ **Suicide**: about 5000 people a year in England take their own lives usually as a result of mental ill health especially, of course, clinical depression. The government's *National Suicide Prevention Strategy* (DH 2002) reports that on average somebody dies from suicide every two hours. It is the commonest form of death in men under 35 and is the main cause of premature death in people with mental illness. The majority of suicides occur in young adult men. Suicide rates are low among Asian men and older people but high in young Asian women. Suicide is far more common in social class V than any other social class. The most common means of suicide are hanging and poisoning with analgesic or psychotropic prescribed drugs. The 5-year progress report on the implementation of the National Service Framework for Mental Health (DH 2004) reported that the trend in suicide was down to a new low of 8.6 per 100,000 population per year.

■ **Criminal justice system**: all forms of contact with the police, courts, prison and probation system are associated with high prevalence rates of mental health problems. For example, 56 per cent of sentenced women and 37 per cent of sentenced men are considered to have a psychiatric disorder. The prevalence of mental health problems is higher for remand prisoners.

Conclusion

Nurses are the professional group in closest contact with mental health service users over lengthy periods of illness and wellness, which provides them opportunity to become involved in many areas of a person's life during different stages of health (Repper 2000). Various models of mental disorder have been described, each of which taps into different aspects of human experience. This emphasizes the importance of mental health nurses embracing an integrated understanding of human experience, through which all models have something to contribute. This is not to say that nurses should avoid specializing in interventions derived from one model, for example, behavioural therapy or psychodynamic counselling. Rather, they should acknowledge the necessary but insufficient basis of such specialist knowledge to describe fully human experience. From this position the profession is better placed to provide holistic, integrated care by either broadening its own perspective, or by enjoining with others who possess complementary specialist knowledge. The profession needs also to develop a theoretical and practical understanding of mental health and well-being (cf. Chapters 1 and 3). The combined evidence base will enable the profession to fully realize the contributions it can make to the well-being and recovery of people who experience a mental disorder. To conclude, we summarize the main points of this chapter below:

■ Mental disorders represent shades in the spectrum of human experience, which comprise a *subjective* and *objective* sense of *self* and a *subjective* and *objective* sense of *community*.

■ Models of mental disorder describe aetiology and treatment implications in relation to different levels of human functioning: biophysiological organism (disease); the unconscious (psychodynamic); thought processes (cognitive); actions (behavioural); and self in context (social).

- The models can be mapped against a four-quadrant framework of human experience (Figure 2.1), demonstrating their partial, though necessary contribution to the treatment and care of people who experience mental disorders.
- Mental health nurses need to develop an integrated understanding of mental disorders, to be demonstrated in collaborative partnerships with service users and professional colleagues.
- The profession needs also to integrate considerations for mental health and well-being into its practice in order to promote comprehensive services to the whole person.

Questions for reflection and discussion

1   Reflect on each of the following and consider how much you feel they contribute to your sense of self: genetic endowment; early childhood experiences; learned behaviour or ways of thinking from parents and peers; and social factors.

2   Reflect on a time in your life when you felt distressed (for example losing a loved one, your job, your self-esteem, or experiencing prolonged periods of stress). Spend a little while familiarizing yourself with the events of that time, what your life looked like and how it felt, and then ask yourself: 'Would others have experienced those events in the same way?' And: 'If not, why not?'

3   Put yourself in the position of a person you have known or nursed who has been diagnosed with a mental disorder. What do you remember or think was their preferred perspective on the nature of their problems and the interventions that they considered most appropriate? Did these differ from the reality of the care they received and, if so, why?

4   Use the framework presented in Figure 2.1 to identify the orientation of the chapters that follow. Are they concerned primarily with the objective or the subjective indicators of health and/or illness at the individual or community level?

Annotated bibliography

- Tyrer, P. and Steinberg, D. (2005) *Models for Mental Disorder: Conceptual Models in Psychiatry* (4th edn). Chichester: John Wiley and Sons. Now in its fourth edition, this text provides a detailed yet accessible explanation of the main models of mental disorder in contemporary practice. We have adopted Tyrer and Steinberg's five basic model structure in this chapter but have pursued a different path to integration. However, we recommend also Tyrer and Steinberg's approach, which in this latest edition includes chapters on integration and application of the models in multi-disciplinary teams.
- Gamble, C. and Brennan, G. (eds) (2005) *Working With Serious Mental Illness: A Manual for Clinical Practice* (2nd edn). London: Baillière Tindall. Though primarily a practice manual as the title suggests, this text devotes a chapter to the stress vulnerability model and a section, comprising eight chapters, to interventions based on a stress vulnerability understanding of serious mental illness. This has been a highly successful text for mental health nurses and is now in its second edition.

■ Mental Health Foundation (2007) *The Fundamental Facts.* London: Mental Health Foundation. This is an invaluable resource that provides a round-up of information on the prevalence and incidence of mental health problems. It also contains an overview of service provision in the UK and of the costs of mental health problems to the nation.

Journal of Psychiatric and Mental Health Nursing Volumes **5:** 3 and **6:** 4. These volumes are dedicated to the contributions of Hildegard Peplau and Annie Altschul to mental health nursing. These pioneers draw upon interpersonal theories of human experience and psychodynamic principles in their work. Papers in these volumes demonstrate the application of Peplau's and Altschul's ideas to contemporary health care practice.

References

American Psychiatric Association (1994) *Diagnostic and Statistical Manual for Mental Disorders, 4th revision.* Washington: American Psychiatric Association.

Brown, G. and Birley, J. (1968) Crises and life events and the onset of schizophrenia. *Journal of Health and Social Behaviour* **9**: 203–14.

Craig, T. (2000) Severe mental illness: symptoms, signs and diagnosis, in C. Gamble and G. Brennan (eds) *Working with serious mental illness: a manual for clinical practice.* London: Baillière Tindall.

Department of Health (1994a) *The Health of the Nation: Key Area Handbook: Mental Illness.* London: HMSO.

Department of Health (1994b) *Working in Partnership: A collaborative approach to care.* London: HMSO.

Department of Health (1999) *A National Service Framework for Mental Health.* London: The Stationery Office.

Department of Health (2002) *National Suicide Prevention Strategy.* London: DH.

Department of Health (2004) *The National Service Framework for Mental Health – Five Years On.* London: DH.

Department of Health (2006) *From Values to Action: The Chief Nursing Officer's review of mental health nursing: Summary.* London: DH.

Drummond, C. (2004) *Alcohol needs assessment research project.* London: DH.

Durkheim, E. (1897) *Le Suicide.* Paris: Alcan.

Ellis, A. (1962) *Reason and Emotion in Psychotherapy.* New York: Stuart.

Falloon, I. (1995) *Family Management of Schizophrenia.* Baltimore: Johns Hopkins University Press.

Gamble, C. and Brennan, G. (2005) *Working with Serious Mental Illness: A Manual for Clinical Practice* (2nd edn). London: Baillière Tindall.

Gournay, K. (1996) Schizophrenia: a review of the contemporary literature and implications for mental health nursing theory, practice and education. *Journal of Psychiatric and Mental Health Nursing* **3**: 7–12.

Gournay, K., Denford, L., Parr, A.-M. and Newell, R. (2000) British nurses in behavioural psychotherapy: a 25-year follow up. *Journal of Advanced Nursing* **32**: 1–9.

Grant, A., Mills, J., Mulhern, R. and Shot, N. (2004) *Cognitive Behavioural Therapy in Mental Health Care.* London: Sage Publications.

Holmes, T. and Rahe, R. (1967) The social readjustment rating scale. *Journal of Psychosomatic Research* **11**: 213–18.

Kinsella, P. and Garland, A. (2008) *Cognitive Behavioural Therapy for Mental Health Workers: A Beginner's Guide.* London: Routledge.

Marks, I. (1987) *Fears, Phobias and Rituals: Panic, Anxiety and Their Disorders.* Oxford: Oxford University Press.

Marks, I., Bird, J. and Lindley, P. (1978) Behavioural nurse therapists: developments and implications. *Behavioural Psychotherapy* **6**: 25–6.

Mental Health Foundation (2005) *Lifetime Impacts.* London: Mental Health Foundation.

Mental Health Foundation (2007) *The Fundamental Facts.* London: Mental Health Foundation.

Meltzer, H., Gill, B., Petticrew, M. and Hinds, K. (1995) *OPCS Surveys of Psychiatric Morbidity in Great Britain, Report 1: the Prevalence of Psychiatric Morbidity among Adults living in Private Households.* London: HMSO.

Morrison, A., Renton, J., Dunn, H. and Williams, S. (2003) *Cognitive Therapy for Psychosis: A Formulation-Based Approach.* London: Routledge.

Office of the Deputy Prime Minister (2004) *Mental Health and Social Exclusion.* London: Office of the Deputy Prime Minister.

Pavlov, I. (1927) *Conditioned Reeves.* London: Oxford University Press.

Pilgrim, D. and Rogers, A. (1999) *Sociology of Mental Health and Illness.* Oxford: Oxford University Press.

Plant, J. and Stephenson, J. (2008) *Beating Stress, Anxiety and Depression.* London: Piatkus Books.

Repper, J. (2000) Adjusting the focus of mental health nursing: Incorporating service users' experiences of recovery. *Journal of Mental Health* **9**: 575–87.

Sainsbury Centre for Mental Health (1998) *Keys to Engagement: Review of Care for People with Severe Mental Illness who are Difficult to Engage.* London: Sainsbury Centre for Mental Health.

Sainsbury Centre for Mental Health (2002) *Breaking the Circles of Fear: A Review of the Relationship Between Mental Health Services and African and Caribbean Communities.* London: Sainsbury Centre for Mental Health.

Scadding, J. (1967) Diagnosis: the clinician and the computer. *Lancet* **ii**: 877–82.

Singleton, N., Bumpstead, R., O'Brien, M., Lee, A. and Meltzer, H. (2001) *Psychiatric Morbidity among Adults Living in Private Households.* London: The Stationery Office.

Skinner, B. (1972) *Beyond Freedom and Dignity.* London: Jonathan Cape.

Soni Raleigh, V. (1995) *Mental Health in Black and Minority Ethnic People: The fundamental facts.* London: Mental Health Foundation.

Sturt, E. (1981) Hierarchical patterns in the distribution of psychiatric symptoms. *Psychological Medicine* **11**: 783–94.

Tyrer, P. and Steinberg, D. (2005) *Models for Mental Disorder: Conceptual Models in Psychiatry* (4th edn). Chichester: John Wiley and Sons.

Whitehead, M. (1992) The Health Divide, in P. Townsend, N. Davidson and M. Whitehead (eds) *Inequalities in Health.* Harmondsworth: Penguin.

World Health Organization (1992) *International Classification of Disease* – 10th edn. Geneva: WHO.

World Health Organization (2001) *The World Health Report 2001: Mental health; New Understanding, New Hope.* Geneva: WHO.

World Health Organization (2004) *Global status report on alcohol 2004.* Geneva: World Health Organization.

Zubin, J. and Spring, B. (1977) Vulnerability – A new view of schizophrenia. *Journal of Abnormal Psychology* **86**: 103–26.

CHAPTER 3

Future directions in mental health promotion and public mental health

Lynne Friedli

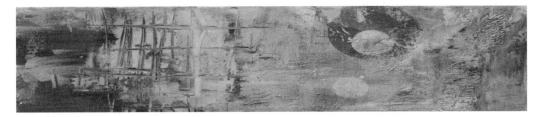

Chapter overview

This chapter covers:

- The emergence of mental health promotion as a discipline;
- Different definitions of mental health promotion;
- Public mental health and population approaches;
- Mental health promotion and recovery.

It concludes by highlighting three key challenges for the future of mental health promotion and public mental health:

- mainstreaming;
- putting inequalities at the centre of the mental health promotion agenda;
- resisting a focus on individual interventions and solutions.

Introduction

Mental health promotion can be described very simply as: *any action to improve mental health*. At the same time, mental health promotion is one of the most complex and contested fields of public health. It is emerging as a topic of considerable policy and public interest, intersecting with current debates about happiness, quality of life and emotional well-being, notably of children (Huppert 2005; Friedli in press). It also prompts challenging questions about the medicalization of sadness, disappointment, anger and frustration (Horwitz and Wakefield 2007).

The literature on mental health promotion reflects broader conflicts about the meaning of mental health, the determinants of mental illness and how society should respond to people experiencing mental health problems. The theory and practice of mental health promotion cannot be separated from how people with mental health problems have been treated, both within the community and by the medical professions and criminal justice system. People's experiences of compulsory admission, detention, medication and other treatments, and mental health services generally, continue to be central to thinking about all aspects of mental health.

The contested nature of mental health promotion and what it means to be mentally healthy echoes similar debates on conformity and diversity within the civil rights movement, the women's, gay and black liberation movements and the disability rights movement. While there may be broad agreement that improving mental well-being is a worthwhile goal, there is far less consensus on the ethics and potential consequences of a prevention agenda. There are concerns about wider civil liberties issues, if the goal of interventions is to eliminate all disorders of the mind, in the same way that the disability rights movement challenges attempts to eliminate all conditions that result in physical disabilities.

As the field of mental health promotion expands to include positive mental health, there are further questions about the relative contribution to mental well-being of individual psychological skills and attributes (e.g. autonomy, positive thinking, self efficacy) and the circumstances of people's lives: housing, employment, income and status. These debates are relevant to all aspects of health and health care and raise challenging questions for the practice of nursing.

Mental illness to mental health: the emergence of mental health promotion as a discipline

Recent years have seen a marked shift in the debates about mental health, from a predominant focus on mental illness to an analysis of the importance of mental health and well-being to overall health (Jane-Llopis and Anderson 2005; Mental Health Foundation 2005). This shift is evident across the UK and in Europe, notably in the World Health Organization (WHO) Europe Declaration[4] and the European Union (EU) Green Paper on Mental Health (European Commission 2006).

This is in part a result of a growing policy acknowledgement of both the economic and public health case for a greater focus on promotion and prevention. The *Wanless Report*, for example, argues that the assessment of population health should move beyond morbidity and mortality data, to the inclusion of measures of positive physical and mental health. 'A health service, not a sickness service' has become an increasingly significant catch phrase for the direction of NHS policy (Wanless 2002, 2004). It is also related more specifically to the costs of mental illness and the limited effectiveness of treatment: it is calculated that the overall cost of mental health problems in the UK amounted to over £110 billion in 2006/7 (Friedli and Parsonage 2007).[5]

---

[4] The WHO European ministerial conference on mental health, in Helsinki in January 2005, brought together all 52 countries in the European region of the WHO. Organized in partnership with the European Union and the Council of Europe, the conference's declaration and action plan will drive the policy agenda on mental health for the coming years (WHO 2005) http://www.euro.who.int/document/mnh/edoc07.pdf; http//www.euro.who.int/document/mnh/edoc06.pdf.

[5] Northern Ireland's share of the total is put around £3.5 billion, reflecting a prevalence rate for mental health problems which is 20-25 per cent higher than in the rest of the UK.

Although the situation across the UK varies, all four countries have a policy commitment to mental health promotion,[6] with perhaps the most comprehensive approach in Scotland, through the National Programme for Improving Mental Health and Well-being, launched in 2001 (http://www.wellscotland.info/mentalhealth/national-programme.html). This includes an ambitious attempt to develop indicators of mental health, to complement existing indicators of mental illness.[7] The Welsh Assembly has published its *Mental Health Promotion Action Plan for Wales: consultation document* (Welsh Assembly 2006), which requires each local health board to develop a mental health promotion strategy by 2007/8. Meanwhile in Northern Ireland, the Bamford Review on mental health promotion (Bamford 2004; DHSSPS 2006), states:

❝   We also want to see a society where everyone plays a role in and takes action to create an environment that promotes the mental health and well-being of individuals, families, organizations and communities

(DHSSPS 2006). ❞

In England, the publication of the National Service Framework for Mental Health (DH 1999) marked a significant turning point. For the first time, health and social services were required to: 'promote mental health for all, working with individuals, organizations and communities' as well as to tackle the stigma, discrimination and social exclusion experienced by people with mental health problems. This commitment was reinforced in the White Paper *Choosing Health* (DH 2004a) and in *Our Health, Our Care, Our Say*:

❝   We will ensure that standard one of the NSF for Mental Health, which deals with mental health promotion, is fully implemented. ❞

❝   We will have delivered if we improve the mental health and well-being of the general population.

(DH 2006) ❞

Guidance to support delivery of mental health promotion, through the development of local mental health promotion strategies, was first published in 2001 (DH 2001), although tackling discrimination and social exclusion has tended to receive a stronger focus than promoting mental health for all (Social Exclusion Unit 2004; NIMHE 2004).

Louis Appleby, National Director for Mental Health remarked on lack of progress on Standard One and in his report *The National Service Framework for Mental Health: Five Years On,* noted: 'We need to broaden our focus from specialist mental health services to the mental health needs of the community as a whole' (DH 2004b).

The launch of *Making it Possible: Improving mental health and well-being in England* (NIMHE 2005) can be seen as an effort to achieve this broader focus and to provide greater leadership and support for a population wide approach to improving mental health. *Making it Possible* sets a framework for action to:

---

[6]   For a review of progress on mental health promotion across the four UK nations, see Friedli, L. (2004) Editorial. *Journal of Mental Health Promotion* **3**(1): 2–6.
[7]   http://www.healthscotland.com/understanding/population/mental-health-indicators.aspx

- raise public awareness of how to look after our own mental health and other people's;
- involve all communities and organizations, across all sectors, in taking positive steps to promote and protect mental well-being.

It argues that improving the mental health of the population will contribute to achieving a wide range of cross-government priorities for children and adults and to meeting Public Service Agreement (PSA) targets in health, education, neighbourhood renewal, crime, community cohesion, sustainable development, employment, culture and sport. The framework sets out nine priorities for action (Box 3.1).

Box 3.1   Public mental health: key areas and measures of success

Action: marketing mental health

People are well informed and motivated to look after their own and others' mental health

People have positive and accepting attitudes to people with mental health problems

Action: equality and inclusion

People have access to a wide range of sources of support for emotional and psychological difficulties

Reduction in inequalities in access to non-pharmacological sources of support, notably for black and minority ethnic communities and older people

Action: tackling violence and abuse

Reduction in prevalence of mental health problems

Reduction in self-harming behaviour

Action: parents and early years

Parents and caregivers have the knowledge, skills and capacity to meet the emotional and social needs of infants and young children

Parents and carers have access to support for themselves and their parenting roles, delivered in a way that is evidence-based and meets their needs

Action: schools

Schools achieving National Healthy Schools Status targets and delivering SEAL

Action: employment

Reduction in mental health related unemployment

Action: workplace

Workplaces adopt HSE stress management standards

Support in place to enable people off work with mental health problems to return to work

Action: communities

Improved quality of life and life satisfaction

Increase in the proportion of local areas with a high 'liveability' score

Action: later life

Improved life satisfaction among older people

Increased opportunities for older people to participate

(NIMHE 2005)

In the European Union, the focus on promotion and prevention has been given a strong impetus by the WHO European Mental Health Declaration and Action Plan and the positive response to the consultation for the EC Mental Health Green Paper, including a warmly supportive Resolution by the European Parliament (European Commission 2006; European Parliament 2006; Stahl et al. 2006).[8] Two important themes emerge:

- The social and economic prosperity of Europe will depend on improving mental health and well-being.
- Promoting mental health, i.e. building communities and environments that support mental well-being, will deliver improved outcomes for people with mental health problems.

This focus on the benefits of *positive* mental health is matched by WHO research demonstrating the value of a focus on assets, as opposed to a deficit model and a call for more studies on the determinants of health, as distinct from studies on the determinants of illness.[9]

WHO Declaration (**2005**) http://www.euro.who.int/document/mnh/edoc06.pdf

66   Mental health and mental well-being are fundamental to the quality of life and productivity of individuals, families, communities and nations, enabling people to experience life as meaningful and to be creative and active citizens.   99

European Commission Social Agenda 2005–2010
http://ec.europa.eu/employment_social/social_policy_agenda/social_pol_ag_en.html

66   The mental health of the European population is a resource … to put Europe back on the path to long-term prosperity.   99

Defining terms: what is mental health promotion?

The difficulty of agreeing a common language and shared definitions of both mental health and mental health promotion is widely acknowledged (Tudor 1996).[10] Mental health, mental well-being, emotional well-being, emotional literacy, well-being and quality of life may be used more or less interchangeably and/or may have very different meanings and significance in different sectors.

---

[8]   The case for promotion and prevention has also been strengthened by the publication of two major WHO reports highlighting emerging evidence of effectiveness (WHO 2004a, 2004b).
[9]   WHO defines a health asset as any factor (or resource) that enhances the ability of individuals, communities, populations etc. to maintain health and well-being. Evidence shows that interventions to maximize and take advantage of health assets can counter negative social and economic determinants of health, especially among vulnerable groups. The result is improved health outcomes (http://www.euro.who.int/socialdeterminants/assets/20050623_1?language=French
[10] See also www.wellscotland.info/uploads/file.php?serve=1147271440-1146844425-conceptsbriefing.pdf&action=download

Mental health promotion is an umbrella term that may include action to promote mental well-being, to prevent mental health problems and to improve quality of life for people with a mental illness diagnosis.

> 66 Mental health promotion is both any action to enhance the mental well-being of individuals, families, organizations and communities, and a set of principles which recognize that how people feel is not an abstract and elusive concept, but a significant influence on health.
>
> (Friedli 2000) 99

Mental health promotion is essentially concerned with:

- how individuals, families, organizations and communities think and feel;
- the factors which influence how we think and feel, individually and collectively;
- the impact that this has on overall health and well-being (Friedli 2000).

> 66 Mental health promotion can be seen as a kind of immunization, working to strengthen the resilience of individuals, families, organizations and communities, as well as: to reduce conditions which are known to damage mental well-being in everyone, whether or not they currently have a mental health problem.
>
> (Health Education Authority 1998) 99

Recognition of the socio-economic and environmental determinants of mental well-being has led to a growing emphasis on models of mental health promotion that work at different levels, for example:

- strengthening individuals – by increasing emotional resilience through interventions designed to promote self-esteem, life and coping skills, e.g. communicating, negotiating, relationship and parenting skills;
- strengthening communities – by increasing social support, social inclusion and participation, improving community safety, neighbourhood environments, promoting childcare and self-help networks, developing health and social services which support mental health, improving mental health within schools and workplaces, e.g. through anti-bullying strategies and mental health strategies.
- reducing structural barriers to mental health – through initiatives to reduce discrimination and inequalities and to promote access to education, meaningful employment, housing, services and support for those who are vulnerable (Health Education Authority 1997; DH 2001).

> 66 Reducing structural barriers to mental health and introducing policies which protect mental well-being will benefit those who do and those who do not, currently have mental health problems, and the many people who move between periods of mental health and mental illness.
>
> (Department of Health 2001) 99

One of the most significant debates about mental health promotion concerns the balance between interventions which focus on strengthening individuals and those which address the wider determinants of mental health. It has been argued that focusing on emotional resilience or life skills, for example, may imply that people should learn to cope with deprivation and disadvantage (Secker 1998).

Current debates: population approaches and public mental health

Public health is concerned with improving the health of the population, rather than treating the diseases of individual patients. *Epidemiology* (from epidemics) is the study of the distribution and determinants of health. Key themes in public health include addressing the root causes of illness, tackling the inequalities which are at the heart of large variations in health and public participation.

What is sometimes called the *new public health* is particularly concerned with the wider determinants of health and overlaps with *ecological public health*, which emphasizes the common ground between health and sustainable development.

Public mental health takes a population wide approach to understanding and addressing risk and protective factors for mental health:

> " Public mental health, (of which mental health promotion is one element), provides a strategic and analytical framework for addressing the wider determinants of mental health, reducing the enduring inequalities in the distribution of mental distress and improving the mental health of the whole population.
>
> (Friedli 2004: 2) "

> " How people feel is not an elusive or abstract concept, but a significant public health indicator; as significant as rates of smoking, obesity and physical activity.
>
> (DH 2001) "

A population wide approach to promoting mental health for all has been used to make the case for the benefits both of improving mental health *and* preventing mental health problems. In addition it has been argued, applying the principle of 'herd immunity', that the more people in a community (e.g. a school, workplace or neighbourhood) who have high levels of mental health (i.e. who have characteristics of emotional and social competence), the more likely it will be that those with both acute and long-term problems can be supported (Stewart-Brown 1998; Blair *et al.* 2003: 143).

Huppert, using the Keyes classification (languishing, moderate mental health, flourishing etc.), applies the work of Rose (1992) to argue for shifting the whole population in a positive direction (Figure 3.1):

- By reducing the mean number of psychological symptoms in the population, many more individuals would cross the threshold for flourishing.
- A small shift in the mean of symptoms or risk factors would result in a decrease in the number of people in both the languishing and mental illness tail of the distribution (Huppert and Whittington 2003; Huppert 2005).

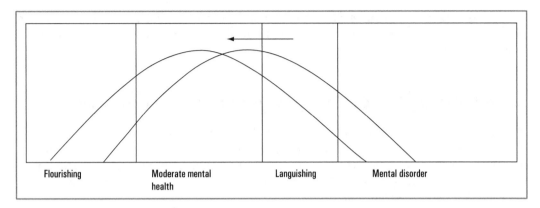

Figure 3.1 Population distribution of mental health
(from Huppert 2005)

This model has been criticized for implying that people with a mental disorder cannot also be flourishing and it is worth noting that Keyes and others have found that individuals who fit the criteria for a DSM mental disorder may have the presence of mental illness plus the absence of mental health, or in some cases may have moderate mental health or be flourishing (Gilleard *et al.* 2005; Keyes 2005). Nevertheless, it does demonstrate the potential of applying public health models to mental health promotion.

A UK population study in 1993 of participants in the Health and Lifestyle Survey found that the prevalence of mental disorders was directly related to the mean number of symptoms in the sub-population (excluding those with a disorder). In a seven-year longitudinal follow-up, Whittington and Huppert showed that the change in the mean number of symptoms in sub-populations (excluding those with a disorder) was highly correlated with the prevalence of disorders (Whittington and Huppert 1996). For this reason, Huppert suggests that population-level interventions to improve overall levels of mental health could have a substantial effect on reducing the prevalence of common mental health problems, as well as the benefits associated with moving people from 'languishing' to 'flourishing' (Huppert 2005).

Keyes argues that when compared with those who are flourishing, moderately mentally healthy and languishing adults have significant psychosocial impairment and poorer physical health, lower productivity and limitations in daily living (Keyes 2004, 2005). Keyes found that cardiovascular disease was lowest in adults who were the most mentally healthy, and higher among adults with major depressive episodes, minor depression and moderate mental health (Keyes 2004). This is consistent with review level evidence that CHD risk is directly related to the severity of depression: a one- to two-fold increase in CHD for minor depression and a three- to fivefold increase for major depression (Bunker *et al.* 2003).

In other words, intermediate levels of mental health are different from mental illness as well as from flourishing. Other research has shown that positive effect and negative effect have a degree of independence in the long term (Diener *et al.* 1995).

In a parallel analysis of adolescents (using measures of emotional well-being, psychological well-being and social well-being as three distinct but correlated factors), Keyes found that prevalence of conduct problems (arrests, truancy, alcohol, tobacco and marijuana use) decreased and measures of psychosocial functioning (self-determination, closeness to others and school integration) increased, as mental health increased. Based on his findings, he argues that children without mental illness are not necessarily mentally healthy. Flourishing youth were found to be functioning better than moderately mentally healthy or languishing youth (Keyes 2006).

What is positive mental health?

There is ongoing debate about what might be called a 'diagnosis of mental health' and what constitutes the necessary or sufficient elements making up positive mental health and well-being, although there is widespread agreement that mental health is more than the absence of clinically defined mental illness (WHO 2004a, 2004b).

Broadly, the literature distinguishes between two dimensions of 'well-being' or 'positive mental health':[11]

- hedonic: positive feelings or positive effect (subjective well-being);
- eudaimonic: positive functioning (engagement, fulfilment, social well-being) (Keyes 2002; Huppert 2005; Lyubomirsky *et al.* 2005; Carlisle 2006; Samman 2007).

Keyes describes the combination of positive feelings and positive functioning as 'flourishing', with individuals exhibiting at least seven of thirteen elements of subjective well-being described as flourishing (Keyes 2002). Others categorize the key elements slightly differently, e.g. a sense of autonomy, a sense of competence and a sense of relatedness (Ryan and Deci 2001). Lyubomirsky *et al.* (2005) focus on the experience of frequent positive emotion and less frequent (but not absent) negative emotion.

Clearly, how positive mental health is defined influences how it is measured. Well-being, for example, may be assessed through either subjective measures (self-assessed, e.g. responses to social survey questions on life satisfaction, quality of life, happiness etc.) and/or objective measures of factors known to influence well-being, e.g. crime, environment, housing, debt. Much of the current debate about well-being is driven by different views on the relative importance of:

- material factors (income, housing, employment);
- psycho-social factors or attributes (relationships, life satisfaction, positive effect, cognitive style);
- the influence of material inequalities on people's subjective well-being (Wilkinson 2005; Eckersley 2006; Pickett *et al.* 2006).

For example, the Sustainable Development Commission proposes indicators of social well-being that include individual subjective well-being, as well as some measure of 'fairness' or social justice (Marks *et al.* 2006).

There is also growing interest in well-being generally (sometimes referred to as the 'happiness debate'),[12] and in how a 'well-being focus' might influence the future direction of UK policy on the economy, health, education, employment, culture and sustainable development (Callard and Friedli 2005; Marks *et al.* 2006). The UK Government's Office of Science and Innovation is conducting a wide-ranging review of *Mental Capital and Mental*

---

[11] The terms 'well-being' and 'positive mental health' are largely synonymous in the literature and are frequently used interchangeably.
[12] cf. Layard 2005; New Economics Foundation 2007.

Well-being as part of its Foresight programme.[13] DEFRA has commissioned a number of major reports on different aspects of well-being, including a review of influences on personal well-being and the relationship between sustainable development and well-being.[14] What all these developments have in common is an interest in the relationship between positive mental health and improved outcomes across a very wide range of domains, including health, health behaviour, education, crime, relationships, employment, productivity and quality of life (Friedli in press).

Beyond stigma – the contribution of mental health promotion to the recovery agenda

Although in practice, mental health promotion interventions often focus on prevention, there is general agreement that mental health is more than the absence of mental illness:

> " Everyone has mental health needs, whether or not they have a diagnosis. These needs are met, or not met, at home, in families, at work, on the streets, in schools and neighbourhoods, in prisons and hospitals – where people feel respected, included and safe, or on the margins, in fear and excluded.
>
> (DH 2001: 28) "

> " Mental health is the emotional and spiritual resilience which allows us to enjoy life and to survive pain, disappointment and sadness. It is a positive sense of well-being and an underlying belief in our own, and others' dignity and worth.
>
> (HEA 1997: 7) "

The definition of mental health as a 'positive sense of well-being' challenges the idea that mental health is the opposite of mental illness. For example, someone with a diagnosis of schizophrenia might feel supported, at ease and optimistic. They might be coping well with life and enjoying a high level of well-being. Equally, many people who are not clinically diagnosed have a poor sense of well-being (Gilleard *et al.* 2005).

The focus on health, rather than illness, and the view that a diagnosis is not inconsistent with mental well-being is one example of the way in which mental health promotion has been informed by, and also contributed to, ideas about recovery. Recovery has been defined as what people need in order to hold on to or regain a life that has meaning for them (Anthony 1993) and aims to enable people with mental health problems to:

■ **maintain existing activities and relationships;**
■ reduce the barriers that prevent people from accessing new things they want to do;
■ gain access to the material resources and opportunities that are their right (Bates 2002; Perkins 2002; Sayce 2002).

---

[13]   www.foresight.gov.uk
[14]   http://www.sustainable-development.gov.uk/what/latestnews.htm#1n210906

Although the reform of mental illness services and addressing the stigma, discrimination and denial of human rights and civil liberties experienced by people with mental health problems remain central, these goals are now also being considered in the context of public mental health. This is an important development because the focus on stigma and discrimination has tended to preclude a wider debate about factors that are toxic to mental health, whether or not one has a diagnosis. We have a wealth of data on public attitudes to mental illness (Braunholtz *et al.* 2007), but very little on public knowledge of what harms and hinders mental well-being: the mental health equivalents of smoking and car exhaust fumes (Friedli *et al.* 2007).

These questions are central in considering some of the potential problems with 'raising awareness' campaigns, which have been at the heart of much mental health promotion activity (Gale *et al.* 2004). At root, these invite the public to adopt a medical explanation for their problems and to seek medical help, while also, usually through case studies or first person accounts, highlighting the consequences of the disorder: stigma and exclusion. They do not invite reflection on economic and environmental causes.

Future opportunities and challenges

The policy environment for mental health promotion has probably never been more favourable as the potential social, economic and environmental costs of not paying greater attention to how people think, feel and relate generate greater interest and debate. Improving mental health, i.e. promoting the circumstances, skills and attributes associated with positive mental health, is now widely seen as a worthwhile goal in itself and also as:

- contributing to preventing mental illness;
- leading to better outcomes, for example in physical health, health behaviours, educational performance, employability and earnings, crime reduction (NIMHE 2005).

There is growing evidence that these beneficial outcomes are not just the result of the absence of mental illness, but are due, wholly or in some degree, to aspects of positive mental health. For example subjective well-being is associated with increased longevity, provides a similar degree of protection from coronary heart disease to giving up smoking, improves recovery and health outcomes from a range of chronic diseases and in young people, significantly influences alcohol, tobacco and cannabis use. Positive effect also predicts pro-social behaviour, e.g. participation, civic engagement and volunteering (Friedli and Parsonage 2007).

Mainstreaming

'Mainstreaming' has long been a holy grail for mental health promotion: gaining cross-sector/cross-government ownership is crucial to securing the long-term investment that public mental health requires. But developments in policy and the prevailing *zeitgeist* suggest that this is already happening.[15] The factors that influence how people think and feel – in

---

[15] See for example David Cameron's speech to Google Zeitgeist Europe 2006 http://politics.guardian.co.uk/conservatives/story/0,1780585,00.html

schools, in the workplace, in the delivery of services, in the built and natural environment and in local communities – are becoming mainstream concerns, even if they are not labelled mental health promotion. There is growing evidence of grass-roots mobilization against global and local trends that are seen as toxic to well-being, often in expressed in concerns about work-life balance, the environment, the neglect of children and older people and the anti-poverty movement (Friedli 2005).

Other issues high on the policy agenda that provide opportunities to call for greater focus on mental health promotion include alcohol, violence, parenting, worklessness, anti-social behaviour and a perceived decline in 'respect'. These issues also provide opportunities to build partnerships with non health sectors – probably the most pressing priority.

Putting inequalities at the centre of mental health promotion theory and practice

Poor mental health is both a cause and a consequence of the experience of social, economic and environmental inequalities (Rogers and Pilgrim 2003; Social Exclusion Unit 2004; Melzer *et al.* 2004). As Rogers and Pilgrim have noted in relation to the oft cited prevalence figures for mental health problems: one in four yes, but not any one in four (Rogers and Pilgrim 2003). Mental health problems are more common in areas of deprivation and poor mental health is consistently associated with unemployment, less education, low income or material standard of living, in addition to poor physical health and adverse life events. Lone parents, those with physical illnesses and the unemployed make up 20 per cent of the population, but these three groups contribute 36 per cent of all those with neurotic disorders, 39 per cent of those with limiting disorder and 51 per cent of those with disabling mental disorders (Melzer *et al.* 2004).

Rogers and Pilgrim (2003) highlight three key issues in understanding the mental health impact of socio-economic inequalities:

- social divisions – mental health problems both reflect deprivation and contribute to it;
- social drift – the social and ecological impact of adversity, including the impact of physical health problems and the cycle of invisible barriers which prevent or inhibit people from benefiting from opportunities;
- social injuries – mental distress as an outcome of demoralization and despair.

A preliminary analysis by Pickett *et al.* (2006) suggests that higher national levels of income inequality are linked to a higher prevalence of mental illness and, in contrast with studies of physical morbidity and mortality, as countries get richer rates of mental illness increase.

Richard Wilkinson's work analyses deprivation as a catalyst for a range of *feelings* which influence health through physiological responses to chronic stress, through the damaging impact of low status on social relationships and through a range of behaviours seen as a direct or indirect response to the social injuries associated with inequalities (Wilkinson 1996, 2005). More recent analysis suggests a significant relationship between inequality and levels of violence, trust and social capital (Wilkinson and Pickett 2007b). Taking the Unicef data on children's well-being as a starting point, Wilkinson and Pickett found that adolescent pregnancy, violence, poor educational performance, mental illness and imprisonment rates were all higher in more unequal countries and states (Pickett and Wilkinson 2007). Unicef looked at 40 indicators (for the period 2000–3) covering material well-being, family and peer relationships, health and safety, behaviour risks, education and sense of well-being. Those at the top of the list: the Netherlands, Sweden, Denmark and Finland were also those with the lowest levels of relative income poverty (Unicef 2007). In the UK, relative poverty for children has doubled since 1979. Wilkinson and Pickett argue that the Unicef data suggest that children's responses to inequality are similar to those found in the adult population and are similarly related to the effects of social status differentiation: greater inequality heightens status competition and status insecurity (and does so across all income groups) (Pickett and Wilkinson 2007; Wilkinson and Pickett 2007a).

In this context, levels of distress among communities are understood not in terms of individual pathology but as a response to relative deprivation and social injustice, which erode emotional, spiritual and intellectual resources essential to psychological well-being: agency, trust, autonomy, self-acceptance, respect for others, hopefulness and resilience (Stewart-Brown 2002; Friedli 2003). In addition, health-damaging behaviours may be survival strategies in the face of multiple problems and despair related to occupational insecurity, poverty and exclusion. These problems impact on intimate relationships, the care of children and care of the self. The 20–25 per cent of people who are obese or continue to smoke are concentrated among the 26 per cent of the population living in poverty, measured in terms of low income and multiple deprivation of necessities (Gordon *et al.* 2000). This is also the population with the highest prevalence of anxiety and depression (Melzer *et al.* 2004). Capacity, capability and motivation to choose health are strongly influenced by mental health and well-being.

Hopelessness and a difficulty in imagining solutions (which are also risk factors for suicidal behaviour) are also factors which may have an important ecological dimension. Mistrust and powerlessness amplify the effect of neighbourhood disorder, making where you live as important for health and well-being as personal circumstances. Poor, socially disorganized neighbourhoods have higher rates of violence and strong norms of violence: risk of violence is constructed by locality. The social variables which predict suicide (which is more strongly associated with social fragmentation than with deprivation) also predict violence to others. Some research suggests clear links between economic deprivation, social disorganization, ethnic inequities and violence (Krueger *et al.* 2004).

Whitehead and Dahlgren (2006) argue that key inequalities in the social distribution of outcomes relate to:

- behaviour;
- health;
- consequences of illness;
- access to services.

(See also Commission on Social Determinants of Health 2007.)

A wealth of existing research exists to suggest that mental health is a significant determinant in each case, influencing:

- capacity and motivation for healthy behaviours;
- risk for physical health (e.g. coronary heart disease);
- chronic disease outcomes (e.g. diabetes);

■ relationship to health services, including uptake and treatment (e.g. patterns of concordance).

Although it is frequently noted that health enables a person to function as an agent and contributes to inequalities in people's capability to function (Anand and Ravillion 1993), it is *mental health* that constitutes the key determinant of agency and helps to explain the relationship between low levels of mental well-being and neglect of self, neglect of others and a range of self-harming behaviours, including self sedation and self medication, e.g. through alcohol, high fat and sugar consumption.

Resisting focus on individual interventions and individual solutions

A focus on social justice may provide an important corrective to what has been seen as a growing over-emphasis on individual pathology. This takes several forms: the expansion of diagnostic categories, as more and more people are exposed to information which suggests they have a mental disorder that needs treatment. When everything from shopping to texting to shyness and lack of interest in sex becomes a site of under-diagnosis and unmet need, the scope for growth appears unlimited. Second, a focus on individual symptoms may lead to a 'disembodied psychology' which separates 'what goes on inside clients' heads' from social structure and context (Smail 2006). The key therapeutic intervention then becomes to 'change the way you think' rather than to refer people to sources of help for key catalysts for psychological problems: debt, housing, benefits. As Joanna Moncrieff observes: 'a society obsessed with its own navel' is unlikely to be able to mount an effective challenge to complex social problems (Moncrieff 2003).

Conclusion

How things are done (values and culture) and how things are distributed (economic and fiscal policy) are probably the key domains that influence and are influenced by how people think, feel and relate (Friedli and Parsonage 2007). Mental health promotion has made and continues to make a significant contribution to our understanding of the wider determinants of mental health and the crucial relationship between social position and emotion, cognition and social function or relatedness (Singh-Manoux and Marmot 2005). Evidence to this effect needs to inform current thinking about how individuals (and children) respond to stressors and appropriate promotion, prevention and treatment strategies across the spectrum of mental health problems.

Questions for reflection and discussion

1 Do you (the reader) have a sense of your own mental health and well-being – and, in what ways do you identify, maintain, develop and promote it?
2 Think about the community in which you live and identify those aspects that have an impact on the mental health of its members.

3 What contributions can the mental health nursing profession make to develop communities and environments that support mental health and well-being?
4 What do you consider to be the key public mental health priorities for your country over the next decade and what role can you play in meeting those challenges?

Annotated bibliography

- Carlisle, Sandra (2007) Series of papers on cultural influences on mental health and well-being in Scotland. http://www.wellscotland.info/publications/consultations4.html. This series of papers provides a valuable introduction to the 'well-being' literature, including perspectives on culture, economics, biology and spirituality. Although written to inform debates in Scotland, they are equally relevant to a wider audience.
- Friedli, L., Oliver, C., Tidyman, M. and Ward, G. (2007) *Mental Health Improvement: evidence based messages to promote mental well-being*. Edinburgh: NHS Health Scotland. http://www.healthscotland.com/documents/2188.aspx. This report, commissioned by NHS Health Scotland, includes an extensive review of the strength of the evidence on what works to improve mental health (e.g. physical activity, diet, arts and creativity), as well as the views of professionals and the public to 'positive steps'. Also included is a helpful case study from British Telecom, describing the response of employees to 'positive mentality', a workplace campaign designed to encourage staff to take care of their mental health.
- Rogers, A. and Pilgrim, D. (2003) *Inequalities and Mental Health.* London: Palgrave Macmillan. Classic and pioneering analysis of the relationship between mental health and inequalities. Essential reading.
- Wilkinson, R.G. and Pickett, K.E. (2006) Income inequality and population health: a review and explanation of the evidence. *Social Science and Medicine* **62**: 1768–84. The extent to which it is inequality, i.e. relative deprivation that has the greatest influence on health remains hotly contested. Richard Wilkinson has made a significant contribution to the evidence and here summarizes the arguments.
- Friedli, L. and Parsonage, M. (2007) *Building an Economic Case for Mental Health Promotion.* Belfast: Northern Ireland Association for Mental Health. This report uses economic analysis to develop the case for greater investment in mental health promotion, outlining the cost effectiveness not only of the prevention of mental illness but also of the promotion of positive mental health. It includes a list of 'best buy' interventions.

References

Anand, S. and Ravillion, M. (1993) Human development in poor countries: on the role of private incomes and public services. *Journal of Economic Perspectives* 7: 133–50.
Anthony, W. (1993) Recovery from mental illness: the guiding vision of the mental health services system in the 1990s. *Psychosocial Rehabilitation Journal* 16(4): 11–23.
Bamford, D. (2004) *The review of mental health and learning disability (Northern Ireland). A strategic framework for adult mental health services: consultation report.* http://www.rmhldni.gov.uk/

Bartley, M. (ed.) (2006) *Capability and Resilience: beating the odds.* ESRC Human Capability and Resilience Research Network. London: UCL Department of Epidemiology and Public Health. www.ucl.ac.uk/capabilityandresilience

Bates, P. (ed.) (2002) *Working for Inclusion: making social inclusion a reality for people with severe mental health problems.* London: Sainsbury Centre for Mental Health.

Blair, M., Stewart-Brown, S., Waterston, T. and Crowther, R. (2003) *Child Public Health.* Oxford: Oxford University Press.

Braunholtz, S., Davidson, S., Myant, K. *et al.* (2007) *Well? What Do You Think? (2006): The Third National Scottish Survey of Public Attitudes to Mental Health, Mental Wellbeing and Mental Health Problems.* Edinburgh: Scottish Government.

Bunker, S.J., Colquhoun, D.M., Esler, M.D. *et al.* (2003) 'Stress' and coronary heart disease: psychosocial risk factors. National Heart Foundation of Australia position statement update *Medical Journal of Australia* **178**: 272–6. http://www.mja.com.au/public/issues/178_06_170303/bun10421_fm.html

Carlisle, S. (2006) *Series of papers on cultural influences on mental health and well-being in Scotland.* http://www.wellscotland.info/publications/consultations4.html

Callard, F. and Friedli, L. (2005) Imagine East Greenwich: evaluating the impact of the arts on health and well-being. *Journal of Public Mental Health* **4**(4): 29–40.

Commission on Social Determinants of Health (2007) *Achieving health equity: from root causes to fair outcomes: interim statement* Geneva: CSDH. http://www.who.int/social_determinants/resources/interim_statement/en/index.html

Department of Health (1999) *National Service Framework for Mental Health.* London: DH.

Department of Health (2001) *Making it Happen: a guide to delivering mental health promotion.* London: DH. www.doh.gov.uk/index.htm

Department of Health (2004a) *Choosing Health: making healthy choices easier.* London: The Stationery Office. http://www.dh.gov.uk/PublicationsAndStatistics/Publications/PublicationsPolicyAndGuidance/PublicationsPolicyAndGuidanceArticle/fs/en?CONTENT_ID=4094550&chk=aN5Cor

Department of Health (2004b) *The National Service Framework for Mental Health: five years on.* London: The Stationery Office.

Department of Health (2006) *Our Health, Our Care, Our Say: a new direction for community services* London: The Stationery Office. http://www.dh.gov.uk/assetRoot/04/12/74/59/04127459.pdf

Department of Health, Social Services and Public Safety (2006) *Mental Health Improvement and Well-being: a personal, public and political issue.* The report of the review of mental health and learning disability (Northern Ireland) on mental health promotion. http://www.rmhldni.gov.uk/mentalhealth-promotion-report.pdf

Diener, E., Smith, H.L. and Fujita, F. (1995) The personality structure of affect. *Journal of Personality and Social Psychology* **69**: 130–41. http://content.apa.org/journals/psp/69/1/130

Eckersley, R. (2006) Is modern Western culture a health hazard? *International Journal of Epidemiology* **35**: 252–8. PDF: http://ije.oxfordjournals.org/cgi/content/full/35/2/252?etoc

European Commission (2006) *Promoting the Mental Health of the Population. Towards a strategy on mental health for the European Union.* http://ec.europa.eu/health/ph_determinants/life_style/mental/green_paper/consultation_en.htm

European Parliament (2006) *European Parliament Resolution on Improving the Mental Health of the Population. Towards a strategy on mental health for the European Union (2006/2058(INI))* http://www.europarl.europa.eu/sides/getDoc.do?pubRef=-//EP//TEXT+TA+P6-TA-2006–0341+0+DOC+XML+V0//EN&language=EN

Friedli, L. (2000) Mental health promotion: rethinking the evidence base. *Mental Health Review* **5**(3): 15–18.

Friedli, L. (2003) Editorial. *Journal of Mental Health Promotion* **2**(4): 1–4.

Friedli, L. (2004) Editorial. *Journal of Public Mental Health* **3**(1): 2–6.

Friedli, L. (2005) Promoting mental health in the UK: a case study in many parts. *Australian Journal for the Advancement of Mental Health* **4**: 2. http://www.auseinet.com/journal/vol4iss2/friedlieditorial.pdf

Friedli, L. (in press) *Mental Health, Resilience and Inequalities.* Copenhagen and London: World Health Organization and Mental Health Foundation.

Friedli, L. and Parsonage, M. (2007) *Building an Economic Case for Mental Health Promotion.* Belfast: Northern Ireland Association for Mental Health.

Friedli, L., Oliver, C., Tidyman, M. and Ward, G. (2007) *Mental Health Improvement: evidence based messages to promote mental wellbeing.* Edinburgh: NHS Health Scotland.

Gale, E., Seymour, L., Crepaz-Keay, D., Gibbons, M., Farmer, P. and Pinfold, V. (2004) *Scoping Review on Mental Health Anti-Stigma and Discrimination – Current Activities and What Works.* Leeds: NIMHE.

Gilleard, C., Pond, C., Scammell, A., Lobo, R., Simporis, K. and Rawaf, S. (2005) Well-being in Wandsworth: a public mental health audit. *Journal of Public Mental Health* **4**(2): 14–22.

Gordon, D., Adelman, L., Ashworth, K., Bradshaw, J., Levitas, R., Middleton, S., Pantazis, C., Patsios, D., Payne, S., Townsend, P. and Williams, J. (2000) *Poverty and Social Exclusion in Britain.* York: Joseph Rowntree Foundation.

Health Education Authority (1997) *Mental Health Promotion: a quality framework.* London: HEA.

Health Education Authority (1998) *Community Action for Mental Health.* London: HEA.

Horwitz, A.V. and Wakefield, J.C. (2007) *The Loss of Sadness: how psychiatry transformed normal sorrow into depressive disorder.* Oxford: Oxford University Press.

Huppert, F. (2005) Positive mental health in individuals and populations, in F. Huppert, N. Bayliss and B. Keverne (eds) *The Science of Well-being.* Oxford: Oxford University Press, pp. 307–40.

Huppert, F.A. and Whittington, J.E. (2003) Evidence for the independence of positive and negative well-being: implications for quality of life assessment. *British Journal of Health Psychology* **8**: 107–22.

Jane-Llopis, E. and Anderson, P. (2005) *Mental Health Promotion and Mental Disorder Prevention: a policy for Europe.* Nijmegen: Radboud University.

Keyes, C.L.M. (2002) The mental health continuum: from languishing to flourishing in life. *Journal of Health and Social Behaviour* **43**: 207–22.

Keyes, C.L.M. (2004) The nexus of cardiovascular disease and depression revisited: the complete mental health perspective and the moderating role of age and gender. *Aging and Mental Health* **8**(3): 266–74.

Keyes, C.L.M. (2005) Mental illness and/or mental health? Investigating axioms of the complete state model of health. *Journal of Consulting and Clinical Psychology* **73**: 539–48.

Keyes, C.L.M. (2006) Mental health in adolescence: is America's youth flourishing? *American Journal of Orthopsychiatry* **76**(3): 395–402.

Krueger, P.M., Bond Huie, S.A., Rogers, R.G. and Hummer, R.A. (2004) Neighbourhoods and homicide mortality: an analysis of race/ethnic differences. *Journal of Epidemiology and Community Health* **58**: 223–30.

Layard, R. (2005) *Happiness: Lessons from a New Science.* London: Allen Lane.

Lyubomirsky, S., King, L. and Diener, E. (2005) The benefits of frequent positive affect: does happiness lead to success? *Psychological Bulletin.* http://www.apa.org/journals/releases/bul1316803.pdf

Marks, N., Thompson, S., Eckersley, R., Jackson, T. and Kasser, T. (2006) *Sustainable Development and Well-being: Relationships, Challenges and Policy Implications. A Report by the Centre for Well-Being, NEF (the New Economics Foundation) for DEFRA (Department of the Environment, Food and Rural Affairs).* London: DEFRA. http://www.defra.gov.uk/science/project_data/DocumentLibrary/SD12007/SD12007_4606_FRP.pdf

Melzer, D., Fryers, T. and Jenkins, R. (2004) *Social Inequalities and the Distribution of Common Mental Disorders.* Maudsley Monographs. Hove: Psychology Press.

Mental Health Foundation (2005) *Choosing Mental Health: a policy agenda for mental health and public health.* London: Mental Health Foundation.

Moncrieff, J. (2003) The politics of a new Mental Health Act. *British Journal of Psychiatry* **183**: 8–9.

National Institute for Mental Health in England (NIMHE) (2004) *From here to Equality: a strategic plan to tackle stigma and discrimination on mental health grounds.* Leeds: NIMHE. http://www.shift.org.uk/mt/archives/blog_12/ FIVE%20YEAR%20STIGMA%20AND%20DISC%20PLAN.pdf

National Institute for Mental Health in England (NIMHE) (2005) *Making it Possible: improving mental health and well-being in England.* Leeds: NIMHE/CSIP.

New Economics Foundation (2007) *European (un)Happy Planet Index: an index of carbon efficiency and well-being in Europe.* London: NEF/Friends of the Earth. http://www.neweconomics.org/gen/uploads/04rix555kx5ws345kbwiox4513072007173920.pdf

Perkins, R. (2002) Are you (really) being served? *Mental Health Today* September: 18–21.

Pickett, K.E. and Wilkinson, R.G. (2007) Child wellbeing and income inequality in rich societies: ecological cross sectional study. *British Medical Journal* **335**: 1080. http://www.bmj.com/cgi/content/full/335/7629/1080

Pickett, K.E., James, O.W. and Wilkinson, R.G. (2006) Income inequality and the prevalence of mental illness: a preliminary international analysis. *Journal of Epidemiology and Community Health* **60**: 646–7.

Rogers, A. and Pilgrim, D. (2003) *Inequalities and Mental Health*. London: Palgrave Macmillan.

Rose, G. (1992) *The Strategy of Preventive Medicine*. Oxford: Oxford University Press.

Ryan, R.M. and Deci, E.L. (2001) On happiness and human potentials: A review of research on hedonic and eudaimonic well-being. *Annual Review of Psychology* **52**: 141–66.

Samman, E. (2007) *Psychological and Subjective Well-being: a proposal for internationally comparable indicators*. Oxford: University of Oxford, Oxford Poverty and Human Development Initiative. http://www.ophi.org.uk/pubs/Samman_Psych_Subj_Wellbeing_Final.pdf

Sayce, L. (2002) Inclusion as a new paradigm: civil rights, in P. Bates (ed.) *Working for inclusion: making social inclusion a reality for people with severe mental health problems*. London: Sainsbury Centre for Mental Health, pp. 71–8.

Secker, J. (1998) Current conceptualisations of mental health and mental health promotion. *Health Education Research* **13**(1): 57–66.

Singh-Manoux, A. and Marmot, M. (2005) Role of socialization in explaining social inequalities in health. *Social Science and Medicine* **60**: 2129–33.

Smail, D. (2006) Implications for practice. *Clinical Psychology Forum* **162**: 17–20.

Social Exclusion Unit (2004) *Mental Health and Social Exclusion: social exclusion unit report*. London: Office of the Deputy Prime Minister.

Stahl, T., Wismar, M., Ollila, E., Lahtinen, E. and Leppo, K. (2006) *Health in all Policies: prospects and potentials*. Helsinki: Ministry of Social Affairs and Health. http://www.stm.fi/Resource.phx/eng/subjt/inter/eu2006/hiap/index.htx.i1153.pdf

Stewart-Brown, S. (1998) Public health implications of childhood behaviour problems and parenting programmes, in A. Buchanan and B.L. Hudson (eds) *Parenting, Schooling and Children's Behaviour: Interdisciplinary approaches*. Aldershot: Ashgate Publishing.

Stewart-Brown, S. (2002) Measuring the parts most measures do not reach: a necessity for evaluation in mental health promotion. *Journal of Mental Health Promotion* **1**(2): 4–9.

Tudor, K. (1996) *Mental Health Promotion: Paradigms and practice*. London: Routledge.

UNICEF Innocenti Research Centre (2007) *Child Poverty in Perspective: an overview of child well-being in rich countries*. Florence: Innocenti Report Card.

Wanless, D. (2002) *Securing our Future Health: taking a long term view*. London: The Stationery Office.

Wanless, D. (2004) *Securing Good Health for the Whole Population: Final Report*. London: HM Treasury. www.hm-treasury.gov.uk/wanless

Welsh Assembly (2006) *Mental Health Promotion Action Plan for Wales: consultation document*. http://new.wales.gov.uk/consultations/currentconsultation/healandsoccarecurrcons/851364/?lang=en

Whitehead, M. and Dahlgren, G. (2006) *Concepts and Principles for Tackling Social Inequities in Health: a discussion paper on levelling up* (Draft). WHO Collaborating Centre for Policy Research on Social Determinants of Health. Copenhagen: University of Liverpool/WHO Europe.

Whittington, J.E. and Huppert, F.A. (1996) Changes in the prevalence of psychiatric disorder in a community are related to changes in the mean level of psychiatric symptoms. *Psychological Medicine* **26**: 1253–60.

Wilkinson, R.G. (1996) *Unhealthy Societies: the afflictions of inequality*. London: Routledge.

Wilkinson, R.G. (2005) *The Impact of Inequality: how to make sick societies healthier*. London: Routledge.

Wilkinson, R. and Pickett, K. (2007a) Income inequality and socioeconomic gradients in mortality. *American Journal of Public Health* **97**: 10.

Wilkinson, R. and Pickett, K. (2007b) The problems of relative deprivation: why some societies do better than others. *Social Science and Medicine* **65**: 1965.

World Health Organization (2004a) *Prevention of Mental Disorders: Effective interventions and policy options. Summary Report*. A report of the World Health Organization, Department of Mental Health and Substance Abuse in collaboration with the Prevention Research Centre of the Universities of

Nijmegen and Maastricht. Geneva: WHO.

http://www.who.int/mental_health/evidence/en/prevention_of_mental_disorders_sr.pdf

World Health Organization (2004b) *Promoting Mental Health: Concepts, emerging evidence, practice. Summary Report.* A Report from the World Health Organization, Department of Mental Health and Substance Abuse in collaboration with the Victorian Health Promotion Foundation (VicHealth) and The University of Melbourne. Geneva: WHO.

http://www.who.int/mental_health/evidence/en/promoting_mhh.pdf

World Health Organization (2005) Helsinki Declaration and Action Plan. WHO, Copenhagen.

CHAPTER 4

Mental health nursing: origins and traditions

Ian Norman and Iain Ryrie

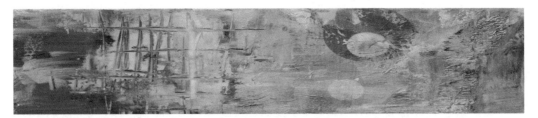

Chapter overview

This chapter seeks to provide a historical perspective on the practice of mental health nursing upon which nurses and other mental health care workers of the future must build. The first part traces the origins of mental health nursing from the eighteenth century to the present day and outlines recent influences on its development. The strength of the old mental hospitals lay in their structure. This structure did not allow mental health nursing to grow and develop, because it did not provide nurses with opportunities for independent thinking and action. But it did provide them with a sense of security and a common shared identity based on a clear sense of their place within the hospital structure, without need to define the nursing role and remit, or the underpinning values or knowledge base of the discipline. Closure of the old hospitals and the development of community-based mental health services meant that these things were to change. Nurses were required to reconsider their roles and responsibilities, their place within multi-disciplinary clinical teams and their relations with mental health service users.

The second part of this chapter traces the history of mental health nursing as an academic and practice discipline and the origins of what we refer to as the interpersonal relations and evidence-based health care traditions within the discipline. Two UK government reviews of mental health nursing, *Psychiatric Nursing: Today and Tomorrow* published in 1968 (Standing Mental Health and Standing Nursing Advisory Committees 1968) and *Working in Partnership* published in 1994 (Mental Health Nursing Review Team 1994), provided some touchstones for the specialty at times of great change. *Working in Partnership*, in particular, reaffirmed that the work of mental health nurses rested fundamentally on their relationships with service users. In this it supported strongly the interpersonal relations tradition of mental health nursing the origins of which are as old as the discipline itself, but which found its clearest expression in Hilda Peplau's seminal work *Interpersonal Relations in Nursing*, first published in 1952. However, the rise of the evidence-based health care movement from the early 1990s challenged mental health nursing in the interpersonal relations tradition and threatened to fragment the discipline into opposing camps. Indeed when the first edition of this textbook was published in 2004 it seemed to many that nursing in the interpersonal relations tradition was in danger of being eclipsed by the increasing dominance of nursing in the evidence-based health care tradition. Five years on, however, these fears appear unfounded. We see today increasing reconciliation between the two traditions of mental health nursing and the debate between their advocates of becoming less relevant as the focus of mental health policy turns to promoting social inclusion recovery and choice; priorities reflected in the third UK government review of mental health nursing *From Values to Action* (CNOE 2006) (discussed in Chapter 35).

In summary this chapter covers:

■   The origins of mental health nursing;
■   Twentieth-century developments, in particular the impact on mental health nursing of the decline of the old mental hospitals and the development of a community-based service;
■   The development of community-based nursing;
■   *Working in Partnership*, the UK Government's second review of mental health nursing (1994);
   Traditions within mental health nursing:
   –   interpersonal relations – Peplau and her legacy;
   –   evidence-based health care;
■   Reconciliation of the traditions in the context of current mental health policy.

Origins

Eighteenth and nineteenth centuries

Throughout the ages people with mental disorder have been the recipients of various forms of care and control. From the twelfth century, the asylum provided a setting for such care, although the importance of the asylum system grew from the late seventeenth century under the influence of the intellectual tradition of the Enlightenment. Notable pioneers were Philippe Pinel in France and the Quaker William Tuke in England who, almost simultaneously, but independently, introduced reforms that unchained the lunatics, and turned the asylums into havens for the insane.

Tuke founded the Retreat at York in 1792 on principles of 'moral treatment'. Chapman (1992) tells us that Tuke believed madness and deranged behaviour to stem from the mode of service provision in eighteenth-century 'madhouses' where 'lunatics' suffered degradation, repression and cruelty. Scull (1981) wrote about care of mentally ill people before the nineteenth century as being a way of solving society's difficulty in knowing how to handle socially disadvantaged groups. Tuke replaced physical constraints with moral constraints based on reason supported by purposeful work and social and educational activities in a normal domestic environment. The 'moral therapists' challenged medical dominance in the treatment of the insane, arguing that medicine had abused care, and medical treatment was unnecessary in moral therapy because carers were selected for their attitude and personality. The moralists considered the newly industrialized society to be the source of mental instability and that cure could be found in calm, productive, non-competitive communities (Scull 1981). The asylum attendants in the Retreat and other similar communities were the first official care agents, and are often regarded as the predecessors of the mental health nurse.

The moral therapy movement marked the start of changing social attitudes towards the insane, which by the first half of the nineteenth century were influenced by a growing social conscience based on a common ethical principle, a belief that the community had a responsibility to the weak (Jones 1960). This found expression in the Lunatics Act 1845, which was a major achievement of the work of the Earl of Shaftesbury as was the construction of a number of Victorian asylums, some of which are still in use today. Changing attitudes to the insane had implications for the role of lunatic attendants who, by the mid-nineteenth century, were expected to set a positive example to patients and to offer them guidance rather than simply be custodians. But, it was difficult to recruit attendants of the right type. Connolly (1992) quotes Dr Browne who, writing in 1897 of male attendants, described them as 'the unemployable of other professions ... if they possess physical strength and a tolerable reputation for sobriety, it is enough; and the latter is frequently dispensed with' (Dr Browne, cited by Connolly 1992: 7). According to Connolly (1992) women attendants of the right type were easier to recruit than men because nursing was widely perceived to be in women's nature.

These recruitment problems are not surprising when one considers working conditions of the time, which were very poor. Records from Springfield Hospital in Tooting, London (then the Surrey Lunatic Asylum) referred to by Connolly (1992), show that in 1842 attendants worked from 6.00 a.m. until 9.00 p.m., and slept in rooms adjacent to the wards. There were nine male and nine female attendants for 350 patients. In a report to Visiting Justices that year, attendants were described as 'the instruments for carrying into effect every remedial measure', the work requiring 'firmness and self control blended with humanity and forbearance' and involving 'many menial Offices'. For this, male attendants working in the Surrey Asylum received between £25 and £30 per year. This compared well with the national average salary of male attendants, which was £26 per year. But attendants were among the lowest paid people in the country, and female attendants were paid substantially less than their male counterparts.

Given the developing role of the asylum attendant beyond a purely custodial function, a number of medical superintendents became convinced of the need for some sort of education and training for attendants. The first course of lectures for attendants was probably given by Alexander Morrison, the Surrey Lunatic Asylum's Medical Superintendent in 1843. This course served as a stimulus for the spread of similar courses of instruction, which culminated in publication of the Handbook for Instruction of Attendants on the Insane, by the Royal Medico-Psychological Association (RMPA) – the Red Handbook – which became a standard text. By 1889 100 hospitals offered programmes of instruction based on the Red Handbook and in 1890 the RMPA established the first register for attendants, who had completed successfully a two-year training programme (Walk 1961). Thus, mental health nursing as a practice discipline represented by qualification is almost 120 years old.

In spite of these positive developments it would be incorrect to interpret the history of mental health nursing as one of progressive improvement in the conditions for patients and their carers in the asylums. Moral treatment, which had heralded positive changes in social attitudes to the insane and the notion of attendants as therapeutic agents, lasted only 50 years in Great Britain (Chapman 1992) because a growing number of patients gradually outstripped the human resource to provide moral treatment to an adequate standard. By the mid-nineteenth century asylums were being built for thousands at a time to, in effect, warehouse madness. These institutions quickly became overcrowded: for example, by 1909 the number of patients in the Surrey Asylum, built originally for 350, had risen to 1235

(Connolly 1992). Bureaucratic organization of patients' lives based on rigid doctor, nurse, patient hierarchies became the norm and attendants were once again relied upon for strength and intimidation, rather than friendliness and common sense (Jones 1960).

The beginning of the nineteenth century also marked the start of a shifting and often uneasy relationship between mental health and general nursing, which continues to the present day. The British Nursing Association (later the Royal British Nursing Association (RBNA)) founded for general nurses in 1887 refused entry to the nursing register to graduates of the Royal Medico-Psychological Association (RMPA) register for attendants.
Mrs Bedford-Fenwick, the RBNA President, set out the reasons for this in 1895 when she pointed to the narrow training received by asylum attendants and concerns about the possible effects of admission on nurses' social status:

> 66 No person can be considered trained who has only worked in hospitals and asylums for the insane … considering the present class of persons known as male attendants, one can hardly believe that their admission will tend to raise the status of the Association.
>
> (Adams 1969: 13, cited by Connolly 1992: 9) 99

The College of Nursing (eventually to become the Royal College), which was established in 1916, maintained the stance taken by the RBNA by continuing to refuse admission to registered attendants. However, the later established General Nursing Council (GNC) started its own course and examination for attendants, thereby introducing an alternative qualification.

Connolly points out that the drive for equal status with general nursing was spearheaded by medical superintendents and senior attendants, and was of little concern to rank and file asylum attendants who, through the National Asylum Workers' Union, were concerned to improve conditions of service and pay, but were not concerned with status or professionalism for many years. Moreover, qualifications, whether registration with the RMPA or the later GNC, carried little weight. Neither was needed to obtain a senior position in an asylum and many asylum matrons had general nursing training only and no experience of asylum work.

Twentieth century

The first half of the twentieth century was marked by renewed optimism in psychiatry. In the inter-war period nomenclature changed, asylums became mental hospitals and male and female attendants became nurses, and the management of mental health was incorporated into the National Health Service (NHS), so providing free care as a right of citizenship. However, mental hospitals remained overcrowded, particularly during both world wars when many staff members were enlisted in the forces or redeployed, so that patients had to be redistributed. Thus the main role of the mental nurses during the first half of the twentieth century remained containment and management of large numbers of patients in overcrowded conditions.

During the early twentieth century allegations of malpractice rose sharply with nurses being the main target for criticism. Such allegations led to calls for a Royal Commission into Lunacy Laws which was established in 1926 and led in turn to the Mental Treatment Act 1930 which introduced categories of 'voluntary' and 'temporary' patients which avoided the pessimistic experience of certification for some patients. The category of 'voluntary patient' was extended and by 1957 this group constituted 75 per cent of admissions. However, admission procedures and rights of patients remained unchanged until the Mental Health Act (1959), which, Connolly (1992) points out, marked the end of the power of magistrates over the asylum system and regain of control by mental health professionals.

During the 1930s many men from depressed areas of the country entered mental health nursing. Ideal entry requirements for nurses from this period into the 1950s were that they should be physically fit, able to take part in organized games or play a musical instrument – criteria that contributed to active sporting and community activities within and between asylums, but did little to improve standards of patient care (Jones 1960). While mental nurses were expected to show kindness and forbearance towards patients and set them a good example, asylum regulations in the early twentieth century governing the conduct of staff were strict and gave little opportunity for the exercise of responsibility or common sense – as envisaged by advocates of moral treatment so many years before. For example, Connolly (1992) cites regulations from Springfield Mental Hospital (formerly the Surrey Asylum) in 1926 which shows that patients had to be counted in and out of the wards and gardens, specified that five rounds be made of the Female Division and six of the Male Division during each period of night duty, and that attendants who were judged negligent, resulting in patients escaping, were required to pay a portion of the expense incurred in recapturing them. In the years immediately following the Second World War Connolly reports that

> 66   all the wards at Springfield Hospital were locked, apart from a few geriatric wards. The gardens were also locked and the hospital as a whole was surrounded by fences. The main block was strictly segregated – male staff and male patients on one side, female staff and female patients on the other. Only maintenance staff and doctors regularly saw both sides. The wards themselves were furnished with hard wooden chairs and long workhouse tables, and there were no curtains between the beds.
>
> (Connolly 1992: 11)   99

From Connolly's account mental nurses of the time, with their general nursing counterparts, were much preoccupied by cleanliness and orderliness to the extent that beds would be lined up with pieces of string to ensure regularity. Task allocation was the dominant form of work organization and time periods were set aside for these tasks to be accomplished – such as bed making, and mealtimes when staff and patients would eat together in the wards. Nursing work was varied, with an emphasis on organizing patients' work: in the wards (for example, cleaning and maintaining the wards, cleaning or feeding other patients), on the farm, in the hospital grounds (for example, rolling the cricket pitch) or in the laundry or tailor's shop where they would make and maintain clothing and bedding. In spite of the emphasis on constructive activity for patients there was little emphasis on preparing patients for return to the world outside hospital.

Psychiatric hospitals in decline

The community had long been considered a brutalizing environment for people with mental health problems (Wing 1990), but in the 1960s a number of factors combined to make it an increasingly attractive care location for local authorities and the government. These factors included:

- gross overcrowding of hospitals, the population of which had reached 150,000 by the mid-1950s, which was more than the buildings could satisfactorily accommodate;
- crumbling building stock which would have required a great deal of money to repair and most of which were unsuitably located to serve the major centres of population;
- escalating NHS labour costs, particularly in the 1960s when the Confederation of Health Service Employees (COHSE), by now the major union for mental health nurses, were awarded major pay increases of 12 per cent in 1959, 14 per cent in 1962 and 5 per cent in 1963 (Nolan and Hooper 2000);
- the majority view that new drugs offered a genuine opportunity for the control of symptoms and, in some cases, cure; and
- the Mental Health Act (1959), which placed a strong emphasis on community involvement in psychiatric care services.

The shift away from the old hospitals to a community-based service was accelerated by other factors, in particular the diminishing power-base of the physician superintendents in the hospitals, which was undermined by new consultant psychiatrists created within the new NHS. The power-base of the consultant psychiatrists was strengthened by the transfer of services such as radiography, pathology and surgery, formerly provided within the mental hospitals to purpose-built general hospitals. Moreover, the consultants were empowered by new drugs on the market, and were free to select their own treatments independent of the physician superintendent's views. As the power of the consultant psychiatrists increased, so the power of the physician superintendents declined until in 1960 the post was declared obsolete.

With the demise of physician superintendents, and the change in the philosophy of psychiatric care away from manual labour as therapy towards therapeutic relationships and environments, the psychiatric hospitals began to change. Wards were unlocked, military-type uniforms (brass buttons, peaked caps) for male nurses were abandoned in favour of white coats, hospital farms which had once provided employment and income were run down and sold off and ancillary staff were employed to carry out the manual tasks once carried out by nurses and patients.

The influence of the anti-psychiatry movement was, in the 1960s, at its peak. Leading figures in the movement – Laing, Szasz, Sedgewick and Foucault – came from very different philosophical and political positions but were united in their mistrust and scepticism of orthodox psychiatry and challenged it to re-examine its *history, origins, claims and achievements* (Nolan 1993: 1). Anti-psychiatrists saw psychiatry as performing a role of social control and so could not claim to be a branch of medicine or a respectable science. The anti-psychiatrists were criticized for underestimating the effectiveness of modern psychiatry in diagnosing and treating mental illness and for overestimating its control function (Chapman 1992). However, their ideas were influential in drawing attention to the coercive aspects of psychiatry in which nurses were perceived to be front-line agents of social control.

Criticism from the anti-psychiatrists was supported by growing evidence about the effects of institutional life on patients. The structure and organization of traditional hospitals was gradually seen to be pathogenic as the new therapeutic regimes at the Cassel, Claybury and Fulbourne hospitals demonstrated the benefits of an 'open-door policy' (Nolan 1993) and a partnership approach to care between staff and patients (Chapman 1992).

Goffman's *Asylums* (1961) is a landmark in the history of care of the mentally ill and of the anti-psychiatry movement. His attack on the 'total institution' in the USA, with its emphasis on block treatment, denial of individuality and social distance between staff and patients, caused the USA and the UK to rethink institutional care (Nolan 1993). Other critics in Britain were also condemning conditions in mental hospitals at the time (Barton 1959; Townsend 1962). Nurses who ran the hospitals felt powerless to respond because they had no decision-making power (Nolan 1993).

The final blow to the mental hospital system came from a series of psychiatric hospital scandals and public inquiries in the 1960s and 1970s that exposed professional neglect and suffering of mentally ill patients, and that seriously weakened psychiatric nursing. In 1961 Enoch Powell, the then Minister of Health, declared that mental hospitals must close and the development of community care for the mentally ill remained a policy of successive governments. Throughout the 1960s and 1970s only limited progress was made in moving patients from the larger hospitals into community settings, and community care itself lacked conceptual clarity. Although overcrowding and the resident population of large psychiatric hospitals had gradually decreased, by 1975, none had closed. Twenty-seven years after his announcement in 1961 that hospitals must close, Enoch Powell reflected on the entrenched bureaucracies of the psychiatric hospitals that prevented even modest changes, let alone closure, being contemplated (Powell 1988, cited in Nolan 1993).

Nevertheless, the Government's White Paper, *Better Services for the Mentally Ill* (DHSS 1975), claimed that the government's policy was working. The development of local services with a shift away from hospital provision towards community-based social services care was still the target although the White Paper declared also that the hospital would remain the centre for mental health care services for the foreseeable future; that is, until adequate community care facilities were in place to prevent 'revolving door' patients, that is, those who needed supervision of their medication, followed by a rapid return to the community, perhaps precipitating readmission. *Better Services for the Mentally Ill* set the tone for the future community-based care of people with mental illness and continues to provide a useful reference point from which current mental health care services can be judged.

Development of community mental health nursing

Closure of the large mental hospitals and their replacement by smaller units attached to local district hospitals, and the development of day hospitals and community-care facilities had a marked impact on the practice of mental health nursing from the 1960s. May and Moore (1963) describe the work of two (later four) nurses seconded from Warlingham Park Hospital in 1954 to visit patients discharged from hospital and now living in Croydon. These 'outpatient' nurses saw ex-patients suffering from schizophrenia and depression, and their duties were to:

- monitor their compliance with medication and attendance at outpatient clinics;
- assess and monitor their mental state;
- monitor difficulties in their personal habits and seek to improve these;
- reassure relatives.

Their role was clinical and investigation and reporting patients' family and social circumstances was not expected; this was the remit of the psychiatric social worker. Each nurse was responsible for a ward of patients. They attended a weekly ward round, and also outpatient clinics and evening aftercare groups.

McNamee (1993) reports that Moorhaven Hospital established what was known as a 'Nursing After-Care' service in 1957. This differed from the Warlingham Park Hospital service in that it involved nurses working both in the wards as well as with patients who had been discharged. It is ironic that more than 40 years later this flexible model of working which offers one approach to bridging the gap between inpatient and community care is rarely seen in practice. Moorhaven Hospital community psychiatric nurses (CPNs) were expected to build relationships with their patients and to use this as a medium for care delivery and for helping patients to cope with the effects of their illness. Thus, the nurse was envisaged as a therapeutic agent, a role that served also to enhance the status of nursing at the time.

The CPN role continued to develop. According to Hunter (1974) their functions in the 1960s included:

- providing practical assistance to patients and their families (for example, help bathing and shaving patients);
- giving advice particularly to patients' families on medication, monitoring its side effects and cooperating with general practitioners and psychiatrists to reduce these;
- acting as a link between the ward and community and facilitating admission in the event of relapse;
- ensuring continuity of care for designated groups of patients (including those with schizophrenia, recurrent depression and organic psychosis);
- supervising patients in outpatient clinics;
- assisting in running social clubs and work groups;
- assisting patients to gain employment and accommodation on discharge from hospital.

The CPN role expanded to assume social and rehabilitative functions particularly from the 1970s following the Local Authority Social Services Act 1970, which abolished specialist social workers for people with mental health problems. CPNs began to offer crisis intervention, group work, psychotherapy and behaviour therapy (Hunter 1974). However, in the 1960s and 1970s CPNs worked primarily within hospital treatment teams, received all referrals from hospital consultants and carried out care programmes that were medically oriented.

A change of emphasis away from medical domination towards a more autonomous social model of care followed attachment of CPNs to general practice in Oxford and elsewhere in the 1970s. These CPNs accepted referrals from many sources (open referral system), including each other, and developed into far more independent practitioners responsible for patient assessment, and also planning and implementing an appropriate care package. Later, though, attachment of CPNs to primary-care teams was criticized (for example, White 1990b; Gournay and Brooking 1994) for deflecting the attention of nurses towards the so-called 'worried well' and away from the needs of people with serious mental illness who are a government priority for mental health care.

In the early 1970s, and particularly following the White Paper *Better Services for the Mentally Ill* (DHSS 1975), there was a growing lobby for specialist community training for mental health nurses. The Joint Board of Clinical Nursing Studies (JBCNS) established a committee to examine requirements for an approved community psychiatric nurse (CPN) course that did not overlap with the requirements for district nurses or health visitors. It was agreed that a separate course was needed to produce highly trained nurses who could meet the specific needs of mentally ill people. In 1974 the JBCNS published the *Outline Curriculum in Community Psychiatric Nursing for Registered Nurses* (JBCNS 1974). This

36–39 week course was designed to prepare Registered Mental Nurses (RMNs) to work in multi-professional environments and to give both rehabilitative and therapeutic care in the community.

The first CPN course was started by Chiswick College in 1973 (White 1990a) and, by the end of the 1970s, CPNs had achieved independent recognition and other colleges and polytechnics were running courses. CPNs worked from general practice clinics or accepted referrals from other agencies, and developed specialist skills to assist and work with care groups and organizations (Simmons and Brooker 1990).

Increased specialization of CPNs and other mental health nurses from the 1970s mirrored and was sometimes forced by increased specialization by their medical colleagues. An important example was the development of training for nurses in behaviour therapy by Isaac Marks at the Maudsley Hospital from 1972 (Simmons and Brooker 1986). This led to the English National Board (ENB) course 650 – 'Short-term Adult Behavioural Psychotherapy', which was the first of a series of post-registration courses to provide community mental health nurses with specialist skills and a specific therapeutic orientation. A more recent example is the Thorn Programme developed and disseminated from the Institute of Psychiatry, King's College London, and the University of Manchester, which trains mental health nurses and other professionals to deliver research-based care and treatment to people suffering from severe and enduring mental illness (Gournay 1997).

The first two UK government reviews of mental health nursing

A major review of psychiatric nursing, *Psychiatric Nursing: Today and Tomorrow* published in 1968 by the then Ministry of Health (Standing Mental Health and Standing Nursing Advisory Committees 1968), focused particularly on inpatient psychiatric nursing, which was the dominant setting for care in that period. This report highlighted the importance of the personal relationship between the nurse and patient as central to the nurse's role. Among other recommendations it identified the need for psychiatric nurses to develop skills in psychotherapy, a view which resonated with Peplau's (1952) interpersonal relations approach to mental health nursing, which was promoted by opinion leaders of the time, such as Altschul (of whom more later). Altschul had endorsed interpersonal skill development for mental health nurses several years previously (Altschul 1964) and had demonstrated its absence in her study of nurse–patient interaction published in 1972 as *Patient–Nurse Interaction in Psychiatric Acute Wards* (Altschul 1972).

A further 26 years were to pass before the next government review of mental health nursing, *Working in Partnership: a Collaborative Approach to Care* (Mental Health Nursing (MHN) Review Team 1994), by which time the context of mental health nursing was much changed. The Thatcher years (1979–90), the *NHS and Community Care Act* 1990, and the development of the internal market in health care with purchaser and provider roles had led to a very different care environment. Marked advances in medical science had led to new drugs (for example, Prozac) and a growing confidence in some psychological therapies (for example, cognitive behaviour therapy), and patients' expectations for care and treatment had risen. In addition there had been major changes in nurse education, consequent upon Project 2000 (UKCC 1986) which had moved education from hospital-based training schools into higher education, and gradual acceptance that nursing should be a research-based profession, leading more nurses to question their existing practice and seek clarification of their role. In the light of these changes, by the 1990s it seemed to many that the review of mental health nursing was both timely and necessary.

The strongest message of *Working in Partnership* was that the relationship between the nurse and service user is at the heart of nursing practice. The report states, 'This review starts from a belief that the work of mental health nurses rests on their relationship with people who use mental health services. This relationship should have value to both parties' (MHN Review Team 1994: 9).

Working in Partnership made 42 recommendations grouped under the following headings: the relationship between nurses and people who use services, the practice of mental health nurses, delivery of services, challenging issues and research and education. The review identified a central role for mental health nurses in the provision of mental health services. Among its recommendations was that nurses should: act as keyworkers, become involved in supervised discharge, and take the lead as providers of information to service-users. The report urged increased opportunities for patients to become involved in their care in partnership with nurses and for nurses to focus their work on the care of people with serious and enduring mental illness. The focus of mental health nurses on this group has strengthened over the past decade and this recommendation is perhaps the most enduring contribution of the report to mental health nursing policy.

The Review Team supported the change in title from 'psychiatric nurse' to 'mental health nurse', on the grounds that this represents the broadening scope of contemporary practice and endorsed continuation of the specialist pre-registration branch of mental health nursing, rather than the creation of a generic nurse and conversion of mental health nursing into a post-registration specialty. The report made recommendations also about the quality and nature of services for patients, including: questioning the value psychiatric units attached to district general hospitals, supporting choice for patients in single-sex accommodation, and gender of key workers.

In summary, *Working in Partnership* contained little that was new, and much of it endorsed conventional wisdom of the time. But it was valued by mental nurses for clarifying their roles at a time of great change in the development of mental health services, and for shoring up the boundaries of the specialty by rejecting generic pre-registration education which would, many feared, dilute mental health nurses' unique identity and contribution to care (Norman 1998). However, it paid too little attention to psychological and other interventions of proven effectiveness delivered by nurses to patients, and the skills required to do this. Although *Working in Partnership* acknowledged the importance of mental health nursing being research based, in the 1990s the specialty had yet to feel the impact of the evidence-based health care movement, and the challenge it was to pose to mental health nursing in the interpersonal relations tradition.

Traditions

In this section we trace the origins of two contrasting traditions within mental health nursing to the influential ideas of Hilda Peplau and the rise of evidence-based health care.

Nursing in the interpersonal relations tradition: Peplau and her legacy

The interpersonal relations tradition of mental health nursing is as old as mental health nursing itself, and has its origins in Tuke's moral treatment. However, it found its first formal expression in the work of Hildegard (Hilda) Peplau who exercised a major influence on mental health nursing from the early 1950s until her death at the age of 89 in 1999. Described by some of her admirers as the 'mother of psychiatric nursing' (Barker 1999: 175) Peplau was the first to coin the term 'nurse–patient relationship' and her book *Interpersonal Relations in Nursing* (1952) became a classic and is still widely read, having been reprinted in London in 1988.

Born in Reading, Pennsylvania in 1909 Peplau graduated as a nurse from Pottsdown, Pennsylvania School of Nursing in 1931. After a varied career as a general nurse Peplau became fascinated by psychiatry and took a BA degree in interpersonal psychology from Bennington College in Vermont in 1943. At Bennington College Peplau studied with Erich Fromm, the foremost post-Freudian analyst of his day; and during this period worked on children's wards in Bellvue Hospital in New York, and also at Chestnut Lodge, a private psychiatric hospital in Rockville, Maryland. It was at Chestnut Lodge that Peplau came into contact with Harry Stack Sullivan, a psychiatrist, who was developing an interpersonal theory of psychiatric illness (Sullivan 1947). For Sullivan psychiatry was not concerned simply with the study of mentally ill people or group processes, but was a broader enterprise concerned with 'the study of what goes on between two or more people, all but one of whom may be completely illusory' (Peplau 1987: 202).

Peplau's major contribution in *Interpersonal Relations in Nursing* was to apply and so develop Sullivan's theoretical perspective to the interpersonal world of the nurse and patient. For Peplau (1987) mental health nursing is an important, therapeutic, interpersonal process characterized by three overlapping and interlocking phases in the nurse–patient relationship – orientation, working and termination. Her study of interpersonal relations revealed for Peplau various roles for the nurse; as, for example, a resource person, teacher, surrogate parent and leader. Later she was to describe these as 'sub-roles' and the role of counsellor or psychotherapist as the heart of psychiatric nursing. Through the medium of their relationships with patients nurses strive to create conditions that aim to promote health and develop patients' ability to engage with those around them.

In 1954 Peplau established the first graduate-level programme for clinical nurse specialists in psychiatric nursing and led this programme until her formal retirement in 1974. During this period, and thereafter, she developed her ideas on interpersonal relations in conference papers and publications (for example Peplau 1987, 1994).

Peplau's influence on UK mental health nursing

Peplau's ideas took a long time to influence academic psychiatric nursing in the UK and it was not until the late 1970s and early 1980s that they gained a secure foothold. A number of mental health nurses contributed to the diffusion of Peplau's ideas in the UK, but we single out two as being particularly influential: Annie Altschul and Phil Barker.

Altschul

Annie Altschul was immediately aware of the importance of *Interpersonal Relations in Nursing* in providing a framework for psychiatric nursing practice, and promoted it. In 1958 Altschul won a Commonwealth Scholarship to study psychiatric nurse education in the USA, in particular psychiatric nurse training for general nursing students. During her trip she was introduced to a nursing curriculum that focused on helping nurses to establish relationships with patients, to use these relationships to move forward patients' recovery and rehabilitation, and terminate these relationships at an appropriate time. Nolan (1999) explains that while this approach presented practical difficulties, such as several nurses being attached to one patient at the same time, Altschul became convinced that this was the way forward for mental health nursing in the UK. Such relationships she believed evolved over time and were fostered by good mentoring, supervision and support of students, and also by nurses being accountable for their actions. Over the next four decades Altschul was well placed to promote her ideas, first as Principal Tutor at the Maudsley Hospital in London and from 1964 at the University of Edinburgh where in 1976 she became the first psychiatric nurse to hold a Chair in Nursing in the UK. She was Emeritus Professor of Nursing at the University of Edinburgh until her death.

Altschul's main contribution to the psychiatric nursing research literature, published in 1972 as *Patient-nurse Interaction*, is her study towards an MPhil degree of how therapeutic relationships between nurses and patients could be established and developed in an inpatient ward. Data collection involved Altschul observing and timing didactic nurse–patient interactions in acute psychiatric wards in the Royal Edinburgh Hospital. For interactions of five minutes' duration or more Altschul asked the nurse what had taken place, on the assumption that these more lengthy interactions were those when a special therapeutic relationship is most likely to develop between nurse and patient, or that interaction would be underpinned by therapeutic principles or intent.

Altschul's study looked for evidence of therapeutic principles underpinning interactions between nurses and patients, but in this she was to be disappointed. She found that nurses in her study did 'not have any identifiable perspective to guide them in their interactions with patients' and the nurses themselves saw mental health nursing as "just common sense" [ts]' (Altschul 1972: 192). She concludes that the relationship between the nurse and the patient was 'irrelevant to psychiatric treatment' (1972: 193). In spite of this, most patients described their relationship with the nurses as helpful; although this finding must be considered in the light of patients' reluctance to criticize nurses, particularly when they are hospitalized and feel vulnerable.

Altschul does not explain clearly the criteria she used for rating interactions for therapeutic content, or her cut-off point of five minutes, rather than four or three. But, a more fundamental limitation of her study, as Macilwaine (1983) points out, is her assumption that the nurses she studied should have based their practice according to theoretical principles, specifically those relevant to forming personal relationships with patients. Although Peplau's writings were popular in the USA, nurse training in the UK in the 1960s did not emphasize nurse–patient relationships. Thus, Altschul's finding that nurses regarded their practice as just common sense could have been confidently predicted. Altschul's study is important, nevertheless, because it was the first British clinical study of mental health nursing carried out by a nurse. Moreover, published only four years after the government's 1968 review of mental health nursing, *Psychiatric Nursing Today and Tomorrow* (Standing Mental Health and Standing Nursing Advisory Committees 1968), it proved a great impetus to UK mental health nurse education being oriented towards providing nurses with knowledge and skills to form relationships with patients and use these therapeutically. *Patient-nurse Interaction* established Altschul's commitment to the study of therapeutic relationships in psychiatric nursing. It also influenced the work of subsequent researchers (for example, Towell 1975; Cormack 1983) and the direction of, in particular, pre-registration nurse education in the UK in the late 1970s and 1980s, which emphasized the acquisition of interpersonal skills (see, for example, ENB and WNB 1982).

An interesting footnote is that towards the end of her life Altschul was to revise her position on the central position of the nurse–patient relationship to nursing practice.

Reflecting on her professional life in 1999 Altschul (1999) writes that although her observations of nurse education in the USA in 1958 convinced her that focusing nurse training around the concept of the therapeutic relationship offered substantial benefits for the nurses, she was 'much less convinced that the patients benefited'. She notes that nursing students of the time who had been well taught to establish and use their relationships with patients constructively, considered that psychiatric nursing could only be conducted under circumstances where it would be possible for nurses to have a well-defined caseload of patients with whom they could have time restricted, intensive one-to-one relationships. In the USA in the late 1950s this could be achieved only if nurses were based in private practice. Altschul reports that she was unconvinced at the time, but had changed her mind. The distinctive contribution of nurses to patient care is often attributed to their continuous presence with patients, in contrast with the sporadic appearance of others such as the psychiatrist, psychologist or occupational therapist. Altschul's position in 1999 appears to be that a continuing presence between the nurse and patient, as occurs in inpatient care, is not conducive to the development and constructive use of therapeutic relationships, since giving attention to a ward of patients is too draining for nurses and relationships with several nurses, simultaneously, is too demanding for inpatients.

Barker

The continuing development of the interpersonal relations orientation within UK mental health nursing literature and practice is well illustrated by the work of Philip (Phil) Barker, currently a psychotherapist and Honorary Professor at the University of Dundee in Scotland.

Unlike Peplau whose *Interprofessional Relations in Nursing* set the agenda for most of her subsequent work, Barker's views on the role and focus of the psychiatric nurse have emerged over time from a series of published papers some of the more important we refer to in the annotated reading list which follows this chapter. His views on the proper focus of psychiatric nursing owe much to his long interest and study of Oriental philosophy and to the influence of writers such as Ed. Podvol (also influenced by Buddhism), psychiatrists such as Thomas Szasz, his long friendship with Hilda Peplau and Annie Altschul, and also first-hand accounts of mental disorder from service users.

Barker's major initiative over the past 15 years, in collaboration with Poppy Buchanan-Barker, has been the development, testing and dissemination of the Tidal Model which is reported to have generated over 100 official projects in the UK, Ireland, New Zealand, Canada, Japan and Australia in a wide range of therapeutic settings, suggesting that the model might be applied to address people's human needs, irrespective of their clinical diagnosis (see http://www.tidal-model.com).

The Tidal Model, which draws upon nautical metaphors, is based upon four closely related ideas:

- Life for us all is a journey on an 'ocean of experience'. Psychiatric crises are one thing, among many, that disrupt people's life journey. The ultimate goal of nursing is to return people to that ocean (within the community) to continue their voyage. So, for Barker mental disorders are 'problems in living' which limit effective functioning of individuals in many aspects of their lives.
- Empowerment is the primary goal of the caring process, so that people are able to take greater control over their lives. This reflects Barker's concept of nursing, developed several years previously, as a social process for facilitating human growth and development, or what he terms 'trephotaxis'.

- Change is a constant feature of the life journey. One aim of interventions within the Tidal Model is to raise people's awareness of the small changes that occur that, ultimately, will have a large effect on their lives.
- Effective nursing involves caring with people rather than for them, or even about them through mutual discussion and understanding between the nurse and the person in care which gives priority to the exploration and development of the person's lived experience. Thus, the Tidal Model eschews standardized protocols and care packages in favour of an individualized approach to nursing care which aims to provide the sort of support that people with problems in living think they need now to take them to the next step of their journey of recovery.

The Tidal Model website highlights research and evaluation as important to the development of the model. But in contrast to the evidence-based health care emphasis on evaluating treatment outcomes (of which more later), the emphasis here is on understanding the processes by which the model has its effect and the changes which occur. So, important questions are how a health care team working within the Tidal Model, doing particular things within a particular care context can achieve a particular set of results. And also how change happens for people, how change impacts on their lives, how other people respond to these changes and the meaning of these changes for the people themselves.

In summary, the interpersonal relations tradition within mental health nursing, particularly as developed by Phil and Poppy Barker and their associates, gives priority to individualized care constructed through dialogue between the nurse and the person with problems in living, which focuses on the lived experience of that person. It is unconcerned about psychiatric diagnosis and eschews standardized packages of care, in favour of decisions about next steps; that is what needs to be done to help the person with problems progress on their life journey and towards recovery. Although the Tidal Model is underpinned by a programme of research, evidence for its effectiveness has not yet been established using research designs which would be acceptable to nurses in the evidence-based health care tradition.

Evidence-based health care

The view that mental health nursing should be evidence based has emerged strongly over the past 20 years. It reflects increasing confidence in scientifically proven methods for treating mental illness and it reflects too certain assumptions about mental health services currently, notably that they either do not provide evidence-based practices, or lack fidelity to evidence-based procedures, and that given resource constraints, patients have a right to treatments with proven efficacy.

Evidence-based health care has a long history dating back, say some authorities, to post-revolutionary Paris, when physicians like Pierre Louis rejected the wisdom of authorities that venesection was good for cholera, and sought answers in the systematic observation of patients (Rangachari 1997). However, it was in 1992 that the term 'evidence-based medicine' was coined by a group led by Gordon Guyatt at McMaster University Medical School in Canada. The term has spread globally since, and 'medicine' has been replaced by 'health care' as other professionals, including mental health nurses, have adopted its principles.

Evidence-based medicine (health care) is defined by Sackett *et al.* (2000) as the integration of three main elements:

■ Best research evidence, i.e. clinically relevant research often in the basic medical sciences but, in particular, clinical research into the accuracy of diagnostic tests, the predictive power of prognostic markers and the efficacy and safety of preventive, therapeutic and rehabilitative treatments (interventions).

■ Clinical expertise, i.e. effective use of clinical skills to assess the risks and benefits of particular interventions for individual patients, given their diagnosis, general state of health.

■ Patient values, i.e. taking into account in making clinical decisions, patients' particular concerns, expectations and values.

Critics of evidence-based health care tend to emphasize the first two of Sackett's elements, but pay little attention to the third, which demonstrates that evidence-based health care is not incompatible with a patient-centred approach. Indeed Sackett *et al.* (2000) point out that when these three elements are integrated in clinical decision-making, the outcome will be a therapeutic alliance between the clinician and the health care professional, which will optimize the patient's clinical outcomes and quality of life.

But why the sudden interest in evidence-based health care? Sackett *et al.*'s (2000) comments in relation to evidence-based medicine apply to evidence-based health care more generally. Sackett and colleagues point to the realization that:

■ busy health care professionals need on-the-spot valid information about diagnosis, prognosis, therapy, prevention and care but can set aside very little time for general reading or study;

moreover

■ traditional sources of this information are inadequate because they are out of date (for example, textbooks), wrong (for example, views of 'experts'), ineffective (for example, didactic continuing professional education), or overwhelming in their volume and diversity (for example, health care journals).

As a result there is an increasing disparity between health care professionals' skills and clinical judgement, which tend to improve over time, and their knowledge base and clinical performance, which decline. Until recently these problems were insurmountable for busy health care professionals, but now several recent developments have enabled this state of affairs to be tackled. The most important of these are:

■ The development of strategies for tracking down and appraising the validity and relevance of evidence. Steps in this process include:
    1   translating information needs into answerable clinical questions;
    2   tracking down the best evidence with which to answer that question;
    3   appraising that evidence for its validity, impact (effect size) and applicability to clinical practice;
    4   integrating this critical appraisal with knowledge of a patient's unique personal circumstances;
    5   evaluating how steps 1–4 were carried out, and identifying how they might be carried out more efficiently and effectively next time.

Steps 1–3, in particular, are the focus of a growing number of evidence-based decision-making in health care courses and manuals (for example, Greenhalgh and Donald 2000; Sackett *et al.* 2000) that are available.

The development of systematic reviews and concise summaries of the effects of health care, many of which have been conducted by groups operating under the umbrella of the Cochrane Collaboration.

The expansion of evidence-based journals of secondary publications (for example, *Evidence-Based Nursing, Evidence Based Mental Health*) that publish around 2 per cent of clinical papers that are considered to offer valid evidence to guide clinical practice.

The development of information technology, which enables almost immediate access to evidence-based journals and systematic reviews.

Increasing emphasis on lifelong learning and better understanding of strategies, which are effective in this and for improving clinical performance; much work in this field has been undertaken by the Cochrane Effective Practice and Organization of Care Group (EPOC).

The methods of evidence-based health care are developed most fully in relation to questions of treatment effectiveness. So, for example, there is a well-established hierarchy of evidence which identifies various types and grades of evidence which relate in turn to the robustness of the evidence source, and so how much it can be trusted to provide a valid answer to questions treatment of effectiveness. The hierarchy of evidence used by the authors of the *NSF for Mental Health* (DH 1999), is shown in Box 4.1.

Box 4.1   Levels of evidence

Type 1 evidence: at least one good systematic review, including at least one randomized controlled trial

Type 2 evidence: at least one good randomized controlled trial

Type 3 evidence: at least one well-designed intervention study without randomization

Type 4 evidence: at least one well-designed observational study

Type 5 evidence: expert opinion, including the opinion of service users and carers

(After *NSF for Mental Health*, DH 1999: 6)

In this hierarchy the randomized controlled trial (RCT) (Type 2 evidence) is considered to offer the highest level of research evidence to answer effectiveness questions, apart from the well-conducted systematic review, which must include at least one RCT (Type 1 evidence). However, by definition, the concerns of evidence-based health care must go beyond the clinical trial because the search is for the best available evidence to answer a clinical question. In the hierarchy readers will note that expert opinion, *including the opinions of service users and carers* is at the bottom of the pile (Type 5 evidence); evidence from this source is to be trusted only in the absence of anything better! This should not always be the case for mental health nurses, however, as we argue later in this chapter.

A leading UK mental health nurse in the evidence-based health care tradition was Kevin Gournay, who retired from his post as Professor of Psychiatric Nursing at the Institute of Psychiatry, King's College London in 2006. Gournay rejected discrete nursing activities in favour of multi-disciplinary approaches to care and treatment. His primary focus was not nurses' relationships with patients, but on 'extending' nurses' roles (to incorporate the roles occupied previously by doctors and psychologists, for example) so that they can contribute fully to delivering evidence-based interventions to patients with recognized mental illness.

Gournay recommended more randomized controlled trials (RCT) to test the efficacy of interventions in which nurses are involved – and has contributed substantially to the research literature in this respect, in collaboration with psychiatrists and psychologists, in particular; for example evaluations of nurses as counsellors (Gournay and Brooking 1994) and the Thorn Programme, a training course for nurses and other health care professionals in the care of people with severe and enduring mental illness (Gournay 1997). Towards the end of his career Gournay, we perceive, was more ready than previously to recognize the practical limitations of the RCT in the complex field of mental health services and as a result more inclined to see the RCT as perhaps the most important, but as only one of several research methods, which can be used to understand nurses' work with patients. Other research designs valued within the evidence-based tradition include epidemiological studies to assess the health needs of populations and also qualitative research methods to examine the nature and experience of mental health nursing interventions. However, in Gournay's view, qualitative studies were best carried out in combination with quantitative research studies and vice versa; a view with which some qualitative researchers would take issue.

In mental health care today the research evidence supports a relatively small set of interventions. A systematic review of RCTs generated a consensus list of ten interventions which were considered important to the role of the mental health nurse and evaluated their effectiveness (Gray *et al.* 2006). Of these there was good evidence for the effectiveness of: cognitive behaviour therapy (CBT) for depression, post-traumatic stress disorder, anxiety and bulimia nervosa; family interventions; psycho-education; assertive community treatment; and counselling, although benefits were only modest and short term. There was equivocal evidence for: medication management; CBT for psychosis, early intervention, deliberate self-harm, anorexia nervosa, and dementia; and physical health promotion. There was evidence for a lack of effect of case management, and a paucity of RCT evidence for the effectiveness of interventions for the management of violence and engagement.

Reconciliation of the two traditions

Fears that the interpersonal relations tradition of mental health nursing would be eclipsed by the rise of the evidence-based health care tradition have not come to pass. Indeed, over the past five years, since publication of the first edition of this book, we have observed increasing consensus that both traditions are integral to the practice of mental health nursing. This was demonstrated by the national consultation conducted as part of the Chief Nursing Officer for England's review of mental health nursing published in 2006 as *From Values to Action* (discussed in Chapter 35) which showed a reasonable consensus of views with, mostly nurses, citing the importance of the nurse's relationship with service users, but also enthusiasm for developing new roles and skills to be applied in non-traditional 'recovery focused' ways in their work (Brimblecombe, personal communication).

Two trends are evident. The first is that the polarized views expressed by individuals from both traditions are becoming less relevant as the focus of mental health care changes towards an emphasis on promoting social inclusion and recovery, reducing social stigma and supporting principles such as choice. Thus, evidence-based practice and interventions are now framed within a recovery-oriented approach (cf. Chapter 5) which emphasizes the central place of the person with mental health problems and the impact of services upon his/her life journey. We discuss the implications of this focus for mental health nurses in Chapter 35.

The second, and related point, is that the polarized views expressed by individuals from both traditions are now less distinct than they might appear. Advocates of evidence-based health care recognize the contribution of 'relationship forming skills' on patients' willingness to engage in psychological treatments and the contribution of relationship factors to treatment outcome (see for example Keijsers *et al.* 2000). Moreover, evidence-based psychosocial interventions for psychosis (disseminated in the form of the Thorn programme, mentioned earlier) are often practised in a 'recovery oriented' way that recognizes the importance of reducing the extent to which remaining symptoms interfere with people's efforts to pursue their goals and interests and emphasizes the importance of how these individuals can be helped to make the most of their lives. A further example of integration is the closer integration of service users' perspectives within the design and conduct of studies to evaluate the effectiveness of mental health care interventions (as for example the formation of the Service Users Research Enterprise (SURE), coordinated by Dr Diana Rose, the Institute of Psychiatry, King's College London) which may have the effect of ensuring that evaluation research focuses on topics which are important to service users and that service user oriented outcomes such as independence, employment, satisfying relationships and good quality of life (the social dimensions of recovery) assume their proper place alongside more traditional outcomes, such as adherence to treatment, relapse or re-hospitalization prevention.

For their part nurses in the interpersonal relations tradition are more inclined than previously to produce evidence of the effectiveness of their work with people in distress. For example, as mentioned previously, Phil and Poppy Barker emphasize that research and development is integral to the Tidal Model, although their emphasis on understanding the processes that lead to the outcome, rather than simply whether or not the Tidal Model 'works', highlights a rather different approach to evaluation than the traditional reliance of nurses in the evidence-based health care tradition on the RCT. Whereas the RCT is the gold standard research method for many in the evidence-based tradition, critics of the RCT argue that it fails to recognize the importance of individual experience, which is crucial to the proper focus of mental health nursing. This argument, as expressed by Rolfe (1996) for example, proposes that unlike medicine and psychology, mental health nurses should not be concerned with putting people into diagnostic categories, providing treatment appropriate to that diagnosis and assessing the effectiveness of this through a well-conducted RCT. Mental health nurses should be concerned with differences between people, rather than similarities between them. The focus of mental health nursing should be on individual presentation of a particular problem, rather than providing *general* interventions to meet *general* problems experienced by people who happen to be in a particular diagnostic category. This is because problems experienced by a group of people generally (for example poor attention span in schizophrenia) is only an approximate guide to the problems experienced by the individual; reduced concentration span might not *be* a problem to the person at all. For Rolfe, the approach to mental health nursing advocated by supporters of the RCT runs the danger of swallowing up the specific needs of particular individuals 'in a general solution to a perceived common problem' (Rolfe 1996: 333).

In response to an article by Gournay advocating the RCT for mental health nursing research Rolfe says, 'Gournay's assertion that we should employ "the rigor of RCTs" is inappropriate and misleading, as are the findings from such studies (see for example, Gournay and Brooking 1994)' … Rolfe concludes, 'The proper focus of nursing is the therapeutic relationship, and we (mental health nurses) must demonstrate on our own terms and not on the terms of medicine that this focus is effective' (Rolfe 1996: 333).

We would accept that some of the outcomes used in existing research have only an indirect relationship with the things that service users value or think important in their lives, and support moves by researchers from the evidence-based health care tradition to incorporate service users' in the design and conduct of evaluations. However, we do not share Rolfe's aversion to the well-conducted RCT, which is the ideal study design to answer questions of treatment effectiveness for groups of people in well-defined categories, because it is the only design which can take account of all those other influences, that are known and unknown, that can influence outcome, other than the intervention. It does present practical problems in the complex world of mental health nursing interventions and services (see Norman and Humphrey 2008 for a discussion of alternative approaches to evaluation and evaluation research) and is probably not the best choice of research method to investigate therapeutic relationships. But therapeutic relationships are not, in our view, the only proper focus for mental health nurses. As the title of this book suggests, mental health nursing is a science as well as an art. The art of nursing is concerned with therapeutic relationships, with a person's internal world and sense of self (with the left-hand quadrants of the framework we introduced in Chapter 1 – see Figure 1.1). The science of nursing, in contrast, is concerned with a person's biophysiological profile and their observable behaviour (with the right-hand quadrants of our framework). Nurses must be concerned with change in all four quadrants in response to pharmacological and psychosocial interventions (covered in Chapters 16 and 14), or different forms of care organization (cf. Chapter 8).

Conclusion

An historical perspective shows that mental health nursing has and continues to be shaped by responses to the challenges presented by people with mental disorder that arise in each succeeding era. It arose under the patronage of the medical profession at a time when philanthropy was fashionable, and its development has been linked closely with developments in psychiatric medicine. A historical perspective shows too that early developments of the nurse's role as a therapeutic agent, as envisaged by advocates of moral treatment, was undermined by social forces which meant that by the early twentieth-century asylums became warehouses for madness, and dumping grounds for socially disadvantaged people who were difficult to manage. Hence, nurses became an essential element in a bureaucratic system for organizing patients' lives, a role that involved operating within rigid doctor/nurse/patient hierarchies to contain large numbers of people in often overcrowded conditions. Nurses throughout this period were, for the most part, poorly educated, undervalued and very poorly paid. However, in spite of the regulation and impersonal procedures that characterized patient care in the old hospitals, accounts from nurses working in the postwar period paint a sense of common purpose between nurses and patients in communities that were self-contained and virtually self supporting (Nolan and Hooper 2000).

The decline and closure of the psychiatric hospitals in the 1960s and 1970s and their replacement by smaller units attached to local district hospitals, day hospitals and community care facilities marked a sea change for psychiatric nursing practice which became community based. Community psychiatric nursing services, which were initially hospital based and medically oriented, developed over the years to encompass broader social approaches to mental health care. Mental health nurses themselves became increasingly specialized and, particularly those working in primary care teams, enjoyed relative autonomy from the psychiatrists. Nolan and Hooper (2000) argue that the breakdown of the old hospitals, the supportive infrastructure they provided and the development of community-based mental health care faced mental health nursing with a crisis of identify from which it has yet to recover.

Two UK government reviews of mental health nursing, the first published in 1968 and the second in 1994, set out the roles and responsibilities of mental health nurses, and in so doing clarified the identity of the discipline at times of great change in society and in mental health services. Both reports, in particular *Working in Partnership*, affirmed that the work of the mental health nurse rests fundamentally on their relationships with patients, so reflecting the major influence of Peplau's ideas, which had become well known in the UK under the influence of Altschul and others during the 1970s and 1980s, and revisions of the pre-registration mental health nursing curriculum (for example ENB and WNB 1982) to emphasize teaching of interpersonal skills. With the benefit of hindsight it is clear that the report paid too little attention to psychological and other interventions of proven effectiveness delivered by nurses to patients, and the skills required to do this. However, it played an important role in re-directing the focus of mental health nurses to the care of people with severe and enduring mental illness, a focus which continues today.

In our distinction between the interpersonal relations and evidence-based practice orientations in mental health nursing we see a long-running debate between those who emphasize the 'art' of mental health nursing and those who emphasize the 'science'. This distinction reflects all left-hand quadrants (artists) and all right-hand quadrants (scientists) in the framework introduced in Chapter 1 (Figure 1.1). The debate between artists and scientists is not unique to nursing, but is present in all practice disciplines. It reflects differing research traditions (phenomenological v. scientific) and differing views about what passes as knowledge (Repper 2000).

For most artists mental health nursing has a distinct and unique identity, which has a clear value base and is readily identifiable in any context. By contrast scientists see nursing as a 'function' that contributes to and is shaped by a multi-disciplinary mental health service. Artists go to great pains to clarify nursing values, roles and activities; to make explicit the particular contribution of nursing to the care of people in emotional distress. Scientists are little concerned with such questions – for them, nurses are there to deliver tried and tested interventions to mentally ill patients. A good relationship between the nurse and patient is taken for granted by scientists. It is important, because without this the patient is unlikely to take advice, but this relationship is simply one aspect of the treatment approach and is not a priority for study in its own right. Artists may formulate or draw upon normative models of nursing (Peplau's interpersonal relations 'model' or Barker's 'Tidal Model' (2003), for instance) that set out ways in which nurses should work with distressed people. For scientists normative models of nursing are to be discouraged because in distinguishing nursing from other care approaches they reinforce a tribal mentality and so can lead to a fragmented and poorly coordinated care approach (Gournay 1997).

The threat that evidence-based health care would eclipse nursing in the interprofessional relations tradition, has not occurred. Over the past few years we have witnessed the growth of consensus among practising mental health nurses who recognize the importance of their relationship with service users, but are enthusiastic also to develop the new roles and skills and to apply these in non-traditional 'recovery focused' ways to help service users make the most of their lives. Mental health nurses today are drawing upon their distinctive traditions to develop a new form of practice to meet the changing focus of mental health care on promoting social inclusion and recovery. In this they are supported by the 2006 Chief

Nursing Officer for England's review of mental health nursing (CNOE 2006), which is the starting point for our discussion of the future of the discipline in Chapter 35.

To conclude we summarize the main points of this chapter below:

- An historical perspective shows that the practice discipline of mental health nursing arose under the patronage of the medical profession and its development has been linked closely with developments in psychiatric medicine.
- The origins of the much discussed therapeutic nurse–patient relationship can be traced to 'moral treatment', which was, however, undermined by asylums becoming dumping grounds for socially disadvantaged people who were difficult to manage.
- The breakdown of the asylum system heralded a period of insecurity but also of opportunity for nursing to grow and develop new ways of working with people with mental health problems in the community.
- UK government reviews of mental health nursing conducted in 1968 and 1994 sought to clarify the identity and remit of mental health nursing at times of great change. The 1994 review, in particular, reaffirmed that the work of the mental health nurse rests fundamentally on their relationship with patients and redirected the role of nurses towards working with people with severe and enduring mental illness.
- We identify two traditions within UK mental health nursing: the interpersonal relations approach (the artists) and the evidence-based practice approach (the scientists). Long represented as in conflict, over the past few years we have witnessed the growth of consensus among practising mental health nurses who recognize the importance of their relationship with service users, but are enthusiastic also to develop the new roles and skills and to apply these in non-traditional 'recovery focused' ways to help service users make the most of their lives.

Question for reflection and discussion

1   Consider the role and responsibilities of mental health nurses today compared with those of their forebears working in mental hospitals in the 1950s and 1960s.

Annotated bibliography

- Nolan, P.A. (1993) *A History of Mental Health Nursing*. London: Chapman & Hall. Probably the most authoritative and comprehensive history of UK mental health nursing yet written.
- *Journal of Psychiatric and Mental Health Nursing*, volumes **5**(3) and **6**(4). These issues are devoted to a consideration of the contribution of Hilda Peplau and Annie Altschul to mental health nursing.
- Peplau, H. (1952) *Interpersonal Relations in Nursing*. New York: G.P. Putman. Peplau was the first to coin the term 'nurse–patient relationship' and her 1952 book was to become a classic. Contemporary ideas about the nurse–patient relationship owe a debt to Peplau's pioneering work. To her supporters Peplau presents an empirically precise theory of nursing that can be verified and developed through further research. To her critics Peplau's theory of nursing, based upon psychodynamic principles, bears little

relation to the work that nurses carry out, contains few operational (empirically testable) definitions and fewer tests of validity. Read Peplau's classic text and judge for yourself.

■ Barker's ideas on the proper focus of mental health nursing are set out in a series of published papers (two of the more important of which are cited below) and also on his The Tidal Model website (http://www.tidalmodel.co.uk).

– Barker, P. (1989) Reflections on the philosophy of caring in mental health. *International Journal of Nursing Studies* **26**(2): 131–41.

– Barker, P.J. (2000) Reflections on a caring as a virtue ethic within an evidence-based culture. *International Journal of Nursing Studies* **37**(4): 329–36.

Follow the debate during the mid-1990s about the proper focus of nursing conducted primarily in a series of commentaries in the *Journal of Psychiatric and Mental Health Nursing*. We list some of the more important contributions below:

– Gournay, K. (1995) What to do with nursing models. *Journal of Psychiatric and Mental Health Nursing* **2**: 352–27.

– Barker, P.J. and Reynolds, B. (1996) Rediscovering the proper focus of nursing: a critique of Gournay's position on nursing theory and models. *Journal of Psychiatric and Mental Health Nursing* **3**: 75–80.

– Rolfe, G. (1996) What to do with psychiatric nursing. *Journal of Psychiatric and Mental Health Nursing* **3**: 331–3.

– Coleman, M. and Jenkins, E. (1998) Developments in mental health nursing: a critical voice. *Journal of Psychiatric and Mental Health Nursing* **5**: 355–9.

– Clarke, L. (1999) *Challenging Ideas in Psychiatric Nursing*. London: Routledge.

– Grant, A. (2001) Psychiatric nursing and organizational power. *Journal of Psychiatric and Mental Health Nursing* **8**: 173–88.

Mental Health Special Issue of the *International Journal of Nursing Studies* 2007; **44**(3). This Special Issue, which is devoted to mental health nursing, includes a number of papers which reflect contemporary mental health nursing practice, including:

– Brooker's Guest Editorial which provides a critique of the Chief Nursing Officer for England's review of mental health nursing (CNOE 2006);

– a paper reporting findings from the national consultation of mental health nurses conducted as part of the review;

– review and discussion papers on: user and carer involvement in training and education of health professionals; interventions delivered by mental health nurses; physical health problems associated with serious mental illness.

References

Altschul, A. (1964) Group dynamics and nursing care. *International Journal of Nursing Studies* **1**: 151–8.

Altschul, A.T. (1972) *Patient–Nurse Interaction: A Study of Interaction Patterns in Acute Psychiatric Wards*. Edinburgh: Churchill Livingstone.

Altschul, A.T. (1999) Editorial. *Journal of Psychiatric and Mental Health Nursing* **6**(4): 261–3.

Barker, P. (1999) Hildegard E. Peplau: the mother of psychiatric nursing: obituary. *Journal of Psychiatric and Mental Health Nursing* **6**: 175–6.

Barker, P. (2003) *The Tidal Model*. http://www.tidalmodel.co.uk

Barton, R. (1959) *Institutional Neurosis*. Bristol: Wright.

Chapman, G. (1992) Nursing in therapeutic communities, in J.I. Brooking, S.A.H. Ritter and B.L. Thomas (eds) *A Textbook of Psychiatric and Mental Health Nursing.* Edinburgh: Churchill Livingstone.

Chief Nursing Officer (England) 2006 *Review of Mental Health Nursing: from values to action.* London: DH.

Connolly, M.J. (1992) History, in J. Brooking, S. Ritter and B. Thomas (eds) *A Textbook of Psychiatric and Mental Health Nursing.* Edinburgh: Churchill Livingstone.

Cormack, D. (1983) *Psychiatric Nursing Described.* Edinburgh: Churchill Livingstone.

Department of Health (DH) (1999) *A National Service Framework for Mental Health.* London: DH.

Department of Health and Social Security (1975) *Better Services for the Mentally Ill.* London: HMSO.

English and Welsh National Boards for Nursing, Midwifery and Health Visiting (1982) *Syllabus of Training: Professional Register – Part 3 Registered Mental Nurse.* London: ENB.

Goffman, E. (1961) *Asylums: Essays on the Social Situation of Mental Patients and Other Inmates.* Harmondsworth: Penguin.

Gournay, K. (1997) Responses to: 'What to do with nursing models' – a reply from Gournay. *Journal of Psychiatric and Mental Health Nursing* **4**: 227–31.

Gournay, K. and Brooking, J. (1994) Community psychiatric nurses in primary healthcare. *British Journal of Psychiatry* **165**: 231–8.

Gray, R., Rance, J. and Robson, D. (2006) *A review of the efficacy of inteventions delivered by mental health nurses.* http://www.nursing.manchester.ac.uk/projects/mentalhealthreview/ (accessed June 2008).

Greenhalgh, T. and Donald, A. (2000) *Evidence Based Health Care Workbook.* London: British Medical Journal Publications.

Hunter, P. (1974) Community psychiatric nursing: a literature review. *International Journal of Nursing Studies* **11**: 223.

Joint Board of Clinical Nursing Studies (1974) *Outline Curriculum in Community Psychiatric Nursing for Registered Nurses.*

Jones, K. (1960) *Mental Health and Social Policy 1945–59.* London: Routledge & Kegan Paul.

Keijsers, G.P.J., and Schaap, D.R., Hoogduin, C.A.L. (2000) The impact of interpersonal patient and therapist behavior on outcome in cognitive-behavior therapy: a review of empirical studies. *Behaviour Modification* **24**(2): 264–97.

Macilwaine, H. (1983) The communication patterns of female neurotic patients with nursing staff in psychiatric units of general hospitals, in J. Wilson-Barnett (ed.) *Nursing Research: Ten Studies in Patient Care.* Chichester: John Wiley and Sons.

May, A.R. and Moore, S. (1963) The mental nurse in the community. *Lancet* **1**: 213–14.

McNamee, G. (1993) A changing profession: the role of nursing in home care, in P. Weller and M. Muijen, *Dimensions of Community Mental Health Care.* London: W.B. Saunders & Co.

Mental Health Nursing Review Team (1994) *Working in Partnership.* London: Department of Health.

NHS and Community Care Act (1990). London: HMSO.

Nolan, P. (1993) *A History of Mental Health Nursing.* London: Chapman & Hall.

Nolan, P. (1999) Annie Altschul's legacy to 20th century British mental health nursing. *Journal of Psychiatric and Mental Health Nursing* **6**(4): 267–72.

Nolan, P. and Hooper, B. (2000) Revisiting mental health nursing in the 1960s. *Journal of Mental Health* **9**(6): 563–74.

Norman, I.J. (1998) Priorities for mental health and learning disability nurse education in the UK: a case study. *Journal of Clinical Nursing* **7**: 433–41.

Norman, I.J. and Humphrey, C. (2008) Evaluation research in R. Watson, H. McKenna, S. Cowman and J. Keady (eds) *Nursing Research: design and methods.* London: Elsevier.

Peplau, H. (1952) *Interpersonal Relations in Nursing.* New York: G.P. Putman.

Peplau, H. (1987) Interpersonal constructs in nursing practice. *Nursing Education Today* **7**: 201–8.

Peplau, H.E. (1994) Psychiatric mental health nursing: challenge and change. *Journal of Psychiatric and Mental Health Nursing* **1**(1): 3–8.

Powell, J.E. (1988) My Years as Health Minister. *The Spectator*, 20 February, pp. 8–10.

Rangachari, P.K. (1997) Evidence-based medicine: old French wine with a new Canadian label. *Journal of the Royal Society of Medicine* **90**: 280–4.

Repper, J. (2000) Adjusting the focus of mental health nursing: incorporating service users' experiences of recovery. *Journal of Mental Health* **9**(6): 575–88.

Rolfe, G. (1996) What to do with psychiatric nursing. *Journal of Psychiatric and Mental Health Nursing* **3**: 331–3.

Sackett, D.L., Straus, S.E., Richardson, W.S., Rosenberg, W. and Haynes, R.B. (2000) *Evidence-based medicine* (2nd edn). Edinburgh: Churchill Livingstone.

Scull, A. (1981) *Madhouses, Mad-doctors and Madmen*. London: Athlone.

Simmons, S. and Brooker, C. (1986) *Community Psychiatric Nursing: A Social Perspective*. London: Heinemann Nursing.

Simmons, S. and Brooker, C. (1990) *Community Psychiatric Nursing: A Social Perspective*. Oxford: Butterworth-Heinemann.

Standing Mental Health and Standing Nursing Advisory Committees (1968) *Psychiatric Nursing Today and Tomorrow*. London: Ministry of Health – Central Health Services Council.

Sullivan, H.S. (1947) *Conceptions of Modern Psychiatry*. Washington, DC: William A. White Psychiatric Foundation.

Towell, D. (1975) *Understanding Psychiatric Nursing: A Sociological Analysis of Modern Psychiatric Nursing Practice*. London: Royal College of Nursing.

Townsend, P. (1962) *The Last Refuge: A Survey of Residential Institutions and Homes for the Aged in England and Wales*. London: Routledge & Kegan Paul.

United Kingdom Central Council for Nursing, Midwifery and Health Visiting (1986) *Project 2000: A New Preparation for Practice*. London: UKCC.

Walk, A. (1961) The history of mental nursing. *Journal of Mental Science* **107**: 466.

White, E. (1990a) The historical development of the educational preparation of CPNs, in C. Brooker (ed.) *Community Psychiatric Nursing: A Research Perspective*. London: Chapman Hall.

White, E. (1990b) *The Third Quinquennial National Survey of Community Psychiatric Nursing*. Manchester, UK: University of Manchester.

Wing, J.K. (1990) The function of asylum. *British Journal of Psychiatry* **157**: 822–7.

CHAPTER 5

Recovery and social inclusion

Rachel Perkins and Julie Repper

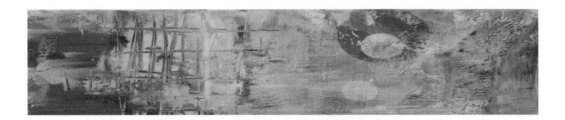

> 66 Recovery refers to the lived or real life experience of people as they accept and overcome the challenge of the disability ... they experience themselves as recovering a new sense of self and of purpose within and beyond the limits of the disability.
>
> (Deegan 1988) 99

> 66 ... a deeply personal, unique process of changing one's attitudes, values, feelings goals, skills, and/or roles. It is a way of living a satisfying, hopeful and contributing life even with the limitations caused by illness. Recovery involves the development of new meaning and purpose in one's life as one grows beyond the catastrophic effects of mental illness.
>
> (Anthony 1993) 99

Chapter overview

Everyone who experiences mental health problems faces the challenge of recovery: the challenge of rebuilding, or, where possible, retaining, a valued and satisfying life. There is no way of going back to the way things were before the difficulties started, but they are not the end of life. Many people who have experienced mental health problems have shown us that there is a way forward: that it is possible to recover meaning and purpose in life. Too often, mental health problems separate a person from the communities that they inhabit. Traditionally this would often have involved physical segregation in remote asylums. With the demise of such institutions, many, perhaps naively, hoped that such social exclusion would be a thing of the past – sadly this was not to be.

> 66   Though a simple aspiration for most people socially isolated by mental
>   illness, the sense of belonging to a community with all that this can imply for
>   mutuality and participation remains stubbornly illusive in spite of community
>   care.
>
>   (Morris 2001)   99

The prejudice and discrimination that constructed the walls of the asylums continue to form
as big a barrier to participation in community life. This social exclusion severely impedes
recovery: it is not possible to rebuild a satisfying and valued life if everywhere you turn you
are debarred from those roles, relationships and activities that give your life meaning.

Traditionally, the primary aim of mental health services and practitioners, has been 'cure':
interventions designed to change the individual so that they 'fit in' by reducing their
symptoms and the attendant deficits and dysfunctions. The success of mental health services
has been judged in terms of the extent to which they have been able to do this and so
discharge people from their care.

Yet symptom reduction is neither a necessary, nor a sufficient condition for recovery.

> 66   One of the biggest lessons I have had to accept is that recovery is not the
>   same thing as being cured. After 21 years of living with this thing it still
>   hasn't gone away.
>
>   (Deegan 1993)   99

For some people, symptoms may continue or recur from time to time but this does not
preclude the possibility of them recovering a meaningful and valued life. Recovery and
inclusion are not contingent on the removal of symptoms, but they do require that we move
beyond changing the individual to changing the world in which they live: increasing the
capacity of communities to accommodate people with mental health problems by providing
the support and adjustments that they need to do the things they want to do.

Nor does the elimination of symptoms guarantee recovery. Prejudice and discrimination
extend beyond the presence of symptoms. People may be excluded because of a history of
such problems – 'once a schizophrenic always a schizophrenic'. While treatments to reduce
distressing and debilitating symptoms are important, they are only a small part of a person's
recovery journey. Rebuilding a meaningful and valued life requires more than the treatment
of symptoms.

Recovery does not mean that all symptoms have been removed, or that functioning has
been fully restored. Instead, it is about reducing the extent to which any remaining symptoms
or problems interfere with the person's efforts to pursue their interests and goals. Recovery
requires that we move beyond 'cure' to thinking about how we can help people to make the
most of their lives. If we are to do this then we must put the individual at centre stage: think
not about 'the patient in our services' but instead about 'the person in their life' and the
impact – for good or ill – that services have on their journey through this life.

In this chapter we will:

- describe the challenge facing people with mental health problems;
- discuss the principles of recovery and social inclusion;
- explore ways in which mental health practitioners can facilitate the individual's recovery
  journey and promote their inclusion and participation in community life.

The impact of mental health problems

Mental health practitioners are accustomed to thinking about the experience of people with mental health problems in terms of their need for different types of interventions and services: medication, inpatient care, outreach services, psychosocial interventions, sheltered accommodation, occupational therapy, medication. This is not the best place to start. We cannot provide appropriate supports and interventions unless we understand the nature of the challenge that they face and what gives their life meaning and value. Only then is it possible to consider how we might help them in their individual journey of recovery.

Having mental health problems is a devastating and life changing experience.

> " When I was diagnosed I felt this is the end of my life. It was a thing to isolate me from other human beings. I felt I was not viable…I felt flawed. Defective.
>
> (cited in Sayce 2000) "

You have to cope with strange and often frightening experiences. Perhaps you find yourself unable to think properly. Perhaps those ordinary, everyday things that you always did without thinking seem impossibly difficult. Perhaps you have experiences that no-one around you believes or understands.

Your confidence and belief in yourself hit rock bottom. You feel very, very alone and very, very frightened. Not only about what is happening to you, but also about the prospect of using mental health services. Everyone knows what it is like to go to their general practitioner or enter a general hospital (whether as patient or visitor). But for most people, psychiatric services remain sinister places cloaked in mystery: images of 'Bedlam' abound.

> " All I knew were the stereotypes I had seen on television or in the movies. To me, mental illness meant Dr Jekyll and Mr Hyde, psychopathic serial killers, loony bins, morons, schizos, fruitcakes, nuts, straightjackets, and raving lunatics. They were all I knew about mental illness and what terrified me was that professionals were saying I was one of them.
>
> (Deegan 1993) "

You are surrounded by people who think you will never amount to very much – views that are too often reinforced by the negative attitudes and prognoses of professionals: 'You have a chronic illness', 'You will not be able to work, have children, live independently …'.

Unthinkable things may happen to you – like being picked up by the police, detained against your will, forcibly medicated – all of which reinforce the frightening stereotypes of madness. And on top of all this, you experience the prejudice and discrimination that, in our society, go hand in hand with mental health problems.

People start treating you differently: as if you are stupid, or dangerous, or both. They start talking about you, rather than to you: 'Is she all right? Is she taking her tablets?'. They behave towards you as if they are walking on eggshells, fearful lest you dissolve into tears or explode into anger.

You risk losing everything that matters to you: your job, college place, friends, even your home and family.

6 6   Out of the blue your job has gone, with it any financial security you may
have had. At a stroke, you have no purpose in life, and no contact with other
people. You find yourself totally isolated from the rest of the world. No-one
telephones you. Much less writes. No-one seems to care if you're alive or
dead.

(cited in Bird 2001)   9 9

Mental health services are replete with people who have lost all that they value in life. And
people with serious mental health problems are at greater risk of losing their lives, both
through suicide and at the hands of heart disease, respiratory disease, stroke, hypertension,
diabetes, bowel cancer, breast cancer and diseases like coronary heart disease. They contract
them earlier and die of them faster resulting in a life expectancy some ten years less than
that of people without mental health problems (Disability Rights Commission 2006).

Too often people are left feeling disconnected from themselves, from friends and family,
from the communities in which they live, and from meaning and purpose in life. For some,
the identity of 'mental patient' eclipses all other facets of personhood and it is all too easy to
lose hope – abandon any belief in the possibility of a positive future – and give up. For
others the prospect of being a 'mental patient' may be so terrifying that the person rejects
any idea that such a label could conceivably apply to them and rejects any help from mental
health services.

For those who experience additional prejudice and discrimination – like those from
minority ethnic communities (including gypsies and travellers), people with physical
impairments or learning difficulties, older people, lesbians/gay men, people from religious
minorities – the exclusion resulting from mental health problems is magnified.

Anyone who experiences a catastrophe in their life – whether it be mental health
problems, the death of someone we love, unemployment or the end of a relationship –
experiences a range of emotions (Kubler-Ross 1969; O'Donoghue 1994). These may include:

- *Denial.* 'It must be a mistake', 'It's not happening to me', 'Everything will be back to
  normal soon'.
- *Anger.* 'Why me?', 'It's not fair'.
- *Grief.* 'My life is over', 'Everything is hopeless'.
- *Shame.* 'Of dear, I hope no-one finds out'.
- *Isolation.* 'Now no one will want to have anything to do with me.'
- *Terror.* 'Now what will happen to me?'

To be diagnosed as having serious mental health problems is a bereavement: it involves loss
of the privileges of sanity; loss of the life the person had or expected to lead; loss of the
person we thought we were or might become. Too often, when practitioners focus solely on
symptoms and cures, such ordinary bereavement responses are seen as pathological –
symptoms of the illness itself. Denial becomes the 'lack of insight' supposedly inherent in the
disorder. Hopelessness, apathy and withdrawal become the 'negative symptoms' and 'lack of
motivation' that are assumed to characterize the 'illness'. Anger becomes a 'symptom' to be
treated or the 'acting out' that may be taken to indicate additional 'personality problems'.

> 66 This has left many people with mental illness feeling devalued and ignored and has resulted in mistrust and alienation from the mental health system.
>
> (Spaniol *et al.* 1997) 99

If we pathologize the ordinary bereavement responses to the multi-faceted catastrophe of mental health problems we risk impeding recovery by alienating people from those very services that are supposed to assist them in their recovery journey.

Principles of recovery and inclusion

People with mental health problems may benefit from a wide range of support and treatment – the critical question is how these enable (or prevent) the person to pursue their ambitions and make the most of their life. In this context the principles and values of services and the aims of interventions are critically important. Recovery is about people's whole lives – not just their symptoms. There are a variety of different ways in which people may gain relief from distressing symptoms: these include medication, psychological therapy, self-help and self-management to enable the person to manage their difficulties themselves, and a range of complementary therapies. However, people's problems extend well beyond the expertise traditionally found within mental health services. Rarely is it a person's ambition in life merely to get rid of distressing and disabling symptoms – they want to do this in order to do the things they want to do and live the lives they wish to lead. This is what recovery is about: enabling people to have the homes, jobs and friends that give everyone's life meaning and via which we get our sense of value. Enabling people to access accommodation, material resources, employment, education, relationships, social and leisure activities is at least, if not more, important in the recovery process as reducing the mental health problems themselves.

It should not be expected that a single practitioner or agency can provide the full range of interventions, supports and assistance that a person needs. First, it is highly unlikely that a single worker/provider can simultaneously be an expert in: welfare benefits; vocational rehabilitation and liaising with employers; individual psychological therapy and family interventions; the impact of various drug treatments; and putting together MFI furniture or making a washing machine work. Second, everyone needs the opportunity to be different people in different relationships and situations. We may be competent at work, delinquent with our friends, inadequate and needy with our nearest and dearest. In a single relationship with a 'key worker' or 'care coordinator' it is not possible for someone to simultaneously address their fears and problems, use/extend their skills and abilities, and achieve the social relationships on which most people rely so heavily for mutual support in their day-to-day lives. However, if a person is receiving help and support from a range of different individuals and agencies – various clinicians, housing and employment workers, friends, family, religious communities, welfare benefits advisors – then effective coordination is required in order to ensure that the person gets all the assistance they need.

Therefore, if they are to facilitate recovery, services need to:

■ *Focus on helping people to do the things that they wish to do in life.* The reduction of symptoms may be a means to this end but it is not an end in itself.

■ *Adopt a team and multi-agency approach.* If responsibility for the provision of all support rests with a single individual or service then the provision of effective support/intervention across diverse domains is jeopardized. It is important where possible to enable people to access mainstream sources of support (like Job Centres, General Practitioners, Citizens Advice Bureaux) where the real expertise lies rather than providing separate segregated services.

■ *Ensure continuity across providers.* If people receive input from multiple agencies and individuals then these must work effectively together.

■ *Foster relationships outside services.* It is the reciprocal relationships with friends, family, neighbours, colleagues (relationships where people can give as well as receive) rather than the one way relationships with mental health practitioners and agencies (where the individual is always on the receiving end of help) that foster self-worth and provide meaning in people's lives.

Recovery is about growth

It is very easy for people with mental health problems to become nothing other than their illness, ceasing to be Fred and becoming 'a schizophrenic' or 'a manic depressive'.

> 66 Schizophrenia is an 'I am' illness, one which may take over and redefine the identity of a person.
>
> (Estroff 1989) 99

If practitioners focus only on deficits and dysfunctions then the identity of 'mental patient', at the expense of all other facets of personhood, is reinforced. People are always more than their 'illness'. Recovery involves redefining identity in a way which includes these difficulties, but enables them to grow, develop and move beyond them.

However, growth is often limited not by characteristics of the person, but by the barriers imposed by discrimination and exclusion.

> 66 My recovery was about how to gain other people's confidence in my abilities and potential ... in my own experience the toughest part was changing other people's expectations of what I could do. Combating a disempowering sense of being undervalued ...
>
> (May 1999) 99

The traditional focus of services is helping the individual to change: reducing their symptoms, helping them to develop new skills, helping them to adjust to what has happened. These may all be important in facilitating recovery, but it is critical that practitioners also attend to reducing the external barriers that they face – increasing the capacity of communities, services and institutions outside the mental health system to accommodate people with mental health problems. Growth is not possible if you are prevented from doing the things you want to do and excluded within the community in which you live.

The mental health world has a lot to learn from the physical disability world. When we think about a person with a broken spine or limited hearing thoughts do not focus on treatment alone. Instead we think about:

■ supports that the person might need – like wheelchairs and personal assistants – to enable them to do the things they do;

■ adjustments in the environment that facilitate access – like ramps and induction loops;

■ changing the attitudes and skills of others in the community in order to remove 'them and us' barriers and enable people to participate as equal citizens.

The challenge for people with mental health problems, and the mental health practitioners who assist them, is to find the psychiatric equivalents of the wheelchair, the induction loop and the disability awareness training. We need to identify the supports and adjustments that the individual might need, and the support and adjustments that others in the community might require if people with mental health problems are to participate fully in community life.

Therefore, if they are to facilitate recovery, services need to:

■ *Focus on a person's strengths and possibilities.* It is a person's abilities, interests, aspirations and assets that constitute the foundations of their recovery: lives cannot be rebuilt on deficits and dysfunctions.

■ *Focus on changing the environment, not simply changing individuals.* A person's ability to access the things they want to do depends on the dynamic interaction between that person, their environment and others who inhabit their world. Changing the environment and providing support is at least, if not more, important as changing the individual to 'fit in'.

Recovery is not an end product or result but an ongoing journey

   ❝ Recovery is a process, not an end point or destination. Recovery is an attitude, a way of approaching the day and the challenges I face. ... I know I have certain limitations and things I can't do. But rather than letting these limitations be occasions for despair and giving up, I have learned that in knowing what I can't do, I also open up the possibilities of all I can do.

(Deegan 1993) ❞

People cannot be 'fixed' as one might mend a television or refurbish a building. If recovery is a continuing journey, then assistance and adjustments often need to be thought of as a continuing process of supporting people in that journey. And this must involve not only helping the person to move forward, but also helping them to maintain what has already achieved. The original work on 'assertive outreach' of Stein and Test (1980) demonstrated that people do not simply require 'training in community living' but ongoing support to sustain their community tenure and the lives they have built for themselves. Likewise, there is now a wealth of evidence which demonstrates that people with mental health problems can be successful in open employment if they are provided not only with help to get work, but also ongoing, time-unlimited support, to sustain their employment (Bond *et al.* 1997, 2001; Crowther *et al.* 2001).

The critical yardstick of success is not whether the person can be discharged and function unaided – this may or may not be possible or desirable – but what they are able to achieve in their life in the presence of support. To again take a parallel with physical impairment the efficacy of, for example, a wheelchair or an induction loop, would never be judged in terms of the extent to which it enabled a person to walk or hear without these aids, but in terms of what it enables the person using it to do.

It is also important to accept that recovery will not be a linear process – there will be problems and set-backs along the way.

> 66 The recovery process is ... a series of small beginnings and very small steps. At times our course is erratic and we falter, slide back, re-group and start again ...
>
> (Deegan 1988) 99

Relapse is not 'failure', but a part of the recovery process – a learning opportunity that can enable a person to move beyond their limitations by identifying the additional support and adjustments that they, or the people around them, may need to successfully pursue their ambitions. However, if a person is not to become dispirited – give up – they need people around them who can 'hold on to hope': believe in them and their possibilities, during those times when they are not able to believe in their own worth and future.

Therefore, if they are to facilitate recovery, services need to:

- *Focus on maintaining, as well as optimizing a person's possibilities.* For some people, problems and symptoms are time limited, but for many they are not. Throughput models are inappropriate in the context of ongoing or recurring problems. The efficacy of an intervention/support should be judged in terms of what it enables a person to achieve, not whether it enables the person to be discharged from the service.
- Adopt a long-term perspective. If recovery is an ongoing process then people may require continuity help and support, and over long periods of time.
- *Offer continuity of support over time.* If support over longer periods of time is to be effective, then it cannot be subject to the presence of a single member of staff. It is inevitable that practitioners will go on holiday, take sick leave, and move on to other jobs. In order to reduce the disruption and discontinuities to which this can lead, it is preferable if people know and trust a number of different team members, so that when one person leaves, some continuity can be preserved. A team approach does not mean that individual relationships are unimportant, merely that everyone needs several such relationships.
- *Accept set-backs and relapse as part of the recovery process.* Practitioners must be willing to help people to persevere. We cannot help a person unless we can continue to believe in their possibilities even when everything seems to be going wrong.

Recovery is not dependent on professional intervention

Recovery is not a professional intervention to which expert professionals hold the key (Anthony 1993). It is an individual journey in which the person's own resources and those available to them outside the mental health system are central. The sources of meaning and satisfaction in most people's lives do not lie within mental health services – they lie in our work, our homes, our relationships, our leisure pursuits, our religion or spiritual beliefs. If people are unable to access the range of ordinary opportunities that other citizens usually take for granted then it is unlikely that they will be able to rebuild lives that they find satisfying and meaningful.

The expertise of experience can also be important. Many people have described the enormous support they have received from others who have faced a similar challenge (May 1999).

> 66 ... the gift that people with disabilities can give each other ... hope, strength and experience as lived through the recovery process ... a person does not have to be 'fully recovered' to serve as a role model. Very often a person who is only a few 'steps' ahead of another person can be more effective than one whose achievements seem overly impressive and distanced.
>
> (Deegan 1988) 99

This may be achieved via self-help groups and user/survivor organizations or more informal friendships and networks within which people can share experiences and support each other's journeys.

Therefore, if they are to facilitate recovery, services need to:

- *Emphasize social integration and re-integration.* Enable people to access and maintain those ordinary relationships, roles, activities and social supports that they value and which provide meaning in their lives.
- *Maximize opportunities for people with mental health problems to support and learn from each other.* People who have 'been there themselves' can often provide enormous encouragement, support or role models to others who face similar challenges.
- Successfully involve service users and their relatives/friends. Tapping the expertise of experience at all levels – individual care planning; the monitoring and operation of individual services; service planning and development – is essential to the development of effective, accessible and acceptable services.

A recovery vision is not limited to a particular theory about the nature and origins of mental health problems

Just as professionals have developed a range of different organic, psychological and interpersonal models for understanding mental distress, so people who have experienced these difficulties understand their difficulties in different ways. Based on the narratives of 30 people with serious mental health problems, Jacobson (1993) identified six frameworks that people have used to understand their difficulties: biological; interaction of biology and environment; abuse or trauma; spiritual or philosophical; political; and the dehumanizing impact of long-term contact with mental health services.

As Anthony (1993) points out, a recovery vision does not commit one to a particular understanding of distress and disability. People need ways of understanding what has happened to them ('Why me?' 'What is the point in my life now?') but whether they choose genes, inter or intra personal problems or the action of various deities, recovery – rebuilding a meaningful and satisfying life is equally important. The critical issue is not veracity of a model or explanation but the extent to which it:

- makes sense to the person: any number of randomized controlled trials are unlikely to persuade a deeply religious person that their lives are wholly determined by their biology;
- enables them to move forward in their life: genetic explanations, for example, may impede growth if characteristics are seen as fixed and immutable; explanations revolving around abuse and trauma preclude the possibility of growth if they are considered to

have done irreparable damage. However, both genetic and traumatic explanations can facilitate growth if they are seen as something over which the person can exercise control or influence and modifiable by social and environmental circumstances.

If mental health practitioners insist that people adopt a single understanding of their difficulties then they are likely to alienate those who prefer alternative explanations.

Therefore, if they are to facilitate recovery, services need to:

- Place the individual at centre stage. If services are to be successful in providing the help that people need, rather than driving them away, their perspectives, wishes and constructions of reality must be heeded.

Everyone's recovery journey is different and deeply personal

There are no rules of recovery, no formula for success.

> Everyone's journey of recovery is unique. Each of us must find our own way and no-one can do it for us.
>
> (Deegan 1993)

> Once recovery becomes systematised, you've got it wrong. Once it is reduced to a set of principles it is wrong. It is a unique and individualised process.
>
> (Deegan 1999)

It is easy for the destructive rigid routines and block treatment of old psychiatric hospitals to spill over into community services (Barton 1959; Goffman 1963; Brown *et al.* 1966; King *et al.* 1971; Ryan 1979).

- There remain community services where a set of rules dictate how people must use them: you cannot have lunch at the day centre unless you attend a group; in order to live in the hostel you have to cook a meal for all residents once a week and attend the community group each day. If a person needs a hot meal it is a waste of their time and scarce resources to insist that they attend a group as well and just how does cooking a meal for eight people train you to cook for yourself at home?
- The 'ladder' models adopted by some services insist that people start at point A and then move in an orderly fashion to point Z: you must start in the rehabilitation ward, and then show that you can manage in a staffed hostel before you can have a flat of your own. It is entirely possible for someone to move directly from hospital to independent accommodation, or be sustained in their own place during a crisis – is this not what home treatment and assertive outreach services are designed to achieve?
- The often implicit assumption that there exists a hierarchy of skills in which you can only move on to more 'advanced' endeavours when you have mastered 'basic' ones: you must be able to wash your socks before you can go to work. Yet it is entirely possible for a person to need help in many aspects of daily life and still hold down a responsible job: how many high flying executives do their own cleaning and cooking?

Such rules inevitably mean that services cannot be tailored to the individual needs and aspirations of the people who use them. Not only is this likely to impede recovery, it is also likely either to de-skill people – prevent them from using their skills/abilities to the full – or alienate them by offering support in a manner that they find unacceptable and infantilizing.

Therefore, if they are to facilitate recovery, services need to:

■ Adopt an individualized approach to assessment and support. People with serious mental health problems are a diverse group and require diverse types of help and support to achieve a range of different goals.

■ Ensure that services respond flexibly to individual needs and wishes. Inflexible 'rules of engagement' and 'block treatment' are not only destructive, they are also ineffective in helping people to rebuild their lives and risk excluding those who cannot, or do not wish to, accede to the regime.

Recovery is possible for everyone

Recovery is not only for those who are more able. It is not contingent on the removal of symptoms or the development of skills. Some people will remain profoundly disabled but with the right kind of support they can find sources of value and meaning in order to move forward in their lives. Some people deny their need for services and reject professional help but they can still achieve the support and encouragement they need to pursue their ambitions outside specialist services: among those friends, family members, and agencies that exist to help all citizens. The critical issue then becomes not whether the individual has appropriate support from mental health practitioners but whether friends, family and community agencies receive the help they need to accommodate the person with mental health difficulties.

It is easy for services to drift 'up market' and focus on those for whom they believe that greatest progress can be made at the expense of those who are more disabled and less willing to accept what is on offer.

Therefore, if they are to facilitate recovery for all, services need to:

■ *Help everyone to identify and make the most of their abilities.* This is especially important when assets and skills are overshadowed by their problems and impairments.

■ *Identify the types and sources of support that are acceptable to the individual.* While evidence-based practice is important, if a person is not willing to accept it can do them no good. Negotiation and compromise on the part of mental health practitioners is critical, as is seeking sources of assistance outside the mental health arena for those who do not think they need such services and do not wish to be associated with them.

Promoting recovery, facilitating inclusion

Promoting recovery and facilitating inclusion requires not only a major change in the guiding philosophy of services – moving away from a focus on minimizing symptoms and reducing dysfunctions towards a focus on enabling people to do the things they want to do and live the lives they want to lead – but also a change in the approach and skills of mental health practitioners. And we must look to the expertise of personal experience for guidance – what people who are recovering from mental health problems have found helpful in their journey.

A brief glance at the accounts of people who have faced the challenge of recovery demonstrates the unique and individual nature of their journeys (see, for example, Leete 1988, 1989; Deegan 1988, 1993, 1996; Spaniol and Koehler 1994; May 1999; Vincent 1999 and Young and Ensing 1999). However, these authors have identified a number of common features that seem to be critically important in the recovery process: hope; relationships; coping with loss; spirituality, philosophy and understanding; taking back control; finding meaning, purpose and opportunity. It is also clear that these do not constitute a recipe for, or set of pre-determined stages of, recovery. They are intimately interlinked and follow no set sequence. For example, some people cannot regain hope, or address what has happened to them, until they have the opportunity to do things they value. Others need to regain a sense of possibility before they are able to think about embarking on the re-building process.

If mental health practitioners are really to support people in their recovery journey then three inter-related components are central: fostering hope and creating hope inspiring relationships, facilitating personal adaptation, and promoting access and inclusion (see Figure 5.1).

Maintaining and fostering hope

Hope has been described as the 'anchor stabilizing our lives in the present and giving life meaning, direction and optimism' (Lindsay 1976). It is critical in recovery and central to the lives of most people (Stotland 1969; Lindsay 1976) – without hope there is no reason to carry on.

There is a considerable body of research into the importance of hope in coping with physical illness (e.g. Hickey 1986). In the mental health arena, hope has long been recognized as key to successful psychotherapy (Menninger 1959; Frank 1968); there is a link between hopelessness and suicide (Drake and Cotton 1986; Beck *et al.* 1990); and the importance of practitioners' hopefulness has been emphasized as central in rehabilitation (Anthony 1993; Woodside *et al.* 1994; Kanwal 1997). Hope may be a generalized sense of some future positive development or related to a specific, valued outcome (like getting a job or getting married) (Dufault and Martocchio 1985).

For people with mental health problems, hope lies at the heart of a person's willingness to take on the challenge of recovery and rebuilding: without hope there is no point. In the face of the prejudice and exclusion that many people with mental health problems have experienced it is very easy to lose hope. And if a person can see no possibility of a positive future then it is all too easy for them to give up trying to do anything at all (Lovejoy 1982; Deegan 1988, 1993, 1996).

But hope does not, and cannot, exist in a vacuum – relationships are central. If everyone around you believes that you have little to offer – that you will never amount to anything very much – then it is difficult (if not impossible) to retain a belief in your own worth. Everyone needs people around who believe in your possibilities. Relationships are important not only as a source of help and support: always to be on the receiving end of support and help from others is a devaluing experience. Giving is as important as receiving and reciprocity in relationships is critical. Relationships in which people can contribute to the well-being of others – help and support them – are an important source of value.

Facilitating personal adaptation
"Over the years I've worked hard to become an expert in my own self care... I've learned different ways of helping myself."
(Deegan 1993)

- Offering a range of acceptable and accessible treatments to reduce distressing and disabling symptoms as much as possible
- Helping people to take control of their own problems and the help they receive
- Enabling people to reach an understanding of what has happened that makes sense to them and allows the possibility of moving forward in life
- Fostering self-belief and mobilising personal resources
- Fostering and promoting peer support and relationships with others who have experienced mental health problems

Promoting access **and inclusion**
"I don't want a CPN, I want a life."
(Rose 2001)

- Facilitating access to material resources (like money, food, housing, transport etc.)
- Helping people to access those roles, activities and resources that other citizens take for granted
- Enabling people to identify and articulate their dreams and aspirations
- Supporting people to maintain valued roles and activities that they value and establish new ones that are in line with their ambitions
- Enabling people to access mainstream sources of support and help wherever possible
- Supporting individuals and agencies outside mental health services (like primary care, employers, colleges, housing authorities, churches ...) to enable them to accommodate people with mental health problems

Fostering hope and hope inspiring relationships
"For those of us who have been diagnosed with mental illness and who have lived in sometimes desolate wastelands of mental health programmes, hope is not just a nice sounding euphemism. It is a matter of life and death." (Deegan 1988)

- Creating hope inspiring relationships with those whom we serve:
  ○ Valuing people for who they are
  ○ Believing in the people's worth
  ○ Having confidence in people's abilities and potential
  ○ Listening to and heeding what they say
  ○ Believing in the authenticity of their experiences rather than dismissing them as merely symptoms
  ○ Accepting and actively exploring their experiences
  ○ Tolerating uncertainty about the future
  ○ Seeing problems and set-backs as part of the recovery process
- Fostering and supporting reciprocal relationships with family, friends, peers, partners and others who are important to the person

Figure 5.1 Promoting recovery, facilitating inclusion

The contribution of people with serious mental health problems often goes unrecognized: family and friends become 'carers' who provide the support and help that people need to survive. Rarely do we recognize the support and help that people with mental health problems offer to those around them – both others with mental health problems and friends, and family outside mental health services. Greenberg *et al.* (1994) have shown that people with a diagnosis of schizophrenia can and do contribute a great deal of practical, social and emotional support to other members of their families. If hope is to be fostered, then we must move beyond ideas about 'carers' and those who are 'cared for' – reciprocal relationships with friends and family in which people support each other are critical to the restoration of hope and self-worth.

This does not mean that relationships with mental health practitioners are unimportant – they can be powerful for good or ill and too many people have described the ways in which contact with such services, and interactions with mental health practitioners, have left them feeling discouraged and dispirited (see Deegan 1990). Both first impressions and ongoing relationships are critical.

The way in which we welcome, or fail to welcome, people when they first arrive in services can either enhance or severely jeopardize the whole experience of services. If no-one explains what will happen, if you are left waiting around, if no-one sits down and reassures you, listens to what has happened, shares your distress, then it is easy to give up hope – both for your own future and the ability of services to assist you. Perhaps we should take a leaf out of the book of hotels and health spas: welcoming customers, making them comfortable, offering refreshments, listening to their problems, asking about our wishes and needs, explaining the services on offer. When the NHS was established a sense of altruism was prominent. Health providers were doing a favour to those who could not afford private care: they should accept that which they were given and be grateful for it! However, ensuing decades have increased expectations and government policy of whatever hue is progressively increasing the choice available to users of public services. In such a climate the jobs of mental health practitioners may well come to depend on the care we offer our customers just as much as those of the staff in hotels and spas.

First impressions also include the way in which mental health problems are presented to the person when they are first diagnosed. Too often this is done in a rather cursory manner – simply telling the person what their diagnosis is – without considering the emotional impact that this will have. As one young woman said to us 'The staff are all very nice, but they don't seem to understand what a big thing this schizophrenia is to me.' People need to have the opportunity to process their diagnosis at both a cognitive and emotional level, but the way in which their problems are presented has a huge impact on the way in which a person deals with them. It is important that a diagnosis of mental health problems is accompanied by both time to talk and ask questions as well as reassurance that recovery is possible, that people can live a decent life with such difficulties rather than a list of symptoms, deficits and the problems likely to ensue.

Russinova (1999) has described a number of practitioner 'relationship skills' that are important in developing effective, ongoing hope-inspiring relationships that can enable people to gain the confidence and self-belief that are critical if they are to rebuild their lives and access the opportunities that they value:

- believing in the person's potential and strength;
- valuing the person as a unique human being;
- accepting the person for who he/she is;
- listening non-judgementally to the person's experiences;
- tolerating the uncertainty about the future developments in the person's life;

■ accepting the person's decompensations and failures as part of the recovery process;
■ tolerating the person's challenges and defeats;
■ trusting the authenticity of the person's experiences;
■ expressing a genuine concern for the person's well-being;
■ using humour appropriately.

This list may sound simple and self-evident, but we should never underestimate how difficult it is to deliver. Most people do not want to need our services and many are too distressed and/or disturbed when they arrive with us to be grateful. Valuing a person, being non-judgemental, expressing genuine concern for their well-being can be hard if someone is angry and abusive or rejects what you offer them, yet these are the core skills of any mental health worker.

But relationships between mental health practitioners and those whom they serve can never be genuinely reciprocal. Workers are paid to be there, have a professional obligation to behave in a certain way, and will move on when it suits them to do so. It is dispiriting to have only relationships with people who are paid to be there, yet as many as 40 per cent of people in community rehabilitation teams have been found to have no contacts other than those with mental health workers (Ford *et al.* 1994). The success of a practitioner/client relationship might best be judged in terms of the extent to which it helps people to maintain and regain those relationships with others – like family, friends, colleagues, other in the community – within which we all derive our sense of value and identity.

Taking back control

Mental health problems are often presented and perceived as uncontrollable – the province of experts. If a person is to take back control over their life they need to both develop ways of understanding and accommodating what has happened to them and ways of taking control over their symptoms and problems, the help they receive and their life and well-being more generally.

As we have already described, the experience of mental health problems constitutes a bereavement: multiple losses that appear to be beyond your control and profoundly change the way you see yourself, your world and your future. In the process of recovery – rebuilding their life and sense of self – people face the task of accommodating what has happened so that they can move on (Perkins and Repper 1996; Repper and Perkins 2002).

■ *Grieving that which has been lost.* People need space and time to grieve, to tell their stories – and to tell them over and over again if necessary: new issues, meaning and understanding can emerge with each telling. In reclaiming a sense of identity and value in the present, it is often necessary for a person to talk of identities and valued roles of the past. And expressing at least some of the anger, fear, despair, resentment, shame that they may feel over what has happened. Sometimes anger and resentment may be directed towards the practitioner and the advantages that they have: we may not feel privileged, but in comparison with many of those with whom we work, we are very fortunate. The process of grieving may be slow. It is difficult to live with mental health problems and there may be little we can do to substantially change the material realities of the person's situation. But we can share the person's burden: understand and accept their distress, help them to feel less alone. An initial sense of profound isolation – being totally alone – is one described by most people who have received a diagnosis of serious mental health problems. And for some this sense of isolation can be ongoing. If people are to feel less alone, contact with others who have shared similar experiences can be extremely important.

■ *Information.* Many of the popular myths and misconceptions that surround mental health problems are inevitably shared by those who experience them, and are regularly reinforced in the popular media. These make the experience even more frightening. Many of those who deny that they have such difficulties do so in order to reject the images of themselves as dangerous and incompetent. It is important that practitioners make active efforts to dispel such myths and in doing this the personal accounts of people who have succeeded in rebuilding their lives can be powerful. There are a number of anthologies in which these can be found (see, for example, Spaniol and Koehler 1994; Read and Reynolds 1996; Simpson 2004) and papers in journals such as *Open Mind* and *Schizophrenia Bulletin* (see, for example, Leete 1989). Information about the many successful people – great painters like Van Gogh, scientists like Einstein, writers like James Joyce, politicians like Churchill – who have had mental health problems can also be useful (see, for example, Jamison 1993, 1995; Post 1994, 1996). It may be helpful to acknowledge that things can be more difficult for people who have serious mental health problems (not only because of the difficulties themselves, but also because of the prejudice and discrimination that exists) but it is not impossible with the right kind of opportunities, help and support.

■ *Understanding what has happened.* As we have already discussed, people need to find a way of understanding what has happened that makes sense to them and allows them a way forward. The experience of serious mental health problems often prompts people to explore broader spiritual and philosophical issues concerning the meaning of their lives: 'Why me?' 'What did I do to deserve this?' 'What's the point?' Without prescribing particular religious and philosophical frameworks, it is important that practitioners enable people to think about these issues as well.

Specialized treatment from professionals – psychological, pharmacological, systemic – can help to control a person's distressing and disturbing symptoms. But if a person is to rebuild their life then it is important that they are able to take back control over both their problems and well-being.

> ❝ To me, recovery means I try to stay in the driver's seat of my life. I don't let my illness run me. Over the years I have worked hard to become an expert in my own self-care. For me, being in recovery means I don't just take medications. Just taking medications is a passive stance. Rather I use medications as part of my recovery process. In the same way, I don't just go into hospital. Just 'going into hospital' is a passive stance. Rather, I use the hospital when I need to.
>
> (Deegan 1989) ❞

There is now a considerable body of knowledge that demonstrates people can develop ways of taking control over the cognitive and emotional difficulties that characterize their mental health problems. People can recognize the early signs of impending problems and take remedial action to avert or minimize a crisis (Breier and Strauss 1983; McCandless-Glincher et al.; Kumar et al. 1989; Mueser et al. 1992; Birchwood et al. 1998; Repper 2000). A number of interventions have been developed to assist people in managing their own symptoms and crises (see, for example, Chadwick et al. 1996; Nelson 1997; Birchwood et al.; Kingdon 1998).

Self-management lies at the heart of the Department of Health 'Expert Patients Programme' (DH 2007). This is a lay-led self-management programme designed to support people living with long-term health conditions such as heart disease, stroke, diabetes and mental illness to increase their confidence, improve their quality of life and better manage their condition.

People who have themselves had experience of dealing with a range of mental health problems have developed a range of different ways of dealing with these (see, for example, the self-management training developed by the Bipolar Organization – formerly the Manic Depression fellowship – www.mdf.org.uk – and Rethink – formerly the National Schizophrenia Fellowship – www.rethink.org.uk). Many of these initiatives are based on the Wellness and Recovery Action Plan (WRAP) developed by Mary Ellen Copeland (1997). WRAP is not a care plan developed by professionals. It is

> ❝ ... a self-management and recovery system developed by a group of people who had mental health difficulties and who were struggling to incorporate wellness tools and strategies into their lives. ❞

WRAP is designed to:

- decrease and prevent intrusive or troubling feelings and behaviours;
- increase personal empowerment;
- improve quality of life;
- assist people in achieving their own life goals and dreams.

WRAP is a structured system to monitor uncomfortable and distressing symptoms and help you reduce, modify or eliminate those symptoms by using planned responses. This includes plans for how you want others to respond when symptoms have made it impossible for you to continue to make decisions, take care of yourself, or keep yourself safe.[16]

It incorporates:

- A daily management plan describing how you feel when you are well and identifies those things you need to do to stay well.
  The identification of
    - triggers: those events and situations that may lead to the onset of uncomfortable symptoms and what you find helpful to do when these occur.
    - early warning signs: the often subtle indications that indicate things are beginning to worsen and what to do when you notice these.
    - symptoms that occur when things have got worse but not yet reached crisis point, and what you can do themselves if these happen.

- A crisis plan that identifies those symptoms that indicate to you that you are no longer able to take make decisions for yourself and keep yourself safe. This tells supporters and health care professionals what you think they should do on your behalf.

- A post-crisis plan describing what you find helpful in working your way out of a crisis and resuming your day-to-day life.

---

[16] www.mentalhealthrecovery.com

Traditional treatments may be one component of the way in which a person can take control over distressing and disturbing symptoms but this might also include self-help, support from friends, and a range of strategies that the person has developed for dealing with particular problems.

> Over the years I have learned different ways of helping myself. Sometimes I use medications, therapy, self-help and mutual support groups, friends, my relationship with God, work, exercise, spending time in nature – all of these measures help me remain whole and healthy, even though I have a disability.
>
> (Deegan 1993)

> … stress does play an enormous part in my illness [schizophrenia]. There are enormous pressures that come with any new experience and environment, and any change, positive or negative is extremely difficult. What ever I can do to decrease or avoid high stress environments is helpful in controlling my symptoms. In general terms all of my coping strategies consist of four steps: (1) recognizing when I am feeling stressed, which is harder than it may sound; (2) identifying the stressor; (3) remembering from past experience what action helped in the same situation or a similar one; and (4) taking that action as quickly as possible after I have identified the source of stress.
>
> (Leete 1989)

People can benefit from the experiences of others who have faced similar difficulties, either individually or within local self-help groups and national networks like the 'Hearing Voices Network' (www.hearing-voices.org.uk) or the various user groups and organizations that exist throughout the country. People can also access the expertise of others who have experienced similar difficulties via their writings (see above) and via self-help 'work books', like *Victim to Victor* (Coleman and Smith 1997a, 1997b). It is important that mental health practitioners actively foster both direct and indirect peer relationships and maximize opportunities for peer support.

However, if people are to take back control over their own lives, then practitioners must give up that control. It is easy to support people in making choices for themselves when they agree with you: the real challenge arises when the person makes choices that the practitioner considers to be wrong (see Perkins and Repper 1998). There are, of course, occasions when it would be unethical or illegal for the practitioner to accede to the individual's wishes: we may not, for example, help people to kill themselves, obtain illegal drugs or put others at risk and all of these things are likely to impede the process of rebuilding a valued and satisfying life. However, such instances are few and far between.

More frequently, people make decisions that the practitioner considers unlikely to be successful. Often from the best of motives, practitioners are eager to help people to avoid failure and its potentially destructive consequences. For example, we may discourage a person going to the Job Centre because we think they are not yet ready for employment; or recommend that they live in sheltered accommodation because we do not think they will be able to look after themselves; or suggest that they do not go out clubbing with their friends for fear that they will get drunk or use drugs and make their problems worse.

Making the most of one's life necessarily involves the risk of failure. Entering relationships involves the risk of rejection; trying to get a job involves the risk of being turned down; studying for qualifications involves risking failure of examinations or assessment. Growth and development necessarily involve the risk of failure. And we can learn as much about ourselves, and our possibilities, from our failures as we can from our successes. It is also the case that people with serious mental health problems are often more expert in coping with failure – because of the numerous losses and disappointments they have experienced – than are the practitioners who are helping them.

Instead of attempting to dissuade people from their chosen course of action we need to:

- offer any support and help that we can to maximize their chances of success;
- endeavour to find ways of circumventing the difficulties that might prevent a person from achieving their chosen goal;
- help them to learn from their experiences and try again if they are unsuccessful (and always avoid saying 'I told you so').

There are a number of ways in which people may be assisted to access the opportunities that they seek. So, for example, even if we think someone is not ready to get a job, we can maximize their chances of doing so by helping them to get to the Job Centre; thinking what they will say when they get there; assisting them to complete application forms or prepare for interviews; and providing ongoing support to retain their job if they are successful. Similarly, if a person wishes to live independently, it is always possible to arrange for support to obtain and maintain the 'home of their own' they desire (obtaining furniture; maximizing welfare benefits and enabling them to obtain any grants to which they may be entitled; arranging home helps, service washes at the launderette, take-away or ready-made meals; introducing the person to inexpensive cafes; helping them to manage money and pay rent). If the person wants to go out clubbing, then we might help them to find someone to go along with them and develop strategies for avoiding the temptations of illegal drugs or limit their alcohol intake.

Promoting access and inclusion

It is impossible for a person to rebuild a meaningful and satisfying life without the opportunity to do the things they value. But prejudice and discrimination frequently limit the access of people with mental health problems to the opportunities that are available to non-disabled citizens.

In order to facilitate recovery, people with serious mental health problems require access to a range of accommodation possibilities; work/education, leisure and social opportunities; and sources of support (see Health Advisory Service 2000). However, Bates (2002) and Repper and Perkins (2002) have outlined things that individual practitioners can do to facilitate inclusion a person's access to valued roles and activities. At a general level, these may include:

- *Information.* Providing people with information about the facilities, opportunities and services available in the local area.
- *Bridge building.* Actively creating links with local facilities to facilitate access. This may involve getting to know key people at the local college, leisure centre, church or job centre; understanding the demands and expectations of these facilities; and the sort of people who use them.

■ *Capacity building.* Increasing the capacity of community facilities to accommodate people who have experienced mental health problems. This typically involves two elements: breaking down myths and misconceptions about people with mental health problems and providing them with the support they feel they need to accommodate people with such difficulties.

At an individual level there are a number of different strategies that practitioners might use to assist a person to access the opportunities and activities that they seek. These include:

■ *Planning and target setting.* Helping people to think about their goals and ambitions, break these down into manageable steps and plan the necessary interim goals and targets on the way.

■ *Practice.* Helping the person to rehearse what they are going to do and practise it until they feel comfortable doing it.

■ *Skills development.* Using a variety of techniques – instruction, prompting, modelling, guided practice, feedback – to help a person to develop the skills they need to engage in their chosen activities.

■ *Graded exposure/return* to help people to overcome fears and anxieties that stop them doing what they want to do or resuming valued activities in which they have previously been involved.

■ *Just visiting* a place or activity beforehand as a way of becoming familiar with how to get there and what to expect.

■ *Time limited experience* (like work experience or college 'taster sessions') in order to try something out before deciding whether it is what they want to do.

■ *Providing transport* to help the person to get to the activity, or actually going with them to help reduce their anxiety.

■ *'Doing with'.* Helping someone to do something by doing it alongside them. This may involve a mental health practitioner, but having your nurse with you in a college class can be stigmatizing. There may be others who are better placed to join the person in the activity and who are less likely to attract negative attention: friends, relatives, volunteers, someone already engaged in the activity, others who experience mental health difficulties.

■ *Subsidy.* Helping to meet the costs of the activity by providing money for things like transport, refreshments, course registration fees and/or exploring other sources of subsidy like bus passes or reduced rates of entry for unemployed or disabled people.

■ *Special groups within ordinary settings.* For example, special groups or classes to introduce people with mental health problems to the local sports centre, college or library.

■ *Staff from different facilities coming into mental health facilities* to introduce them to familiarize people with the activities involved before going to the community facility.

■ *Mentoring.* Arranging for someone who is already involved in the setting/activity to provide information about what will be expected before they go, introduce them to the activity and provide advice and encouragement when they are there.

■ *Helping people to make new friends.* Often people lack the friendships and relationships on which most of us rely so heavily. Practitioners can help people to increase their social networks and contacts by, for example, enabling them to access activities where they are likely to meet people who share their interests; accessing internet chat-lines and e-groups (some of which are designed specifically for people with mental health problems like the Yahoo 'uksurvivors' e-group); placing or replying to advertisements in 'lonely hearts'/'contact' columns of local newspapers and listings magazines; befriending; or facilitating contact between service users who share interests/aspirations.

■ *Help and support when difficulties arise.* The fluctuating nature of mental health problems often means that it is important to ensure that assistance is readily available when difficulties arise.

■ *Working out ways of coping with symptoms/difficulties in the setting.* Leete (1989), for example, offers numerous examples of strategies that she has found useful in coping with the symptoms of her schizophrenia in a work setting.

■ *Self-help and support groups* where people with mental health problems who are engaged in similar activities (e.g. working, going to college) can get together and gain encouragement and support from each other.

■ *Negotiating adaptations and adjustments on the part of the provider.* These involve changing the physical or social environment, and/or the expectations on the person, so that they are able to engage in the activity. The UK 1995 Disability Discrimination Act not only outlaws discrimination against people with mental health problems but also requires that employers and providers of education, goods and services make 'reasonable adjustments' to ensure that people with such difficulties can access the opportunities they offer.

■ *Helping people to obtain their rights under the law.* As indicated above, the 1995 Disability Discrimination Act covers people with mental health problems and has been used by people with such difficulties to good effect (see Sayce 2001). Sayce (2001, 2002) has suggested that mental health practitioners should:

  – Be aware of the rights and protection that the Disability Discrimination Act provides for people with mental health problems and inform people with whom they work of these. Such information can be obtained from the Disability Rights Commission Help Line or website.

  – Provide information about the assistance available from the Disability Rights Commission Help Line[17] and case-work team and helping them to access this.

  – Help employers, colleges, and the providers of goods and services to decide what 'reasonable adjustments' a people with mental health problems might need to facilitate access (either on an individual basis or as part of a more general 'capacity building' initiative – see above).

  – Provide advocacy in relation to employment, education, leisure and other services.

There are many ways in which practitioners can enable people to access opportunities that they seek, but it is important that any such assistance is tailored to the needs/preferences of the person concerned. In choosing an appropriate approach practitioners might consider (Repper and Perkins 2002):

■ *Individual acceptability.* What sort of help does the person want?

■ *Social acceptability.* What sort of help would draw least negative attention to the person?

[17] Disability Rights Commission Help Line: Telephone: 08457–622633, Text phone: 08457–622644. Disability Rights Commission Website: www.drc-gb.org

- *Amount and availability.* How much help does the person need and what support might be available?
- *Existing abilities and resources.* How can the person's abilities, social contacts and other resources be used to best effect?
- *Issues of control.* How far can the person themselves control the amount, timing and nature of the help they receive?
- *Evidence of past effectiveness.* What sorts of help has been effective/ineffective in the past?
- *The research evidence.* For example, skills development and practice are more effective when conducted in the setting in which the skills will be used because things learned in one setting do not always generalize to other situations (Shepherd 1977, 1978; Appelo *et al.* 1992; Ekdawi and Conning 1994). Similarly, Bond *et al.* (1997, 2001) have identified a number of factors important in the success of programmes to facilitate access to employment including rapid job-search and minimal pre-vocational training; the availability of time-unlimited workplace support and the integration of clinical treatment with vocational rehabilitation.

Images of possibility

Perhaps the most important factor in both recovery and rehabilitation is a belief in possibility. If a person is to embark on the task of rebuilding a valued and satisfying life with mental health problems then they must believe in the possibility of a positive future. If a practitioner is to be able to assist the person in this process then they too must believe in the person's possibilities.

The traditional focus of mental health practitioners on the remediation of symptoms, dysfunctions and shortcomings is not helpful in generating a framework that engenders such images of possibility in either practitioners or the people whom we serve. As Peter Chadwick (1997), a lecturer in psychology who himself has a diagnosis of schizophrenia, has described:

> " Deficit-obsessed research can only produce theories and attitudes which are disrespectful of clients and are also likely to induce behaviour in clinicians such that service users are not properly listened to, not believed, not fairly assessed, are likely treated as inadequate and are also not expected to be able to become independent and competent individuals in managing life's tasks. "

If rehabilitation is to be effective in facilitating recovery then practitioners must extend their role beyond that of 'therapists who alleviate symptoms' to one of 'facilitators who assist people to rebuild lives'. We may hold a variety of theories about the nature and origins of mental health problems, but our primary role is to identify people's assets and possibilities and help them to recognize and exploit these themselves. If we are to be successful in these endeavours we must respect both the worth of people who experience serious mental health problems, but also the expertise of their experience.

A commitment, and ability, to learn from people with mental health problems, as well as their friends and relatives is essential, as is an openness and willingness to be corrected by experience. Expertise does not mean never making mistakes but the ability to learn from those mistakes. Those whom we serve are our most important teachers.

Conclusion

It is not possible to promote recovery unless we understand both the nature of the challenge facing people with mental health problems and the ways in which they are responding to this challenge. Recovery is all about the individual's experiences and aspirations:

- Recovery is about whole lives, not just symptoms, so services must focus on helping people to do the things they wish to do by adopting a whole team, multi-agency approach with clear coordination and continuity, and by fostering relationships outside services.
- Recovery is about growth so services must focus on a person's strengths and possibilities and change the environment rather than the individual.
- Recovery is not an end point but an ongoing journey so services must maintain, as well as optimizing a person's possibilities, adopting a long-term perspective and continuity of support over time.
- Recovery is not a professional intervention but an individual's journey towards a meaningful life so services need to emphasize social integration and maximize opportunities for people with mental health problems to support and learn from each other.
- Recovery is not limited to any particular theory about mental health, it is based on the perspectives, wishes and aspirations of each individual.
- Everyone's recovery is different and deeply personal so services need to adopt an individual approach to assessment and support, and respond flexibly to individual needs and wishes.
- Recovery is possible for everyone; services need to help everyone identify and make the most of their abilities, and identify the types and sources of support that are acceptable to each individual.

If services are to promote recovery and facilitate recovery, then three inter-related components are essential:

- Facilitating personal adaptation through a range of acceptable and accessible treatments to reduce distressing and disabling symptoms, and enabling people to reach an understanding of what has happened to them, and fostering peer support and relationships.
- Maintaining and fostering hope, and creating hope inspiring relationships with the individual and those important to them.
- Promoting access to material resources, roles, relationships, activities and sources of support, and supporting agencies outside the mental; health system to accommodate people with mental health problems.

Questions for reflection and discussion

1   The concept of recovery is not confined to mental health problems. Consider an event that has had an impact on your life (such as losing a job, the death of a loved one, serious illness, moving house ...) and think about the effect this had on you, ways in which you coped, what helped you and what did not help. If possible discuss this with another person and note the similarities and differences in your experiences of recovery. How has the experience changed you/your life in the long term?

2   Recovery is only possible if service providers understand the impact of mental health problems on them: what they have lost through having mental health problems, what they risk losing and what they want in order to give their life meaning. Does the current system of assessment that you use facilitate this understanding? Consider ways in which it could be developed to facilitate a more user-centred approach that is ongoing, well communicated and well coordinated.

3   Access to roles and relationships that are valued, both by the individual and within their society, is an essential part of recovery; facilitating such access is a critical component of rehabilitation. All mental health teams need to consider ways in which this 'socially inclusive work' could become a more integral and effective part of the service they provide. As a team, it might be useful to consider 'general level' strategies that might be introduced or strengthened within the team. Each one of these will need to be considered in some depth, and an action plan developed.

   (a)   How could information about facilities, opportunities and services within the local area be collected, compiled, maintained and presented?

   (b)   How could bridge building be organized and facilitated within the service?

   (c)   How might your team increase the capacity of community facilities to accommodate people who have experienced mental health problems through education, information and support?

Annotated bibliography

■   Repper, J. and Perkins, R. (2003) *Social Inclusion and Recovery. A Model for Mental Health Practice.* Balliére Tindall, London. This text provides a more detailed analysis of recovery and inclusion by the authors of this chapter. It draws on service users' experiences of living with mental health problems, and their accounts of recovery to construct a model for practitioners seeking to promote recovery and inclusion.

■   Leete, E. (1989) How I perceive and manage my illness, *Schizophrenia Bulletin* **15**: 197–200. Although this paper is somewhat dated, it still provides an inspirational account of the ways the author has developed to cope with the effects of her cognitive and emotional difficulties. Diagnosed with schizophrenia, Ms Leete now maintains her employment and social relationships through carefully considered and implemented strategies to cope with, for example, her anxiety, tendency to misinterpret situations, difficulties in concentrating and inability to respond quickly. Over 20 different coping strategies are described along with descriptions of the types of situations that are likely to be distressing or difficult.

■ Sayce, L. (2000) *From Psychiatric Patient to Citizen. Overcoming Discrimination and Social Exclusion*, London: Macmillan. An in-depth analysis of the discrimination and exclusion experienced by people who have mental health problems with reference to extensive US and UK literature, research and personal contact. Various ways of overcoming this exclusion are debated through practical examples and theoretical debate.

■ Perkins, R.E. and Repper, J.M. (1996) *Working Alongside People with Long Term Mental Health Problems*. Cheltenham: Stanley Thornes. Again, somewhat dated, but this remains one of very few texts available for direct care workers about the process of rehabilitation – facilitating access to socially valued roles, relationships, opportunities and facilities. It examines a range of different approaches that might be useful, and draws attention to the challenges that (still) remain.

References

Anthony, W.A. (1993) Recovery from mental illness: The guiding vision of the mental health system in the 1990s. *Innovations and Research* **2**(3): 17–24.

Appelo, M.T., Woonings, F.M.J. and Van Nieuwenhuizen, C.J. (1992) Specific skills and social competence in schizophrenia. *Acta Psychiatrica Scandanavica* **85**: 419–22.

Barton, R. (1959) *Institutional Neurosis*. Bristol: Wright.

Bates, B. (2002) A-Z of Socially Inclusive Strategies. Unpublished text. First presented at 'Piece of Mind' Conference, New College, Nottingham, January 1999.

Beck, A.T., Brown, G., Berchick, J., Stewart, L.B. and Steer, R.A. (1990) Relationship between hopelessness and suicide: A replication with psychiatric outpatients. *American Journal of Psychiatry* **147**(2): 11–23.

Bird, L. (2001) Poverty, social exclusion and mental health: A survey of people's personal experiences. *A Life in the Day* **5**: 3.

Birchwood, M., Smith, J., Macmillan, F. and McGovern, D. (1998) Early intervention in psychotic relapse, in C. Brooker and J. Repper (eds) *Serious Mental Health Problems in the Community: Policy, Practice and Research*. London: Baillière Tindall.

Bond, G.R., Becker, D.R., Drake, R.E. *et al.* (2001) Implementing supported employment as an evidence based practice. *Psychiatric Services* **52**(3): 313–22.

Bond, G.R., Drake, R.E., Meuser, K.T. and Becker, D.R. (1997) An update on supported employment for people with severe mental illness. *Psychiatric Services* **48**: 335–46.

Breier, A. and Strauss, J. (1983) Self control in psychiatric disorders. *Archives of General Psychiatry* **40**: 1141–5.

Brown, G.W., Bone, M., Dalison, M. and Wing, J.K. (1966) *Schizophrenia and Social Care*. Oxford: Oxford University Press.

Chadwick, P., Birchwood, M. and Trower, P. (1996) *Cognitive Therapy for Delusions, Voices and Paranoia*. Chichester: John Wiley and Sons.

Chadwick, P.K. (1997) *Schizophrenia: The Positive Perspective. In Search of Dignity for Schizophrenic People*. London: Routledge.

Coleman, R. and Smith, M. (1997a) *Working with Voices*. Gloucester: Handsell Publishing.

Coleman, R. and Smith, M. (1997b) *Working with Self Harm*. Gloucester: Handsell Publishing.

Copeland, M.E. (1997) *Wellness Recovery Action Plan*. Dummerston, VT: Peach Press.

Crowther, R.E., Marshall, M., Bond, G.R. and Huxley, P. (2001) Helping people with severe mental illness to obtain work: Systematic review. *British Medical Journal* **322**: 204–8.

Deegan, P. (1988) Recovery: The lived experience of rehabilitation. *Psychosocial Rehabilitation Journal* **11**(4): 11–19.

Deegan, P. (1989) A letter to my friend who is giving up. Paper presented at the Connecticut Conference on Supported Employment, Connecticut Association of Rehabilitation facilities, Cromwell, CT.

Deegan, P. (1990) How recovery begins. Paper presented at the eighth Annual Education Conference Alliance for the Mentally Ill of New York State, Binghamton, New York.

Deegan, P. (1993) Recovering our sense of value after being labeled. *Journal of Psychosocial Nursing* **31**(4): 7–11.

Deegan, P. (1996) Recovery as a journey of the heart. *Psychosocial Rehabilitation Journal* **19**(3): 91–7.

Deegan, P.E. (1999) Recovery: an alien concept. Paper presented at Strangefish Conference 'Recovery: An Alien Concept' at Chamberlin Hotel, Birmingham.

Department of Health (2007) *The Expert Patients Programme.* London: DH.

Disability Rights Commission (2006) *Equal Treatment – Closing the Gap. The Disability Rights Commission Formal Investigation into Physical Health Inequalities Experienced by People with Learning Disabilities and/or Mental Health Problems.* London: DRC.

Drake, R.E. and Cotton, P.G. (1986) Depression, hopelessness and suicide in chronic schizophrenia. *British Journal of Psychiatry* **148**: 554–9.

Dufault, K. and Martocchio, B. (1985) Hope: its spheres and dimensions. *Nursing Clinics of North America* **20**(2): 379–91.

Ekdawi, M. and Conning, A. (1994) *Psychiatric Rehabilitation – A Practical Guide.* London: Chapman and Hall.

Estroff, S.E. (1989) Self, identity and subjective experiences of schizophrenia: in search of the subject. *Schizophrenia Bulletin* **15**: 189–96.

Ford, R., Beadsmore, A., Norton, P. *et al.* (1994) Developing case management for the long term mentally ill. *Psychiatric Bulletin* **17**: 409–11.

Frank, J. (1968) The role of hope in psychotherapy. *International Journal of Psychiatry* **5**: 383–95.

Goffman, E. (1963) *Stigma: Notes on the management of spoiled identity.* Harmondsworth: Penguin.

Greenberg, J.S., Greenley, J.R. and Benedict, P. (1994) Contributions of persons with serious mental illness to their families. *Hospital and Community Psychiatry* **45**: 475–80.

Health Advisory Service (2000) *Review of Adult Mental Health Rehabilitation Services in Wandsworth, Merton, Sutton, Kingston and Richmond.* London: HAS.

Hickey, S.S. (1986) Enabling hope. *Journal of Cancer Nursing* **9**(3): 133–7.

Jacobson, N. (1993) Experiencing recovery: A dimensional analysis of recovery narratives. *Psychiatric Rehabilitation Journal* **24**(3): 248–55.

Jamison, K.R. (1993) *Touched with Fire: Manic-depressive Illness and the Artistic Temperament.* New York: The Free Press.

Jamison, K.R. (1995) Manic depressive illness and creativity. *Scientific American* February, 46–51.

Kanwal, G.S. (1997) Hope, respect and flexibility in psychotherapy. *Contemporary Psychoanalysis* **33**(1): 133–50.

King, R., Raynes, N. and Tizard, J. (1971) *Patterns of Residential Care.* London: Routledge.

Kingdon, D. (1998) Cognitive behaviour therapy for severe mental illness: strategies and techniques, in C. Brooker and J. Repper (eds) *Serious Mental Health Problems in the Community: Policy, Practice and Research.* London: Baillière Tindall.

Kubler-Ross, E. (1969) *Death and Dying.* London: Macmillan.

Kumar, S., Thara, R. and Rajkumar, S. (1989) Coping with symptoms of relapse in schizophrenia. *European Archives of Psychiatric Neurological Science* **239**: 213–15.

Leete, E. (1988) The treatment of schizophrenia: A patient's perspective. *Hospital and Community Psychiatry* **38**(5): 486–91.

Leete, E. (1989) How I perceive and manage my illness. *Schizophrenia Bulletin* **15**: 197–200.

Lindsey, H. (1976) *The Terminal Generation.* Old Tappan, NJ: Fleming-Revel.

Lovejoy, M. (1982) Expectations and the recovery process. *Schizophrenia Bulletin* **8**(4): 605–9.

May, R. (1999) Routes to Recovery – the roots of a clinical psychologist. Paper presented at Strangefish Conference 'Recovery: An Alien concept' at Chamberlin Hotel, Birmingham.

McCandless-Glincher, L., McKnight, S., Hamera, E., Smith, B.L., Peterson, K. and Plumlee, A.A. (1986) Use of symptoms by schizophrenics to monitor and regulate their illness. *Hospital and Community Psychiatry* **37**: 929–33.

Menninger, K. (1959) Hope. *American Journal of Psychiatry* **116**(12): 481–91.

Morris, D. (2001) Citizenship and community in mental health: A joint national programme for social inclusion and community partnership. *The Mental Health Review* **6**: 21–4.

Mueser, K.T., Bellack, A. and Blanchard, J. (1992) Comorbidity of schizophrenia and substance abuse: implications for treatment. *Journal of Clinical and Consulting Psychology* **60**: 845–55.

Nelson, H. (1997) *Cognitive Behavioural Therapy with Schizophrenia*. London: Nelson Thornes.

O'Donoghue, D. (1994) *Breaking Down the Barriers. The Stigma of Mental Illness: A User's Point of View*. Aberystwyth: US, the All Wales User Network.

Perkins, R.E. and Repper, J.M. (1996) *Working Alongside People with Long Term Mental Health Problems*, Cheltenham: Stanley Thornes.

Perkins, R.E. and Repper, J.M. (1998) *Dilemmas in Community Mental Health Practice. Choice or Control*. Oxford: Radcliffe Medical Press.

Post, F. (1994) Creativity and psychopathology: A study of 291 world-famous men. *British Journal of Psychiatry* **165**: 22–34.

Post, F. (1996) Verbal creativity, depression and alcoholism: an investigation of one hundred American and British writers. *British Journal of Psychiatry* **168**: 545–55.

Read, J. and Reynolds, J. (1996) *Speaking Our Minds*. London: Macmillan.

Repper, J. (2000) Adjusting the focus of mental health nursing: Incorporating service users' experiences of recovery. *Journal of Mental Health* **9**(6): 575–87.

Repper, J. and Perkins, R. (2003) *Social Inclusion and Recovery: A Model for Mental Health Practice*. London: Ballière Tindall.

Rose D (2001) User-focused monitoring. *Mental Health and Learning Disabilties Care* 4(6): 207–210

Russinova, Z. (1999) Providers' hope-inspiring competence as a factor optimizing psychiatric rehabilitation outcomes. *Journal of Rehabilitation* **16**(4): 50–7.

Ryan, P. (1979) Residential care for the mentally disabled, in J.K. Wing and R. Olsen (eds) *Community Care for the Mentally Disabled*. Oxford: Oxford University Press.

Sayce, L. (2000) *From Psychiatric Patient to Citizen. Overcoming Discrimination and Social Exclusion*. London: Macmillan.

Sayce, L. (2001) Not just users of services, but contributors to society: The opportunities of the Disability Rights Agenda. *Mental Health Review* **6**(3): 25–8.

Sayce, L. (2002) *Beyond Good Intentions: Making anti-discrimination strategies work*. London: Disability Rights Commission.

Shepherd, G. (1977) Social skills training: The generalisation problem. *Behaviour Therapy* **8**: 100–9.

Shepherd, G. (1978) Social skills training: The generalisation problem – some further data. *Behaviour Research and Therapy* **116**: 287–8.

Simpson, T. (ed.) (2004) *Doorways in the Night. Stories from the threshold of recovery*. Local Voices: Yorkshire Arts Circus.

Spaniol, L. and Koehler, M. (eds) (1994) *The Experience of Recovery*. Boston: Center for Psychiatric Rehabilitation.

Spaniol, L., Gagne, C. and Koehler, M. (1997) Recovery from serious mental illness: What it is and how to assist people in their recovery. *Continuum* **4**(4): 3–15.

Stein, L.L. and Test, M.A. (1980) Alternative to mental hospital. I. Conceptual model, treatment programme and clinical evaluation. *Archives of General Psychiatry*. **37**: 392–7.

Stotland, E. (1969) *The Psychology of Hope*. San Francisco: Jossey-Bass.

Vincent, S.S. (1999) Using findings from qualitative research to teach mental health professionals about the experience of recovery from psychiatric disability. Presentation at the Harvard University Graduate School of Education Fourth Annual Student Research Conference, Cambridge, MA.

Woodside, H., Landeen, J., Kirkpatrick, H., Byrne, C., Bernardo, A. and Pawlick, J. (1994) Hope and schizophrenia: Exploring attitudes of clinicians. *Psychosocial Rehabilitation Journal* **8**: 140–4.

Young, S.L. and Ensing, D.S. (1999) Exploring recovery from the perspective of people with psychiatric disabilities. *Psychiatric Rehabilitation Journal* **22**(3): 219–31.

Part 2

Contexts

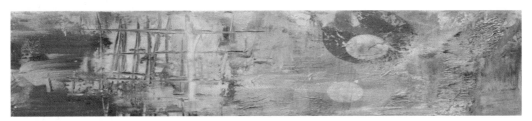

Chapter contents

CHAPTER 6

The policy and service context for mental health nursing

Andrew McCulloch and Richard Ford

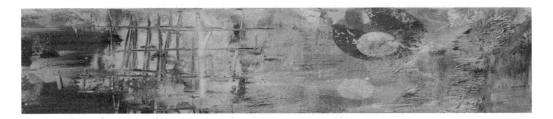

Chapter overview

In this chapter we chart the history of mental health service development over the last 60 years and describe current mental health service provision, and the associated roles of mental health nurses. Current mental health policy, including the *National Service Framework (NSF) for Mental Health* (DH 1999) is examined, as is the *Capable Practitioner* Framework (Lindley *et al.* 2001) and the *Ten Essential Shared Capabilities* (NHSU 2005) for contemporary practice. We conclude by forecasting the impact of current developments on the mental health nursing roles of the future.

This chapter covers:

- Principles of mental health care;
- A brief history of mental health service provision since 1950;
- Current services and workforce;
- Current mental health policy;
- The required competencies and capabilities of the mental health nurse;
- Future practice.

Principles of mental health care

The mental health user and survivor movement has grown substantially over the last two decades. There are now hundreds of groups across the UK. In particular they were able to influence the implementation of the *NSF for Mental Health* (DH 1999). It is the NSF that has set out the principles for contemporary mental health care in England in the first decade of the twenty-first century. There is little dispute about these principles (Table 6.1) although the extent that they have been put into practice is variable. For example *Users' Voices* (Rose

2001) found that a majority of users did not receive all the information they required and did not know if they had a care plan or a key worker in line with the Care Programme Approach (CPA). It is now clear that people who use public services, including mental health services, must be enabled to become 'capable users'. A capable or expert user is well informed about mental health and mental health services, is at the centre of their care, working in partnership with staff, and can exercise choice.

People with mental health problems can expect that services will:
- involve service users and their carers in planning and delivering care;
- deliver high quality treatment and care which is known to be effective and acceptable;
- be well suited to those who use them and non-discriminatory;
- be accessible so that help can be obtained when and where it is needed;
- promote their safety and that of carers, staff and the wider public;
- offer choices which promote independence;
- be well coordinated between staff and agencies;
- deliver continuity of care for as long as this is needed;
- empower and support staff;
- be properly accountable to the public, service users and carers.

Table 6.1 National Service Framework for Mental Health Guiding Values and Principles (DH 1999)

A brief history of mental health service provision since 1950

Until the 1960s/1970s mental health care was organized around the old asylums, which were built mainly in the period 1840–1920. From the end of the 1950s onwards, the asylum population started to decline significantly because of the introduction of new medication, and changes in care and the thinking surrounding mental health. This process became recognized by the government and it was Enoch Powell, then Health Minister, who announced that the asylums would decline in his famous 'water tower' speech. Almost all of the old long-stay beds have now disappeared.

As the total number of psychiatric beds for people of all ages declined from about 140,000 in the early 1950s to around 28,000 (depends on which categories of bed are included in the count) at the time of writing, the utilization of acute beds became much more intensive. This increase in the intensity of use has been due not just to the loss of beds, but also to an increase in demand (McCulloch *et al.* 2000). In parallel with the reduction in bed numbers, the level of community provision for people with mental health problems has increased steadily. However, most community mental health teams do not deliver comprehensive care packages either because they are too heavily loaded or because they are spending too much time dealing with patients whose condition does not require continued secondary care interventions. More specialized community teams, such as assertive outreach and crisis intervention teams were slower to develop, but the *NSF for Mental Health* (DH 1999) and *NHS Plan* (DH 2000a) have stimulated such developments, and assertive outreach in particular – a system of intensive support for people with severe mental health problems who have difficulty in engaging with other services – has developed rapidly and hit national targets set for development. Crisis resolution and early intervention teams have now also hit target numbers although late in relation to NSF milestones. Some 60 people per 100,000 adult population now receive assertive outreach and some 280 per 100,000 adults receive crisis resolution each year (Association of Public Health Observatories 2007) and there are some 700 specialized mental health teams consisting of 252 assertive outreach teams, 343 crisis resolution teams and 118 early intervention teams (Appleby 2007). However, not all of these teams meet the required criteria set out in either English policy or the international literature (McCulloch *et al.* 2003; DH 2004a).

The development of services on the ground has been reflected by the development of national policy. In the 1970s the replacement model for the old asylums was seen to consist of acute psychiatric units in district general hospitals, coupled with multi-disciplinary community mental health teams. This vision has since been elaborated within the NSF to include a comprehensive system of care embracing:

- inpatient care;
- crisis care;
- assertive outreach;
- community teams;
- 24-hour nursed care;
- residential care;
- supported housing;
- daytime activities;
- social support.

The *NHS Plan* set specific targets for the introduction of intensive community teams such as assertive outreach. The protection of the public has become an increasing part of the mental health policy agenda and has led to difficulties for staff in terms of paperwork and risk assessment and in knowing whether their function is to care for individuals or to protect others.

Current services and workforce

Although the UK has a national health service, adult mental health care is delivered by a large number of relatively autonomous NHS trusts including Foundation Trusts, local authority social services departments (whether in partnership with the NHS or as part of more integrated services), and independent for profit and voluntary sector organizations. To add to this complex organizational picture, health services are commissioned by local NHS primary care trusts and social care services are commissioned by social services departments (now part usually of wider local authority adult service directorates), either from their own in-house providers or from independent sector agencies (these are the English organizational arrangements – Scotland, Wales and Northern Ireland have different structures). There are also various joint commissioning and sub-contracting processes in operation across the country and sometimes children's and older people's mental health care have different commissioning and provision arrangements. An overview is provided by strategic health authorities, which represents the local headquarters for the NHS. It is, therefore, not easy to establish what services are being provided by which groups of staff.

In 2006/7 the NHS in England spent £9.125 billion on hospital and community mental health care. This figure does not include primary mental health care but for the same year the King's Fund estimated that all health and social care services for people with mental disorder as £22.5 billion (McCrone *et al.* 2008). In 2002/3 spending on mental health accounted for 11.8 per cent of health and social services expenditure, 82 per cent of this being spent by the NHS.

The number of admissions to psychiatric beds fell by about 10 per cent to 122,260 in the four years to 2002/3. Many admissions involve detention under the Mental Health Act. During 2004/5 there were 46,700 detentions under the Act (some people may be detained more than once during a year).

Department of Health returns indicate that on 30 September 2004 there were 41,586 whole-time equivalent qualified nursing posts in the mental health field (14 per cent of all qualified nursing posts). Most nurses continue to work in hospital or residential settings with only one third (13,627) working in the community. However, community services have continued to expand as described above.

Mental health policy under New Labour

The White Paper *Modernising Mental Health Services* (DH 1998a) was the first comprehensive statement from the government about the future direction of mental health policy since *Better Services for the Mentally Ill* in the 1970s (DHSS 1975). *Modernising Mental Health Services* emphasized three key aims of the government's vision for mental health:

- safe services: to protect the public and provide effective care for those with mental illness at the time they need it;
- sound services: to ensure that patients and service users have access to the full range of services that they need;
- supportive services: working with patients and service users, their families and carers to build healthier communities.

It also laid down the principles for modernization, which would be implemented through the *NSF for Mental Health* (DH 1999). The modernization agenda was to be delivered through a number of mechanisms including:

- *Additional investment in mental health services.* There was to be an additional £300 million each year for mental health services for working-age adults coming on stream in 2002/3 and targeted mainly on the development of specialist community teams. However, this money was not ring-fenced to be spent on mental health and there is evidence that much of this money was spent elsewhere.
- *Legal framework.* In July 1998, ministers announced a root and branch review of the Mental Health Act to ensure that the legislative framework supports modern mental health care. An independent expert group prepared initial proposals for consultation early in 1999 and following a Green Paper, a White Paper was published at the end of 2000. In 2002 a draft bill was published for further consultation. This did not prove satisfactory

and a new draft bill was produced in 2004 and eventually received royal assent in 2007. The final Act still has not been fully implemented at the time of writing and many commentators see the resulting legislation as inferior to what was originally proposed. It has very little support from within the mental health community which is one reason why the path to new legislation has been so tortuous.

■ *Organizational framework.* The new policy environment emphasized the need for integrated and multi-agency partnerships in care and requires more coherent and effective management of the interfaces and boundaries of services and functions. In the ten years since 1998 good progress has been made in integrating health and social care in mental health but less progress has been made in creating a wider 'joined up' approach to mental health issues.

The national service frameworks

The *NSF for Mental Health* (DH 1999) was the first national service framework, and seeks to implement the government's agenda to drive up quality and reduce unacceptable variations in health and social services. The government's strategy for delivering core standards for the NHS has now been working for some time and consists of standards:

■ set by the National Institute for Health and Clinical Excellence, Social Care Institute for Excellence and national service frameworks;
■ delivered by clinical governance, underpinned by professional regulation and lifelong learning;
■ monitored by the Healthcare Commission.

The *NSF for Mental Health* (DH 1999) addressed the mental health needs of adults of working age. It sets out national standards and national service models, specified approaches to implementation at national and local levels, and set a series of milestones and performance indicators to assure progress. It also identified an organizational framework for providing integrated services and for commissioning across the spectrum of care.

The *NSF for Mental Health* set standards in seven areas, each based on the evidence and knowledge base available and supported by service models and examples of good practice. These are set out in Table 6.2.

Standard 1 aims to ensure health and social services promote mental health and reduce the discrimination and social exclusion associated with mental health problems.

Health and social services should:
■ promote mental health for all, working with individuals and communities;
■ combat discrimination against individuals and groups with mental health problems, and promote their social inclusion.

Standards 2 and **3** aim to deliver better primary mental health care, and to ensure consistent advice and help for people with mental health needs, including primary care services for individuals with severe mental illness.

2 Any service user who contacts their primary health care team with a common mental health problem should:
■ have their mental health needs identified and assessed;   ⇨

■ be offered effective treatments, including referral to specialist services for further assessment, treatment and care if they require it.

3 Any individual with a common mental health problem should:

■ be able to make contact round the clock with the local services necessary to meet their needs and receive adequate care;

■ be able to use NHS Direct, as it develops, for first-level advice and referral on to specialist helplines or to local services.

Standards 4 and **5** aim to ensure: that each person with severe mental illness receives the range of mental health services they need; that crises are anticipated or prevented where possible; prompt and effective help if a crisis does occur; timely access to an appropriate and safe mental health place or hospital bed, including a secure bed, as close to home as possible.

4 All mental health service users on CPA should:

■ receive care which optimizes engagement, anticipates or prevents a crisis, and reduces risk;

    have a copy of a written care plan which:

– includes the action to be taken in a crisis by the service user, their carer and their care coordinator,

– advises their GP how they should respond if the service user needs additional help,

– is regularly reviewed by their care coordinator,

– is able to access services 24 hours a day, 365 days a year.

(*Note*: Standard 4 reinforced the Care Programme Approach (CPA) which was first introduced in 1990.)

5 Each service user who is assessed as requiring a period of care away from their home should have:

■ timely access to an appropriate hospital bed or place which is:

– in the least restrictive environment consistent with the need to protect them and the public,

– as close to home as possible;

■ a copy of a written care plan agreed on discharge which sets out the care and rehabilitation to be provided, identifies the care coordinator, and specifies the action to be taken in a crisis.

Standard 6 aims to ensure health and social services assess the needs of carers who provide regular and substantial care for those with severe mental illness, and provide care to meet their needs.

6 All individuals who provide regular and substantial care for a person on CPA should:

■ have an assessment of their caring, physical and mental health needs, repeated on at least an annual basis;

■ have their own written care plan which is given to them and implemented in discussion with them.

Standard 7 aims to ensure that health and social services play their full part in the achievement of the target in *Saving Lives: Our Healthier Nation* to reduce the suicide rate by at least one fifth by 2010.

Local health and social care communities should prevent suicides by:

■ promoting mental health for all, working with individuals and communities (Standard 1);

■ delivering high quality primary mental health care (Standard 2);

■ ensuring that anyone with a mental health problem can contact local services via the primary care team, a helpline or an A&E department (Standard 3);

■ ensuring that individuals with severe and enduring mental illness have a care plan which meets their specific needs, including access to services around the clock (Standard 4);

■ providing safe hospital accommodation for individuals who need it (Standard 5);

■   enabling individuals caring for someone with severe mental illness to receive the support which they need to continue to care (Standard 6);

and in addition:

■   support local prison staff in preventing suicides among prisoners;

■   ensure that staff are competent to assess the risk of suicide among individuals at greatest risk;

■   develop local systems for suicide audit to learn lessons and take any necessary action.

Table 6.2 The National Service Framework for Mental Health standards (DH 1999)

For the first time government policy on mental health was accompanied by an explicit standards-based implementation framework. It also specified what is required from all those working in mental health services at various levels to deliver effective mental health services. This carries with it a clear requirement that training and professional development is oriented towards the implementation of the strategy and the achievement of the standards.

Each local health and social care community was required to prepare for implementing the NSF by establishing a local implementation team, which would then produce a local implementation plan.

The NHS Plan

The NHS Plan (DH 2000a) added significantly to the specific proposals set out in the NSF and detailed the specific service components required. All of these had and still have major implications for the workforce, and they are summarized in Table 6.3.

The NHS Plan, like the *NSF for Mental Health*, recognized that implementation would only succeed if staff were available in the right numbers, and were well trained and motivated. The Plan considerably raised the demand for staff implied in the *NSF for Mental Health*. In addition to the NSF another 3300 staff, 435 community teams, about 100 day centres and 200 secure beds were promised. In combination this implied that an additional 8000 staff were required: a 12 per cent addition to the workforce, and many of them requiring new or specific specialist skills on top of basic training. It would appear that at least some of the required workforce expansion has indeed taken place at the time of writing, but it is hard to track this at a detailed level.

Mental health policy implementation guide

The flurry of policy guidance did not end with the *NHS Plan*. The original strategy gave the overall framework, the *NSF for Mental Health* put into place national standards, and the *NHS Plan* then detailed some of the service models. This was then reinforced by detailed policy guides on a range of issues including:

■   effective care coordination;

■   mental health promotion;

■   workforce action team report;

■   talking therapies;

■   assertive outreach;

■   crisis resolution;

■   early intervention in psychosis;

- acute inpatient care and psychiatric intensive care;
- community mental health teams;
- carers and families.
- dual diagnosis (coexisting mental health and substance misuse problems);
- suicide prevention strategy;
- primary mental health care;
- mental health needs and care for people from black and minority ethnic communities;
- personality disorder

(all available from www.csip.org.uk).

It is difficult both to get an overview of these guides and to understand what they mean in terms of developing a whole systems approach to mental health locally.

Mental health policy development since the NHS Plan

While the NSF and NHS Plan continue to set the broad direction for mental health policy there have been a number of significant developments since. It is not possible to list all of these but key concerns of Government have included social exclusion and specifically employment, the development of talking therapies and public mental health. Each of these are discussed below.

Other important areas where we are seeing developments include services for people from black and ethnic minorities, services for vulnerable families, health promotion for people with mental health problems, direct payments, choice, care pathways, prisons and personality disorder. These cannot be reported in full here for reasons of space but the CSIP and DH websites cited below can be used to locate all the relevant policy documents.

Social exclusion

In 2004, the Social Exclusion Unit, part of the Office of the Deputy Prime Minister, published a major report on *Mental Health and Social Exclusion* (ODPM 2004). This is perhaps the strongest, evidence-based, policy report to appear since the first edition of this book. It highlights the key role mental ill health – both severe mental illness and chronic common mental health problems – have in creating social inclusion. It set out a 27 point action plan as a basis for a joined up approach across Government to tackle this problem. Action falls under six key themes:

- stigma and discrimination – a sustained programme to challenge negative attitudes and promote awareness of people's rights;
- the role of health and social care in tackling social exclusion – implementing evidence-based practice in vocational services and enabling reintegration into the community;
- employment – giving people with mental health problems a real chance of sustained paid work reflecting their skills and experience;
- supporting families and community participation – enabling people to lead fulfilling lives the way they choose;
- getting the basics right – access to decent homes, financial advice and transport;
- making it happen – clear arrangements for leading the programme and maintaining momentum.

■ Money for the National Service Framework (2003/4)	£300 million
Primary care	
■ Help for GPs on common mental health problems (2004)	1000 new graduate primary care mental health workers to help 300,000 people; 500 community mental health staff to help 500,000 people
■ Help for primary care teams, NHS Direct and A&E departments for people who need immediate help (2004)	
Community services	
■ Treatment and support for young people and their families (2004)	50 early intervention teams to help all young people who experience first episode of psychosis – around 7500 a year
■ Crisis resolution (2004)	335 teams, treating around 100,000 people a year and reducing pressure on acute inpatient units by 30 per cent
■ Assertive outreach (2003)	50 teams, in addition to the target of 170 for April 2001, helping 20,000 people
■ Services for women (2004)	Women-only day centres in every health authority
Carers	
■ Respite care (2004)	700 more staff to increase breaks for carers, helping about 165,000 carers
High secure hospitals	
■ Reduction in places (2004)	Move 400 patients to more appropriate accommodation
■ Long-term secure care (2004)	200 extra beds
■ After discharge support (2004)	400 more community staff to provide intensive support
Prisons	
■ Better health screening and support for prisoners (2004)	300 more staff to identify and provide treatment. Everyone with severe mental illness will receive treatment and none should leave prison without a care plan and a care coordinator
Personality disorders	
■ Secure accommodation and rehabilitation (2004)	140 new secure places, 75 specialist rehabilitation, hostel places and almost 400 extra staff for people with severe personality disorder who pose a high risk to the public

Table 6.3 Mental health clinical priorities in the NHS Plan

This report could have been the start of a major change process for service users, their families and for services. Sadly it would appear that little has happened in direct response to this report. This may have occurred for a variety of reasons including the waning influence and eventual disappearance of the Office of the Deputy Prime Minister, lack of buy in and action by other Departments, and other policy developments such as incapacity benefit reform overshadowing the report. However, we have seen useful activity by the Care Services

Improvement Partnership and by local services in developing more socially inclusive services (e.g. by modernizing day services) and there is still some hope that a substantial national effort to tackle stigma might emerge in England following an announcement of substantial lottery funding, albeit this is not a Government initiative, particularly as there is now evidence of success in this regard in Scotland.

Talking therapies

A current policy development that has great potential to change the way that primary care can provide effective mental health services is the Improving Access to Psychological Therapies (IAPT) programme. It is also related in some ways to the Social Exclusion Unit report.

In December 2004, Lord Layard, a health economist, presented data to a Downing Street seminar, on the association between mental illness and unemployment. He drew on the following evidence and arguments:

- There are 1 million people receiving incapacity benefit who have a mental health problem.
- 90 per cent of those are not in contact with specialist mental health services, and suffer from depression and/or anxiety.
- Effective interventions exist for depression and anxiety, including medication, and cognitive behaviour therapy (CBT).
- A number of programmes run by the Department of Work and Pensions (DWP) have shown that CBT, and programmes related to CBT such as condition management programmes, can support people to return to work.
- The CBT service is best delivered through a treatment team or treatment centre approach, which can ensure high quality psychological assessments and interventions.

Lord Layard proposed that new treatment centres be created to provide CBT and employment advice to people whose long-term employment was at risk because of mental health problems. Funding for these centres would come from the savings generated by people returning to work earlier. Savings would be generated from reduced health care costs (both physical and mental health costs), reduced payments on benefits, and increased taxation revenue, as people return to work earlier, and reduced social costs through improved outputs.

Pilots were conducted in Doncaster and Newham that were designed to test not only the applicability of the CBT treatment centre approach, but to understand and quantify the economic gains that could fund this programme nationally. Following success of the pilots the Government announced in late 2007 national roll out, and at the time of writing regional contracts to provide the training required to skill up the workforce have been let. The training phase is likely to last about three years and nurses as well as psychologists will be in the front line of those delivering CBT.

Public mental health

Public mental health has only recently emerged as a policy priority within the UK. In 2004 the Department of Health (2004b) published *Choosing Health: Making healthy choices easier*, which set out a new approach to public health that reflected the rapid and radical transformation of English society in the latter half of the twentieth century. Though there was much hope and anticipation in the mental health field for this document it did little to further the cause of public mental health and even less for the lives of those people whose mental health was at risk. Its overarching priorities included improving diet and nutrition and increasing exercise, both of which are known to also promote and sustain mental health, but neither of which made reference to their associated mental health benefits.

Improving mental health was included as a priority but its justification was expressed in relation to physical health '… because mental well-being is crucial to good physical health and making healthy choices'. The reverse is also true but the policy document missed this integral understanding and thus an opportunity to mainstream public mental health promotion. Indeed the latest evidence suggests that mental health is the key mediating factor between social stressors such as poverty and health outcomes.

More recently Lord Darzi's Next Stage Review of the NHS *High Quality Care for All* (DH 2008) placed far greater emphasis on public mental health and the actions that are necessary to improve it. Every primary care trust is required to commission personalized well-being and prevention services in partnership with their local authorities. These services will initial focus on six key goals one of which is improving mental health and two others deal with conditions related to mental health (alcohol harm and drug addiction). At the time of writing PCTs are consulting with their communities to identify which services should be commissioned for these purposes and how they should be delivered. It is too early to judge the impact of this work but it does herald a greater understanding and integration of mental health within the public health paradigm.

Other elements of the Next Stage Review that have implications for the mental health field include:

- a new Fit For Work service will help people who want to return to work but are struggling with ill health including those who experience mental health problems.
- an NHS constitution will give people rights to choose treatment and providers, which may have implications for people suffering from mental health problems who want therapies that are not widely available. Mental health is explicitly mentioned within the constitution.
- personal health budgets are to be piloted, which may be particularly relevant to people suffering from long-term mental health problems.
- new integrated care organizations will be developed, which bring together health and social care staff and build on successful initiatives to integrate local authority services with Mental Health Trusts.

National Service Framework for Older People

There is little in the way of health and social care policy that specifically addresses the needs of older people with mental health problems. However, the *National Service Framework for Older People* (*NSFOP*) (DH 2001a) has eight standards with one specific standard for mental health care: **Standard 7** which covers the promotion of good mental health in older people and the treatment and support of older people with dementia and depression (cf. Chapter 24).

" Standard 7: Older people who have mental health problems have access to integrated mental health services, provided by the NHS and councils to ensure effective diagnosis, treatment and support, for them and for their carers. "

This standard is broad. The *NSFOP* also refers to key interventions under Standard 7. It points out that improving prevention, care and treatment depend on promoting good mental health, the early recognition and management of mental health problems in primary care with the support of specialist old age mental health teams, and access to specialist care. In this way the structure of the *NSFOP* is similar to that for working age adults. The emphasis is on mental health promotion and supporting primary care and only where necessary providing direct care within specialist services. The *NSFOP*, like the *NSF*, puts an emphasis on comprehensive, multi-disciplinary, accessible, responsive, accountable and systematic services. However, there is little evidence that mental health promotion and early intervention for older people has developed in practice (see for example, NAO 2007).

The other standards of the *NSFOP* also apply to older people's mental health services. Particular note should be given to:

Standard 1 which aims to ensure that older people are never unfairly discriminated against in accessing NHS or social care services as a result of their age.

" Standard 1: NHS services will be provided, regardless of age, on the basis of clinical need alone. Social care services will not use age in their eligibility criteria or policies, to restrict access to available services. "

Standard 2 which aims to ensure that older people are treated as individuals and that they receive appropriate and timely packages of care which meet their needs as individuals, regardless of health and social services boundaries.

" Standard 2: NHS and social services treat older people as individuals and enable them to make choices about their own care. This is achieved through the single assessment process, integrating commissioning arrangements and integrated provision of services, including community equipment and continence services. "

Although Standard 2 of the *NSFOP* is clear about the organizational model of integrated commissioning and provision there is no further guidance on the service models. On the one hand this gives services greater freedom to develop models that are responsive to local need. On the other hand, where resources and expertise are limited poor models may develop, for example, where one ward attempts to meet the needs of people with dementia and those with functional mental illness within the same setting. The development of a national dementia strategy is currently underway and this is likely to have a beneficial impact on dementia services albeit no new resources will be attached to the strategy.

Child and adolescent mental health services

The 2003 Green Paper *Every Child Matters* (HM Treasury 2003) started the creation of a new policy framework for children and young people which made mental health an explicit part of the agenda and emphasized early intervention and support for families. This new policy agenda started to energize the development of Child and Adolescent Mental Health Services (CAMHS) which had long been a 'cinderella within a cinderella'. The following year saw the publication of the *National Service Framework for Children, Young People and Maternity Services* (NSFCYPM) (DfES/DH 2004) and within this a specific framework for addressing the mental health and psychological well-being of children and young people – the CAMHS Standard (DfES/DH 2004).

Almost all the standards of the NSFCYPM have some relevance for CAMHS but the most important are 1–5 and the CAMHS standard 9 itself:

Standard 1: Promoting health and well-being, identifying needs and intervening early

The health and well-being of all children and young people is promoted and delivered through a coordinated programme of action, including prevention and early intervention wherever possible, to ensure long-term gain, led by the NHS in partnership with local authorities.

Standard 2: Supporting parenting

Parents or carers are enabled to receive information, services and support which will help them care for their children and equip them with the skills they need to ensure their children have optimum life chances and are healthy and safe.

Standard 3: Child, young person and family-centred services

Children and young people and families receive high quality services which are coordinated around their individual and family needs and take account of their views.

Standard 4: Growing up into adulthood

All young people have access to age appropriate services which are responsive to their specific needs as they grow into adulthood.

Standard 5: Safeguarding and promoting the welfare of children and young people

All agencies work to prevent children suffering harm and to promote their welfare, provide them with the services they require to address their identified needs and safeguard children who are being or who are likely to be harmed.

Standard 9: The mental health and psychological well-being of children and young people

All children and young people, from birth to their 18th birthday, who have mental health problems and disorders have access to timely, integrated, high quality multi-disciplinary mental health services to ensure effective assessment, treatment and support, for them, and their families.

The NSF acknowledges that around 40 per cent of children with a mental disorder do not currently receive a specialist service, although this figure may be conservative. It refers to the pre-existing commitment, set out in the 2002 planning and priorities guidance to achieve comprehensive CAMHS by 2006. While it is clear that CAMHS are still not comprehensive across every health and social care economy in England it is also clear that large investment in CAMHS has occurred because of these policy commitments. Expenditure on CAMHS rose by 80 per cent from 2002/3 to 2005/6. However, there has not been much evidence of any developments in mental health promotion and prevention although in late 2007 Government announced increased resources for mentally healthy schools and a strategic review of CAMHS which is currently under way.

It is interesting that while in some respects recent policy on children's mental health sets out a quite radical vision – with a shift in emphasis to mental health promotion, prevention and early intervention, the CAMHS delivery system remains unreformed. CAMHS remains delivered by a variety of different agencies, according to local history and local developments, and continues to be conceptualized as working at four levels:

Tier 1: A primary level of care.
Tier 2: A service provided by specialist individual professionals relating to workers in primary care.
Tier 3: A specialized multi-disciplinary service for more severe, complex or persistent disorders.
Tier 4: Essential tertiary level services such as day units, highly specialized outpatient teams and inpatient units.

It is important to recognize that this model is merely conceptual. In many areas one or more of these service elements either do not exist or rely on ill-equipped or ill-trained generic services, e.g. GPs or sometimes adult mental health services. Few, if any, areas have CAMHS which are integrated vertically (between the tiers) and horizontally across other relevant services such as education, housing and adult mental health. For example, the authors are only aware of two primary mental health care services for young people nationally that integrate in this way. It is hoped that the current review of CAMHS can address these issues.

Effectiveness: a service that achieves its aims

A modern effective mental health service will be orientated towards the needs of users and underpinned with:

- high levels of expertise;
- correct targeting;
- timely and accessible delivery;
- evaluation and review, supporting both internal and external continuous quality improvement.

It is acknowledged that achieving quality in mental health care is not just about clinical effectiveness, but about improving health and social outcomes for people who use the service. Aspirations to improve services and deliver a sustained quality service have not, in the past, had systems and structures to enable them to succeed. A range of new structures and systems has been established to ensure that quality is continually improved and sustained. There are three main mechanisms.

Defining the right treatments and services

The National Institute for Health and Clinical Excellence (NIHCE) is a special health authority with the remit of coordinating the production and dissemination of evidence-based clinical and public health guidelines. Although many practitioners and managers in the field believe that the evidence base is poor, the real picture is more complicated. Although research on mental health is often weak, and much of it focuses on clinical not social outcomes, there is still a significant body of research within the UK and from the USA and Europe that needs to be disseminated and operationalized. NIHCE guidelines cover a wide range of mental health issues with guidelines on antenatal and postnatal mental health, anxiety, bipolar disorder, dementia, depression, depression in children and young people, eating disorders, obsessive compulsive disorder, post-traumatic stress disorder, schizophrenia, self-harm and violence, already published, and more in the pipeline. There are also some influential appraisals of drugs and technology in the mental health field most notably of anti-dementia drugs and atypical anti-psychotics.

Local implementation of high quality services

Clinical governance lies at the heart of local structures for improving quality, supported by moves to strengthen professional self-regulation and the development of values and structures that support lifelong learning. Clinical governance needs to be seen as a major opportunity for developing an effective quality framework. It has been suggested that an organization with a successful clinical governance framework will be characterized by:

- clinical staff with different attitudes and behaviour, including greater openness and willingness to address quality issues in a corporate way;
- managers who see themselves as responsible for quality of care, who are committed to a team approach to quality improvement, and who are willing to allow clinical leadership and responsibility to be developed. Changes in clinical governance will require similar changes in managerial governance.

One major problem with the concept of clinical governance is that the term itself implies a technical approach to improving quality focused on NHS services and does not describe the inclusive, often democratic nature of the quality process in the modern mental health environment. The very term 'clinical' can be seen as missing the practical and problem oriented responses which patients and families want. Partnerships with service users, carers and staff in local authority social services and other departments, and local community sector agencies, all have a part to play in delivering a quality mental health service. It is clear, in particular, that the National Performance Assessment Framework for Social Services and the Best Value quality regime serve the same purpose as clinical governance in social care. What is important here is that the underlying aim of delivering effective, quality services is seen as a partnership issue and that local quality systems are harmonized across and between the agencies to define local standards.

Lifelong learning

Lifelong learning is a concept which was originally used in industry, which recognizes the accelerating pace of change in technology, skills and society. As the nature of the work changes, so does the nature of employment. Skills quickly become obsolete at a time of great technological change. The government's strategy for lifelong learning was set out in *Working Together, Learning Together: a framework for lifelong learning for the NHS* (DH 2001b).

Continuing professional development

These developments set the context for the NHS human resources strategy *Working Together: securing a quality workforce for the NHS* (DH 1998b) and subsequently for the *Improving Working Lives Standard* (DH 2000b), *HR in the NHS Plan* (DH 2002) and *Learning for Change in Healthcare* (DH 2006a). Continuing professional development (CPD) has a significant role to play in supporting the developing human resources (HR) strategy. National policy sends a clear message that maintaining profession specific isolation within CPD is not consistent with lifelong learning approaches. Integrated care for patients will rely on models of training and education that give staff a clear understanding of their own roles, those of others within both the health and social care professions and how they inter-relate.

A developing framework for practice

Modern mental health services now require staff who can cope with:

- heavy demand for emergency psychiatric admissions and crisis care often from patients with multiple issues including substance misuse;
- working across settings and agencies in both health and social care;
- formal integration of CPA and care management currently evolving into new forms of person-centred planning often with a recovery ethos;
- new evidence-based psychological, social and pharmacological interventions;
- high levels of severity of illness and disability;
- the new policy context;
- changes to the legal context arising from the Mental Capacity Act and the shortly to be enacted Mental Health Act 2007;
- assertive outreach for people with severe mental illness who do not engage with other services;
- home treatment and crisis-intervention services providing emergency psychiatric care in the community;
- early intervention;
- psycho-educational and cognitive behavioural approaches to family work;
- working in partnership with carers and users.

The capable practitioner

The current situation

From an older style institutional system of care has emerged a more open but complex community-based system of care delivery. The vision of the comprehensive, integrated community mental health service with specialized functional teams of multi-disciplinary practitioners providing an array of evidence-based medical, psychological and social interventions based on user and carer need, represents a quantum leap in organizational development (cf. Chapter 8).

The Workforce Action Team

Following publication of the NSF, DH set up the Workforce Action Team (WAT) to advise on the workforce implications. The WAT set out some 'guiding principles' for positive change. These include the following:

- The education and training provided must ensure that the workforce is competent to understand the evidence base of their work (and its limits) and be able to take this into account in delivering services.
- Pre- and post-qualifying education and training must provide the competencies required to deliver the *NSF for Mental Health*.
- Lifelong learning and continuing professional development should be actively promoted, with staff given the necessary supervision and support to enable them to ensure their continuing fitness for practice.
- The workforce should be trained to deal with the emotional impact of their work and actively to seek lifelong support and supervision within the framework of an appropriate human resources policy.
- Staff involved in the delivery of training and supervision in the workplace should be trained and supported in these roles.
- Staff involved in the delivery of education and training should have an understanding and experience of contemporary practice.
- Service users and carers should be involved in planning, providing and evaluating education and training.
- Education and training provided must ensure that the workforce can operate collaboratively and effectively in multi-professional and multi-agency contexts.

The Capability Framework

A key component of the WAT Report is the work completed by the Sainsbury Centre for Mental Health, *The Capable Practitioner* (Lindley *et al.* 2001). This document describes a framework of capabilities, which encompass the requisite skills, knowledge, values and attitudes of the multi-disciplinary mental health workforce to effectively deliver the type of services envisioned in the *NSF for Mental Health*.

Capability as a concept not only includes the element of competence or skill, but in addition captures the more fundamental requirements of effective practice, namely appropriate attitudes, values and relevant knowledge. Moreover, the concept of capability emphasizes the necessity of the transfer of acquired learning into the workplace.

To be capable in mental health care practitioners need:

- the ability effectively to implement evidence-based interventions within the service configurations specified in the *NSF for Mental Health*;
- judgement and decision-making capacity to apply appropriate effective interventions under complex, potentially stressful conditions, which adhere to agreed performance levels in the workplace;
- the ability to manage their own learning in the workplace, and to learn from experience, so as to build in the capacity for continuous improvement through lifelong learning;
- awareness of ethical considerations which integrate awareness of culture and values into professional practice; and

- the ability effectively to problem-solve and remove barriers to effective practice in the workplace, and to develop a working environment more conducive to the delivery of effective interventions.

Parameters

Development of the framework included an analysis of the requirements both professional and professionally non-affiliated staff needed to fulfil in order to deliver effective care to all working-age adults (not just those with severe long-term mental illness) within the new services outlined within the *NHS Plan* and *NSF for Mental Health*. This included all the key professional disciplines of psychiatry, nursing, occupational therapy, social work and clinical psychology along with those workers described as non-professionally aligned.

There was no attempt within the framework to differentiate levels of expertise between the disciplines. This is rightly a matter for the accrediting and professional bodies to determine. However, there is a clear message with the framework that while it is essential that the various multi-disciplinary groups have some common foundation of capability or core competencies, there is also a need for specialization and development of higher levels of capability among the multi-disciplinary groups.

Underlying principles and structure

This section provides a summary of the underlying principles and structure of the Capability Framework. For a full description please refer to *The Capable Practitioner* report (Lindley *et al.* 2001).

The purpose of the framework is to ensure that interventions are 'capable' across the comprehensive range of settings that, within the specifications of the *NSF for Mental Health*, constitute an integrated mental health service. This encompasses primary care, acute inpatient care, community-based crisis resolution teams, assertive outreach, residential and day care, and specialist secure and forensic settings.

The Capability Framework can perhaps be best seen as a broad inclusive 'map' of the knowledge, skills values and attitudes required of the mental health workforce that will enable it to deliver such effective interventions, in this complex array of different settings. These domains of the framework include:

- ethical practice;
- knowledge;
- process of care;
- interventions.

Table 6.4 summarizes the content outlines of the framework. The *NSF for Mental Health* was critically studied to ensure that all the standards were carefully and comprehensively covered. The second column in Table 6.4 indicates for each domain of the Capability Framework the NSF standards it is designed to apply to. There is also a final component, which is the application of these domains to a variety of mental health settings or systems.

Domains of Capability Framework	NSF standards	Indicative content
Ethical practice	1–7	Attitudes, values and codes of practice
Knowledge	1–7	Policy and legislation; models of mental health, evidence-based practice and mental health services
Process of care	14–16: NSF (1–7) 17–18: NSF (6) 19: NSF (1–7) 20: NSF (4, 5, 7) 21: NSF (4, 5) 22: NSF (22–25)	Effective communication; partnerships with users and carers; teamwork and team liaison; comprehensive assessment; care planning, care coordination and review; supervision, professional development and lifelong learning; clinical and practice leadership
Interventions	26–30: NSF (1–7) 31–34: NSF (2–7) 35–36: NSF (1)	Medical and physical care Social and practical Psychosocial interventions: ■ Early intervention ■ Early signs monitoring and relapse prevention ■ Psycho-education ■ Crisis intervention ■ Cognitive behavioural individual and family interventions ■ Therapeutic strategies for alcohol or drug misuse ■ Psycho-education

Table 6.4 Summary of content outline of the capability domains

Ethical practice

The framework of capabilities for modern mental health work makes basic assumptions about the underlying *NSF for Mental Health* values and principles of care (Table 6.1). Such standards are at the core of mental health practice and are seen as cross-cutting themes throughout all the domains of the Capability Framework. For the purpose of this model it is assumed that as a starting point, all mental health workers will base their practice on these values.

Knowledge

Knowledge is the foundation of effective practice. The capability of a single practitioner involves constant interplay between knowledge and the practical application of mental health skills. The framework suggests the need for four kinds of specialized knowledge: policy and legislation, current understandings of mental health and mental illness, research evidence on effective care and treatment to optimize recovery, and models of mental health service delivery.

This includes knowledge of the policy outlined in this chapter and knowledge of any new legislation once enacted. A good understanding of the CPA and its operation would also be required. Other important components of knowledge include the various explanatory models of mental health and the evidence which underpin them, and knowledge of mental health and mental illness in terms of causation, incidence, prevalence, description of disorders and the impact on individuals, families and communities. Understanding of the evidence base for effective interventions, including medical, psychological, social and environmental interventions along with service delivery models is also essential.

The statements in the framework for this domain denote the knowledge required by *most* of the mental health workforce.

Process of care

The process of delivering mental health care involves working within a social system (the NHS, Social Services, the community at large), a legal system (such as the Mental Health Act and Mental Capacity Act), within policy frameworks (the Care Programme Approach and clinical governance) and with the range of services available in the community and resources and expertise that exist within teams of multi-disciplinary practitioners.

Specific capabilities are required to optimize the relationship with carers and families and the network of care available to the service user. Finally, the relationship with the service user must encourage user participation and utilize the understanding of each individual's experience.

The capabilities for effective care coordination in the Capability model are divided as follows:

1 effective communication;
2 effective partnership with users and carers;
3 effective partnership in teams and with external agencies;
4 comprehensive assessment;
5 care planning, coordination and review;
6 supervision, professional development and lifelong learning;
7 clinical and practice leadership.

The statements in the framework for this domain denote the process of care capabilities required by *some* of the mental health workforce.

Interventions

The *NSF for Mental Health* undertakes its own 'evidence-based review' of psychosocial interventions, on the basis of which it recommends the implementation of those interventions. The review for each particular intervention is brief and far from comprehensive. The interventions and services described by the *NSF for Mental Health* with respect to people with severe mental illness include:

- early intervention;
- early signs monitoring and relapse prevention;
- cognitive behavioural interventions;
- behavioural family intervention;
- assertive outreach;
- crisis resolution and home treatment;
- medication adherence;
- dual diagnosis.

The Capability Framework recognizes that part of effective care coordination is the capability to deliver these evidence-based interventions for facilitating recovery and meeting the needs of mental health service users, their carers and families.

Historically, this has been the domain of professional specialists, where specific interventions were linked to professional groups. This model outlines a range of interventions that need to be delivered, but does not specify which group of practitioners should deliver them. The capabilities described in the framework offer a range of interventions beyond the standard psychological models:

- medical and physical health care;
- psychological interventions;
- social and practical interventions;
- mental health promotion.

The statements for this domain reflect the increasing specialization of the framework and denote interventions required by *only a few* of the mental health workforce.

Applications

The provision of mental health care in the UK has moved towards the development of comprehensive services. The mental health workforce will need to draw on values, knowledge, process skills and a range of interventions that will enable them to practise effectively. But in reality, this practice will relate to specific service settings.

While the model attempts to map a broad brush of capabilities not specific to any setting or professional level, the final section of the model addresses the specific applications required for each of these areas that are distinct from the essential capabilities described in the previous section. These are:

1   primary care;
2   community-based care coordination (CMHT);
3   crisis resolution and early intervention;
4   acute inpatient care;
5   assertive outreach;
6   continuing care;
7   services for complex needs (such as dual diagnosis clients).

The Capability Framework is best understood as a conceptual map with sufficient detail to define the skills development agenda established by the NSF. Ethical practice is seen as the underpinning domain that *all* mental health workers must possess. Most workers should have good knowledge of mental health issues, such as policy and legislation, and models of mental health. Capabilities to deliver effective care coordination (i.e. process of care) should be applied by *some* workers, and interventions, perhaps the realm of the more specialist worker, should be practised by *only a few* workers. The final domain in the framework describes the specific service settings in which practice takes place (i.e. their application).

The ten essential shared capabilities

Building on the Capable Practitioner, the NHS University, the National Institute for Mental Health, and the Sainsbury Centre for Mental Health in 2005 produced a learning pack for mental health practice: *The Ten Essential Shared Capabilities* (NHSU 2005). This takes on board more recent policy developments such as the Social Exclusion Unit report together also with the momentum that has developed around the concept of 'recovery'.

The ten essential shared capabilities are:

1. working in partnership
2. respecting diversity
3. practising ethically
4. challenging inequality
5. promoting recovery
6. identifying people's needs and strengths
7. providing service user-centred care
8. making a difference
9. promoting safety and positive risk taking
10. personal development and learning.

These are broadly reflected in the National Occupational Standards for Mental Health which were published shortly afterwards.

From values into action

From the point of view of mental health nursing the most important document of recent years has been the Chief Nursing Officer's review of mental health nursing (DH 2006b).

The Chief Nursing Officer carried out the review in order to address the question: How can mental health nursing contribute to the care of service users in the future?

The recommendations of the review covered three key domains:

Putting values into practice:

■ Mental health nursing should incorporate the principles of the Recovery Approach into every aspect of their practice. This means working towards aims that are meaningful to service users, being positive about change and promoting social inclusion for mental health users and carers ...

■ All mental health nurses need to do what they can so that all groups in society receive an equitable service ...

Improving outcomes for service users:

■ Developing and sustaining positive therapeutic relationships. should form the basis of all care.

■ Mental health nursing should take a holistic approach, seeing service users as whole people and taking into account their physical, psychological, social and spiritual needs.

■ Inpatient care should be improved.

■ Mental health nurses need to be well trained in risk assessment and management. They should work closely with service users and others to develop realistic individual care plans.

A positive, modern, profession:

■ Mental health nurses should (focus) on working directly with people with high levels of need and supporting other workers to meet less complex needs.

■ Pre-registration training courses should be reviewed to ensure that essential competencies are gained.

■ Career structures should be reviewed according to local needs and a range of new nursing roles should be developed.

■ The recruitment and retention of mental health nurses needs to be improved.

Future practice

By way of a conclusion to this chapter we summarize its content and examine its implications for mental health nurses. Mental health problems are common and affect all of us in one way or another. In the past the psychiatric hospital was the only place for specialist mental health care and all qualified nurses worked in these hospitals. Gradually hospital care has become less prominent. Mental health nurses have for many years been working in community settings and more recently in community mental health teams with other professionals. From 1998 onwards there has been a flood of policy initiatives that are beginning to influence care. Nurses need to know about current policy as part of the knowledge base towards becoming capable practitioners. Equally, they will need to practise ethically and be skilled at delivering effective interventions within the framework of a sound process of care delivery. The presentation of mental health problems is also beginning to change, with a massive increase in drug dependency problems in the last decade.

For mental health nurses there are massive implications, as our crystal ball shows:

■ **User-centred practice**: nurses of tomorrow will be expected to work in partnership with people who use mental health services, their families and their communities, possibly using a recovery model as proposed in the recent review of mental health nursing;

■ **Specialization**: there is already an array of different types of mental health care service based in many varied settings. Nurses will no longer be able to shift effortlessly from one service type to another. They will develop highly specialized skills in their chosen service area and they may identify more with this service area and the other professionals they work alongside than with the nursing profession;

■ **Public mental health**: there is an increasing policy drive to develop services and interventions that support public mental health. This trend is set to continue in the coming decades and mental health nurses will need to contribute their specialist knowledge to this agenda. For some this will require a shift in orientation from individualized care to developing a community awareness and its associated public level interventions.

■ **New staff groups**: as mental health services expand they will continue to recruit a more varied workforce who do not hold traditional qualifications. Nurses will more often become enablers, facilitators, educators, supervisors and consultants, rather than being expected to deliver most of the hands-on care;

- **Continuous development and change**: nurses can expect their roles and the world around them to keep changing. The expectation of lifelong learning has emerged. Also, services need to keep improving and change management has become a core skill for nurses working at all levels. A good example is the way that dual diagnosis interventions for people with coexisting mental health and drug and alcohol problems have moved from a specialist service to a core skill for all mental health staff;
- **Information management and technology** (**IM&T**): all nurses will be expected to use IM&T not just to maintain patient data, but also to manage patient care and access and use the knowledge base;
- **Primary mental health care:** nurses may increasingly work in primary and intermediate care delivering assessment together with variety of interventions including talking therapies.

Acknowledgements

This chapter draws on our work while at the Sainsbury Centre for Mental Health (both authors) and the Mental Health Foundation (Dr McCulloch), much of which was undertaken collaboratively with colleagues.

Questions for reflection and discussion

1   What are the three biggest challenges posed by policy to my personal practice or to my team?
2   How in my personal practice can I both empower users and improve public safety at the same time, or do occasions arise when this is impossible?
3   Is current government policy feasible and if not what elements of it need to go on hold?
4   How do my skills, knowledge and attitudes relate to the Capable Practitioner Framework and/or to the Ten Essential Shared Capabilities?

Annotated bibliography

- Department of Health (1999) *National Service Framework for Mental Health.* London: The Stationery Office. The main policy document relating to mental health services in England, the NSF for Mental Health contains not only the standards but a wealth of readable information as a rationale for each standard.
- www.csip.org.uk and www.dh.gov.uk: The Department of Health and the Care Services Improvement Partnership websites carry all the policy guidance. In particular the implementation guides are relevant to all people connected with the mental health field.
- www.scmh.org.uk: The Sainsbury Centre for Mental Health (an independent charity) website has a number of topic guides relating to issues such as primary care, assertive outreach and crisis resolution.
- The Mental Health Foundation (2007) *The Fundamental Facts: The Latest Facts and Figures on Mental Health.* London: Mental Health Foundation. A favourite of both the

authors. This report is attractively presented and gives headline information on mental health problems and associated socio-economic factors. The MHF website is at www.mentalhealth.org.uk.

■ Singleton, N., Bumpstead, R., O'Brien, M., Lee, A. and Meltzer, H. (2000) *Psychiatric Morbidity among Adults Living in Private Households*: *Summary Report*. London: Office for National Statistics (available for download from www.statistics.gov.uk). Straight facts and figures. A range of further reports have been published from this large scale survey.

References

Appleby, L. (2007) *Breaking Down Barriers*. London: DH.

Association of Public Health Observatories (2007) *Indications of Public Health in the English Regions: 7: Mental Health*. York: Association of Public Health Observatories.

Department for Education and Skills/Department of Health (2004) *National Service Framework for Children, Young People and Maternity Services*. London: DH.

Department of Health (1998a) *Modernising Mental Health Services: Safe, Sound and Supportive*. London: DH.

Department of Health (1998b) *Working Together: Securing a Quality Workforce for the NHS*. Wetherby: DH.

Department of Health (1999) *A National Service Framework for Mental Health*. London: The Stationery Office.

Department of Health (2000a) *The NHS Plan: A Plan for Investment, A Plan for Reform*. London: DH.

Department of Health (2000b) *Improving Working Lives Standard*. London: DH.

Department of Health (2001a) *National Service Framework for Older People*. London: DH.

Department of Health (2001b) *Working Together, Learning Together, A Framework for Lifelong Learning for the NHS*. London: DH.

Department of Health (2002) *HR in the NHS Plan*. London: DH.

Department of Health (2004a) *The National Service Framework for Mental Health – Five Years On*. London: DH.

Department of Health (2004b) *Choosing Health: Making healthy choices easier* London: DH.

Department of Health (2006a) *Learning for Change in Healthcare*. London: DH.

Department of Health (2006b) *From Values to Action: The Chief Nursing Officer's review of mental health nursing*. London: DH.

Department of Health (2008) *High Quality Care for All*. London: DH.

Department of Health and Social Security (1975) *Better Services for the Mentally Ill*. London: HMSO.

HM Treasury (2003) *Every Child Matters*. London: HMSO.

Lindley, P., O'Halloran, P. and Juriansz, D. (2001) *The Capable Practitioner*. London: Sainsbury Centre for Mental Health.

McCrone, P., Dhanasiri, S., Patel, A., Knapp, M. and Lawton-Smith, S. (2008) *Paying the Price: the cost of mental health care in England to 2026*. London: King's Fund.

McCulloch, A., Muijen, M. and Harper, H. (2000) New developments in mental health policy in the United Kingdom. *International Journal of Law and Psychiatry* **23**(3–4): 261–76.

McCulloch, A., Glover, G. and St John, T. (2003) The National Service Framework: Past, Present and Future. *Mental Health Review* **8**(4): 7–17.

National Audit Office (2007) *Improving Services and Support for People with Dementia*. London: The Stationery Office.

NHS University (2005) *The Ten Essential Shared Capabilities*. London: NHS University.

Office of the Deputy Prime Minister (2004) *Mental Health and Social Exclusion*. London: Office of the Deputy Prime Minister.

Rose, D. (2001) *Users' Voices*. London: Sainsbury Centre for Mental Health.

CHAPTER 7

Law and ethics of mental health nursing

Philip Fennell, Toby Williamson and Victoria Yeates

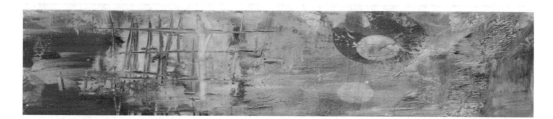

Chapter overview

Mental ill health and learning disability nursing pose more acute legal and ethical issues than any other branch of medicine. The vast majority of mentally disordered people consent to their treatment, and their decisions about their health care pose no threat to their own health or safety or the safety of other people. However, a minority of people with mental disorders cannot or will not accept that they are ill and may need treatment in their own interests or those of others. Some may even be so afflicted by mental disorder that they lack the capacity to make basic decisions about their care, to consent to treatment, or indeed to complain when they are the victims of abuse. Explanations and understandings of mental disorder can vary significantly between different professions and individual practitioners, as well as between practitioners, service users and carers. These factors set mental disorder apart from other illnesses and result in difficult ethical and legal tensions. Overshadowing all is the stigma attached to mental disorder. This chapter will focus on the law of England and Wales although reference will also be made to the law in Scotland.

Our aim is to provide relatively detailed coverage of the legal aspects of mental health nursing practice. While it is not feasible to do this within the word constraints of a single chapter, the launch of the *Art and Science of Mental Health Nursing* (ASMHN) website to support this textbook provides us with this opportunity. Our approach is to cover the key issues here and to refer readers to more detailed coverage of the same material and additional supplementary material on the website, which can be accessed at www.openup.co.uk/normanryrie.

There are three main sources of legal rules governing good clinical practice in mental health nursing:

- the common law developed by the decisions of the judges;
- specific mental health and mental capacity legislation enabling patients to be deprived of their liberty and treated without consent; and
- international obligations under the European Convention on Human Rights, and other international Conventions such as the UN Convention on the Rights of the Child.

In legal terms mental disorder is given special status. This is reflected in the arrangements which exist to detain and treat mentally disordered patients without consent, both under specific mental health legislation and under mental capacity legislation. However, different legislative regimes operate within the United Kingdom. The Mental Health Act (MHA) 1983 and the Mental Capacity Act 2005 apply to England and Wales. Northern Ireland has its own Mental Health Order and no specific mental capacity legislation. Scotland has the Mental Health (Care and Treatment) (Scotland) Act 2003 and the Adults with Incapacity (Scotland) Act 2000. Each has its own accompanying Code of Practice accessible at www.scotland.gov.uk. In England and Wales the Mental Health Act 1983 has been amended by the Mental Health Act 2007, most of which came into force in October 2008. Subsequent references to the MHA 1983 or 'the 1983 Act' are to the Mental Health Act 1983 as amended by the Mental Health Act 2007. The 1983 Act allows for the detention and forcible treatment of patients suffering from mental disorder of a sufficiently serious nature or degree to warrant treatment in the interests of their own health or safety or for the protection of others. Nurses have various statutory powers and functions under the 1983 Act. They may detain patients who are seeking to leave hospital using the nurse's holding power; or they may use reasonable force to administer treatment which a detained patient or community patient is required to accept under the MHA 1983. Suitably qualified nurses are eligible to act as responsible clinicians (RCs). Treatment without consent under the MHA 1983 is only possible if the treatment is for mental disorder, if the patient is detained and subject to Part IV, or is a community patient when treatment may be given in limited circumstances subject to new Part IVA. Compulsory treatment of a detained patient is lawful provided it is sanctioned by a second opinion doctor, regardless of the patient's capacity to consent (MHA 1983, s 58).

Specific legislation in England, Wales and Scotland also allows for adults who lack mental capacity to make decisions about treatment they may require to be given any treatment for their physical or mental illness which is necessary in their best interests (Northern Ireland at present does not have specific legislation and is therefore reliant upon the judge-made common law). In England and Wales the Mental Capacity Act 2005 applies and in Scotland the relevant legislation is the Adults with Incapacity (Scotland) Act 2000. Both pieces of legislation establish principles, procedures and safeguards for supporting people to make decisions for themselves, including ways in which people can plan for a situation where they may lack the capacity to make decisions in the future. They also provide for situations where decisions need to be made on a person's behalf because they lack the capacity to make the decision themselves. However there are also significant differences between the two pieces of legislation – this chapter will consider the law in England and Wales. (For more information on the law in Scotland see www.scotland.gov.uk for relevant Codes of Practice.) In Northern Ireland mentally incapacitated patients may be treated under common law without their consent, and reasonable force may be used to administer treatment which is necessary in the patient's best interests.

Issues of confidentiality also loom large in psychiatric nursing, and there is a considerable body of case law both of the English Courts and the European Court of Human Rights on the circumstances where patient confidentiality may be breached to protect health or the rights and freedoms of others. Nurses have other common law powers and duties. They owe a duty of confidentiality to patients not to disclose personal information about patients unless there is some overriding public interest. This duty of confidence is reinforced by terms in nurses' contracts of employment, and in *Ashworth Hospital v Mirror Group Newspapers* (2002) it was held that hospitals may, in certain cases, obtain an order that a journalist disclose the identity of any member of their staff who breaches professional confidence.

For the purposes of the Human Rights Act 1998 a nurse exercising powers to detain or restrain a patient would be likely to be found to be acting as a public authority – 'any person or body certain of whose functions are of a public nature'. Section 6 of the Human Rights Act 1998 makes it unlawful for a public authority to act in a way which is incompatible with a Convention Right, unless the public authority was required to act in that way by legislation. It is therefore important for nurses to understand the basic requirements of the European Convention on Human Rights.

This chapter covers:

- The sources of ethical guidance and legal rules and their interrelationship;
- Ethical guidance and the powers of the Nursing and Midwifery Council;
- The nurse's duty of care and the common law of negligence;
- The powers of nurses to restrain a patient from leaving hospital under the Mental Health Act 1983;
- Treatment of adults who lack capacity under the Mental Capacity Act 2005, including powers of restraint and detention;
- Treatment of detained patients for mental disorder without consent;
- Confidentiality and the duty to disclose information;
- The influence of the Human Rights Act 1998;
- Brief consideration of wider ethical issues.

Omitted from this chapter, but covered in supplementary material on the ASMHN website www.openup.co.uk/normanryrie is:

- special legal arrangements to address the interface between the Mental Health Act 1983 and the Mental Capacity Act 2005, which exist, in part, to ensure that the Mental Capacity Act is not used inappropriately to detain people for a mental disorder;
- treatment of children under mental health legislation.

The Mental Health Act 1983 and the Mental Capacity Act 2005

In England and Wales there are two relevant statutory regimes for mental health and learning disability nurses, the Mental Health Act 1983 and the Mental Capacity Act 2005.

1. Treatment of mental disorder under the Mental Health Act 1983 as amended by the Mental Health Act 2007

The Mental Health Act 1983 as amended by the Mental Health Act 2007 provides for the detention and treatment of people who suffer from mental disorder, either as inpatients or subject to supervised community treatment (SCT). This chapter provides an overview of these powers and how they should be used. To be subject to compulsory powers a person must be suffering from mental disorder. Mental disorder is widely defined as 'any disorder or disability of the mind' and so is an umbrella term covering mental illness, personality disorder, autistic spectrum disorder, and learning disability.

Personality disorder

The Diagnostic and Statistical Manual of the American Psychiatric Association (DSM-IV) describes personality disorder as 'an enduring pattern of inner experience and behaviour that deviates markedly from the individual's culture' (cf. Chapter 26). The enduring pattern must be inflexible and pervasive across a wide range of personal and social situations, and must lead to clinically significant distress or impairment in social, occupational or other important areas of functioning. The pattern must also be stable and of long duration and its onset must be traceable back at least to adolescence or early adulthood.

Learning disability

The application of the MHA to learning disability is limited. New s 1(4) of the MHA 1983 defines learning disability as 'a state of arrested or incomplete development of the mind which includes significant impairment of intelligence and social functioning'. There must be a state of arrested or incomplete development of the mind, and it must include significant impairment of intelligence and social functioning.

Addiction or sexual deviancy

'Dependence on alcohol or drugs is not considered to be a disorder or disability of the mind' (Section 1(3) of the MHA 1983). This does not mean that addicts are excluded entirely from the scope of the MHA 1983. A person may have a mental disorder which is completely unrelated to their dependence on alcohol or drugs. Excess consumption of alcohol or drugs may precipitate recognized forms of mental illness such as Korsakoff's Syndrome, drug induced psychoses, delirium consequent on withdrawal, or depression.

The removal of the exclusion in relation to sexual deviancy in the 1983 Act is intended to remove obstacles to detention under the Mental Health Act of paedophiles, since paedophilia is a form of sexual deviancy but it is also classified as paraphilia in the Diagnostic and Statistical Manual IV of the American Psychiatric Association.

Mental disorder of a nature or degree warranting compulsory powers

Not only must a person be suffering from mental disorder but it must be of a kind or degree warranting confinement, reception into guardianship or a community treatment order. Determining whether mental disorder is of the relevant nature or degree warranting treatment in hospital depends on whether the relevant admission criteria (necessity for own health or safety or for the protection of others and availability of appropriate treatment) are met. The disorder must be of a nature or degree making it appropriate for the person to receive treatment in hospital. Treatment in hospital must be necessary in the interests of the person's own health or safety or for the protection of other persons.

The MHA has an accompanying Code of Practice (DH 2008) to provide statutory guidance to anyone using the powers in the MHA 1983. Nurses should be familiar with the Code; if a nurse does not follow the Code they must be able to give convincing reasons why not. The Welsh Assembly will be issuing its own Code of Practice, which at the time of writing has yet to be published.

2. Treatment of mental or physical disorder in people who lack capacity because of mental disability

The Mental Capacity Act (MCA) 2005 provides a framework for making decisions of behalf of people who lack mental capacity because of mental disability and to enable a person to plan ahead for the day when he or she may lose decision-making capacity. Under s 3 of the MCA 2005 a person's capacity is to be assessed by asking whether there is any mental disability (disturbance or disability of mind or brain) which renders him or her unable to communicate a decision, unable to understand and retain relevant treatment information, or unable to use and weigh that information in the balance as part of the process of arriving at a decision. Mental disability is wide enough to include learning disability without abnormally aggressive or seriously irresponsible conduct. It is also wide enough to include mental illness. The MCA provides a defence to anyone (D) who carries out an act of care or treatment if they take reasonable steps to ascertain whether the person (P) has capacity, reasonably believes that P lacks capacity and reasonably believes that the act is in P's best interests. Such acts can include treatment for mental or physical disorder, although for serious treatments extra safeguards apply. However, there are limitations placed upon this regarding the use of restraint with someone who lacks capacity, such as physically guiding someone who is not safe to move around independently. Any form of restraint including physical restraint can only be used if it is reasonably believed it is necessary in order to prevent the person from coming to harm and the action is in proportion to the seriousness and the likelihood of the potential harm.

The MCA also provides procedures to deprive incapacitated adults of their liberty where necessary in their best interests. The MCA applies to anybody over the age of 16 (with a few exceptions). It includes important principles which should be applied in any situation involving mental capacity issues covered by the Act. These include always starting from an assumption of capacity, supporting someone to make and communicate their decision, and not assuming a lack of capacity just because the person's decision appears unwise or eccentric. The Act establishes a simple legal test of capacity, and the assessment of capacity must only be in relation to the specific decision that needs to be made (the 'functional test'). This test could apply to any decision including simple decisions about daily care as well as more serious decisions in relation to consent to treatment. The Act does not require specific professions to assess a person, so in many situations nurses, as they do now, would carry out the assessment, though where more serious decisions were involved it may be necessary to involve a more senior clinician.

Section 2 of the MCA 2005 states that a person lacks capacity if they are unable to make a decision, and s 3(1) sets out the test to be met if a person is to be found unable to make the relevant decision. The person must be unable because of a temporary or permanent impairment or disturbance in the functioning of mind or brain:

1. to understand the information relevant to the decision;
2. to retain that information;
3. to use or weigh that information as part of the process of making the decision; or
4. to communicate his decision (whether by talking, using sign language or any other means).

Relevant treatment information includes information about the reasonably foreseeable consequences of deciding one way or another, or failing to make the decision.

If a person is assessed to lack capacity any decision made or action taken on behalf of the person must be done in their best interest and the Act provides a 'checklist' of how to determine best interests. This includes taking into account the wishes, feelings, beliefs and values of the person (including any written statements they may have made) and consulting with family members and others involved in the person's care where practicable and appropriate. Where a person has no-one else with whom it is appropriate to consult and the decision concerns serious medical treatment or a change in hospital or residential care for the individual an Independent Mental Capacity Advocate (IMCA), a new role established under the Act, must be involved and consulted with by the decision-maker when determining the person's best interests.

The Act also provides a way of enabling people to plan ahead should they lose capacity in the future. People over the age of 18 can make an advance decision to refuse treatment (referred to elsewhere as a 'living will' or 'advance directive') whereby they can specify particular treatments they would not want to have and in what circumstances, should they lose the capacity to refuse it in the future. To be valid the decision has to be made while the person still has capacity to make the treatment decision, it must specify clearly the treatment being refused, and must be clear about the circumstances in which it is to apply. This means that a patient can refuse specified treatment for mental disorder, or to be admitted to hospital for treatment of mental disorder, and if the decision is valid and applicable it will prevent the person being admitted or given the relevant treatment under the Mental Capacity Act should they later lose capacity. However, an advance decision refusing admission and medication for mental disorder may be overridden by detention and treatment under the Mental Health Act. Unless it is immediately necessary to save the patient's life or to prevent serious deterioration in his or her condition, electroconvulsive therapy (ECT) may not be given to a patient who has made a valid and applicable advance decision refusing the treatment, even if the patient is detained under the MHA 1983.

The MCA 2005 also allows a person over the age of 18 to make a Lasting Power of Attorney (LPA) whereby they choose someone (the 'attorney') to make decisions on their behalf should they lose capacity in the future. These could be decisions about the person's money, property, health or personal welfare.

The MCA 2005 also establishes a new Court of Protection to deal with any mental capacity issues covered by the Act. The Court will be able to resolve complex or disputed cases and can make declarations about whether someone has capacity or not, make decisions on behalf of someone who lacks capacity, or appoint a deputy where a series of decisions need making. The deputy would have to make those decisions in the person's best interest and together with LPAs, it is therefore possible that nurses may find themselves having to respect the decision of a deputy or attorney regarding consent to treatment for a person who lacks capacity (though the powers and deputies and attorneys are limited for people detained under the Mental Health Act).

The MCA 2005 has an accompanying Code of Practice to provide statutory guidance; anyone acting in a professional or paid role and working with a person who may lack capacity has a legal duty to have regard to the Code (Department for Constitutional Affairs 2007). This means nurses should be familiar with it and if a nurse does not follow the Code they must be able to give convincing reasons why not. The MCA also includes sections on research involving people who lack capacity, and a new criminal offence of ill treatment or wilful neglect.

The influence of the Human Rights Act 1998

The coming into force of the Human Rights Act 1998 has prompted a considerable body of case law in which the English Mental Health Act 1983 has been tested in various ways for its 'Convention compliance'.

The case law can be divided into two groups: first, cases concerning detention and its review which mostly involve the protections against arbitrary detention in Article 5 of the European Convention on Human Rights (ECHR); and second, cases concerning the general rights of detained inpatients, engaging *inter alia* the right to life under Article 2, the protection against inhuman and degrading treatment in Article 3, the right to respect for correspondence, privacy and family life under Article 8, and the right to an effective remedy for human rights infringements under Article 13. In Convention terms the use of the nurse's holding power is a detention on grounds of unsoundness of mind under Article 5(1)(e). For a psychiatric detention to be lawful, unless it is an emergency there must be (1) objective medical evidence before a competent authority of a true mental disorder which is (2) of a kind or degree warranting confinement and (3) opportunities for review to ensure that conditions justifying initial detention continue to be met. Most detentions using the nurse's holding power will be emergency measures to prevent immediate threat to the patient or to others, and so it will be sufficient for the medical evidence to be obtained immediately after detention. The nurse will need to ensure that detention is necessary in the circumstances.

Sources of ethical guidance and their interrelationship with legal rules

There are several principal sources of ethical and policy guidance for nurses:

1   the *Code of Professional Conduct* of the Nursing and Midwifery Council (NMC 2008), and the Guidance issued by the Council on issues relevant to mental health nursing;
2   the *Code of Practice on the Mental Health Act 1983* published by the Department of Health and the Welsh Office;
3   the *Mental Health (Care and Treatment) (Scotland) Act 2003 Codes of Practice Volumes 1–3* (2005) published by the Scottish Executive;
4   the *Mental Capacity Act 2005 Code of Practice* (2007) published by the Ministry of Justice (formerly the Department for Constitutional Affairs);
5   the *Adults with Incapacity (Scotland) Act 2000: Code of Practice for Persons Authorized to carry out Medical Treatment or Research under Part 5 of the Act* (2008) published by the Scottish Executive.

The Nursing and Midwifery Council *Code of Professional Conduct* (2008) requires nurses to treat people in their care kindly and considerately, without discrimination as individuals, respecting their dignity, and acting as an advocate to help them access relevant health and social care, information and support. The Code emphasizes collaboration with the person being cared for, sharing with them information about their condition, listening to their concerns, meeting any language and communication needs, and responding to those concerns and preferences. The Code also requires respect for confidentiality. Disclosure may be justified on a need to know basis to other members of the care team and in such a case an explanation should be given to the service user about how and why information is shared by those who will be providing their care. Nurses have a duty to disclose information if they believe someone may be at risk of harm. The Code lays great emphasis on ensuring that nurses obtain consent for any course of treatment or care, respecting and upholding the right of a person with capacity to be fully involved in decisions about their treatment or care, and be aware of mental capacity legislation, ensuring that people who lack capacity remain at the centre of decision-making and are fully safeguarded. Where emergency care is provided or where care is provided under mental capacity legislation, a nurse must be prepared to demonstrate that he or she has acted in the patient's best interests. Nurses must maintain clear professional boundaries, particularly sexual boundaries, with people in their care, their families and carers.

The nurses' duty of care and the common law of negligence

Common law is the law developed through case-by-case precedent by the judges. Nurses owe a common duty of care to their patients, to avoid causing them injury by wrongful acts or omissions. The standard of care expected of a nurse is that of responsible practitioners skilled in the specialty. In order for a nurse to be liable in negligence, the patient or other person suing them must establish three basic elements:

1   that the nurse owed them a duty of care;
2   that the nurse breached that duty;
3   that the breach of duty caused them injury.

The first question is who is owed a duty of care. Nurses owe a duty of care to people who they should reasonably foresee as being likely to be injured by their acts or failure to act. This means that patients and clients are owed a duty of care, as are work colleagues. So the nurse in charge owes a duty of care to a vulnerable elderly mentally ill client who lacks mental capacity and who is seeking to leave the ward late at night in freezing temperatures. Equally, a nurse who is told by a patient that he or she intends to assault another member of staff would owe a duty of care to that colleague, to take reasonable steps to avoid that risk coming to pass.

The second issue in a negligence action is whether the nurse broke the duty, that is, fell short of the standard of care to be expected of a nurse. This means that expert witnesses are called to state what they would have considered to be acceptable nursing practice. In the hypothetical example of the frail elderly person with mental illness seeking to leave the ward in freezing temperatures, it would be hard to imagine any responsible body of nursing opinion coming forward to support allowing him or her to leave.

When a client needs inpatient care for mental disorder this may take place following informal admission, following detention under the Mental Health Act, or if the patient lacks capacity to consent to informal admission and deprivation of liberty is in their best interests, via the deprivation of liberty safeguards in the Mental Capacity Act 2005. Patients may be admitted informally. *The Mental Health Act Code of Practice* says that: 'On admission, all patients should be assessed for immediate and potential risks of going missing, suicide, self-harm and possible harm to others, and individual care plans should be developed including actions to be taken should any of these occur'(DH 2008: para. 15.3).

Patients who 'persistently and purposefully' attempt to leave a ward, whether or not they understand the risk, should be considered for formal detention under the Act. A registered mental health/learning disability nurse may hold the patient for up to six hours so that an assessment of the need to detain him or her may be made. Other nurses have the power to use reasonable force to restrain a mentally incapacitated patient where it is necessary to prevent harm to the patient, thus the need for nurses in carrying out their duty under the NMC *Code of Professional Conduct* to keep their knowledge and skills up to date, and to ensure that they possess the knowledge, skills and abilities required for lawful, safe and effective practice. Basic knowledge of the relevant law and ethical guidance is a requirement for lawful nursing practice.

The third issue in a negligence claim is whether the claimant has suffered injury as a result of the breach of duty. This means that the claimant must establish that his or her injury resulted from the negligence of the nurse and was not attributable to some other cause. Moreover the injury must be of a kind recognized by the law, which allows claims for recognized psychiatric illness or injury resulting from negligence, as well as for physical injury. The injury suffered must also be of a reasonably foreseeable kind. A whole vista of dire consequences would be reasonably foreseeable in the case of the frail elderly woman allowed to leave the ward late on a freezing cold night. If the woman died as a result of hypothermia, or falling into a river, the nurse could be sued for negligence. The employing hospital would be liable to meet the damages claim under the doctrine of vicarious liability whereby an employer is liable for the acts or omissions of his or her employee in the course of employment duties. In addition to suing for negligence, the relatives could ask the Health Service Commissioner (the Health Ombudsman) to investigate and report, and they could complain to the Nursing and Midwifery Council that the nurse was guilty of professional misconduct.

The Mental Health Act 1983

The main source of statutory powers and duties for mental health nurses is the Mental Health Act 1983, which governs the care and treatment of people suffering from mental disorder. The Mental Health Act 2007 has significantly amended the 1983 Act. The 2007 Act introduces a broader definition of mental disorder, recasts the criteria for compulsory admission, establishes new powers of Supervised Community Treatment. The 2007 Act creates the statutory roles of Approved Mental Health Professional (AMHP) (to replace the Approved Social Worker (ASW), Responsible Clinician (RC) (to replace the Responsible Medical Officer (RMO), as well as the completely new role of Independent Mental Health Advocate (IMHA). Nurses are eligible to seek qualification to perform the statutory functions of AMHPs. Appropriately qualified nurses are eligible to become Approved Clinicians, and an Approved Clinician (AC) is eligible to become a Responsible Clinician. The 2007 Act also introduces into the MCA 2005 new procedures to authorize deprivation of liberty of mentally incapacitated people.

The *Mental Health Act Code of Practice* (DH 2008) provides guidance to doctors, approved clinicians, managers and staff of hospitals, and approved mental health professionals on how they should undertake their duties under the Act, as well as on 'aspects of medical treatment for mental disorder more generally'.

Professional roles

Approved Mental Health Professionals

Applications for compulsory admission may be made by either the patient's nearest relative or an Approved Mental Health Professional (AMHP). Competent registered mental health/learning disability nurses may seek approval to act as an AMHP.

Responsible Clinicians and Approved Clinicians

The MHA 2007 replaces the role of Responsible Medical Officer (who had to be a doctor) with that of Responsible Clinician (RC). The RC in the case of a patient who is liable to be detained for assessment or treatment or who is a community patient is defined as 'the approved clinician with overall responsibility for the patient's case' (MHA 1983, s 34). The RC has significant powers such as the power to renew detention of a patient detained under s 3 for treatment, the power to send a patient on extended leave and to recall from leave, and the power to initiate Supervised Community Treatment. A Responsible Clinician must be an Approved Clinician.

The Approved Clinician Directions provide that not only doctors, but also social workers, nurses, chartered psychologists and occupational therapists, are eligible to seek approval as ACs from the Strategic Health Authority in England. In addition to the professional qualification, candidates for approval will have to demonstrate competencies in identifying the presence and severity of mental disorder and determining whether the disorder is of a kind or degree warranting compulsory confinement. They will also have to have completed the necessary approved clinician training. The responsibilities of an Approved Clinician are considerable and it is likely that only experienced senior clinicians will be able to meet the competencies required.

Informal and detained patients

Of the approximately 250,000 admissions to psychiatric hospitals which take place every year over 90 per cent are informal. Informal admission is appropriate for patients who have capacity and who consent to admission. In theory an informal patient is entitled to leave hospital at any time, but they may be prevented from doing so if staff decide that they need to remain in hospital and invoke the holding power under MHA 1983, s 5. The order of preference applicable to mental health admission is as follows: informal admission if the patient is capable and consents; admission under the MCA deprivation of liberty safeguards if the patient lacks capacity and deprivation is in his or her best interests; with detention under the Mental Health Act 1983 as a last resort where the patient is refusing treatment and there is danger to self or to others. Hence, although the Mental Health Act and the Mental Capacity Act both allow for detention and treatment without consent, a guiding principle of both Acts is the least restrictive alternative.

Detention under the Mental Health Act 1983

In order to be liable to detention or Supervised Community Treatment under the 1983 Act, a person must be suffering from mental disorder within the meaning of the Act, that is from 'any disorder or disability of the mind'.

Section 2 Admission for assessment

A person suffering from mental disorder may be detained under the 1983 Act for assessment for up to 28 days on the application of the patient's nearest relative or an AMHP, supported by two medical recommendations, one of which must be from a doctor approved under section 12 of the 1983 Act as having special expertise in the diagnosis or treatment of mental disorder (MHA 1983, s 2). A diagnosis of mental disorder is not enough on its own to justify detention. The disorder must be 'of a nature or degree which warrants detention for assessment with or without medical treatment'. Moreover, detention must be necessary in the interests of the patient's health *or* safety *or* for the protection of others. A mentally disordered person does not have to be behaving dangerously to self or others to be compulsorily admitted. They could be detained because it is necessary for their own health, including mental health.

There is an emergency procedure under section 4 of the MHA 1983 for admission for assessment where only one medical recommendation is necessary. The conditions for admission for assessment under section 2 must be met, and detention may continue for a maximum of 72 hours unless a second medical recommendation is furnished within that time to convert the emergency admission into a full 28-day admission for assessment. Until the second medical recommendation is furnished, the patient may not be given treatment without consent unless he or she lacks capacity to consent and the treatment is immediately necessary in his or her best interests.

Section 3 Admission for treatment

Section 3 of the 1983 Act provides for compulsory admission for treatment for up to six months, renewable for a further six months and thereafter at 12-monthly intervals. An application may be made by either the nearest relative or an AMHP and must be supported by medical recommendations given by two medical practitioners. Treatment for mental disorder includes nursing and also psychological intervention and specialist mental health habilitation, rehabilitation and care.

A patient who is detained under s 3 has the right to apply to the Mental Health Review Tribunal (MHRT) for discharge once within the first six months following admission, and once in each period for which the detention is renewed.

Section 5 The nurse's holding powers

A patient who initially consents to admission but later seeks to leave hospital may be restrained from doing so using the doctor's, approved clinician's or nurse's holding power under s 5 (4) of the MHA 1983.

The nurse's holding power enables a registered mental health or learning disability nurse to hold an inpatient in a psychiatric ward or hospital for not more than six hours. During that time the doctor or AC in charge of the patient's treatment or his or her deputy should attend to determine whether the managers should be furnished with a report.

The Mental Health Act Code (DH 2008: para. 12.25) emphasizes that: 'The decision to invoke the power is the personal decision of the nurse who cannot be instructed to exercise this power by anyone else.' The nurse's holding power can only be used *where the patient is receiving treatment for mental disorder as an inpatient*. The grounds for its use are:

1. that the patient is suffering from mental disorder to such a degree that it is necessary for his or her health or safety or for the protection of others that he or she be immediately restrained from leaving hospital; and
2. that it is not practicable to secure the immediate attendance of a practitioner (or clinician) for the purpose of furnishing a report.

In carrying out an assessment the Mental Health Act Code (DH 2008) para. 12.28 states that the following factors should be taken into account:

■ the patient's expressed intentions;
■ the likelihood of the patient harming themselves or others;
■ the likelihood of the patient behaving violently;
■ any evidence of disordered thinking;
■ the patient's current behaviour and, in particular, any changes in their usual behaviour;
■ whether the patient has recently received messages from relatives or friends;
■ whether the date is one of special significance for the patient (e.g. the anniversary of a bereavement);
■ any recent disturbances on the ward;
■ any relevant involvement of other patients;
■ any history of unpredictability or impulsiveness;
■ any formal risk assessments which have been undertaken (specifically looking at previous behaviour);
■ any other relevant information from other members of the multi-disciplinary team.

The nurse must record in writing on a statutory form the fact that the statutory criteria are satisfied, and must deliver the completed form to the managers or their appointed officer as soon as possible after completion but the six hours detention starts to run from the time when the nurse signed the form (Mental Health Act Code of Practice (DH 2008), para. 12.23). The reasons for invoking the power must be entered in the patient's nursing and medical notes. It is worth emphasizing that this power can be used only where an informal patient is receiving treatment as an inpatient for mental disorder; it cannot, for example, be used on a general hospital ward where the patient is receiving treatment for a physical disorder. A nurse invoking s 5(4) is entitled to use the minimum force necessary to prevent the patient from leaving hospital.

The nurse's holding power may only be used to restrain the patient from leaving hospital. The common law allows for reasonable force to be used in self-defence, for the defence of others, or to prevent a breach of the peace. These powers apply regardless of whether the person has capacity. They can only be used to justify detention or restraint within the hospital insofar as it is reasonably necessary, and only for so long as the risk of breach of the peace or crime persists. Hence, they would not authorize any restraint or seclusion to continue after the risk had passed.

Sections 5 and 6 of the MCA 2005 provide a legal defence for anyone who takes action that is in the best interests of a person who lacks capacity in relation to the decision to remain in hospital. This includes reasonable restraint where the restraint is imposed to prevent harm to the patient and is a proportionate response both to the likelihood of harm and the severity of the harm. In order for the action to be lawful the person taking it must have taken reasonable steps to determine whether the person has capacity in relation to the relevant decision, must reasonably believe that the person indeed lacks capacity, and must reasonably believe that what they are doing is in the person's best interests.

Supervised community treatment

The MHA 2007 introduced the new 'community treatment orders' or supervised community treatment (SCT). To be eligible for SCT the patient must be liable to be detained in hospital under section 3 or, if a Part 3 offender patient, be subject to a hospital order, a hospital direction or a transfer direction *without restrictions*. A patient who is subject to SCT is known as a 'community patient'.

The RC must be of the opinion that:

1.   the patient is suffering from mental disorder (any disorder or disability of mind) of a nature or degree which makes it appropriate for him or her to receive medical treatment;
2.   it is necessary for his or her health or safety or for the protection of other persons that he or she should receive such treatment;
3.   subject to his or her being liable to be recalled, such treatment can be provided without his or her continuing to be detained in a hospital;
4.   it is necessary that the responsible clinician should be able to exercise the power to recall the patient to hospital;
5.   appropriate medical treatment is available for him or her.

All of the above criteria must be satisfied for a patient to be eligible for SCT. The order will be made by the patient's Responsible Clinician (RC), who in the future could be a suitably qualified nurse.

A community treatment order must 'specify conditions to which the patient is to be subject'. Any conditions must be agreed between the RC and the AMHP. The only limitation on the scope of the conditions is that the RC and AMHP must agree that they are 'necessary or appropriate' for:

1.   ensuring that the patient receives medical treatment;
2.   preventing risk of harm to the patient's health or safety;
3.   protecting other persons (MHA 1983, s 17B).

A patient who is on s 17 leave from a hospital may have their leave revoked and be recalled to the hospital where they were detained if the RC considers it necessary in the interests of the patient's health or safety or for the protection of other persons. Revocation and recall are by the RC giving notice in writing 'to the patient or to the person for the time being in charge of the patient'.

A community patient may be recalled to any hospital if in the RC's opinion:

1.   the patient requires medical treatment in hospital for his or her mental disorder;

2. there would be a risk of harm to the health or safety of the patient or to other persons if the patient were not recalled to hospital for that purpose.

A patient may also be recalled for breach of a condition of a CTO, although this is not a necessary condition of recall.

The RC may also recall a community patient to hospital if the patient fails to comply with a condition of the CTO.

Self-determination and the right to be respected as an individual

Respecting the client as an individual is a core principle of the nursing *Code of Professional Conduct* (NMC 2008). It reflects the underlying function of the European Convention on Human Rights, the maintenance and promotion of the dignity of the individual. It is also reflected in the long title of the Council of Europe Convention on Human Rights and Biomedicine (1996) the convention for the protection of human rights and the dignity of the human being with regard to the application of biology and medicine (Beyleveld and Brownsword 2002). Other contributors to this book have emphasized the importance of treating the service user as a whole person, not just treating their mental disorder. Good mental health nursing is distinguished by its ability to respect personhood, to achieve the delicate balance between three aspects of respect for persons: respect for the service user's choices; respect for the service user's welfare, and respect for the rights and freedoms of other persons. At the same time there is a need to balance the choices of the sufferer against the rights of others, since mental disorder may impel sufferers, for example, through command hallucinations or severe depression to commit criminal acts. Respect for choices reflects the value placed on personal autonomy or the right of self-determination. Respect for welfare has connotations of paternalism or what some have sought less pejoratively to describe as 'parentalism'. Here emphasis is placed on making the treatment decisions that will promote the welfare and best interests of the person. Finally, respect for the rights and freedoms of others essentially means protecting the public against risks to their safety. Increasingly, government policy lays emphasis on risk assessment and risk management, and the goal of mental health policy is the management of the risk of suicide, self-harm, and violence to others.

A fundamental principle of all health care law is that adult patients with mental capacity have the right of self-determination, to determine what shall be done with their own body. But the right of self-determination is not absolute. Under the European Convention the relevant aims that may justify interference with personal autonomy are the protection of public safety and health and the protection of the rights and freedoms of others. Where we afford more respect to the patient's welfare than we do to their wishes and intervene for the protection of the individual's own health we are acting in a paternalist or parental fashion. Intervention for the public safety or for the protection of the rights for freedoms of others is based on what Cavadino (1989) has called police powers. Both types of intervention are justified under English Law.

Before proceeding to examine the legal possibilities to treat a person without consent it is important to emphasize that consent seeking is afforded high value as an ethical and legal principle. It enables patients to weigh up for themselves in accordance with their own value system the risks and benefits of proposed treatment and make their own decisions about what is in their interests. When treating mentally disordered patients whether or not detained, it is important to remember that though they are mentally disordered or are detained under the Mental Health Act it does not necessarily mean that they are incapable of giving a valid consent to treatment. The NMC *Guidelines for Mental Health and Learning Disabilities Nursing: A Guide to Working With Vulnerable Clients* (1998) stresses that nurses 'should not assume that patients are incompetent merely because they belong to a particular care group' and that it is 'important to devote as much time as necessary to explaining issues to clients in order to explore fully the consequences for them'.

Treatment for mental disorder is defined very widely in the Mental Health Act 1983, s 145(1) which provides that 'medical treatment' includes nursing, and also includes psychological intervention and specialist mental health habilitation, rehabilitation and care. The list in s 145 is non-exhaustive and treatment for mental disorder also includes such interventions as ECT and the administration of drugs, but it also includes basic nursing and care, as well as anything geared towards equipping or re-equipping the client with basic social and living skills.

The Code of Practice emphasizes that it is essential for patients being treated under the Mental Health Act to have a written treatment plan. This should be recorded in their notes, which should form part of a coherent care plan under the Care Programme Approach, and should be formulated by the multi-disciplinary team in consultation where practicable with the client. The treatment plan should include a description of the immediate and long-term goals for the patient and should give a clear indication of the treatments proposed and the methods of treatment. Wherever possible, the whole treatment plan should be discussed with the patient. Patients should be encouraged and assisted to make use of advocacy support available to them, if they want it. Where patients cannot (or do not wish to) participate in discussion about their treatment plan, any views they have expressed previously should be taken into consideration. If it is intended carers are to be involved in providing care during the currency of the care plan, plans should not be based on any assumptions about the willingness or ability of carers to support patients, unless those assumptions have been discussed and agreed with the carers in question.

There are three circumstances where English law allows a person to be treated without their consent. They are:

1   Where an adult lacks capacity to make the treatment decision they may, subject to certain limits, be given any treatment for mental or physical disorder which is necessary in their best interests under the Mental Capacity Act 2005.
2   Where a person is liable to be detained or subject to Supervised Community Treatment under the Mental Health Act 1983 the Act specifies the circumstances in which they may be given treatment without their consent, regardless of their capacity or lack of it, as long as the treatment is for mental disorder and it is appropriate for the treatment to be given.
3   A child who is incapable of consenting or is refusing treatment may be given any treatment which is necessary in their best interests provided there is consent from a person with parental responsibility for the child or from the Family Division of the High Court. Children requiring inpatient or outpatient treatment may be detained under the Mental Health Act.

Treatment of mentally incapacitated adults under the Mental Capacity Act 2005

The Mental Capacity Act provides that all adult patients who suffer from no mental incapacity have the right of self-determination, to determine whether to accept or refuse medical treatment, even if the result of refusal may be the patient's own death. It is for those alleging that a patient is incapable to establish on the balance of probabilities (that it is more likely than not) that the patient lacks capacity. The more serious (life-threatening) the decision, the greater the level of capacity required.

Under the common law, the defence of necessity applied to anyone carrying out an act of care or treatment on behalf of a mentally incapacitated adult provided that intervention was necessary in the person's best interests. The position is now governed by the Mental Capacity Act 2005, which provides a defence against a battery action to anyone carrying out an act of care and treatment where they have taken reasonable steps to establish whether the patient lacks capacity, they reasonably believe the person lacks capacity and they reasonably believe that what they are doing is in the patient's best interests.

The Mental Capacity Act 2005 sets out five statutory principles. They are:

1   a person must be assumed to have capacity unless it is established that they lack capacity;
2   a person is not to be treated as unable to make a decision unless all practicable steps to help him or her to do so have been taken without success;
3   a person is not to be treated as unable to make a decision merely because he or she makes an unwise decision;
4   an act done, or decision made, under this Act for or on behalf of a person who lacks capacity must be done, or made, in his or her best interests;
5   before the act is done, or the decision is made, regard must be had to whether the purpose for which it is needed can be as effectively achieved in a way that is less restrictive of the person's rights and freedom of action.

A patient lacks capacity in relation to a matter if, at the material time he or she is unable to make a decision for himself or herself in relation to the matter because of a temporary or permanent impairment of, or disturbance in the functioning of, the mind or brain. Note that a person lacks capacity 'in relation to a matter', making capacity task specific. People are not to be treated as incapable because they have a particular diagnosis. Incapacity is to be established on the balance of probabilities, the standard of proof in civil proceedings.

Incapacity

The person must be unable because of a temporary or permanent impairment or disturbance in the functioning of mind or brain:

1   to understand the information relevant to the decision;
2   to retain that information;
3   to use or weigh that information as part of the process of making the decision; or
4   to communicate his decision (whether by talking, using sign language or any other means).

Relevant treatment information includes information about the reasonably foreseeable consequences of deciding one way or another, or failing to make the decision.

The test of being unable to comprehend and retain material treatment information means that a person will lack mental capacity if they cannot understand a simple explanation of the fact that the doctors think they are ill and that the treatment proposed is intended to alleviate the symptoms or cure the illness. Capacity should always be assessed in relation to the actual treatment being proposed, and the 'broad terms' explanation of the treatment and its likely effects should be tailored to the level of mental ability of the client.

A person may comprehend the treatment information, but if they are unable to retain the information in their mind long enough to arrive at a decision they will lack mental capacity. This element in assessing incapacity is particularly evident in the mental illnesses of old age, Alzheimer's and other dementias. The person may understand the information at the time it is imparted, but be nevertheless unable to hold it in their head long enough to make a decision.

A person who is able to understand and retain the treatment information may still be incapable if they are incapable of using the information and weighing it in the balance as part of the process of arriving at a decision. An example would be a person reacting to the shock of a relationship breakdown who takes an overdose. That person may be perfectly capable of understanding the need for treatment by stomach wash or neutralizing drug, perfectly capable of believing that information and perfectly capable of understanding and believing that they will die if they do not have the treatment. But, if they say that life is not worth living because they have lost their partner or their job, are they capable of weighing the information in the balance to arrive at a decision? The effects of the shock and trauma of the relationship breakdown or of the depressive illness may be so disturbing their mental processes that they are unable to weigh the information in the balance to arrive at a decision. If they were to have treatment for their condition their decision might be very different. In such a case the doctors in the emergency department would assess the person as lacking mental capacity, and would administer the life-saving treatment as being necessary in the patient's best interests, using reasonable force if necessary. The person making the assessment of capacity must not make it merely on the basis of the person's age or appearance, or condition or an aspect of behaviour, which might lead others to make unjustified assumptions about his/her capacity to make decisions.

Best interests

It is a principle of the MCA 2005 that any act or decision, for or on behalf of a person who lacks capacity, must be done, or made, in his best interests.

Section 4 of the MCA 2005 sets out the approach to be adopted in assessing best interests. The person making the determination must not make it merely on the basis of the person's age or appearance, or condition, or an aspect of behaviour, which might lead others to make unjustified assumptions about what might be in his or her best interests. The assessor must take into account all the circumstances of which he or she is aware and which might reasonably be regarded as relevant. He or she must consider whether it is likely that the person will at some time have capacity in relation to the matter in question, and, if this appears likely, when that is likely to be.

The person making the best interests determination must, so far as reasonably practicable, permit and encourage the person to participate, or to improve his or her ability to participate, as fully as possible in any act done for him or her and any decision affecting him or her. If practicable and appropriate the decision-maker must consider the views of anyone named by the person to be consulted, any carer or person interested in his or her welfare, any donee of a lasting power of attorney granted by the person, and any deputy appointed by the Court of Protection.

Where the determination of best interests relates to treatment which those providing health care consider to be necessary to sustain life, the decision-maker must not, in considering whether the treatment is in the best interests of the person concerned, be motivated by a desire to bring about his or her death. As long as the processes and requirements of s 4 have been fulfilled, and the balance sheet test applied, there is sufficient compliance with the best interests requirement if the decision-maker reasonably believes that what he or she does or decides is in the best interests of the person concerned.

Defence in relation to acts of care, treatment and restraint done in the best interests of people who lack mental capacity is covered in supplementary material to this chapter which is available on the ASMHN website www.openup.co.uk/normanryrie.

Treatment under Part 4 of the Mental Health Act 1983

Part 4 of the MHA 1983 introduced a framework of powers to administer treatment for mental disorder without consent, subject to a system of second opinion safeguards. A patient's responsible clinician is in overall charge of the management of the case of a detained patient. If that RC is not a doctor, it is likely that for the purposes of treatment by medicines or ECT under Part 4 of the MHA 1983 the person in charge of the treatment will be another Approved Clinician who has the power to prescribe.

Section 57 Psychosurgery and surgical implants of hormones to reduce male sex drive

Section 57 specifies the treatments, psychosurgery and surgical hormone implants for the reduction of male sex drive, which cannot be given without both the patient's valid consent and a second opinion that the treatment is appropriate. This procedure must be observed whether or not the patient is detained.

Section 58 Medicines for Mental Disorder

Section 58 authorizes treatment without consent. Section 58 applies only to patients who are liable to be detained under powers authorizing detention for more than 72 hours, and who are not conditionally discharged restricted patients, or remand patients subject to s 35. Section 58 treatments (currently medicines for mental disorder) require either the patient's consent or a certificate from a second opinion appointed doctor stating that the patient is either (a) incapable of consenting, or (b) capable and refusing, but that the treatment ought to be given. Section 58 applies to medicines for mental disorder, but the patient only becomes eligible for a second opinion if 'three months or more have elapsed from the first occasion in that period [of detention] when medicine was administered to him by any means for his mental disorder' (MHA 1983, s 58(1)(b)). Medication does not necessarily have to be administered continuously throughout the three months.

Paragraph 23.37 of the Mental Health Act Code of Practice states: 'Although the Mental Health Act permits some medical treatment for mental disorder to be given without consent, the patient's consent should still be sought before treatment is given, wherever practicable. The patient's consent or refusal should be recorded in their notes, as should the treating clinician's assessment of the patient's capacity to consent.' Capacity and consent to treatment under s 58 may be certified either by the AC in charge of treatment or an SOAD.

If the patient is incapable of consenting or refuses, a second opinion is required. The SOAD may decide that the patient is capable and consents. In deciding whether drug treatment ought to be given without consent, the SOAD must be satisfied that 'it is appropriate for the treatment to be given'. Before making the decision the SOAD must consult two other people who have been professionally concerned with the patient's medical treatment, one of whom must be a nurse, and the other neither a nurse nor a doctor. Neither may be the RC or a doctor.

The Mental Health Act Commission's Guidance Note entitled *Nurses, the administration of medicines for mental disorder*, and the Mental Health Act 1983 GN 2/2001, draws attention to the three-month rule and states that it is the responsibility of the nurse administering the prescribed medication to patients detained under the 1983 Act to ensure that he or she is legally entitled to administer the medication. A copy of the form on which the patient's consent is certified and a description of the treatment is given, or the form on which the SOAD certifies that the treatment outlined on the form should be given should be kept with the medicine card. The nurse administering the treatment should:

- check the medicine card for date of entry of prescription for the medicine, its dose and route of administration;
- ensure that the three-month period has not been exceeded by checking the date of the first administration;
- ensure that where the patient has consented to medication beyond the three-month period, the form 38 is in place and correctly completed;
- ensure that where a second opinion has been obtained the Form 39 is in place and correctly completed;
- ensure that the administration of medicine is consistent with NMC professional guidance.

The Guidance Note also refers to PRN or 'as required' medication and states that this should be authorized on the statutory form if a second opinion has been obtained.

Section 62 Emergency treatment

Section 62 is intended to allow treatment to be given if a second opinion cannot be arranged sufficiently speedily to cope with an emergency, while at the same time protecting patients against hazardous or irreversible treatments.

Irreversible means having unfavourable irreversible physical or psychological consequences, and hazardous means entailing significant physical hazard. Moreover urgent treatment under these sections can continue only for as long as it remains immediately necessary. If it is no longer immediately necessary, the normal requirements for certificates apply.

Section 58A Electroconvulsive therapy

The MHA 2007 introduces a separate provision to deal with electroconvulsive therapy under new s 58A. This provides that, except in an emergency threatening life or serious deterioration in the patient's condition, ECT may not be given to a capable patient who is refusing the treatment.

As with medicines, the AC in charge of treatment certifies that an adult patient is capable and has consented. Section 58A means that ECT will no longer be able to be given without consent to an adult patient with capacity or a competent child patient who is refusing the treatment, unless it is an emergency covered by s 62(1A). Whether or not the patient is capable s 62(2) authorizes ECT in an emergency where immediately necessary to save life or prevent serious deterioration in the patient's condition.

Section 63 Other treatment for mental disorder

Section 63 of the Act provides that any medical treatment for mental disorder not specifically identified as requiring a second opinion may be given to a detained patient without consent, if it is given by or under the direction of the AC in charge of treatment. Treatment, which is broadly defined may include force-feeding, any treatment for the symptoms and sequelae of the mental disorder as well as treatment for the core disorder itself. So a stomach wash for a detained patient who had attempted suicide as a result of a depressive illness could be treated under s 63 as treatment of the sequelae of mental disorder.

Part 4A of the Mental Health Act 1983

Part 4A regulates treatment for mental disorder of mentally capable, mentally incapable and child patients who are subject to CTOs and who have not been recalled to hospital. The basic principle is that a patient with capacity (or competence if a child) may only be given treatment in the form of medicine for mental disorder if they consent and there is a certificate authorizing the treatment from an SOAD. If the patient is capable treatment may only be given without consent by recalling the patient.

Within one month of being placed on a CTO, a patient should be visited by an SOAD who authorizes the treatment which can be given while the patient is in the community and also specifies what treatment may be given if the patient is recalled to hospital. The requirement of authorization by an SOAD is called 'the certificate requirement', which is covered in supplementary material on the ASMHN website www.openup.co.uk/normanryrie.

Covert administration of medication

The NMC issued its most recent position statement in 2007 covering the covert administration of medicines, disguising medicine in food and drink. Since this involves treatment without consent, this may be authorized under the Mental Capacity Act 2005 if the patient lacks mental capacity and the treatment is necessary in their best interests, or under Section 58 of the Mental Health Act 1983 if the administration of medication covertly is expressly authorized by a certificate from an SOAD.

The position statement states that the NMC recognizes that there may be 'exceptional circumstances' in which covert administration may be considered to prevent a patient/client from missing out on essential treatment. In such circumstances and in the absence of informed consent, the following considerations may apply:

- The best interests of the patient/client must be considered at all times.
- The medication must be considered essential for the patient's/client's health and well-being, or for the safety of others.
- The decision to administer a medication covertly should not be considered routine, and should be a contingency measure. Any decision to do so must be reached after assessing the care needs of the patient/client individually. It should be patient/client-specific, in order to avoid the ritualized administration of medication in this way.
- There should be broad and open discussion among the multi-professional clinical team and the supporters of the patient/client, and agreement that this approach is required in the circumstances. Those involved should include carers, relatives, advocates and the multi-disciplinary team (especially the pharmacist). Family involvement in the care process should be positively encouraged. The method of administration of the medicines should be agreed with the pharmacist. It is very important that the method of administration be agreed with a pharmacist, since crushing tablets or dissolving them may alter the bio-availability of certain drugs.
- The decision and the action taken, including the names of all parties concerned, should be documented in the care plan and reviewed at appropriate intervals.

Regular attempts should be made to encourage the patient/client to take their medication. This might best be achieved by giving regular information, explanation and encouragement, preferably by the team member who has the best rapport with the individual. There should be a written local policy, taking into account the professional practice guidelines (NMC 2007).

Confidentiality and the duty to disclose information

Doctors and nurses owe a duty of confidentiality to keep private information which they have obtained in the course of treating patients. This is a general duty which is reinforced by nursing contracts of employment, and by the Code of Professional Conduct. Article 8 of the European Convention on Human Rights guarantees the right of respect for home, correspondence, privacy and family life. The right of respect for privacy includes the right of medical confidentiality. Information which is the subject of medical confidentiality may be disclosed with the consent of the patient if competent. Otherwise it can only be disclosed if it is in accordance with the law, and necessary in a democratic society for (*inter alia*) the protection of public safety, health or morals, or the protection of the health and rights of others. So a breach of confidentiality might involve a breach of the nurse's common law duty, a breach of the contract of employment, breach of the Human Rights Act, and professional misconduct.

The duty of confidence is not absolute. Under the European Convention Article 8(2) it may be interfered with if the interference is in accordance with law and necessary in a democratic society. As a matter of English law, the duty of confidence may be overridden if disclosure is necessary in the public interest. Disclosure must be for one of the following purposes: national security, public safety, economic well-being of the country, prevention of crime or disorder, the protection of health or morals, or the rights and freedoms of others. Moreover, the disclosure must be 'proportionate', that is, it must be only to the extent necessary and to the proper officials necessary to achieve the legitimate purpose.

Take the example of a Responsible Clinician considering the discharge of a detained patient, and that patient has told a nurse that he intended to kill his mother if discharged to her care. The nurse owes a duty of confidence to the patient, to keep confidential information obtained in the course of the nurse–patient relationship. However, there is also a duty under the Code of Professional Conduct to cooperate with others in the team and to act to identify and minimize risk to patients and clients.

Moreover, there is a duty of care owed to the mother who is an identifiable foreseeable victim of the patient if he or she is discharged. In such a case the nurse would be justified in passing this information to the RC, and if the RC did not take it seriously, to the hospital managers. The important aspect of decision-making in these circumstances is to ensure that disclosure is justified under one of the above purposes of public interest, that the public interest cannot be served without disclosure, and that disclosure is only to those who need to know to avert the threat to the public interest.

Inpatients' rights

States have a duty under Article 2 not to kill people by the use of force. They also have positive duties under Article 2 to take steps to protect the right to life. Those detaining psychiatric patients owe a duty to take reasonable care to prevent them from committing suicide.

The European Court of Human Rights has held that in respect of a person deprived of his or her liberty, recourse to physical force, which has not been made strictly necessary by his or her own conduct, diminishes human dignity and is in principle an infringement of Article 3. Treatment of a mentally ill person could be incompatible with the standards imposed by Article 3 in the protection of fundamental human dignity, even though that person might not be capable of pointing to any specific ill-effects in terms of physical injury or psychiatric illness. Detaining hospitals owe a duty to patients to carry out a risk assessment and to take reasonable care to avoid placing patients in a situation where they are at risk of suicide or being killed by others.

Control and treatment

Once detained, patients may be subject to a regime of control and treatment, which may vary in strictness according to the assessed level of risk. However, there could be inhuman or degrading treatment contrary to Article 3 if medical treatment, control, restraint or seclusion (1) causes physical or mental injury or (2) infringes human dignity by being more than strictly necessary to control the patient's behaviour. Medical treatment deemed necessary by responsible medical opinion will not in principle infringe Article 3. Nevertheless, treatment which is not severe enough to be inhuman or degrading may still breach Article 8 which states that everyone has the right to respect for his or her home, his or her correspondence, his or her family life and private life.

Policies

In a series of cases the English courts have been asked to review different hospital policies towards detained patients. Restrictions on children's visits to offender patients in special hospitals were held to be justified in a democratic society for the protection of the rights of children. Ashworth Hospital's policy on random monitoring of phone calls was held not to breach Article 8 as it was necessary to pursue a legitimate aim, and the hospital's refusal to issue condoms to patients was held not to breach Articles 2 or 8.

The decision to treat forcibly can engage the right of respect for privacy under Article 8, with the consequence that decisions to treat without consent must be proportionate and must be of the minimum interference necessary in order to achieve a legitimate aim such as health (including the health of the individual), or for the protection of the rights of others. Moreover, reasons must be given by RMOs and second-opinion doctors that explain which justification under Article 8(2) (health, the rights of others, etc.) applies to the treatment authorized.

Seclusion

The Code of Practice on the Mental Health Act 1983 (para. 15.43) defines seclusion as 'the supervised confinement of a patient in a room, which may be locked to protect others from significant harm. Its sole aim is to contain severely disturbed behaviour which is likely to cause harm to others.' Seclusion can engage Article 3 if the conditions or duration reach a minimum level of severity causing physical or recognized psychological injury. Article 8 can also be engaged. However, neither Article 3 nor Article 8 can be breached merely by the fact of general segregation from the hospital population. The *Mental Health Act Code of Practice* (2008: Chapter 15) provides guidance on when seclusion may be permitted, and how it is to be reviewed by nurses and doctors. NICE (2005) has also issued guidance on the short-term management of disturbed/violent behaviour in inpatient psychiatric settings and emergency departments (cf. Chapter 33).

Wider ethical issues

Legal safeguards, codes of practice, and professional guidance are essential to help ensure nurses practise ethically, within the law. Nevertheless, unlike nursing people with physical disorders, providing nursing care and treatment to people with mental disorder may often involve the use of legal powers to make decisions and carry out actions on their behalf including detaining and treating them against their will. This is partly a reflection of the nature of mental disorders, where the person themselves may consider that there is nothing wrong with them and view all care or treatment interventions as unnecessary, intrusive and possibly highly oppressive. This poses very real challenges for nurses and other mental health practitioners in maintaining or developing a relationship with the person that is still positive and therapeutic. At times this may not even be possible yet the nurse still must act professionally and ethically towards the individual, showing respect for their views and beliefs, but always trying to negotiate a more constructive relationship. This reflects the diversity of values that often exist between people who use mental health services and those who provide them. This diversity may also occur between different professional disciplines, and between professionals, service users and family carers. What is 'good' or 'right' for a service user may appear to be very 'wrong' if not 'bad' for that person (or possibly others) in the eyes of a nurse treating them. Over the last few years there has been greater recognition of this diversity in values, partly stimulated by the voices of service users themselves (as well as carers), and partly because of the differences of opinion that frequently occur between mental health practitioners. While there are no simple answers to the problems these issues pose, there is an increasing body of literature, as well as practical guidance and training available to help nurses, among others, to develop both their thinking and practice to be better equipped in dealing with these ethical challenges (e.g. Woodbridge and Fulford 2004).

Conclusion

To conclude, the main points made in this chapter are summarized below:

■ Mental health and learning disability nursing pose more acute legal and ethical problems than any other branch of medicine.
■ In the UK there are different legal regimes for mental health and mental capacity issues, particularly in Scotland.
  There are three principal sources of ethical and policy guidance for nurses in England and Wales:
  – the *Code of Professional Conduct* of the Nursing and Midwifery Council, and the Guidance issued by the Council on issues specific to mental health nursing;
  – the *Mental Health Act 1983, Code of Practice* published by the Department of Health and the Welsh Office;
  – the *Mental Capacity Act 2005 Code of Practice* published by the Department for Constitutional Affairs.

  There are three main sources of legal rules governing good clinical practice in mental health nursing:
  – the common law developed by the decisions of judges over the years;
  – Parliamentary legislation which confers statutory rights and duties;
  – the European Convention on Human Rights.
■ Nurses owe a duty of care to their patients, to avoid causing them injury by wrongful acts or omissions. Case law demonstrates the need for nurses in undertaking their duty of care to keep knowledge and skills up to date, and to ensure that they possess the knowledge, skills and abilities required for lawful, safe and effective practice.
■ In England and Wales the main source of statutory powers and duties for mental health nurses is the Mental Health Act 1983, which governs the care and treatment of people suffering from mental disorder, but consideration must also be given to the Mental Capacity Act 2005 and the circumstances where treatment and admission may take place under that Act.

■ Respecting the patient as an individual is a core principle of the Nursing Code of Professional Conduct; this is reflected in the underlying function of the European Convention on Human Rights, which is the maintenance and promotion of the dignity of the individual. Recognizing the individuality of a patient requires that their role as a partner in their care be respected.

■ The important issue for mental health nurses and all those who exercise statutory functions under mental health legislation is that they are aware of the legal and ethical context in which they operate; that they are aware of the circumstances where the different Convention rights, common law rights, statutory rights and ethical principles may be engaged, and of how to ensure that their decision-making achieves a fair balance between protecting those rights and the need to detain, control and treat mentally disordered people. This may have to take into account a diversity of values between practitioners, family carers and the mentally disordered person.

Questions for reflection and discussion

1 When considering the circumstances where you should use your statutory powers to override a person's decision to reject treatment for mental disorder reflect on how you would feel in such a situation if you were that service user. What steps would you want those making decisions on your behalf to take to find out your values, views and preferences? What decision would you expect a competent professional carer to make in your best interests?

2 Reflect on the circumstances when you would be entitled to communicate confidential medical information about a service user to a third party. Reflect on the balance required by Article 8 of the European Convention on Human Rights between the right of respect for privacy and the need to protect health or morals or the rights and freedoms of others. Reflect on the fact that if information should be divulged it should only be to the extent necessary to remove the risk, and to the proper authorities.

3 Reflect on the need for careful use of language when discussing decisions about care and treatment, on the fact that psychiatric diagnoses carry with them a degree of fear and stigma, and on the fact that insensitive remarks about diagnosis or prognosis may add greatly to the burden of carers and service users. How would you go about negotiating a relationship with a service user where they were clearly very fearful or suspicious of you, or flatly denying they had a mental disorder at all?

Annotated bibliography

■ Fennell, P. (2007) *Mental Health: the New Law*. Bristol: Jordans. A full account of the Mental Health Act 1983 as amended by the Mental Health Act 2007.

■ Jones, R.M. (2008) *Mental Health Act Manual* (12th edn). London: Sweet and Maxwell. The Mental Health Act 1983 as amended by the 2007 Act and the accompanying rules, regulations and Code of Practice. The materials are annotated and the explanations are comprehensive and informative on all the key practical issues.

■ Supplementary material to this chapter is available on ASMHN website www.openup.co.uk/normanryrie.

Conventions

■ Council of Europe, European Convention on Human Rights and Fundamental Freedoms (1950).
■ Council of Europe, Convention for the protection of human rights and the dignity of the human being with regard to the application of biology and medicine (the Oviedo Convention (1996)).
■ United Nations, UN Convention on the Rights of the Child 1989.

Statutes

■ Adults with Incapacity (Scotland) Act 2000
■ Children Act 1989
■ Family Law Reform Act 1968
■ Human Rights Act 1998
■ Mental Capacity Act 2005
■ Mental Health (Care and Treatment) (Scotland) Act 2003
■ Mental Health Act 1959
■ Mental Health Act 1983
■ Mental Health Act 2007
■ The Mental Health (Approved Mental Health Professionals) (Approval) (England) Regulations 2008 SI 2008 No 1206
■ The Mental Health (Nurses) (England) Order 2008 SI 2008 No 1207

References

American Psychiatric Association. *Diagnostic and Statistical Manual of Mental Disorders of the American Psychiatric Association* (DSM-IV-R).
Beyleveld, D. and Brownsword, R. (2002) *Human Dignity in Bioethics and Biolaw.* Oxford: Oxford University Press.
Cavadino, M. (1989) *Mental Health Law in Context: Doctor's Orders.* Aldershot: Dartmouth Publishing.
Department for Constitutional Affairs (now the Ministry of Justice) (2007) *Mental Capacity Act 2005 Code of Practice.* www.dca.goc.uk
Department of Health, Ministry of Justice, Welsh Assembly Government (2007) *Mental Health Act 2007 Explanatory Note.*
Department of Health (2008) *Mental Health Act 1983 Code of Practice.* www.dh.gov.uk.
Mental Health Act Commission (2006) Nurses, the Administration of Medicine for Mental Disorder and the Mental Health Act 1983. Guidance note. London: Mental Health Act Commission.
Ministry of Justice (2007) *The Mental Capacity Act 2005 Code of Practice.* London: Ministry of Justice.
Nursing and Midwifery Council (1998) *Guidelines for Mental Health and Disability Nursing: A Guide to Working With Vulnerable Clients.* London: NMC.
Nursing and Midwifery Council (2007) *Position Statement on the Covert Administration of Medicines – Disguising Medicine in Food and Drink.* London: NMC.
Nursing and Midwifery Council (2008) *Code of Professional Conduct.* London: NMC.

Scottish Executive (2005) *Mental Health (Care and Treatment) (Scotland) Act 2003 Codes of Practice Volumes 1–3.* Edinburgh: SE.

Scottish Executive (2008) *The Adults with Incapacity (Scotland) Act 2000: Code of Practice for Persons Authorized to carry out Medical Treatment or Research under Part 5 of the Act.* Edinburgh: SE.

Woodbridge, K. and Fulford, K.W.M. (2004) *Whose Values? A workbook for values-based practice in mental health care.* London: Sainsbury Centre for Mental Health and Warwick Medical School.

CHAPTER 8

Functional teams and whole systems

Steve Onyett

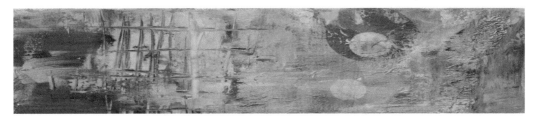

Chapter overview

This chapter defines 'functional teams' and 'whole systems' before then describing the teams in question and looking briefly at the research on what they can achieve for users. It then considers team working itself before looking at the whole service system and how teams within it need to interrelate. The penultimate section considers how to achieve effective whole systems working before looking at some of the specific implications for nurses.

I describe what the *Mental Health Policy Implementation Guide* (MHPIG) (DH 2001, 2002a, b) says about various forms of teams but from a critical perspective, since the guide itself is an excellent reference with which readers should be familiar.

The chapter covers:

■ the meaning of functional team;
■ types of mental health teams;
■ key issues about the operation of all teams;
■ effects of team provision on outcomes for service users;
■ engaging service users and their social networks;
■ whole systems thinking and inter-team relationships;
■ service integration and improvement;
■ implications for mental health nursing.

What do we mean by 'functional teams'?

The phrase 'functional teams' does not appear in the MHPIG or the *NSF for Mental Health* (although the rather alarming word 'functionalized' appears once). Nonetheless, the phrase has emerged to distinguish teams that are established to fulfil a specific function. The implication is that 'functional teams' are different from existing community mental health teams (CMHTs). This itself could be seen as fairly damning, implying that CMHTs either have no function or are 'dysfunctional'. This was perhaps true of many CMHTs of the 1980s and

1990s (Onyett 2003), although many CMHTs had learned the lessons of the international case management and assertive community treatment literature prior to the *NSF for Mental Health* and had accordingly become more targeted and clear about their operations. The MHPIG was also keen to dispel the notion that the newer teams are to usurp existing CMHTs.

The full range of interventions referred to in the MHPIG covers 'early intervention; assertive outreach; home treatment; the needs of those with comorbidity; black and minority ethnic communities; homeless people; or mentally disordered offenders'. The guidance refers also to rehabilitation teams focusing on the housing, income, occupational and social needs of people with 'serious disabilities resulting from their mental illness'.

This functional approach is helpful in thinking about team design in a locality. The overriding imperative to bear in mind is that whatever the fashion for new teams may be, our task is to ensure that the right functions are fulfilled for the right people. In parts of the Avon area the *Developing Individual Services in the Community* framework (DISC) (H. Smith 1998) was used to provide an even more comprehensive approach to local needs assessment and service development. The use of such a framework with a broad range of stakeholders serves to establish some key values and a shared language about what mental health services should be achieving for people. Team functions explored using the DISC framework are listed in Box 8.1. Finding a common language for the mission of the locality service is also promoted by such an approach and can form the bedrock of other process-based approaches to improvement such as process mapping (see www.csip.org.uk/resources/directory-of-service-improvement.html) and the development of care pathways.

Box 8.1   The functions explored using the DISC framework

With respect to the following key functions, how are the needs of local people currently being met, and how might they be better met:

- Needs for equitable and fair access and good information
- Needs for individual planning
- Meeting needs in crisis
- Needs for treatment and support with mental distress
- Needs for ordinary living and long-term support, for example regarding employment, housing and money
- Needs for personal growth and development

It is important to consider how teamworking *across the patch* provides the right range of functions for service users. This teamworking within the locality will include a range of service configurations, the design of which needs to be informed by local needs assessment, existing strengths in local provision, and the unique history, geography and demography of the patch.

The newer teams may be the key to achieving this range of functions. However, we should not be dazzled by novelty. Rather we should build on existing strengths, particularly on those parts of the existing system where mental health service users have built strong and effective relationships with staff. Since the earlier edition of this chapter, strengths-based approaches to organizational development have emerged to support such work, including appreciative enquiry (Srivastva and Cooperrider 1999) and a solution-focused approach (Jackson and McKergow 2002).

It is unhelpful to restrict the term 'functional teams' to the newer service models only. All local teams need to be functional, including inpatient teams. The existing research evidence reviewed below suggests that even the most intensive community service will not completely eliminate the need for inpatient care. The principles of effective team design and teamworking are applicable equally to inpatient teams, and indeed it may be at admission and discharge that effective whole systems working is *most* essential to promote continuity of care, least restrictive and controlling interventions and effective communication with all the stakeholders involved. Continuity of practice between the hospital and the community is critical, and it is encouraging to see the emergence of teams (often crisis-resolution teams) that span inpatient and community care by having members that provide both.

Whole systems working demands 'whole systems thinking', a term that highlights the need to design, plan and manage organizations as living, independent systems while working to achieve 'seamless' care for those they aim to serve. Complex health and social problems lie beyond the ability of any one practitioner, team or agency to resolve. Whole systems thinking emphasizes also the need to develop shared values, purposes and practices within and between organizations, and uses large group interventions to bring together the perspectives of a wide range of stakeholders across a wider system (Iles and Sutherland 2001).

Types of mental health team

This section outlines policy guidance and research findings with respect to the different types of mental health team featured in the *NSF for Mental Health and NHS Plan* (DH 2001a) and described in detail in the MHPIG.

'Assertive outreach' teams

These are teams aiming to serve people with 'a severe and persistent mental disorder (for example, schizophrenia, major affective disorders) associated with a high level of disability' (DH 2001), who are heavy users of inpatient or intensive home-based care, and who have difficulty also in maintaining lasting and consenting contact with services. These people are likely to have multiple complex needs including risk of harm to others or themselves, persistent offending, concurrent substance misuse and unstable accommodation or homelessness. The MHPIG identifies key aspects of service design and implementation as the critical ingredients of assertive outreach teams. These teams should:

- be self-contained and responsible for providing a wide range of interventions (these are specified in detail in the MHPIG);
- have a single responsible medical officer who is an active member of the team;
- provide treatment on a long-term basis with an emphasis on continuity of care;
- deliver most services in community settings;
- emphasize maintaining contact and building relationships with service users;
- provide care coordination by the team;

■ maintain small caseloads of no more than 12 service users per staff member.

A DH/CSIP (2005) research seminar highlighted the possibility that 'fidelity' to the assertive model was based upon US research and therefore a UK version was needed. In general however the UK National Forum for Assertive Outreach (NFAO 2005) endorsed these key requirements and further described the following key features of assertive outreach as critically important:

■ Most services provided directly by the team and not brokered out.
■ Caseloads shared across clinicians. Staff know and work with the entire caseload, although a Care Programme Approach (CPA) care coordinator is allocated to and responsible for each client.
■ Highly coordinated, intensive service with brief daily handover meetings and weekly clinical review meetings.
■ Extended hours, seven day a week service with capacity to manage crises and have daily contact with clients where needed. This function is also advocated for crisis resolution teams below and so will need to be negotiated locally.

Some teams have sought to avoid the term 'assertive' because it overemphasizes the potentially coercive nature of intensive community treatment. Words such as 'intensive' or 'active' community treatment have been proffered as alternatives. It is also unhelpful that these teams are described as 'assertive outreach' teams in the Guidance. Assertive outreach has been used to describe the practice of taking services to where people need them in their own environment, regardless of the type of team. It is also a key feature of the crisis resolution and early intervention teams described below. The more commonly used term in the international literature on these kinds of teams is 'assertive community treatment' (ACT). The defining characteristic of ACT is not the location of care but the intensity of service provision provided in community settings in order to achieve effective working relationships with people with whom this can be a challenge (in line with the emphasis of the key features highlighted by the NFAO above). The acronym 'ACT' will therefore be used here because of its widespread currency.

The efficacy of ACT in a UK context remains contested and large UK studies of service structure are under way. The prevailing view appears to be that the successes of ACT as practised in the USA have not been replicated in Europe (DH/CSIP 2005) although there are examples of successful services, as described below. This failure is attributed on the one hand to a failure to implement ACT with sufficient fidelity to the model, and on the other to the fact that standard mental health care in Europe is far superior, therefore making the contrast with ACT less measurable (Tyrer 2000). Reviews of ACT (Marshall & Lockwood 2000; Mueser et al. 1998) conclude that well-designed teams achieve better engagement, reduced hospital admissions, increased independent living and increased user satisfaction. In particular, the team approach where the team as a whole manages the caseload was seen as a key feature associated with better outcomes.

The effectiveness of assertive outreach teams relies heavily on their capacity to achieve effective engagement and this appears to be an area of particular achievement (Wright et al. 2003; Killaspy et al. 2006). Priebe et al. (2005) found that the key factors promoting engagement were (i) social support and engagement without a focus on medication, (ii) time and commitment from the staff, and (iii) a therapeutic relationship based on a partnership model. Disengagement was associated with three key themes: (i) a desire to be an independent person, (ii) a lack of active participation and poor therapeutic relationship, and (iii) a sense of loss of control due to medication and side effects.

The UK experience, as elsewhere, has shown that when ACT is discontinued improvements are lost, for example in social functioning and reduced time in hospital (Audini *et al.* 1994). This has important implications for when and how a step down to less intensive provision takes place. Burns and Firn (2002) suggest that ACT teams need to reduce support gradually to that which users will receive in step-down care. They ensure that service users are stable on one contact per month for at least three months, and their experience is that the whole discharge process usually takes around six months.

The conclusions of the DH/CSIP (2005) research seminar stressed that while assertive outreach was successful in achieving effective engagement and high levels of satisfaction among users and staff, the implementation of effective psychosocial interventions was deemed to be lacking (Wright *et al.* 2003). They advocated consideration of the range of disciplines who should be considered as able to deliver such interventions.

Crisis resolution (or 'home treatment') teams

These teams provide a 24-hour service to users in their own homes to avoid hospital admissions where possible and provide the maximum opportunity to resolve crises in the contexts in which they occur. Their role in the mental health system is to ensure that individuals experiencing severe mental distress are served in the least restrictive environment and as close to home as possible.

Although the MHPIG advocates local flexibility regarding client groups, crisis teams are most commonly targeted on people with severe mental distress who might require hospital admission. These teams therefore need to sit in the pathway between community-based referrers and inpatient care and be able to act as a point of assessment and as a gatekeeper to other parts of the mental health system for people in severe distress. They will therefore usually need the capacity to provide immediate home treatment 24 hours a day, 7 days a week.

Clients will often be people with an existing diagnosis of severe mental disorder such as schizophrenia, manic depressive disorder or severe depressive disorder. The guidance recommends excluding people with mild anxiety disorders, a primary diagnosis of alcohol or other substance misuse, an exclusive diagnosis of personality disorder, and a recent history of self-harm in the absence of a diagnosis of psychosis. It also advocated not responding to crises related solely to relationship issues. In reality applying these exclusion criteria out of hours and in crisis may be challenging. A national survey of CRTs (Onyett *et al.* in press) found teams to be pragmatic in their inclusion criteria with nearly half accepting people with substance misuse disorders and a high proportion not excluding people diagnosed with personality disorder. The MHPIG highlights the following key principles of care:

- a 24-hour, 7-day a week service;
- rapid response following referral;
- intensive intervention and support in the early stages of the crisis;
- active involvement of the service user, family and carers;
- an assertive approach to engagement (i.e. assertive outreach as described above);
- time-limited intervention with sufficient flexibility to respond to differing service user needs;

■ an emphasis on learning from the crisis with the involvement of the whole social support network.

Joy et al.'s (2001) review of crisis intervention reported only a limited effect on admissions. However, they can substantially reduce length of stay (Audini et al. 1994; Johnson et al. 2005) and rates of admission where teams provide out of hours cover (Johnson et al. 2005; Glover et al. 2006). Joy et al.'s (2001) review found home care to be as cost effective as hospital care with respect to loss of people to local services, deaths and mental distress. Crisis services reduced the burden on families, and were preferred by both users and families (Johnson et al. 2005; Joy et al. 2001), and staff.

The English national survey (Onyett et al. in press) found only 40 per cent of teams saw themselves as fully set up with lack of staffing highlighted as the key obstacle to effective operation; a finding corroborated by the survey data. Teams were composed largely of nurses and support workers rather than providing the full range of multi-disciplinary skills advocated by the MHPIG. In particular teams lacked and sought adequate senior medical cover.

The majority of CRTs were urban teams and these operated with greater fidelity to the MHPIG, and took on a larger proportion of referrals for ongoing work. Overall, fidelity to the MHPIG was variable and compromised by the finding that around a third of teams were not involved in gatekeeping and just over half offered a 24-hour, seven-day per week home visiting service. Routing all referrals for inpatient care through the crisis service is critical to their success in offering a realistic alternative to admission through offering 24-hour cover with sufficient intensity to provide a realistic alternative to inpatient care. Our national survey (Onyett et al. in press) found that support from those practitioners who can circumvent the system by making direct admissions to inpatient care was seen as critical to CRTs being able to adopt their gatekeeping role. This and other field experience has led to refreshed DH/CSIP (2007) guidance.

Early intervention teams

These teams work proactively to serve people in the early stages of developing psychotic symptoms to reduce their longer-term dependency on services and promote better outcomes. They are targeted on people aged between 14 and 35 with a first presentation of psychotic symptoms, and people aged 14 to 35 during the first three years of psychotic illness.

Increased delay between the first onset of psychotic phenomena and receiving treatment produces negative longer-term consequences (Drake et al. 2000). It may also be that the early stages of psychotic experience are a critical phase during which key psychological and biological changes occur (Birchwood et al. 1998). The first few years of psychosis carry the highest risk of social disruption and suicide. It therefore follows that providing help as soon as possible should have a positive longer-term impact. The guidance highlights that it can take up to two years after the first signs of psychosis for an individual to begin receiving help. Lack of awareness, ambiguous early symptoms and stigma all contribute to the delay in appropriate help being offered. Service systems need to be able to identify people early in the course of their distress by working closely with primary care, ACT teams, and other people who are likely to encounter young people with psychotic experiences (for example, college counsellors, police, agencies for homeless people).

Garety and Jolley (2000) highlighted encouraging early evidence for the efficacy of psychological interventions in the early phases of psychotic experience. Subsequent randomized controlled trials have found that clients of early intervention teams report reduced readmissions, improvement in symptoms and better quality of life (Craig *et al.* 2004).

In summary, the guidance suggests that an early intervention service should:

- reduce the stigma associated with psychosis and improve professional and lay awareness of the symptoms of psychosis and the need for early assessment;
- reduce the length of time young people remain undiagnosed and untreated;
- focus on managing symptoms rather than the diagnosis;
- develop meaningful engagement, provide evidence-based interventions, and promote recovery during the early phase of psychotic experience;
- increase stability in the lives of service users, facilitate personal development and provide opportunities for personal fulfilment (for example, through education and meaningful employment);
- provide a seamless service for those aged 14–35, that integrates child, adolescent and adult mental health services and works in partnership with primary care, education, social services, youth and other services;
- provide culture, age and gender sensitive family-orientated services in the least restrictive and stigmatizing setting. This will include separate, age-appropriate facilities for young people;
- at the end of the treatment period, ensure that the care is thoughtfully and effectively transferred.

The maintenance and re-establishment of the integration of young people with age-appropriate, mainstream services is an ongoing aim of early intervention services. Therefore, there is a need to establish a wide range of links, for example, with primary care, education, youth agencies, leisure providers and other relevant services across the voluntary and statutory sectors.

Despite a rapid growth in EI teams, a national survey in 2005 (Pinfold *et al.* 2007) found marked regional variations in implementation with many teams barely viable. Around a third of the population in England were judged to have no local early intervention service. Of 117 teams, 86 had funding and 63 were operational and only three teams met all the relevant features of early intervention teams. Just over half the teams cited lack of funding as limiting development.

Community mental health teams

CMHTs appear to be that crucial part of the whole service system that is left when the other newer service models have become operational. The MHPIG update on CMHTs (DH 2002a) is, therefore, not prescriptive about team structure but rather focuses on the functions that the team should achieve. However, it also stresses that even these functions may be fulfilled in other ways. It highlights three major functions:

1. giving advice on the management of mental health problems by other professionals – in particular advice to primary care and a triage function enabling appropriate referral;
2. providing treatment and care for those with time-limited disorders who can benefit from specialist interventions;
3. providing treatment and care for those with more complex and enduring needs.

The guidance acknowledges that the first two functions above may be fulfilled by CMHTs in the form of primary care liaison teams. There are also a rich variety of other primary care or community-based services that may fulfil this function, not least the UK government's own plans for 1000 new graduate workers in primary care to help GPs manage common mental health problems, and the 500 new 'Gateway' workers to respond to people requiring immediate help. The NHS Plan required that both types of worker were to be trained and deployed by 2004.

The MHPIG also highlights that 'rehabilitation and recovery teams' may fulfil the third function. Where there are complex issues such as difficulty establishing effective working relationships with users, and multiple diagnoses this function is also likely to be fulfiled by the local ACT team.

We are, therefore, left in a problematic situation regarding social policy on teams. We have recommendations for CMHTs that acknowledge that many of their functions will be carried out in other ways, and recommendations for newer team models that key commentators continue to suggest are already carried out by existing CMHTs (Tyrer et al. 2001). Some have felt it nonsensical to reconfigure already effective services to accord with newer service models where existing teams have already evolved to fulfil the required functions (for example, Tyrer 1998; Thornicroft et al. 1999; Simmonds et al. 2001).

In this context it has to be questioned whether it is helpful to restrict the term CMHT to a specific *type* of team since in practice it may be impossible to reliably define and recognize from one locality to the next. It is notable that mature UK ACT teams tend to stress their continuity of practice with existing CMHTs rather than differences (Burns and Firn 2002) and this has been substantiated by Simmonds et al.'s (2001) review of CMHTs which found them to be achieving many of the functions claimed for the newer service models, such as reducing inpatient treatment, reducing costs, less dissatisfaction with care, better engagement and fewer suicides. Any team providing coordinated multi-disciplinary input in community settings through a team process is by definition a 'community mental health team'.

The MHPIG describes the CMHT 'function' as being to: increase capacity within primary care through collaboration, reduce stigma, ensure that care is delivered in the least restrictive and disruptive manner possible, and stabilize social functioning and protect community tenure. However, there is nothing in the description of how CMHTs work that gives them a privileged role in achieving these functions. It is questionable whether involvement in a dedicated team process is the best way to serve such individuals. *Our Health, Our Care, Our Say* (Department of Health 2006) identified a range of approaches to the support of people with mental health problems by primary care. At the core of these approaches is the notion of 'stepped care'. This approach operates on the principle that the first recommended intervention should be the least restrictive of those currently available that is likely to provide significant health gain. The model also advocates self-correction through systematic monitoring of the results of treatments and decisions about treatment provision so that changes can be made expediently ('stepping up') (Bower and Gilbody 2005). Although there is some supportive evidence for the use of stepped care, rigorous evaluations of the underlying assumptions are scarce, and a substantial research on the optimal content and organization of stepped care has yet to be done.

The MHPIG also describes a 'substantial minority' of CMHT caseloads as requiring 'ongoing treatment, care and monitoring for periods of several years'. This includes people with:

- severe and persistent mental disorders associated with significant disability (such as schizophrenia and bipolar disorder);
- longer-term disorders of lesser severity but which are characterized by poor treatment adherence requiring proactive follow-up;
- a significant risk of self-harm or harm to others;
- needs for a level of support that exceeds that which a primary care team could offer (for example, chronic anorexia nervosa); and
- disorders requiring skilled or intensive treatments (for example, CBT, vocational rehabilitation, medication maintenance requiring blood tests) not available in primary care.

The guidance makes efforts to describe a valued role for CMHTs as a separate service from the new 'functional' teams. However, it is easy to see how CMHT staff may come to feel devalued and demoralized. They are being described as the place where primary care addresses its capacity problems regarding people with more minor mental health problems, while simultaneously being the repository for all the community-based clinical provision that the newer teams decline; and in many cases offering stepdown care where these teams feel they have fulfilled their role. CMHTs may also have least control over their caseloads while continuing to serve very challenging clients.

Issues of definition and lack of fidelity in implementation make outcome research on CMHTs as with any teams problematic. CMHTs are also so ubiquitous it is difficult to envisage a site where a standard care would not include CMHT provision of some kind. As described above the systematic review of CMHTs by Simmonds *et al.* (2001) found that they achieved some of the benefits of ACT but to a lesser extent. For example, the impact on reducing inpatient bed use was interpreted by the authors as less than ACT but greater than case management. As with much of the ACT literature (for example, Marshall and Lockwood 2000) Simmonds *et al.* found no evidence of gains in social functioning and clinical symptomatology. Again, as with the ACT reviews, definition problems abound in that some of the teams covered may, in practice, be as close to ACT teams as many of the teams covered in ACT reviews. For example, the team described by Merson *et al.* (1992) (which used to be managed by the author) included many of the features of an ACT team, including home visiting and clinical co-working with colleagues within and outside the team.

Operational considerations

Whatever type of team we are thinking about there are some key issues about the operation of any team that need to be considered. In the past team working was seen merely as what people do in teams. Ovretveit (1986) noted how 'Just calling a group of practitioners a team has become a way in which managers and planners avoid the real problems and work needed to coordinate an increasingly complex range of services in the community'.

Whenever thinking about team design we need to keep in mind why and if team working is needed. Shea and Guzzo describe a work group as 'three or more people employed by an organization who see themselves as a group, are seen by others in the organization as a group and *who depend on each other for resources to accomplish a task or set of tasks*' (1987: 327, emphasis added). Teams need to look hard at this issue of interdependence between team members to get the job done. It bears on what types of decisions can be best made within the user–staff member relationship alone by pooling their shared expertise and experience, which require the involvement of others in the team or beyond, and which require the involvement of the whole team. These detailed issues are explored in detail in Onyett (2003).

We need to look to the broader social psychology literature to identify the requirements of good teamworking. Reviews (e.g. Onyett 2007; Mickan and Rodger 2005) highlight the following features as critical:

- a clear and motivating vision among the host organizations based on explicit human values;
- clear, shared and motivating objectives, that are aligned with this vision and value set;
- membership that comprises the minimum number of people required to achieve these outcomes;
- a need among members to work together to achieve team objectives;
- diverse, differentiated and clear roles. productive difference within the team can be maintained through a positive sense of identification with one's profession or discipline where objectives are aligned at a professional, team, organizational and individual practitioner level. Professional distinctiveness can comfortably coexist with team identification in contexts where the teams' super-ordinate goals are salient and meaningful to those involved and where team members can see their particular contribution to these goals (Haslam and Platow 2001);
- cohesion and a positive sense of team identification but not to the extent of creating impermeable boundaries around the team or demonizing other local services;
- mutual respect within the team and beyond;
- effective communication, characterized by a depth of dialogue wherein people are able to suspend assumptions and judgements, while promoting active and attentive listening and individual and collective reflection;
- ambition manifest in an expectation of excellence;
- the necessary authority, autonomy and resources to achieve these objectives;
- time out for the team to review what it is trying to achieve, how it is going about it and what needs to change. this also requires that the team collects information in an ongoing way about what it is doing, who it is serving, and how;
- clear leadership both within and around the team to promote the features listed above.

In sum, we cannot assume such teams will work well because of a magical 'synergy' that arises when people are organized into groups. Good team working can be achieved only through premeditated design and good team process that both take thorough account of the context of the team's work. This in turn requires a clear understanding of the tasks that the team has to perform for the people it is established to serve, and some consideration of the knowledge, skills and experience that individuals need to bring to the team. Thus, teams must be designed to work well and to recruit and train their members accordingly.

Outcomes for users

We have seen above how the outcomes of different team models remain contested because of uncertainty about the fidelity of implementation to specific models, the different contexts in which teams are implemented and the extent to which they constitute an improvement on the existing local service system.

Determining the effect of team provision on outcomes for users is problematic because of the user's involvement with other services and other 'uncontrolled' aspects of their lives. To judge services properly we need to take account of the net benefit of running the service in a way that encompasses outcomes for users, the effects on their social supports, service use, hospitalization, involvement in the criminal justice system and other indicators of community mental health. Very few studies have achieved such comprehensive evaluation although the Madison experiment (Stein and Test 1980) and the study of the Crisis Intervention Service in New South Wales (Hoult 1986) provide notable exemplars. Both supported the development of intensive community interventions. Provan and Milward (1995) also looked at the whole system of community support. They examined the 'network effectiveness' of four community mental health services. Networks were evaluated rather than specific organizations, recognizing that outcomes for users will depend on the actions of a range of agencies. This study found that integration of providers was unlikely to improve outcomes unless the network was stable, resourced adequately and centrally and directly controlled.

In the USA evaluations of several national service demonstrations have shown that although reforms in the system occurred the impact on individual service users was very limited (Goldman *et al.* 1994; Ridgely *et al.* 1996). These changes have been seen as necessary but insufficient for improving the lives of people with severe mental distress and attention has shifted to content and quality of services (Goldman *et al.* 2001).

Sashidharan *et al.* (1999) argued, from the perspective of an experienced clinician informed by the existing research, that it is common sense to expect more intensive and targeted community services to make a difference but that different team types should, therefore, be evaluated in terms of the extent to which they provide an effective platform for the delivery of care (Gournay 1999). The achievement of positive outcomes for users will be determined by the quality of that care. In order to get the care at all, users need to remain effectively involved with teams. It, therefore, makes sense to evaluate teams principally in terms of the extent to which they successfully involve users and their social networks in change and where possible use bespoke approaches to measuring outcomes that relate specifically to their aspirations.[18]

Engaging users and their networks

The working alliance between users and staff has a substantial impact on outcomes for people with severe mental health problems (see Onyett 2000 for review and Chinman *et al.* 2000). This is more likely to be achieved if they are getting a service they want.

People receiving ACT, case management and crisis resolution services are more likely to remain in contact with services than people receiving standard community care (Marshall and Lockwood 2000; Marshall *et al.* 1998; Joy *et al.* 2001; Wright *et al.* 2003). Intensive

---

[18] See for example the 'Social Inclusion Web' developed by Peter Bates of the National Development Team http://www.ndt.org.uk/projectsN/SI.htm

community teams are also better able to ensure that difficult-to-serve people maintain contact following discharge from hospital (Ford *et al.* 1995; Holloway and Carson 1998; Johnston *et al.* 1998). This may be explained by the balance of evidence which suggests that these services are preferred by users and their social networks (Hoult *et al.* 1983; Merson *et al.* 1992; Marks *et al.* 1994; Holloway and Carson 1998; Joy *et al.* 2001; Johnson *et al.* 2005). This tends to be because of the high quality of their relationships with staff (McGrew *et al.* 1996; Killaspy *et al.* 2006). McGrew *et al.* (2002) found that even when asked specifically about aspects of ACT that users disliked least 44 per cent were unable to identify a negative aspect. However, such research needs to be interpreted in light of the obvious power relationships that exist between staff and users. Another 21 per cent expressed concern about home visits and intrusiveness, although others complained about the lack of intensity of contact.

Overall, it can be concluded that where teams are intensive, proactive and focus on developing good working relationships by providing support to achieving outcomes valued by users themselves, they can effectively engage them, keep them out of hospital and in many cases improve important aspects of their lives. However, there is a risk that these good working relationships will become soured if intensive approaches are implemented insensitively or are too strongly identified with a coercion and control.

Smith *et al.* (1999) warn against the more coercive aspects of ACT as practised in parts of the USA and Canada becoming manifest in the UK, in particular the withholding of welfare payments unless users accept treatment. Deci *et al.* (1995) found that 82 per cent of the 303 US ACT teams they surveyed provided 'financial management' of users' income.

Spindel and Nugent (1999) also criticized ACT teams' role in collaborating with other agencies to enforce treatment, particularly medication, and expressed concern about ACT staff collaborating with probation and parole officers to reincarcerate users when they were found to be non-compliant. Diamond also expressed concern about the nature of some inter-agency working and communication:

> " This communication, even when done with the client's permission, allows enormous pressure to be applied for the client to take medication, stay in treatment, live in a particular place, or 'follow the plan' in any number of ways. This pressure can be almost as coercive as the hospital in controlling behaviour, but with fewer safeguards.
>
> (1996: 58) "

The *NSF for Mental Health* tended to frame ACT as part of a risk reduction and crisis prevention strategy rather than as a way of providing users with better quality care on their own terms. Indeed, the most explicit *NSF for Mental Health* standard for ACT concerns suicide prevention. It is too early to draw firm conclusions about the advantages or disadvantages of ACT with respect to risk of harm to users themselves or to others (Marshall and Lockwood 2000). Burns and Firn caution against ACT's role in reducing risk being 'overplayed' stating that 'teams work best when they engage patients collaboratively rather than attempting to control them' (2002: 295). While not neglecting the important role that ACT can have in helping to assess and manage risk they also make the point that untoward incidents happen in the contained environment of a hospital ward and so it would be an unrealistic 'hostage to fortune' to suggest that ACT represents a panacea for risk management.

There is a risk for all of us that the advantages of working actively and intensively with individuals and agencies can become oppressive because they are embedded in ideologies and practices that fail to pay enough respect to users' views, aspirations and rights. In this context the emphasis being paid by the National Institute of Mental Health for England on the recovery approach and an explicit set of values to underpin mental health work is very welcome (see Chapter 5, this volume).

'Whole systems thinking'

'Whole systems thinking' has a high profile within the policy rhetoric within the *NSF for Mental Health* and the subsequent MHPIG. At its most prosaic, whole systems thinking is about ensuring that all the component parts of a mental health system are in place and 'in balance' (*NSF for Mental Health*, DH 1999: 7). The MHPIG emphasizes: 'the need for whole systems development which will address the most conspicuous gaps in service provision. We cannot afford to focus on any single aspect of the mental health system and hope that this will provide a solution' (1999: 3). Achieving the stated 'balance' referred to in the *NSF for Mental Health* requires new priorities, new investment and reinvestment of existing resources. Unacceptable variations in service use, for example, in the use of hospital beds, are interpreted as 'a sign that not all mental health services are operating a whole systems approach' (1999: 49).

This demands high levels of joint working and communication both between individuals in teams, and across teams working in different settings. The MHPIG also makes clear the requirement for new information systems to improve both direct care and our overall understanding of the quality of care being delivered. This will also be needed to inform and monitor the *de facto* rationing that goes on through team referral and allocation processes (Griffiths 2001).

As soon as we begin to think about what is required to achieve a high level of joint working between elements of the whole service system, we need to acknowledge the complexity of the system involved. Systems are embedded within each other. Koestler (1967) proposed that nested systems, such as teams, or users and their support networks, are represented as complex strata of 'holons'. The 'holon' is a part-whole combining the Greek 'holos' meaning whole and the suffix 'on' which, as in proton or neutron, suggests a particle or part. The idea was invoked to reconcile the tension between parts of a system being both parts and wholes depending on your perspective.

The nested quality of holons is depicted in Figure 8.1 where the various organizational levels are presented as a series of holons in relation to each other. In a mental health context these strata could represent the relationship between a nurse and a service user, the users support network, the team, the management support to ensure effective teamworking, and the organization culture within which teams can flourish. These strata also connect horizontally with other holarchies that form part of the individual's life such as their work environment, their local community and society in general.

Figure 8.1 illustrates the key feature of this conceptualization: the 'transcend-and-include' principle; the way in which the holons represent emergent processes where complex systems include and add to the qualities of the systems that comprise them. Edwards (2005) states, for example, that 'work teams include, but are more than (transcend), the sum of interactions between pairs of individuals (dyads); organizational departments include, but are more than, the sum of interactions between teams and dyads; organizations include, but are more than,

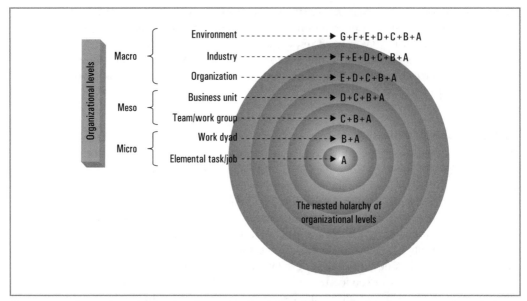

Figure 8.1 An ecological holarchy of organizational levels/holons showing the transcend and include relations between levels/holons

the sum of interactions between departments, teams and dyads' (2005: 271). The use of the holon provides a way of conceptualizing emergent culture and also provides insights into why sometimes things go wrong. For example, an organization (such as a large specialist mental health trust) can become so large that nested systems within it, such as tiers of management or teams, become dissociated from it and lose all sense of organizational identification. Alternatively where teams become extremely internally cohesive they can become dissociated from management and the wider work of the organization with the result that they end up denigrating almost everything outside the team. It is a sad reality of organizational life that teams often build a positive sense of identity by demonizing other parts of the system that are not them.

The nature of complex systems is such that a change in one element has implications for many other elements. Taking the obvious need for service elements to work effectively together means looking at the system of care at the individual level – the level described by the integrated care programme approach (or 'care coordination'). Care coordinators should be the glue that binds the system together in a coherent way for service users and their supports.

Guidance stressed that: 'It is critical that the care co-ordinator should have the authority to co-ordinate the delivery of the care plan and that this is respected by all those involved in delivering it, regardless of agency of origin' (NHSE/SSI 1999: 22). This has never been robustly and widely achieved, and has since become an ambition that is shared with more recent approaches such as the deployment of Community Matrons to work across agencies in the interests of older adults with mental health problems.

Achieving coordinated care delivery is supported by strong inter-agency agreements between health and social care on the use of pooled budgets and partnership agreements to support the implementation of integrated care plans. Care coordinators need to work with families and other natural supports, as well as liaising with other agencies such as employers, housing providers, primary care, inpatient facilities (for both physical and mental health care), education providers, leisure services, benefit agencies and criminal justice agencies. The role should also include 'inreach' into inpatient settings and prisons. Indeed, the multi-agency nature of the work is such that the MHPIG states: 'No one service or agency is central [to the system of relevant agencies involved]. Service users themselves provide the focal point for care planning and delivery' (DH 2000: 3). It therefore follows that teams need to be built around their needs to support the exercise of care coordination and that these teams need to be commissioned as part of a coherent whole system. This imperative has been given a renewed importance with the 'personalized care' agenda evident in the social care White Paper (DH 2006).

MHPIG guidance on inter-team relationships

For care coordinators and other team members to work effectively across teams there needs to be clarity about who is being served and how and when they can achieve access. The alarming Figure 8.2 describes *only* those direct referral relationships described in the MHPIG. In reality the referral network will be even more complex. Figure 8.2 captures just some of the complexity at service level and the need for clarity about how parts of the system will interrelate. It highlights also the importance of an inter-team care coordinator role that will smooth transitions and ensure continuity.

The central importance of inter-team relationships was highlighted by Richter *et al.*'s (2006) survey of 53 health care teams within five PCTs. Teams whose leaders identified strongly with both their team and the PCT, and had frequent contact with members of other teams, displayed more harmonious and more productive relationships with other teams.

Box 8.2 describes the respective service responses that the MHPIG advocates from the different teams. Extended hours, rather than a 24-hour response is advocated for ACTs. Burns and Firn (2002) found the introduction of a seven-day working week particularly valuable in that it covered weekend periods when users were particularly vulnerable to relapse arising from lack of activity, contact and increased substance misuse. Contrary to expectations, these periods are not used for dealing with crises and mainly comprise planned visits and phone calls.

The MHPIG envisaged that crisis resolution teams will usually provide the crisis response for clients of the ACTs and early intervention teams out of hours. However, it is important to stress that the MHPIG does not propose that crisis response work would be restricted to the crisis resolution service. Where the ACT team is involved with the individual concerned they should offer the community-based response within working hours. Where continuing input is needed following a crisis the ACT team, crisis resolution team and the other parts of the local service system should work together to ensure that the least restrictive and stigmatizing setting for care is arranged. The whole system should work together to avoid hospitalization and restrictive care wherever possible, and opportunities to provide care in the community or in the service user's own home should be grasped.

The MHPIG stresses that effective joint working requires links to be established between the teams within a locality so that:

- Handover and referrals are made easily.
- Crises are anticipated and contingency plans are known to all involved in care.
- Early intervention and assertive outreach service users are aware of whom to contact out of hours.

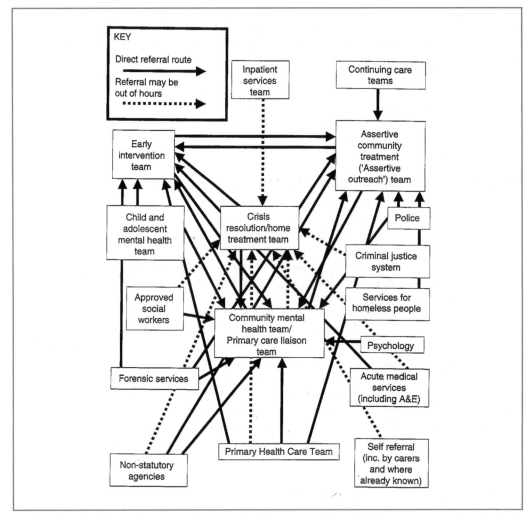

Figure 8.2 Direct referral relationships described in the Mental Health Policy Implementation Guide: Community Mental Health Teams (DH 2002a)

- Staff from the assertive outreach team and/or early intervention team can participate in the crisis resolution/home treatment team out of hours rota. It may be advantageous to also involve inpatient staff in these rotas so that they do not feel like an excluded part of the wider system and are able to contribute their skills, expertise and knowledge of the user to promote continuous and effective care.
- If inpatient care is needed for ACT clients, the team can maintain contact during the user's stay, contribute to decision-making concerning discharge planning and ensure that the home environment is ready for discharge. Regular joint, formal reviews should aim to promote transfer to the least stigmatizing and restrictive environment as soon as clinically possible.
- Local arrangements are made between the crisis resolution team, the early intervention team and child and adolescent mental health services to ensure rapid access to an out-of-hours crisis service for users under 16 years old.

Box 8.2   Mental Health Policy Implementation Guidance (DH 2002a) on service responses around the clock

Team type	Core working hours	Out of hours response
Assertive community treatment	8 a.m. to 8 p.m., 7 days a week	One member of staff on call for phone advice.
		No provision for home visits. If visits are required, referral should be made to the crisis resolution team.
Early intervention	8 a.m. to 8 p.m., 7 days a week	A member of staff on call for phone advice, or alternatively from staff at a linked community respite facility (either by telephone or by visiting the unit).
		No provision for home visits. If visits are required, referral should be made to the crisis resolution team or the CAMHS out-of-hour service.
Crisis resolution/ home treatment	A shift system is required to ensure a minimum of two trained caseworkers available 24 hours a day, 7 days a week.	
Home visits to known service users require two caseworkers. The 24-hour assessment team for assessment of new referrals should also include a senior psychiatrist.	The evening/through the night service is usually accessed through an on-call system.	
The medical on call rota should allow a senior psychiatrist to undertake home visits 24 hours a day.		
CMHT/primary care liaison team (for example, evening work for a relative support group).	9 a.m. to 5 p.m. weekdays with flexible out-of-hours working for specific tasks.	⇨

Team type	Core working hours	Out of hours response
Some teams may chose to work with moderately extended hours, for example, 8 a.m. to 7 p.m. to accord with GP surgery times. This is strongly recommended for improved primary care liaison.	No crisis provision is made out of hours by the CMHT and patients and carers would access the local emergency services (crisis resolution teams, help lines, A&E etc.).	

Service integration and improvement

One feature of complex systems is that you can define them as narrowly or as widely as you wish. It is a question of utility in terms of the issues you need to address and just how much you and your colleagues can hold in your heads and work with effectively.

Capturing the whole complexity of 'whole systems'

Figure 8.3 illustrates a local whole system. At the centre are users themselves and their social networks. The latter phrase is used advisedly. Bainbridge (2002) provides a powerful critique of how the term 'carers' makes a range of assumptions about the role of relatives, friends and others in users' lives while also making unhelpful assumptions about how they define their role with respect to the user concerned. In the main it is this social system that teams should be working with rather than taking an overly individualistic view (see M. Smith 1998).

Working outwards, there is then the question of how practitioners relate to that complex social system and how in turn they are supported in their work by the team (or teams) of which they are a member. There is then the question of how the team fits into the local service system which in turn is influenced by how other interconnected systems concerned with the relationship between health and social care, primary and specialist care, the statutory and voluntary sector and hospital and community care interact. For many service users there are then issues concerning how they transfer to or from related systems of care for children and adolescents or older adults. All this is similarly embedded within other systems concerned with the provision of housing, employment, benefits, and, in many cases, a range of other specialist services. These systems themselves operate in ways that are influenced by wider societal perceptions of people with mental health problems.

The evolution of one system influences and is influenced by other systems. For example, tabloid scandalmongering and misrepresentation has fed social concerns about risk of violence from service users, which have almost certainly influenced politicians, and, in turn, social policy and new legislation. At a team level this has influenced the profile of risk assessment and management for clinicians and increased personal anxieties about responsibility and accountability. More positively, the disability rights movement and the political rhetoric of social inclusion has influenced the mental health user movement, academic debate and those working in mental health services and has helped shaped the

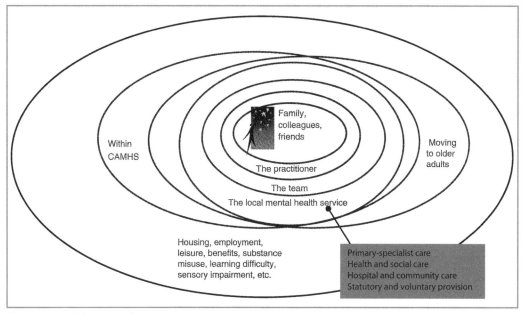

Figure 8.3 A local whole system

new recovery-orientated ideology of care promulgated vigorously by the National Institute of Mental Health for England. These developments in turn influence practice in ways that lead to tensions and paradoxes that can never be fully resolved. For example, team members are likely to find themselves working in contexts that are concerned with risk reduction while advocating an ideology of care that gives primacy to issues of self-determination, independence, autonomy and choice. Working with mental health systems requires that practitioners seek to understand them. This is not easy since changes in complex systems cannot be attributed simply to the actions of individuals and the rules they follow. Systems are best understood by observing them over time, to see what works and what does not.

Working with complexity

Change gurus such as Senge *et al.* (1999) use observations of biological growth as a metaphor for organizational change. For example, a growing tree develops through a reinforcing process of water and nutrients allowing root systems to expand to draw in more water and nutrients while simultaneously being constrained by limiting factors such as the availability of space and the effect of population and insects. New limitations may emerge as the growth gets to different levels. Observing and understanding the world as it is, rather than imposing reductionist, linear, mechanistic models is a key feature of working effectively with complexity. As Leonardo da Vinci said, 'Those who take for their standard anyone but nature – the mistress of all masters – weary themselves in vain.' You cannot make a tree grow through encouragement or threats, and you need to attend to removing the limiting factors as much if not more than promoting those factors that reinforce change and growth. Moreover, growth and change take time; achieving one stage of development is a requirement to achieving the next stage of development.

The certainty-agreement diagram in Figure 8.4, derived from Stacey (2000), provides a useful guide. It describes continua of certainty about how things are and agreement about how things should change. Most of the time we are somewhere in the middle of these continua which defines a 'zone of complexity' (Plsek and Greenhalgh 2001). Here it is not obvious what to do, as in the simple zone, but there is not so much disagreement and uncertainty as to throw the whole system into chaos.

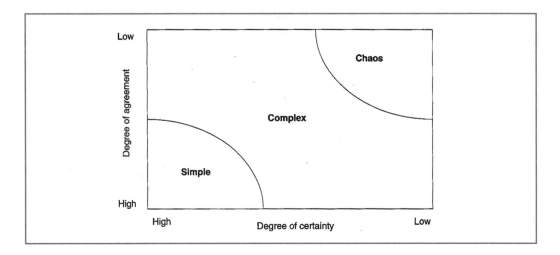

Figure 8.4   Certainty-agreement

If the aim is to move the system more towards the simple zone where groups of stakeholders can jointly partake in planned action, then measures to increase certainty about the current situation and agreement about what should be done are desirable. The first stage in planned developments involving a range of partners, whether they are agencies working to implement strategy, or team members working together, is to develop a shared vision of how things could be. There is, therefore, a need to focus explicitly on articulating basic values about what services should be achieving for people and developing effective local needs assessment at the individual, service and locality level.

Having described a preferred future it is then important to understand the current situation, and this is where the all-important user perspective is critical. As the MHPIG states, 'All elements have to interact as a system, so that the service user experiences continuity during their pathway through care, with each element offering added value' (DH 2001: 86–7). Process redesign (Locock 2001) is a method for exploring this experience with users and front-line staff in a systematic manner (see http://www.csip.org.uk/resources/directory-of-service-improvement.html for guidance). All such approaches need to start with the experience of users as the foundation from which to develop services.

Equipped with a vision for a preferred future and a clear sense of how things currently are it is then important to capture the strengths, assets and achievements that have got the service to where they are now, even if it does not feel as if much progress has been achieved. A solution-focused approach to systems change (Jackson and McKergow 2002) provides an accessible and effective range of approaches to help services describe their preferred future, explore where they are now, and capture the strengths that have got them there before then considering how those strengths and positive experiences can inform action.

Working in the zone of complexity places a high value on intuition and imagination. It requires multiple approaches that make effective use of experience, experimentation, freedom to innovate and working at the edge of knowledge and experience. Tools for this include the use of action learning (Smith 2001) and the plan-do-study-act cycle of quality improvement (Berwick 1998). Increasingly, these take place in the context of improvement work that involves large groups of participants with a strong emphasis on working bottom-up so that the involvement and influence of users, their networks and front-line staff is maximized (cf. Chapter 9).

Another feature of working with complexity is the need to use only minimum specifications for change that allow maximum freedom for creativity. This contrasts somewhat with the highly specified approach embodied within the MHPIG and the performance management that accompanies it. This bears on the issue of local commissioning, which requires performance managers to support local innovation by allowing local solutions to emerge that both achieve the functions sought by centrally prescribed models while not over-specifying the means such that local ownership, interest and commitment is sacrificed.

Carrots are more powerful than sticks in influencing practitioners' behaviour. The achievement of meaning in one's work through feeling clinically effective appears to be a central source of personal reward and job satisfaction for staff (Onyett 2003). The benign exploitation of the positive meaning that people attach to their work underpins solutions focused approaches (Jackson and McKergow 2002) and other novel approaches to change, such as 'appreciative inquiry' (Srivastva and Cooperrider 1999). Being able to engage hearts and minds through showing personal interest in colleagues is also a key leadership skill that has been shown to impact positively on a range of outcomes including admission rates to hospital for crisis resolution teams (see forthcoming publications from Sainsbury Centre for Mental Health on 'Leadership and Performance of Crisis Resolution Teams', www.scmh.org.uk). A wide range of people in leadership and management roles have a key role to play in developing work contexts where staff can stay effective and feel that their work has social value. Team effectiveness research (e.g. West and Markiewicz 2004) provides practical guidance on how this can be achieved. Our work at CSIP has sought to bring leadership and teamwork together at local level through action-learning processes as part of local improvement work. This approach underpins the Effective Teamwork and Leadership Programme which was positively evaluated (Rees and Shapiro 2005) and continues to evolve (see http://icn.csip.org.uk/leadership/). The RCN's Clinical Teams Programme (CTP) works on similar action learning based principles. It has been particularly successful with newly formed teams especially where teams have been or are going through a process of integration. It has also been successful when several teams share a common client pathway. The structure and content of the CTP is based on the evaluations of the Clinical Teams Project which delivered the CTP to 105 health and social care teams across England. Evaluation (RCN 2006, see www.rcn.org.uk) highlighted the challenge of implementing such programmes but also the considerable benefits for example increased openness and critical reflection within the team, and the creation of a local group of proactive change agents as a resource for the host organization.

NIMHE has also developed 'The Creating Capable Teams Approach'; an 'off the shelf', five step approach to support the integration of new ways of working and new roles, within existing resources, into the structures and practices of a multi-disciplinary team. The programme aims to provide a clearer understanding of the needs of their service users and carers and of the capabilities that exist within the team. Participants review the team skill mix and consider the introduction of new ways of working and new roles. Completion of the team profile and workforce plan enables the team to influence and contribute to the organization's workforce planning process. For further information see www.newwaysofworking.org.uk.

What does it all mean for nursing, and for nurse education?

Community mental health nurses (CMHNs) were at the forefront of more intensive approaches to community teamworking before the advent of the *NSF for Mental Health* and the MHPIG. Home visiting ('assertive outreach' by another name) has been central to this. Thus, CMHNs have been working more holistically and autonomously than some other staff in the past. In some cases autonomous working has been associated with increased morale (Collins *et al.* 2000), and clinical experience suggests that it has resulted in greater self-confidence within the discipline leading to a more egalitarian and productive dialogue with other disciplines (Burns and Firn 2002). In common with other mental health disciplines, a greater focus on the operational management of more tightly designed teams has also been experienced by nurses as a threat to their professional autonomy and identity.

However, greater emphasis on operational management may prevent the frequency of poor practice that has been associated with freedom and lack of accountability (Morrall 1997). The role of inpatient nurses, hitherto neglected, is now also being given the attention that such a central and skilled role demands (DH 2002c). However, counter to the move towards strengthening professional identification and practice, the *NSF for Mental Health* and subsequent *New Ways of Working* initiative (see www.newwaysofworking.org.uk) has stressed the need to recruit and retain staff with the right range of competencies, regardless of their background. Features such as their attitudes and life experiences, and whether they reflect the diversity of the communities being served are coming to be seen as equally important as the individual's professional training. Indeed, Holmes (2001) argues that we are in a 'postdisciplinary' world where people have hitherto unimaginable access to knowledge and technical skills leading to increased specialization and an erosion of the link between one's profession or discipline and the actual work activity undertaken. Complexity requires 'solutions accommodating the unpredictability, irrationality and serendipity of everyday life' (Holmes 2001: 232) which have to be achieved collaboratively by a range of parties each bringing particular and specific insights and skills. Holmes criticizes as reactionary nurses' desire to protect and strengthen professional identify while embracing inter-professional collaboration and extended roles. He argues for purposefully designed generic mental health worker roles.

This proposal was rejected by the *Pulling Together* review conducted by the Sainsbury Centre for Mental Health (Sainsbury Centre for Mental Health 1997) and perhaps for good reason. Blanket genericism may erode the diversity that is needed to ensure effective multi-disciplinary team working. While it is important that some core aspects are shared across disciplines (such as basic human values, an ability to form effective working relationships and skills in assessment), the elements that separate us as disciplines should be celebrated in the interests of promoting a wide and flexible skills mix. In CMHTs the best outcomes in terms of staff morale are achieved when staff can simultaneously feel a valued sense of belonging (or 'identification') with both their team and their discipline (Onyett 1997). This is not to argue against new roles that address gaps in provision that have been identified, or changes in professional training to provide more interprofessional work experience and exposure to different cultures and mental models.

With increased professional self-determination and diversity of role comes an imperative for nurses to place greater emphasis on lifelong learning. The increasingly inter-dependent nature of education and training requires a focus in increasing whole systems' capability to improve. Fraser and Greenhalgh (2001) describe a range of education and training interventions aimed at developing systems. They tend to be self-directed, team focused, and based upon story telling and other narratives, particularly from users of the service.

Conclusion

In summary, the key points that emerge from this chapter are as follows:

- We need to be mindful of, but not dazzled by, the guidance on functional teams and the research to support it. This information needs to be integrated with what we know to be local needs and circumstances and the existing strengths within the local context – particularly those that build positive relationships around users and their supports. The principles of stepped care should be borne in mind when considering service design at a local level.
- All teams need to be functional. Not just the new models.
- If we can achieve effective team working and the full implementation of care coordination many of the complex issues of how local teams interrelate would be solved. Effective team working requires clear objectives, effective leadership and management, support for change, an expectation of excellence and good team member participation in decision-making.
- Whole systems working is more than a way of thinking about how services work together. It requires bottom-up approaches that take full account of the complexity of systems, the nature of change, recognition of where power lies to make things different, and incorporates the experience of a wide range of stakeholders.
- Education and training for mental health staff needs to reflect this postmodern environment in which disciplines become less defined, increased collaboration is required, there is an increased emphasis on learning by experience, and recognition that change is best achieved from the bottom up by focusing on the experience of users, their social networks and staff.

Questions for reflection and discussion

1   What types of mental health teams operate in your work context and what are their defining characteristics?
2   How 'functional' is the current organization of teams in your area of work? How far do they ensure that the right functions are fulfilled for the right people?

3 How 'functional' is the multi-disciplinary team within which you currently work? Where does the power lie within the team? What might be done to improve the ability of the team to meet service users' needs?

4 With reference to service users that you know in receipt of community mental health services, consider the benefits or otherwise of adopting the 'team approach'.

Acknowledgements

I am grateful to Becky Dewdney-York, Project Manager CSIP SW Improving Access to Psychological Therapies – Primary Care Mental Health – Workforce Research for an invaluable update on primary care and mental health service developments.

Annotated bibliography

- Department of Health (2001–2) *Mental Health Policy Implementation Guide.* London: DH. As the definitive government guidance on teams this is required reading. The astute reader will embed it within an informed view of what is important for local service development and implementation.
- Onyett, S.R. (2003) *Teamworking in Mental Health.* London: Palgrave. This text takes a deeper look at team working itself, regardless of the service model in which it takes place. It has a strong emphasis on practice within teams as well as giving a historical perspective and further guidance on the leadership, management and improvement of teams.
- Burns, T. and Firn, M. (2002) *Assertive Outreach in Mental Health: A Manual for Practitioners.* Oxford: Oxford University Press. Although about ACT this book can be read as a grounded, accessible and commonsense guide about working in any mental health team context. Its big strength is that it draws directly from the experience of running a mature ACT team. Highly recommended even if you do not agree with their position on compulsion.

References

Audini, B., Marks, I.M., Lawrence, R.E., Connolly, J. and Watts, V. (1994) Home-based versus out-patient/in-patient care for people with serious mental illness. Phase II of a controlled study. *British Journal of Psychiatry* **165**: 204–10.

Bainbridge, M. (2002) Carers are people too. *Mental Health Today* June: 24–7.

Berwick, D.M. (1998) Developing and testing changes in delivery of care, *Annals of International Medicine* **128**: 651–6.

Birchwood, M., Smith, J., Macmillan, F. and McGovern, D. (1998) Early intervention in psychotic relapse, in C. Brooker and J. Repper (eds) *Serious Mental Health Problems in the Community: Policy, Practice and Research.* London. Baillière Tindall.

Bower, P. and Gilbody S. (2005) Stepped care in psychological therapies: access, effectiveness and efficiency. Narrative literature review. *British Journal of Psychiatry* **187**: 189.

Burns, T. and Firn, M. (2002) *Assertive Outreach in Mental Health: A Manual for Practitioners.* Oxford: Oxford University Press.

Chinman, M.J., Rosenheck, R. and Lam, J.A. (2000) The case management relationship and outcomes of homeless persons with serious mental illness. *Psychiatric Services* **51**: 1142–7.

Collins, K., Jones, M.L., McDonnell, A., Read, S., Jones, R. and Cameron, A. (2000) Do new roles contribute to job satisfaction and retention of staff in nursing and professions allied to medicine? *Journal of Nursing Management* **8**: 3–12.

Craig, T.K.J., Garety, P., Power, P. *et al.* (2004) The Lambeth Early Onset (LEO) team: randomised controlled trial of the effectiveness of specialised care for early psychosis. *British Medical Journal* **329**: 1067–70.

Deci, P.A., Santos, A.B., Hiott, D.W., Schoenwald, S. and Dias, J.K. (1995) Dissemination of assertive community treatment programs. *Psychiatric Services* **46**(7): 676–8.

Department of Health (1999) *National Service Framework for Mental Health: Modern Standards and Service Models*. London: DH.

Department of Health (2000) *The NHS Plan*. London: DH.

Department of Health (2001) *Mental Health Policy Implementation Guide*. London: DH.

Department of Health (2001a) *Mental Health National Service Framework* (and the NHS Plan). *Workforce Planning, Education and Training Underpinning Programme: Adult Mental Health Services. Final Report by the Workforce Action Team*. London: DH.

Department of Health (2002a) *Mental Health Policy Implementation Guide: Community Mental Health Teams*. London: DH.

Department of Health (2002b) *Mental Health Policy Implementation Guide: Dual Diagnosis Good Practice Guide*. London: DH.

Department of Health (2002c) *Mental Health Policy Implementation Guide: Adult acute in-patient care provision*. London: DH.

Department of Health (2006) *Our Health, Our Care, Our Say: a new direction for community services*. London: DH.

Department of Health/CSIP (2005) *Assertive Outreach in Mental Health in England. Report from a day seminar on research, policy and practice*. London: DH.

Department of Health/CSIP (2007) *Guidance Statement on Fidelity and Best Practice for Crisis Resolution Teams*. London: DH.

Diamond, R.J. (1996) Coercion and tenacious treatment in the community: applications to the real world, in D.L. Dennis and J. Monahan (eds) *Coercion and Aggressive Community Treatment. A New Frontier in Mental Health Law*. New York: Plenum Press.

Drake, R.J., Haley, C.J., Akhtar, S. and Lewis, S. (2000) Causes and consequences of duration of untreated psychosis in schizophrenia. *British Journal of Psychiatry* **177**: 511–15.

Edwards, M.G. (2005) The integral holon. A holonomic approach to organizational change and transformation. *Journal of Organizational Change Management* **18**(3): 269–88.

Ford, R., Beadsmore, A., Ryan, P. *et al.* (1995) Providing the safety net: case management for people with a serious mental illness. *Journal of Mental Health* **1**: 91–7.

Fraser, S.W. and Greenhalgh, T. (2001) Coping with complexity: educating for capability. *British Medical Journal* **323**: 799–803.

Garety, P. and Jolley, S. (2000) Early intervention in psychosis. *Psychiatric Bulletin* **24**: 321–3.

Glover, G., Arts, G. and Babu, K.S. (2006). Crisis resolution/home treatment teams and psychiatric admission rates in England. *British Journal of Psychiatry* **189**: 441–5.

Goldman, H.H., Morrissey, J.P. and Ridgely, M.S. (1994) Evaluating the program on chronic mental illness. *Millbank Quarterly* **72**: 37–48.

Goldman, H.H., Ganju, V., Drake, R.E. *et al.* (2001) Policy implications for implementing evidence-based practices. *Psychiatric Services* **52**(12): 1591–7.

Gournay, K. (1999) Assertive community treatment – why isn't it working? *Journal of Mental Health* **8**: 427–9.

Griffiths, L. (2001) Categorisation to exclude: the discursive construction of cases in CMHTs. *Sociology of Health and Illness* **23**(5): 678–700.

Haslam, S.A. and Platow, M.J. (2001) The link between leadership and followership: how affirming social identity translates vision into action. *Personality and Social Psychology Bulletin* **27**(11): 1469–79.

Holloway, F. and Carson, J. (1998) Intensive case management for the severely mentally ill: controlled trial. *British Journal of Psychiatry* **172**: 19–22.

Holmes, C.A. (2001) Postdisciplinarity in mental health-care: an Australian viewpoint. *Nursing Inquiry* **8**(4): 230–9.

Hoult, J. (1986) Community care of the acutely mentally ill. *British Journal of Psychiatry* **149**: 137–44.

Hoult, J., Reynolds, I., Charbonneau-Powis, M., Weekes, P. and Briggs, J. (1983) Psychiatric hospital versus community treatment: The results of a randomized controlled trial. *Australian and New Zealand Journal of Psychiatry* **17**: 160–7.

Iles, V. and Sutherland, K. (2001) *Organizational Change*. London: NCCSDO.

Jackson, P.Z. and McKergow, M. (2002) *The Solutions Focus*. London: Nicholas Brealey Publishing.

Johnson, S., Nolan, F., Hoult, J. *et al.* (2005) Outcomes of crisis before and after introduction of a crisis resolution team. *British Journal of Psychiatry* **187**: 68–75.

Johnston, S., Salkeld, G., Sanderson, K. *et al.* (1998) Intensive case management in Australia: a randomized controlled trial. *Australian and New Zealand Journal of Psychiatry* **32**: 551–9.

Joy, C.B, Adams, C.E. and Rice, K. (2001) Crisis intervention for those with severe mental illness, in *The Cochrane Library*, Issue 4, Oxford: Update Software.

Killaspy, H., Bebbington, P., Blizard, R. *et al.* (2006) The REACT study: randomised evaluation of assertive community treatment in north London. *British Medical Journal* **332**: 815–20.

Koestler, A. (1967) *The Ghost in the Machine*. London: Arkana.

Locock, L. (2001) *Maps and Journeys; Redesign in the NHS*. Birmingham: Health Services Management Unit, University of Birmingham.

Marks, I.M., Connolly, J., Muijen, M. *et al.* (1994) Home-based versus hospital based care for people with serious mental illnesses. *British Journal of Psychiatry* **165**: 179–94.

Marshall, M. and Lockwood, A. (2000) Assertive community treatment for people with severe mental disorders. *Cochrane Database Syst Rev* 2000;(2):CD001089.

Marshall, M., Lockwood, A. and Green, R. (1998) Case management for people with severe mental disorders (Cochrane review), in *The Cochrane Library*, Issue 4, Oxford: Update Software.

McGrew, J.H., Wilson, R.G. and Bond, G.R. (1996) Client perspectives on helpful ingredients of assertive community treatment. *Psychiatric Rehabilitation Journal* **19**(3): 13–21.

McGrew, J.H., Wilson, R.G. and Bond, G.R. (2002) An exploratory study of what clients like least about assertive community treatment. *Psychiatric Services* **53**: 761–3.

Merson, S., Tyrer, P., Onyett, S. *et al.* (1992) Early intervention in psychiatric emergencies: a controlled clinical trial. *The Lancet* **339**: 1311–14.

Mickan, S. and Rodger, S. (2005) Effective health care teams: a model of six characteristics developed from shared perceptions. *Journal of Interprofessional Care* **19**(4): 358–70.

Morrall, P.A. (1997) Professionalism and community psychiatric nursing: a case study of four mental health teams. *Journal of Advanced Nursing* **25**: 1133–7.

Mueser, K.T., Bond, G.R., Drake, R.E. and Resnick, G. (1998) Models of community care for severe mental illness: a review of research on case management. *Schizophrenia Bulletin* **24**(1): 38–73.

NFAO (2005). Annual report 2004–05. London: NFAO.

NHSE/SSI (1999) *Effective Care Coordination in Mental Health Services: Modernising the Care Programme Approach*. London: DH.

Onyett, S.R. (1997) Collaboration and the community mental health team. *Journal of Interprofessional Care* **11**(3): 257–67.

Onyett, S.R. (2000) Understanding relationships in context as a core competence for psychiatric rehabilitation. *Psychiatric Rehabilitation Skills* **4**: 282–99.

Onyett, S.R. (2003) *Teamworking in Mental Health*. London: Palgrave.

Onyett, S. (ed.) (2007) *Working Psychologically in Teams*. London: BPS/CSIP.

Onyett, S.R., Kinde, K., Glover, G., Floyd, S., Bradley, S., and Middleton, H. (in press) Implementation of crisis resolution home treatment teams in England: findings of a national survey 2005–2006. *Psychiatric Bulletin* **32**: 374–7.

Ovretveit, J. (1986) *Organization of multidisciplinary community teams*, BIOSS Working paper. Uxbridge: Brunel University.

Pinfold, V., Smith, J. and Shiers, D. (2007) Audit of early intervention in psychosis service development in England in 2005. *Psychiatric Bulletin* **31**: 7–10.

Plsek, P.E. and Greenhalgh, T. (2001) The challenge of complexity in healthcare. *British Medical Journal* **323**: 625–8.

Priebe, S., Watts, J., Chase, M. and Matanov, A. (2005). Processes of Disengagement and Engagement in Assertive Outreach Patients: Qualitative Study. *British Journal of Psychiatry* **187**: 438–43.

Provan, K.G. and Milward, H.B. (1995) A preliminary theory of interorganizational network effectiveness: a comparative study of four community mental health systems. *Administrative Science Quarterly* **40**: 1–33.

Rees, A. and Shapiro, D. (2005) Effective Team Working and Leadership in Mental Health Programme. Evaluation Feedback Report to the NHS Leadership Centre. NHS Evaluation Group. University of Leeds.

Richter, A.W., West, M.A., van Dick, R. and Dawson, J.F. (2006) Boundary spanners' identification, intergroup contact and effective intergroup relations. *Academy of Management Journal* **49**: 1252–69.

Ridgely, M.S., Morrissey, J.P., Paulson, R.I., Goldman, H. and Calloway, M.O. (1996) Characteristics and activities of case managers in the RWJ Foundation Program on Chronic Mental Illness. *Psychiatric Services* **47**(7): 737–43.

Royal College of Nursing (2006) *Developing Effective Teams, Delivering Effective Services.* Executive Summary. London: RCN.

Sainsbury Centre for Mental Health (1997) *Pulling Together. The Future Role and Training of Mental Health Staff.* London: SCMH.

Sashidharan, S.P., Smyth, M. and Owen, A. (1999) PRiSM Psychosis Study: Thro' a glass darkly: A distorted appraisal of community care. *British Journal of Psychiatry* **175**: 504–7.

Senge, P., Roberts, C., Ross, R. *et al.* (1999) *The Dance of Change.* London: Nicholas Brealey.

Shea, G.P. and Guzzo, R.A. (1987) Groups as human resources. *Research in Personnel and Human Resources Management* **5**: 323–56.

Simmonds, S., Coid, J., Joseph, P., Marriott, S. and Tyrer, P. (2001) Community mental health team management in severe mental illness: a systematic review. *British Journal of Psychiatry* **178**: 497–502.

Smith, H. (1998) Needs assessment in mental health services: the DISC framework. *Journal of Public Health Medicine* **20**(2): 154–60.

Smith, M. (1998) Social systems intervention. *Nursing Standard* **13**(1): 35–6.

Smith, M., Coleman, R., Allott, P. and Koberstein, J. (1999) Assertive outreach: a step backward. *Nursing Times* **95**(30): 46–7.

Smith, P.A.C. (2001) Action learning and reflective practice in project environments that are related to leadership development. *Management Learning* **32**(1): 31–48.

Spindel, P. and Nugent, J. A. (1999) The Trouble with PACT: Questioning the increasing use of assertive community treatment teams in community mental health. http://www.peoplewho.org/readingroom/spindel.nugent.htm.

Srivastva, S. and Cooperrider, D. (1999) *Appreciative Management and Leadership. Rev.* Euclid, OH: Lakeshore Communications.

Stacey, R.D. (2000) *Strategic Management and Organizational Dynamics* (3rd edn). Harlow: Pearson Education.

Stein, L.I. and Test, M.A. (1980) Alternative to mental hospital treatment, I. *Archives of General Psychiatry* **37**: 392–7.

Thornicroft, G., Becker, T., Holloway, F. *et al.* (1999) Community mental health teams: evidence or belief? *British Journal of Psychiatry* **175**: 508–13.

Tyrer, P. (1998) Cost-effective or profligate community psychiatry? *British Journal of Psychiatry* **172**: 1–3.

Tyrer, P. (2000) Effectiveness of intensive treatment in severe mental illness. *British Journal of Psychiatry* **176**: 492–3.

Tyrer, P., Simmonds, S., Coid, J., Mariott, S. and Joseph, P. (2001) A defence of community mental heath teams (letter). *British Journal of Psychiatry* **179**: 268.

West, M.A. and Markiewicz, L. (2004) *Building team-based working.* Blackwell: BPS.

Wright, C., Burns, T., James, P. *et al.* (2003) Assertive outreach teams in London: models of Operation Pan-London Assertive Outreach Study, Part 1. *British Journal of Psychiatry* **183**: 132–8.

CHAPTER 9

Service improvement

Jean Penny and Iain Ryrie

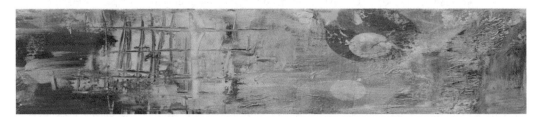

Chapter overview

Mental health services in the UK have undergone a period of unprecedented change in recent decades. This trend is set to continue and nurses should anticipate that their roles and the world around them will keep changing. Consequently, service improvement and change management are now core skills for nurses working at all levels. Traditionally however, service improvement as a discrete discipline, with its own evidence base and skills set, has not been an integral part of curricula for health care professionals in training or practice.

In 2005 the Department of Health established the NHS Institute for Innovation and Improvement, which aims to support the NHS to transform health care for patients and the public by rapidly developing and spreading new ways of working, new technology and world class leadership. To support this aim the NHS Institute's 'Improvement in Pre-registration Education' programme has worked with partners in the NHS and higher education to develop improvement capability in the NHS workforce by engaging with pre-registration health care students during their professional education. The programme aims to develop health care professionals who actively seek to improve their service, are receptive to new ideas and can use a variety of tools and techniques to bring about improvement.

In this chapter we present the case for improvement, introduce the Discipline of Improvement and report on the work of the NHS Institute to demonstrate the value and impact of a systematic approach to service improvement in practice. The first part of the chapter outlines contemporary drivers for improvement, describes the origins of the Improvement Discipline and presents its four key elements which draw heavily from the industrial and commercial sectors and from psychology. The second part of the chapter describes how the discipline has been woven into curricula for nurses in training. We include a case study to demonstrate its impact in practice and its potential to equip health care professionals with the knowledge and skills they need to develop first class services based on the needs of service users and their carers.

In summary this chapter covers:

■ Contemporary drivers for service improvement;
■ the origins of service improvement;
■ The Discipline of Improvement;
■ Service improvement in pre-registration education;

■   The NHS Institute's 'Improvement in Pre-registration Education' programme.

Contemporary drivers for service improvement

The National Service Framework for Mental Health (DH 1999) set a challenging agenda for the development of mental health services (cf. Chapters 6 and 35). Subsequent generic policy documents including *Our Health, Our Care, Our Say* (DH 2006a) and the NHS *Next Stage Review* (DH 2008) have reiterated the direction of travel, which involves closer partnership working with service users and the public in the design, development and governance of services. This position is reinforced further by *World Class Commissioning* (DH 2007) which identifies a role for service users and the public in all stages of the commissioning cycle.

These are key drivers for service improvement that speak to the responsibilities of organizations and the strategic objectives they should pursue. What has been less evident in the literature are guidance and examples of how individual, qualified practitioners or student nurses can contribute to these strategic objectives. It is not unusual to find reports of clinical governance projects that have used audit methods to improve service quality and safeguard high standards in the mental health field (Taylor and Jones 2006), and there is an increasing recognition of the need for clinical management skills among the workforce, which might typically include workload and clinical information management (Lloyd *et al.* 2008). Typically these are high level skills exercised by experienced staff often working in a strategic or managerial role once removed from the direct delivery of care.

There is less information available to guide individual practitioner contributions to the service improvement agenda through their routine work with service users and carers. Rarely is this subject included in pre-registration educational curricula and the Chief Nursing Officer's review of mental health nursing does not make the role explicit within its recommendations (DH 2006b). Nevertheless, the NHS *Next Stage Review* calls for greater freedom for front-line staff to find ways to deliver better and safer services to service users and their families (DH 2008). Service improvement capability needs therefore to be part of the professional development of all NHS staff. The mental health nursing profession must position itself within this vision and provide methods for students, qualified staff or managers to make meaningful contributions to the improvement agenda. The Discipline of Improvement provides such a method.

Origins of service improvement

NHS modernization and service improvement began in earnest in the late 1980s and early 1990s when two industrial, corporate led and organization wide change concepts predominated: Business Process Reengineering and the all-encompassing Total Quality Management (McLeod 2005). While both have similarities including an emphasis on experimentation and the need to design and operate a seamless value adding system (Senge *et al.* 1994), there are fundamental differences. The objective of Business Process Reengineering is to achieve massive gains by forcing organizations to fundamentally rethink their basic processes, while Total Quality Management puts an emphasis on continuous and incremental improvement and tries to keep functional hierarchies intact (Gadd and Oakland 1996). It is these two change models that have shaped the move for service improvement in health care today.

In the early 1990s the literature was bullish and defined Business Process Reengineering as 'the fundamental rethinking and radical redesign of business processes to achieve dramatic improvements in measures of performance such as cost, quality, service and speed' (Hammer and Champy 1993: 2). This created the appeal of a top down opportunity to radically transform existing structures and patterns of working and was heralded as the new approach to change management. The emphasis was on starting from scratch with a strong focus on customers by changing traditional departments and reorganizing along work processes (Coulson-Thomas 1994; Stroetmann et al. 1994). However, the literature of the late 1990s begins to report flaws with industries using Business Process Reengineering techniques identifying problems in implementation and realizing the predicted results. It is said that 70 per cent of Business Process Reengineering projects failed with the biggest obstacles being lack of sustained commitment and leadership, unrealistic expectations and resistance to change (Malhotra 1998).

The model of Business Process Reengineering therefore evolved over time by integrating incremental process change methods and incorporating various other philosophies, concepts, methods and tools, similar to Total Quality Management (Malhotra 1998; Blanton 1999). The key difference in this evolution is the integration of learning and the empowerment of staff in a bottom up approach to change.

Although the risks of large-scale change programmes were well documented, the Leicester Royal Infirmary became a national pilot site for this change methodology, which was an innovation in English health care in 1992 (McNulty and Ferlie 2002). In an evaluation that was completed ten years after the Leicester Royal Infirmary pilot, Thomas et al. (2002) reflected on the state of readiness for whole systems change and the effect of professional and organizational boundaries. They concluded that the NHS is unused to the idea of systematic change since it is full of linear structures that inhibit learning across boundaries.

A need was therefore realized for strategies to support a fundamental change of thinking and behaviour so that the knowledge and skills of health care improvement would become firmly embedded in NHS culture (Fillingham 2004). This was the beginning of the movement to build service improvement capability in the NHS with the recognition that alongside the tools and techniques, there was also the need to understand the attitudes and behaviours necessary for change to happen.

Much has been written on how this could be achieved. Berwick (1998a, b, c) and colleagues from the Institute for Healthcare Improvement (IHI) in the USA produced a series of papers on improvement in health care. The focus of these papers included physician involvement, measurement and data collection, developing and testing changes in the delivery of health care and the importance of cooperation. At the same time the NHS in England was working with clinical teams to use and adapt improvement methods and thereby add to the body of improvement knowledge (Bevan et al. 2000; Kerr et al. 2002). Yet improvement was not generally considered part of a professional's development, causing Bevan (2005) to ask: 'How can we build on the current NHS leadership, learning and improvement capabilities so that all levels of the health care workforce, across all parts of the system can deliver the new agenda?'

The Discipline of Improvement

The Discipline of Improvement incorporates the knowledge, skills, attitudes and behaviours used by experienced NHS improvers to make effective sustainable improvements (Penny 2002; Penny *et al.* 2004). The discipline draws on models and theories from multiple sources many of which are well established. It is the way in which connections are made between these components that offers a new approach to understanding change within the complex world of health care provision (Clarke *et al.* 2004). These established models and theories are all underpinned by research evidence, yet often these areas of expertise are owned by individuals, teams or professions who rarely meet to join their knowledge and skills for the benefit of improving NHS services and care.

The evidence base for service improvement is organized into a framework that includes four key domains: understanding user needs and experiences, processes and systems, people and cultures, and initiating and sustaining improvements. Box 9.1 summarizes these domains and poses a series of questions for each to elaborate their meaning. Many of these elements are familiar to experienced practitioners such as the psychology of involvement and change and project and programme management but to many the industrial models of processes and systems, and how they are applied to health care, are new.

The knowledge and skills of improvement start with a willingness to listen to and understand the issues that face service users, their carers and staff. By first really listening and then looking in detail at how current processes and systems impact on their experiences, safety and outcomes, improvement ideas can be generated.

Mapping the journeys or processes that service users have to navigate as they go through complex health care systems is a good way to begin to understand their experience. This is a team activity that should include the people involved in the service under review as well as other key stakeholders. Process maps have an agreed start and end point such as 'service user is referred for assessment' to 'service user completes a treatment programme'. Then all the steps and actions the service user encounters between these two points are written down. The areas that cause problems for the service user, their carers or staff such as delays, duplication of work or lack of communication are identified and, through discussion, ideas for improvement captured.

While understanding what is most likely to be the problem and generating improvement ideas is a first step, understanding how to test improvement ideas and implement those that are likely to work requires another set of skills. Individual preferences and the culture of a team, department and entire organization can have a big impact. What seems a good idea to one person in one part of the service may not seem so great to others elsewhere for a variety of reasons. Testing an idea to generate measurable evidence is therefore an important part of the improvement process. A key tool in this respect is Langley *et al.*'s (1996) Model for Improvement. This model asks three key questions:

- **What are you trying to achieve?** – this question requires an improvement leader to work with those involved in the service under review as well as other key stakeholders to discuss and agree the aim for the improvement.
- **How will you know a change is an improvement?** – this question leads to an agreement of the four or five key measures that will indicate whether the aim has been achieved and if it really is an improvement.

Box 9.1   The service improvement framework

User needs and experiences

- Do you really know what happens to users and their carers as they use your service?
- Do you know what is important to them?
- Do you know what they need to make their experience better?
- Do you know what they would like more of and what they do not want?
- How do you involve them in ideas to improve your service? Do you really listen to them?

People and cultures

- Do you like change yourself? What would encourage you to do things differently? Do your colleagues and leaders like change?
- Are there always lots of ideas and encouragement to do things differently or are people generally reluctant to move from the status quo?
- What is the culture like in your team or organization? Does it embrace change or is it reluctant to do things differently?
- Are there identifiable factors in your team culture that facilitate or inhibit the adoption of change?

Processes and systems

- Have you ever mapped the processes in your service?
- Do you know how users arrive at your service and where they go to when they leave you?
- Do you know where and why users experience frustrations or where their care may be delayed? Do you know how long they have to wait at different stages of their journey?
- Do you understand how your part of the system impacts on others?

Initiating and sustaining

- What do you measure about your service? Are they the things that matter to your users and their carers?
- Do you know how to test your idea before implementing?
- If your improvement idea has been tested and shown to be an improvement, do you know what to do? How does your improvement idea fit with the business plan of your organization?
- What factors influence the sustainability of the improvement and how would you know that a change is actually a sustainable improvement?

- **What changes can you make that will result in the improvements that you seek?** – if those involved in the service and other key stakeholders are asked for ideas to achieve the aim, expect a variety of ideas from a variety of sources. All improvement ideas should be considered and those thought to be most likely to achieve the aim are tested and studied before implementation.

Small scale testing of selected improvement ideas is undertaken using the plan, do, study, act (PDSA) cycle. The testing of each selected idea is planned including where, how and who will test and what are the expected effects in terms of the measures of improvement. Test results are then studied to understand what happened and how it compares with what was expected. Subsequent actions are considered according to this assessment. If the effects were positive a bigger test of the same idea for a longer period would be advisable. If the effects were not as good as expected it may be possible to repeat the test by modifying the improvement idea or it may be necessary to try another of the improvement ideas. PDSA cycles are repeated until an effective improvement idea has been identified which receives support from all key stakeholders. This model not only promotes a continuous approach to improvement but supports the development of an improvement culture. The method encourages people to get involved, to understand user experiences and the processes and systems they encounter. It tests improvement ideas, measures their effects and captures the learning.

Improvement is therefore an all-embracing discipline, drawing on models, frameworks and learning from industry and commerce as well as from other health care systems around the world. A valuable literature has started to accrue. One source is the 16 short texts that form the Improvement Leaders' Guides (NHS Institute for Innovation and Improvement 2006). These are written by NHS improvers who have passed on their experiences and advice, and provide a valuable source of information for anyone wanting to know more about the knowledge and skills of improvement.

Service improvement curricula for nurses

In 2007 the NHS Institute for Innovation and Improvement commissioned a piece of work that reviewed the extent to which a sample of English universities (n=15) include the Discipline of Improvement in their pre-registration courses of education (NHS Institute for Innovation and Improvement 2007).

Only one university felt they were delivering formalized service improvement learning. This was embedded in a Professional Development module that ran from year 1 throughout a student's training. Among the other universities there was a fairly even divide between those that did not deliver service improvement learning and those that included aspects of the discipline but not as part of a formal or explicit service improvement module or learning experience. Elements of service improvement were included in a range of modules including 'change management', 'service re-design' and 'leadership and management'. Typically this involved a stand-alone lecture rather than a consistent theme that was revisited throughout the modules.

Plans to develop or formalize service improvement activities into discrete modules or units of learning were not evident across this sample of universities. A number of barriers were reported. Some universities felt that pre-registration students' focus should not include service improvement. They felt that students were familiarizing themselves with clinical environments and could not appreciate the value of service improvement learning. One respondent described a defensive, risk averse culture in which the university must strive to make students fluent and literate in their clinical areas. Service improvement was seen as being beyond this initial literacy.

The long lead-in times required to develop curricula were seen as a barrier as was the jam-packed nature of existing curricula. One university representative felt they were asked to do everything with little flexibility. There was also recognition that service improvement learning requires clinically credible staff. For some universities being clinically credible remained an ongoing challenge.

It would appear that the service improvement discourse has started to enter higher education for health care practitioners but often in ad hoc ways with few universities drawing their strands of work together into coherent whole units or modules of learning. There does appear to be a willingness among some universities to explore further development of this discipline with calls for support from the NHS Institute to:

- work with clinical representatives, educational leads and patients to build business cases;
- support universities to bring innovation and curricula together in coherent strategic plans;
- support the development of clinically credible teaching staff;
- contribute to the curriculum validation process.

The NHS Institute's 'Improvement in Pre-registration Education' programme

A strategy for building improvement capability in NHS staff in England was initiated by the NHS Modernisation Agency and continued by the NHS Institute for Innovation and Improvement and underpins section 4 (Service Improvement) and section 5 (Quality) of the Knowledge and Skills Framework (DH 2004). The NHS Institute has been working with higher education institutions (HEI) and their NHS partners to develop, pilot and spread short courses in service improvement for pre-registration health, social and medical care students. Phase 1 ran until March 2007 and involved three universities who developed, implemented and refined the short courses. Phase 2 began in May 2007 and consisted of two elements; further development and implementation of the learning by the original three partner organizations; and extending their implementation to include six new partner organizations. This section draws from an external evaluation of Phase 2 commissioned by the NHS Institute (NHS Institute for Innovation and Improvement 2008). We specifically report detail of the learning experience and evidence of its impact on students' knowledge and their practice.

Service improvement learning

The curricula incorporated the four components of service improvement into a core day during which students were introduced to the subject and to a number of improvement tools including the plan, do, study, act (PDSA) cycle, process mapping and the model for improvement (Langley *et al.* 1996). During this core day students were also exposed to the experiences of service users and patients from which opportunities for service improvement could be identified. This was achieved by having service users present in the 'classroom' or using specifically designed case studies based on real scenarios. Some universities developed DVDs with patients that recounted in imaginative ways their experiences with health and social care systems.

Each programme required students to further develop and apply their improvement learning in a clinical or related setting. This was achieved in different ways. Typically the core day was broken down into a number of sessions with students encouraged to apply the learning between each session, e.g. 3 x 2 hour sessions. This provided students with time to reflect on practice, on the service improvement opportunities they had identified and their proposed approaches to address those needs.

The opportunity to practise or implement learning between sessions was considered critical by the phase 2 partners but also necessitated close working with and development of practice partners, facilitators and mentors. Delivery of the core day to these staff ahead of students undertaking the learning was a successful strategy in these respects. Partners also used abridged workshops and produced hard copy briefing materials. Importantly this cross-fertilization between practice and education staff was reported to bring increasing clinical credibility to the participating universities.

Students were encouraged to undertake small improvement projects as part of the learning or to draft abstracts of improvement ideas detailing the steps that could be taken. Some universities summatively assessed the learning, others did not. However, the value of summative assessments was recognized across the field and those students who were not summatively assessed as part of this learning were encouraged to apply it to other modules in which summative assessments were made.

University partners variously described the improvement product as both a framework and a process or as a series of principles and a set of actions. As a framework it brings together elements of practice that are not unfamiliar to students but which are focused in a tighter way enabling them to see a whole that is greater than the sum of its parts. As a process it was felt to focus students' understanding of improvement as an everyday task rather than a high level activity, and provide them with confidence and permission to reflect on practice and to question how health care is delivered. The process was characterized as developmental in nature allowing students an opportunity to try things out and to develop knowledge and experience through practice. Importantly, this experiential knowledge complements the theoretical components of the improvement framework. It was felt that these dual elements provided students with 'a capacity and ability to look with a fresh eye at the experience of service users, how their experience arises and how it can be improved' (NHS Institute for Innovation and Improvement 2008: 9).

Impact of learning

A mixture of complementary methods was used by the evaluation team to identify evidence for the impact of the learning in practice. These included a cross-sectional survey of students to capture their knowledge and attitudes towards service improvement, any opportunities they had to undertake service improvement while on placement, and their anticipated future use of the learning. Additionally there was space for students to describe the key lessons they had taken from the learning. The survey was administered to students on completion of their learning experience by HEI staff. Evaluation staff also collected case vignettes from students and staff to document evidence of the application of learning in practice. These followed a loose structure that described the improvement opportunity or problem, the actions taken by students and the impact of any actions.

Across the field 15 professional disciplines received the improvement learning, which included occupational therapists, physiotherapists, doctors, nurses (four branches), midwives, operating department practitioners, dieticians, radiographers, social workers, social carers, psychologists and dentists. In total, this included 2235 students of which 1135 completed the cross-sectional survey. The data were presented in aggregate form making it difficult to pick out results for individual disciplines.

Following the learning a majority of students were keen to be involved in service improvement work (81 per cent) with a significant proportion feeling confident about being involved (67 per cent). A majority reported that the service improvement learning was important for their professional development (88 per cent) and 85 per cent believed it would enhance their future job prospects. The survey invited students to list the key lessons they had taken from their service improvement learning experience. A summary of that learning is presented below.

Service improvement tools

Students consistently reported that PDSA cycles and process mapping were the key service improvement tools they had taken from the learning. They were variously described as easy to use, simpler and less time consuming than expected.

Patients and service users

Students emphasized the importance of patient safety and involving service users and carers in the identification of potential service improvements. This involvement was underpinned by a need to listen carefully so that their perspective and experience could be understood properly. Students also reported the importance of patient and service user perspectives to evaluate whether any change had been successful.

Communication

Effective communication was seen by many as being the crux of service improvement. There was particular emphasis on the need to improve communications between all professionals and for all professionals to be aware of its importance. Listening, reflecting and feeding back were thought to be vital. A key lesson some respondents took away in these respects was the relationship between feedback and change. They learned how non-judgemental, timely feedback can actually encourage change. As well as communicating with others, students emphasized the importance of honest communication with themselves, being aware of their own actions, taking time to reflect and developing the capacity to show empathy.

Whole systems

A number of students gained a better understanding of the contexts and systems within which health and social care are delivered. Implications for identifying and planning service improvements included a need to consider the whole picture, to plan across whole systems, to facilitate complex multi-disciplinary involvement and to involve as broad a range of people as possible.

Improvement and change

Students consistently reported that they had learned there is always room for improvement, that it is a constant need and that there is no reason to fear change. They also expressed optimism about the student's role bringing a fresh view, being well placed to identify what needs improving and feeling confident enough to suggest improvements. They were realistic about the improvement process and recognized that small steps can make a big difference and that simple ideas are often the most effective and easiest to implement.

Career

A number of students emphasized the value of this knowledge when applying for their first post qualification position and attending interviews. In at least two cases when the survey was completed the students' demonstration of their service improvement knowledge was key to securing their first qualified posts. Many others believed that the learning would have a positive impact on career opportunities, give them a confidence boost as they approached qualification and provide them with a knowledge base and skill set to become a useful member of clinical and social care teams. Among those students who received this learning toward the end of their training a number requested that it should be introduced much earlier in the curricula from year 1 onwards.

In addition to these reported survey results a number of case vignettes were captured that demonstrate application of the improvement learning in practice. An example is provided in Box 9.2.

Box 9.2   Case vignette of impact in practice

A student was on placement with a mental health physiotherapy team that had use of a gym. They provided sessions for women with common mental health problems such as anxiety and depression. Some of the women attended spasmodically and some had been attending for many months. Although the hour-long session was well structured there was no real sense of progression. It was not possible to tell whether pieces of equipment or specific activities were too hard or whether they should be progressed to an increased level or amount of time. The student identified the need for some objective markers so that a client's progress can be monitored and appropriate adjustments made to their programme.

The student reviewed a number of available indicators and selected a 60 metre walk test and use of the BORG scale. The latter provides a rating of perceived exertion for different activities and pieces of equipment. Completing these simple tests over time would then provide an indication of progress.

The student implemented the approach as a pilot with two women who agreed to participate. The tests were unobtrusive, easy to administer and worked well within the gym context. Test results revealed where the women were having difficulty with equipment or activities and where they were ready to progress. It was concluded that this approach ensures exercises are suited to the needs of the individual and provides participants with measure of their progress across time. It also provides a systematic way for staff to ensure throughput of women over time, thereby freeing spaces for other women who could benefit from this service. The student has written up this work and provided a protocol and pro-forma for ongoing use by the mental health physiotherapy team.

In another reported case study an improvement facilitator who supported students on their placement reported an intention to use subsequent cohorts of service improvement students to continue the work that had been initiated. This suggests the emergence of a mechanism that will help sustain and further embed service improvement work in practice.

The case vignettes presented in the Phase 2 evaluation report do provide an indication of the outcomes that can be achieved as a result of introducing the discipline of service improvement into pre-registration education. The report also acknowledges that many other factors affected the perceptions and performance of these health and social care students besides the service improvement learning, and that the evaluation was not designed to test cause and effect relationships. The results should therefore be interpreted with some caution.

Nevertheless, the evaluation does capture a range of data to build a case for the benefits that service improvement learning can bring. There is a clear relationship between the positive ratings and qualitative comments on the student survey and the case vignettes. Students appear able to apply this learning in practice in systematic ways that produce demonstrable benefit. The following quotations from students further support these inferences.

> 66 I am beginning to witness the positive outcomes of my suggestions on placement now, which prior to this module I would not have felt confident in suggesting let alone researching, process mapping, explaining and justifying to others and indeed implementing these improvements. 99

> 66 My previous perception was that the organization in the NHS was all set by government legislation and NHS management. The truth is that small improvements developed by all workers in the health service can be put in place to change services for the better.
>
> (NHS Institute for Innovation and Improvement 2008: 17–18) 99

Conclusion

Change is a constant in our world that is driven by a quest for improvement. Public services are now subject to this principle more than ever before. The emancipation of service users from passive recipients of care to active partners in the design and delivery of services heralds a new era. While 'trust me I'm a doctor' was once the mantra, today 'trust me I'm a service user' is equally valid.

Mental health nurses need an approach to engage with this agenda as part of their routine contact with users and carers. Improvement and change management skills are no longer the sole responsibility of higher managers and strategy planners. They are now needed as integral parts of service delivery by all levels of the workforce.

The heavily conceptualized and radical discipline of business process reengineering and its softer derivative, total quality management, have tended to raise the subject to a level that is off-putting or even impenetrable for some. However, from this work a simpler, more practical model for improvement has been forged, which can be adopted and used by all levels of health care personnel including students.

The work of the NHS Institute and its partners has been central to these developments. The improvement product described in this chapter marries theory with practice, principles with action and provides both a framework and a process. Evaluative data from the NHS Institute demonstrate a clear link between improvement learning and positive changes in practice. Students are able to develop a strategic awareness of service delivery that takes into account individual patient need and the wider context of health and social care. It equips them with skills and confidence to identify improvement opportunities and engage qualified staff in improvement activity.

These findings are in marked contrast to those universities who felt their students were unable to appreciate the value of service improvement learning or that it was beyond their initial literacy requirements as health care practitioners. The NHS Institute's work reports an appetite among students for this skills and knowledge base. At the time of writing the Institute is initiating Phase 3 of its improvement in pre-registration education programme. A total of 26 universities are scheduled to deliver the improvement learning to more than 5000 students. It may now be possible for improvement in health and social care to become everybody's business.

In summary the main points are:

- The pace of change in health and social care is set to continue and nurses should expect their roles and the context of care to continue to evolve.
- Change management and service improvement have typically been the responsibility of senior staff with managerial, operational and strategic roles.
- Current policy requires greater freedom for front-line staff to find ways to deliver better and safer services to service users and their families. Consequently service improvement and change management are now core skills for nurses working at all levels.
- From business process reengineering and total quality management activities in the NHS a simpler, more practical model for improvement has emerged with the potential for use by all levels of health care personnel including students.
- The Discipline of Improvement incorporates the knowledge, skills, attitudes and behaviours necessary to make effective sustainable improvements and is organized into a framework that includes four key domains: understanding user needs and experiences, processes and systems, people and cultures, and initiating and sustaining improvements.
- Over the last two years the NHS Institute for Innovation and Improvement has been working with nine university partners to introduce improvement learning into pre-registration education for health, social and medical care students.
- Evidence to date indicates that improvement learning can facilitate positive changes in practice. Students are able to develop a strategic awareness of service delivery, taking account of the experiences of service users, and feeling more confident to identify improvement opportunities and engage qualified staff in improvement activity.

Questions for reflection and discussion

1   If you were a service user receiving community mental health care, what might you want improved?
2   As a student nurse, how confident are you about raising opportunities for service improvements when you are on placement? What facilitates or frustrates your ability to do this?
3   Think of an improvement idea that would enhance the quality of the care you deliver:

- How would you go about testing the idea?
4 What data would you collect to determine whether it really is an improvement?
5 Which of the four parts of the Discipline of Improvement do you feel least comfortable with? What can you do to find out more and develop your skills?

Annotated bibliography

- NHS Institute for Innovation and Improvement (2006) *Improvement Leaders' Guides* (previously branded for NHS Modernisation Agency) available online from www.institute.nhs.uk/improvementguides. A boxed set of 16 short texts written by experienced NHS improvers about different aspects of improvement. They present a range of models, frameworks and ideas to try and learn from. Invaluable for anyone who wants an introduction to the knowledge and skills of improvement.
- Goldratt, E. and Cox, J. (1993) *The Goal.* Aldershot: Gower. An easy to read introduction to system, processes and constraints written in the form of a novel.
- Lloyd, C., King, R., Deane, F. and Gournay, K. (2008) *Clinical Management in Mental Health Services.* Chichester: Wiley-Blackwell. Although the focus of this book is on clinical management it deals with a number of issues relevant to improvement including leadership, change, evidence-based practice, communications and public relations. It offers a practical guide to improve prevention, care and recovery for people who have mental health problems.

Useful websites:

- http://www.institute.nhs.uk/
- http://www.improvementfoundation.org/
- http://www.ihi.org/ihi
- Websites in England and USA all providing useful information and opportunities to develop improvement knowledge and skills.

References

Bevan, H. (2005) Functionality for the future: a strategy for building leadership, learning and improvement capability for the new NHS. Unpublished paper for the NHS Institute for Innovation and Improvement.

Bevan, H., Penny, J. and Layton, A. (2000) A breakthrough approach to reducing delays and patient waiting times. *Clinician in Management* **9**: 27–31.

Berwick, D. (1998a) Physicians as leaders in improving health care. *Annals of Internal Medicine* **128**: 289–92.

Berwick, D. (1998b) Developing and testing changes in delivery of care. *Annals of Internal Medicine* **128**: 651–6.

Berwick, D. (1998c) Cooperation: the foundation of improvement. *Annals of Internal Medicine* **128**: 1004–9.

Blanton, G.A. (1999) Total quality management, in J. Juran and A. Blanton Godfrey (eds) *Juran's Quality Handbook* (5th edn). London: McGraw-Hill.

Clarke, C., Reed, J. and Wainwright, D. (2004) The discipline of improvement: something old, something new? *Journal of Nursing Management* **12**: 85–96.

Coulson-Thomas, C. (1994) *Business Process Reengineering: myth and reality.* London: Kogan Page.

Department of Health (1999) *A National Service Framework for Mental Health.* London: DH.

Department of Health (2004) *The NHS Knowledge and Skills Framework and the Development Review Process.* London: The Stationery Office.

Department of Health (2006a) *Our Health, Our Care, Our Say: a new direction for community services.* London: The Stationery Office.

Department of Health (2006b) *From Values to Action: The Chief Nursing Officer's review of mental health nursing.* London: DH.

Department of Health (2007) *World Class Commissioning: Vision.* London: DH.

Department of Health (2008) *High Quality Care for all, NHS Next Stage Review Final Report.* London: DH.

Fillingham, D. (2004) Modernisation Ideas. *Health Service Journal* 22 January.

Gadd, K. and Oakland, J. (1996) Chimera or culture? Business process reengineering or total quality management? *Quality Management Journal* **96**: 20–38.

Hammer, M. and Champy, J. (1993) *Reengineering the Corporation: a manifesto for business revolution.* London: Nicholas Brealey.

Kerr, D., Bevan, H., Gowland, B., Penny, J. and Berwick, D. (2002) Redesigning cancer care. *British Medical Journal* **324**: 164–6.

Langley, G., Nolan, K., Nolan, T., Norman, C. and Provost, L. (1996) *The Improvement Guide: a practical approach to enhancing organizational performance.* San Francisco: Jossey Bass.

Lloyd, C., King, R., Deane, F. and Gournay, K. (2008) *Clinical Management in Mental Health Services.* Chichester: Wiley-Blackwell.

Malhotra, Y. (1998) Business Process Redesign: an overview. *Engineering Management Review* **26**: 3.

McLeod, H. (2005) A review of the evidence on organizational development in healthcare, in E. Peck (ed.) *Organizational Development in Healthcare.* Oxford: Radcliffe.

McNulty, T. and Ferlie, E. (2002) *Reengineering Healthcare: the complexities of organizational transformation.* Oxford: Oxford University Press.

NHS. Modernisation Agency Management Board. October.

NHS Institute for Innovation and Improvement (2006) *Improvement Leaders' Guides* (previously branded for NHS Modernisation Agency). Available online from www.institute.nhs.uk/improvementguides

NHS Institute for Innovation and Improvement (2007) University survey of improvement curricula. Unpublished paper for the NHS Institute for Innovation and Improvement.

NHS Institute for Innovation and Improvement (2008) Evaluation of the improvement in pre-registration education programme: final report. Unpublished paper for the NHS Institute for Innovation and Improvement.

Penny, J. (2002) Building the discipline of improvement for health and social care: next steps for NHS improvement, the early vision and way forward. Unpublished paper. MA Management Board. November.

Penny, J., Bevan, H., Swaby, V. and Wilcock, P. (2004) Building the discipline of improvement in health and social care. Unpublished paper.

Senge, P., Ross, R., Smith, B., Roberts, C. and Kleiner, A. (1994) *The Fifth Discipline Field Book.* London: Brearley.

Stroetmann, K., Maier, M. and Schertler, W. (1994) Business process reengineering – a German view, in Coulson-Thomas, C. (ed.) *Business Process Reengineering: myth and reality.* London: Kogan Page.

Taylor L. and Jones S. (2006) Clinical governance in practice: closing the loop with integrated audit systems. *Journal of Psychiatric and Mental Health Nursing* **13**: 228–33.

Thomas, P., McDonnell, J., McCulloch, J. and Ferlie, E. (2002) Facilitating learning and innovation in primary care organizations. Unpublished paper. Imperial College London Business School, Brent NHS PCT.

Interventions

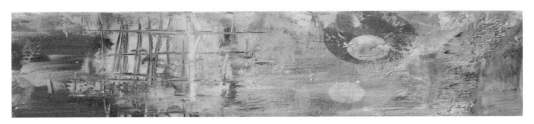

CHAPTER 10

Assessment

Iain Ryrie and Ian Norman

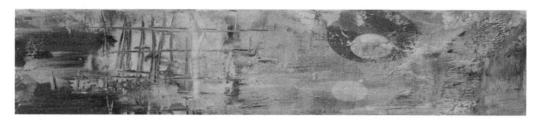

Chapter overview

Assessment is a cornerstone of mental health nursing and permeates all aspects of professional work. It can be difficult to comprehend the breadth of activity that represents assessment, and even harder to disentangle different approaches and their associated methods. We draw on the work of Barker (2004) to provide a 'map' of assessment that allows all its 'bits and pieces' to be understood collectively. Each is accorded its legitimate place in the framework, allowing each to be judged for its utility in relation to the person being assessed. The chapter is divided into two sections. The first deals in general with the principles and practice of assessment, from which the framework is developed. The second provides specific examples of selected assessment strategies. Further detail on the assessment of people with specific mental health problems can be found in relevant chapters of this book.

This chapter covers:

- defining assessment;
- the purpose of assessment;
- the scope of assessment;
- methods of assessment;
- assessing the whole person.

Defining assessment

In its broadest sense assessment permeates all aspects of nursing care. It is not just a discrete activity that initiates the 'nursing process' or 'problem-solving cycle', leading to a plan of care, which is implemented and evaluated. The preferences people have for different health care options (planning) necessitate assessment, as do their abilities to engage meaningfully with the intervention itself (implementation), and evaluation requires still further assessment activity. Even then, it would be incorrect to suggest that assessment occurs only at these key points in the nursing process. It is an ongoing cycle of activity that all nurses perform in all nursing situations.

Assessment may be implicit or explicit, informal or formal. It may involve simply noting a person's appearance and behaviour during a home visit or observing someone who is deemed to be at risk over extended periods. It can involve structured instruments that specify the type or severity of problem that someone experiences, or it may take the form of a seemingly casual conversation. Common to all types of assessment is the collection of information.

The information we collect as nurses must be meaningful and necessary. Assessment data traditionally describe a person's appearance and behaviour, or their presentation and performance, or again, the form and function of their thoughts and feelings. Barker (2004) emphasizes the importance of these two viewpoints and their use by nurses to better understand a person. However, Barker cautions also against simply collecting data on the form and function of a person's thoughts and feelings, which can contribute to the formation of a medical diagnosis but will tell us little else about the person in the broader context of their life. Diagnosis is therefore one 'bit' of assessment, which focuses typically on problems, deficits and abnormalities. More broadly, assessment information encompasses a person's overall sense of self and their position in life, including not only problems and diagnoses but also their assets and strengths (Barker 2004).

The collection of information is only one part of the assessment process. Savage (1991) and Barker (2004) point to the inferences nurses draw from the available data, and the decisions they make regarding a person's need for care. Assessment is therefore a two-stage process. It is not enough to only gather information; we must be able to do something useful with it, and that use is nursing's purpose. Hence, assessment is central to all nursing activity.

Barker has defined mental health nursing assessment as 'the decision-making process, based upon the collection of relevant information, using a formal set of ethical criteria, which contributes to an overall evaluation of a person and his circumstances' (Barker 2004: 7). This definition is useful since it implies the ongoing nature of assessment by referring to 'the decision-making process', which we take to be continuous and ever present in the activities of a nurse. Barker highlights also the importance of a '… formal set of ethical criteria', referring to such issues as confidentiality, note keeping, our style of interaction, how we ask questions, what we ask and why.

We would add to Barker's definition by stating that evaluations can be made also of groups, communities and the public. Group programmes may involve assessment of the group's cohesion, the balance of its members or their aggregate characteristics. Community assessments are increasingly important in contemporary care. For example, knowledge of a locality's geography, social structures, deprivation and resources is important for outreach teams that work with drug users or with those who experience severe symptoms of mental disorder. The mental health of the public is also increasingly recognized as an important mediator of individual health for which assessment of relevant indicators is needed (Wilkinson *et al.* 2007).

The purpose of assessment

We have emphasized two assessment stages, the collection of information and the use of that information to infer the need for nursing or other health care interventions. Though medical diagnosis is an important part of assessment, and one we fully acknowledge, mental health nursing is interested not in medical diagnoses per se, but in the way a person functions as a result of their condition. We need to comprehend their life problems (and strengths), and to understand the context within which these problems arise. Nursing diagnoses have been advocated for this purpose, which describe the nature of a person's problem and the effect it has on their functioning (Ward 1992). For example, 'I feel under threat and am angry with everyone I encounter.' This nursing diagnosis could be present in several medical diagnoses however, including paranoid schizophrenia or generalized anxiety disorder. Better then to deal with the nature of the problem and its implications, than with overlapping categories.

We have to confess that neither of us have been strong advocates of the term 'nursing diagnosis', preferring to use other, non-medical, terms to describe nurses' activity. But we agree fully with Ward (1992) and Barker (2004) that the exploration of relationships between a person's thoughts, feelings and behaviour is a diagnostic process, and one that nurses perform. Whether this procedure is referred to as nursing diagnosis, problem identification or functional analysis may be less important to the person in care.

Barker (2004) identifies four assessment objectives (summarized in Table 10.1), the products of which provide the basis for nursing diagnoses. The information in Table 10.1 provides an assessment overview; it tells us something about the quality, content and context of a person's health concern, its relationship to contributing factors and its effect on the person's and others' functioning. These data allow us to make judgements about why a problem exists and the factors that seem to be associated with it. In turn we are able to identify areas of need and so plan interventions. As a simple example consider the following problem statement: 'Arguments with my parents mean I don't like to be at home, so I spend my time alone in public parks where I smoke cannabis to make the day more interesting.' We can make several judgements about this person's need for care. The relationship between family tensions and personal isolation represents one possible area of need, and the lack of meaningful daily activity another. We might consider an opportunity to reflect on the positive and negative consequences of cannabis smoking to be a further need.

Objectives	Outcome
Measurement	Key questions such as how often a person experiences a problem or exhibits a behaviour provide information on the scale or size of the problem
Clarification	Key questions such as where, with whom and under what circumstances problems arise provide information on the context or conditions associated with the problem
Explanation	Key questions such as the effects of a person's behaviour, their own and others' interpretation of its meaning provide evidence for the possible purpose or function of the problem
Variation	Key questions such as how the person's problem varies over time and in different situations provide evidence for its seriousness and the degree to which it dominates their life

Table 10.1 Assessment objectives and outcome
(After Barker 2004)

The concept of 'needs led' assessment is an underlying principle of the NHS and Community Care Act (1990) and the *National Service Framework for Mental Health* (*NSF*) (DH 1999). What is accepted as a need will vary across and within professional groups and, more importantly, between professionals and the people in their care. Bradshaw's (1972) definitions of need are till often cited to understand these differences:

■ *Normative needs* are defined by an expert or professional. This may involve a standard below which a person is considered to be 'in need'. For example, a community nurse who deems an isolated person to be in need of social skills training is making a normative assessment of their need.

■ *Comparative needs* are identified by comparing the service provision received by one community or population, with the levels of provision received elsewhere. This approach may provide objective evidence for unmet needs in specific areas or localities.

■ *Felt needs* are identified by the users of services and their carers. They are subjective and specific to them, for example the felt needs of a family or user group.

■ *Expressed needs* represent the translation of felt needs into action. For example, an individual who feels isolated may attend a drop-in service, or the close family of a person who experiences a psychotic breakdown may attend a carers' group.

These different needs can conflict, for example normative and felt need and there will be occasions where identified needs have to be balanced against available resources. Thus, as Pickin and St. Leger (1993) point out, a need may only be considered to exist in health care terms if there are the necessary resources to meet it. The possible relationships between these types of need and between need and resource are therefore far from perfect. But this is not true only of health care, it seems a good metaphor for life in general if we consider our own felt needs against the resources we have at our disposal. As Barker states, 'There is no obvious solution to this conflict. This is just one nettle of the assessment process that we must grasp without too much trepidation' (2004: 88).

The scope of assessment

Increasing emphasis is placed on assessment of the 'whole person', by which different authors may mean different things. We have suggested that mental health nursing assessments are concerned with how people function in relation to health problems as well as in relation to the broader context of their lives. This focus on functioning provides one way of understanding the whole person and thereby the potential scope of assessment.

Barker (2004) draws out a number of different levels on which people function or live simultaneously including their physiological self, biological self, behavioural self, social self and spiritual self. Actions as well as thoughts and feelings are included in Barker's 'behavioural self'. These levels reflect the four-quadrant framework we introduced in Chapters 1 and 2 to provide explanations of mental health and disorder respectively (Figure 1.1). By so doing we proposed that human experience is made up of a *subjective* and *objective* sense of *self* and a *subjective* and *objective* sense of *community*. We employ these dimensions again to represent the whole person, and reproduce the framework in Figure 10.1.

	Subjective	Objective
Self	Thought	Brain function
	Feelings	Autonomic nervous system function
	Self-acceptance	
	Cognitive style	Physiological balance
	Emotional intelligence	Exercise
	Spirituality	Diet
	Creativity	Alcohol and drug use
	Talking	Rest
	I	IT
	WE	ITS
Community	Relationships	Legislation
	Belonging	Policy
	Inclusion	Services
	Social support	Employment
	Social capital	Material wealth
	Community participation	Built environment
	Tolerance	Nature
		Public health indicators

Figure 10.1 The Scope of Mental Health Assessment

Figure 10.1 presents an overview of the scope of assessment. Consideration of each of the quadrants is necessary to understand and assess the whole person. The upper left quadrant (*subjective–self*) reflects a person's inner thoughts and feelings. It is concerned with the subjective meaning a person attributes to their life and/or their problems. We would position Barker's (2004) spiritual self and the thought and feeling components of his behavioural self in this quadrant. The upper right quadrant (*objective–self*) reflects a person's quantifiable, observable, external attributes. We would include the action component of Barker's (2004) behavioural self in this quadrant, along with the physiological and biological self. Similarly, we would place psychiatric diagnoses in this quadrant for their attempt to categorize people according to external, normative criteria.

The lower left quadrant (*subjective–community*) captures a person's collective sense of self. Their relations with family members and significant others are important here, as are their cultural roots and identity. But there is another side to our sense of self in community and this is reflected by the lower right quadrant (*objective–community*). As well as the inter-subjective experiences of culture and kinship there are inter-objective social phenomenon in the form of health and social care systems, legislation, financial and other community resources that impact on our sense of self and thus on our sense of health or illness.

We would place nursing diagnoses or problem statements that deal with a person's thoughts, feelings or beliefs (written in the first person and using their words) in the upper left (*subjective–self*) quadrant. Those that deal with external, observable behaviour or actions are upper right (*objective–self*). In reality, problem statements can straddle both quadrants (or all quadrants) dealing with thoughts and behaviours in relation to self and community. This is to be expected since human experience is made up of all four quadrants. To repeat our earlier example, 'Arguments with my parents mean I don't like to be at home, so I spend my time alone in public parks where I smoke cannabis to make the day more interesting.'

Figure 10.1 therefore represents our framework for assessment of the whole person upon which all assessment approaches and methods can be mapped. However, we must also consider in general terms the focus of any assessment in each of the quadrants, which might focus on indicators of health or illness.

Health and illness

Mental health and mental illness are inseparable, relational terms, and the reality they describe is human experience. This is not to say that we only feel ill because *previously* we have felt healthy, but rather we feel ill against a background sense of health, we feel the two *simultaneously*. We can say we are ill because we experience limitations in our health, but it would be incorrect to say that we are ill because we have no health. Assessment therefore encompasses 'health' and 'illness', or 'mental health' and 'mental illness'. With some notable exceptions that we will come to, mental health nursing has focused largely on 'illness' in assessment practice. By this we mean deficits, problems, abnormalities, negative risks and so on. Their correlates (strengths, solutions, commonalities, positive risks) have received far less attention.

Health remains a poorly understood concept and is frequently used as a euphemism for illness. For conceptual ease we equate illness with diagnoses, dysfunctions, problems and abnormalities at both the individual and community level. Correspondingly we equate health with strengths, solutions, assets and skills at both the individual and community level. The following case study of Tom in Box 10.1 emphasizes the importance of health for an individual with a debilitating illness.

> ### Box 10.1   Case study: Tom
>
> Tom is an 80-year-old man with dementia whose mobility is limited, but who insists on a twice-daily walk. His insistence is borne of an inner belief that his ability to walk connects him with life as he has always known it, despite the fact that his mind seems to be deserting him quite literally. His morning walk connects him with the local newsagent where he buys a daily paper, which connects him with the wider world. Throughout his working years as a commuter he attempted to complete the crossword in this daily paper and he feels it is more important than ever to maintain that activity. His walks also expose him to society in general. He comes across people and does what he has always done, says hello, comments on the weather, strokes a dog or simply talks nonsense at the supermarket checkout. He has always been like this, outgoing and happy. He is also very proud of these abilities, these markers of himself, particularly as he knows something is terribly wrong.
>
> In fact, Tom is fast progressing in his dementia. His short-term memory has been virtually destroyed and he can no longer comprehend complex tasks. He has severe arterial restriction in his lower limbs and on two occasions Tom was found lying by the side of the road that leads from his home into town. Someone saw him fall once and commented that they thought he was drunk as he staggered up the road. At the time this hurt Tom deeply, he began to panic and refused any help.
>
> Now it is true that Tom is facing a progressively debilitating disease that will ultimately kill him (if he doesn't stagger into the path of traffic before then!). But what is far more apparent is his sense of health, those things that he can still do in spite of his illness. He may have lost his short-term memory to a ravaging, organic, pathological process, but Tom is still very much alive in his habits, his long-established routines and fundamental interactions with the world. Tom's community psychiatric nurse was an integral thinker who, while acknowledging the disease and its associated problems, set about assessing Tom's health with a view to preserving what was important to him.
>
> Tom now leaves the house with an urban version of a traditional shooting stick which allows him to rest when necessary. The nurse also asked one of Tom's children to write a message for him, which the nurse had laminated, and which now hangs on the back door next to his shooting stick. It simply asks Dad to remember to take his stick, and to enjoy his walks. Both his children's names are printed at the bottom of the message. On occasion Tom can now be found on the road leading back to his house, sitting on his stick and bothering anyone who passes with stories about his useless legs.

Although Tom's nurse was aware of his problems/illness (limited mobility and dementia) she was aware also of his strengths/health (outgoing and social). More importantly, in the second stage of assessment she used this information to promote Tom's independence, and sense of self, irrespective of his illness. Tom might have been discouraged from leaving the house alone and offered transport to attend a day hospital where he could mix with others. In this case the information gathered from the assessment would have been used with his limitations (illness) very much in mind.

We can relate Tom's case study to Figure 10.1 to clarify the four quadrants. His 'inner belief that his ability to walk connects him with life as he has always known it' is an example of upper left, *subjective–self* information. His diagnosis of dementia and his limited mobility due to arterial restriction are upper right, *objective–self* data. The value Tom places on his social connections reflects the lower left quadrant, or *subjective–community*. Finally, the nurse's knowledge of Tom's family structure and the production of a laminated message by his family is evidence of lower right or *objective–community* awareness.

When considering what to assess we need then to take account of the context, the person's background sense of health, within which an experience of illness is felt. As well as gathering information on a person's problems and deficits we need to know something of their strengths and personal ideals. We need, in short, to develop an understanding of the whole person.

The scope of nursing assessment

We turn now to our vision for nursing assessment within this framework. We advocate the principle of holistic care and have presented a framework that we believe maps, in general terms, all that is the experience of being human. It follows that holistic nursing care, or assessment of the whole person, requires familiarity with, and assessment of all quadrants in relation to both health and illness. Nurses are in an ideal position to champion this perspective given that they may have contact with service users over extended periods, which in turn provides opportunities to become involved in many areas of a person's life during different stages of health (Repper 2000). From this position nurses are well placed to provide holistic, integrated care which can be enhanced by enjoining with other workers who possess complementary specialist knowledge and skills. Thus, the case for multi- and interdisciplinary assessments in which nurses embrace the contributions of others to develop a holistic understanding of the person and their difficulties.

Methods of assessment

This section gives an overview of the main methods by which assessment information can be gathered. Selected assessment strategies for each of the quadrants are presented in the final section of the chapter. Information gathering for assessment can be more or less formal and explicit. Whether a formal or less formal approach is preferred depends on the circumstances. Take for example a person who is talkative and eager to communicate their experience. An informal approach that allows the person free expression would be recommended, particularly in the early stages of their contact with services. On the other hand, a withdrawn individual who finds it difficult to communicate may benefit from a more structured, formal approach. In both cases the information provided (or the information that is sought) is documented and arranged in a systematic way that tells us something about the person, the problems they encounter in relation to their condition and life in general, and the strengths or attributes they may possess.

Taking our cue from the person to be assessed, and the reason for assessment, methods are usually selected to increase specificity as the assessment procedure progresses. Thus, a broad overview of an individual leads to the collection of information regarding the nature and implications of a specific problem.

We outline three main data collection methods for mental health nursing assessments: interviews; questionnaires, rating scales and structured pro forma; and observations.

Interviews

The interview is a means of eliciting information by questioning people. Typically this will involve the person in care but may also include others who know the person well including their relatives, friends and other health care professionals. There is little benefit in asking questions if we are unable to listen properly to the answers that are provided. A good interviewer requires good listening skills.

Barker (2004) states that a good listener is someone who helps a person to elaborate and qualify what they have to say, and who is able to curb any desire to offer premature interjections or summaries. Active or reflective listening is an important skill in this respect. Reflective listening can involve repeating key words used by the interviewee, perhaps with an inflection in tone, which invites them to elaborate their point. It may be more appropriate to simply ask if someone could elaborate on a topic, or ask them to explain the meaning an issue has for them. Open questions that invite elaboration rather than closed questions, which need only a single categorical answer, are crucial for reflective listening. Summarizing at discrete points during an interview to check for understanding is another example of reflective listening.

Each of these techniques communicates accurate empathy in so far as they convey an interest in, and an understanding of, the person's experience. Research demonstrates that therapeutic change, and the necessary relationship between therapist and client for this to occur, is dependent on the manifestation of accurate empathy by the therapist (Rollnick *et al.* 2008). This is a fundamental tenet of the therapeutic alliance.

Reflective listening is only beneficial if it is accompanied by appropriate non-verbal behaviour. It is no good asking someone to elaborate while we fumble to read a text, or sit with our arms crossed admiring the view from a window, or position ourself in a room with constant interruptions. Interest can be conveyed as much through our non-verbal behaviour and the environment in which we choose to interview someone, as it can by what we say (or don't say). The verbal and non-verbal interpersonal skills that underpin effective listening and interviewing are thoroughly reviewed by Barker (2004) and have been described in dedicated texts such as Egan (1994) and Newell (1994). The latter having been written specifically for nurses.

Interviews may be more or less structured depending on their purpose and the type of information to be collected. Following Barker (2004), Table 10.2 represents a summary of the possible goals and aims of the interview, with the aims reflecting interpersonal functions between the nurse and the person receiving care.

Questionnaires, rating scales and structured pro formas

Questionnaires and rating scales generate quantifiable measures of human experience. They stem from the objective right-hand quadrants in Figure 10.1 and therefore complement, but cannot replace, the subjective left-hand quadrants. Instruments of this type may invite simple categorical responses (for example, yes or no) to a question or statement. Many also invite the rating of a statement according to a series of possible responses that reflect different degrees of agreement with the statement.

Goal		Aim
Descriptive	Collecting information to form a broad overview or picture of the person and to develop a therapeutic, trusting relationship	Relationship building
		Trust building
Diagnostic	Investigation of a problem area in which relationships between a person's thoughts, feelings and behaviour are explored, and from which nursing or medical diagnoses can be formed	Professional collaboration
		Problem identification
Therapeutic	Ongoing face-to-face meetings to help the person through the process of care by clarifying problems, identifying solutions and reflecting with the person on their progress/response	Problem resolution

Table 10.2 Interview goals and aims
(After Barker 2004)

These approaches can generate quantified summaries of the person in care. We may say that Tom's dementia is severe following administration of a questionnaire, on which he scored poorly. We could reduce this further by saying he scored 2 out of a possible 20, thereby indicating severe dementia. Such an approach can be advantageous. Questionnaires and rating scales are usually developed through extensive research during which the instruments are refined to enhance the accuracy (validity) and consistency (reliability) with which they measure a concept of interest. A well-researched instrument can assess comparative or normative needs, and provide a quantifiable basis to judge progress. However, to say that Tom's dementia questionnaire score was 2 tells us very little about the person behind this numeric.

We include various pro formas in this section, such as logbooks and diaries, which allow people to document specific experiences in a structured way (Barker 2004). A simple example is the 'antecedent', 'behaviour', 'consequence' framework, against which the context of a behavioural problem can be mapped. By substituting 'behaviour' for 'belief' in this framework we can map the context of a cognitive problem. Barker (2004) offers a further example using the headings 'action', 'emotion', 'thought', while Fox and Conroy (2000) advocate the acronym 'FIND' (frequency, intensity, number and duration of a problem).

Observations

Observation is a continuous form of data collection within the context of nursing care. It may be relatively informal, such as an overall assessment of a person's appearance and behaviour or the assessment of interactions within a ward environment. Structured observation methods include the prospective use of pro formas such as those described in the previous section. These can be completed by the person receiving care or by nursing staff. Observation schedules can yield important information but can also present a challenge to those who complete them. They require more or less continuous attention or good recollection in order to capture a representative set of data. This can be difficult for a person with a mental health problem and for their nurse who may not be available during periods when a problem is present.

Mental health care involves another type of observation that is concerned with documenting biochemical and physiological indices. Barker (2004) acknowledges this aspect of assessment but does not pursue it as a legitimate activity for the mental health nurse. We take a more integral view given that the *objective–self* is a part of human experience and would encourage nurses to familiarize themselves with the rationale and meaning of these observations (see, for example, McConnell 1998).

Plant and Stephenson (2008) emphasize the importance of physiological indices in the assessment of mental health problems. For example, deficiencies in zinc, magnesium, iron, omega-3 fatty acids and the B vitamins are not uncommon following childbirth and these deficiencies are implicated in depression. Therefore the assessment of postnatal depression in women should always include physiological screening for these deficiencies. Other examples, as indicated in Chapter 1, are the levels of key neurotransmitters which have a role to play in the experience of mental health problems. Although not widely used in the UK at present, methods are available to analyse urine or blood samples to determine whether specific neurotransmitters are too high or too low. Plant and Stephenson (2008) argue that these should be routine observations undertaken in the course of a mental health assessment, especially if there is an intention to prescribe medication that affects neurotransmitter levels.

Assessing the whole person

In this section we provide some examples of assessment strategies for each of the quadrants in Figure 10.1. We begin with an exploration of the breadth of personal and social information that needs to be collected when people first enter a health care system. Those who are already known to services may have extensive past medical or nursing notes. Though the information contained within these notes may be useful they are not a substitute for the collection of contemporary data regarding a person's presenting problem, or for the opportunity to elicit someone's personal history in their own words.

Presenting problem and personal history

Gamble and Brennan (2006) identify four core elements of the information gathering process that describes a person's presenting problem and history (Table 10.3). The core elements in Table 10.3 reflect predominantly the right-hand quadrants of Figure 10.1 (*objective–self* and *objective–community*). They are concerned with external, quantifiable attributes and phenomena, with the exception of 'personal insights'. This is not to say that Gamble and Brennan (2006) are uninterested in a person's subjective feelings, as their work testifies. However, their main approach, in terms of identifying health-related need, tends towards objective assessment.

Barker (2004) provides a more integrated approach that begins with the generation of an admission profile and description of the presenting problem. By admission profile Barker refers to any point of entry into health or social care services, whether these be residential or community based. Tables 10.4 and 10.5 contain the key components of an admission profile and a presenting problem inventory.

Core element	Examples
History of psychiatric disorder and past physical history	■ family and social background ■ past treatments, contacts with services and risk levels ■ current medication and any side effects
Current financial, social functioning and environmental factors	■ personal relationships ■ employment
Psychiatric diagnosis and current symptoms	■ to include effects of symptoms on behaviour
Personal insights	■ evidence of the person's awareness and understanding of their difficulties

Table 10.3 Core elements of the information gathering process (After Gamble and Brennan 2000)

Component	Examples
Name, age, sex, marital state	
Family	■ whether any dependants and who they live with ■ siblings ■ whether part of an active extended family
Domestic	■ living alone or with significant others
Occupation	■ employment status ■ nature of employment
Socialization	■ close friends and other acquaintances ■ membership of clubs or organizations including church
Financial status	■ access to hard cash or other funds ■ record of outstanding bills or debt
Medical cover	■ name and contact details of any physician/social worker ■ current medication

Table 10.4 Admission profile (After Barker 2004)

It is evident that Barker's (2004) initial assessment draws on all four quadrants, incorporating both subjective and objective data of self and community. However, these data are firmly oriented toward problems, which Barker acknowledges. He believes it may be inappropriate to consider a person's strengths or assets at this stage, particularly as it may indicate a fear on behalf of the nurse to deal with a person's problems. We agree, but with one exception; evidence of exceptions to the presenting problem. We have found it useful to ask people early in an assessment process whether there are ever any exceptions to the presenting problems they describe. If so, we would encourage exploration of those exceptions since this often uncovers potential solutions to the problem.

Component	Examples
Functioning	■ changes in bodily functions including limbs, speech and memory
Behaviour	■ changes in behaviour including behaviours that might be upsetting the person or others
Affect	■ specific feelings associated with problems
Cognition	■ specific thoughts about the problems, including ruminations and recurring thoughts
Beliefs	■ the meaning the problems have for the person
Physical	■ physical problems associated with the difficulty for example pain, loss of appetite, listlessness
Relationships	■ any changes in usual relations and whether associated with the problem
Expectations	■ what the person thinks will happen to them now they are in touch with services

Table 10.5 Inventory for presenting problem
(After Barker 2004)

Having elicited an admission profile and inventory of the presenting problem Barker (2004) then recommends the development of this thumbnail sketch. Specific topic headings are provided, which expand the available information to include past history, present circumstances and the way a problem interferes with the person's life experience (Table 10.6).

During this stage of the assessment process Barker (2004) places much greater emphasis on a person's strengths, assets and preferences while maintaining an interest in all four quadrants of human experience, as evidenced in Table 10.6. Barker (2004) also draws attention to exploring a person's hopes for the future having examined their past in some detail. Questions pertaining to their aspirations, their expectations and hopes, and their future plans are important in this respect. Through these enquiries a more holistic picture of the person begins to emerge, from which it is possible to identify areas where further investigation may be needed. This investigation may follow any one of the specific strategies we describe in the following sections.

Subjective–self

The upper left quadrant of Figure 10.1 represents a person's inner world, their thoughts feelings and beliefs. The psychodynamic model and its therapeutic approach (cf. Chapter 2) tap into this quadrant with their interest in assessing the ideas and feelings behind the words and actions that constitute human behaviour. Though some mental health nurses specialize in this tradition, the profession as a whole does not practise according to psychodynamic principles. Nevertheless, assessment of the *subjective–self* is a necessary component of holistic nursing practice.

Barker (2004) refers to this as 'learning from the person', which necessitates listening to a person's life story or personal narrative. It is true that a personal narrative may allude to behaviours or social structures, which are external, observable attributes that belong elsewhere in Figure 10.1. But we can still ask for the meaning they hold for the person. This orientation lies at the heart of *subjective–self* assessments. It focuses on a person's thoughts, feelings, personal values and beliefs, which describe their sense of self and the meaning they attribute to their life experience.

Topic	Example
Education	■ description of schooling at basic and advanced level
	■ attitudes towards schooling and adult learning
Occupation	■ past and present occupations
	■ feelings towards present job
	■ any work aspirations
	■ degree to which present problems interfere with work
Social network	■ does the person enjoy going out?
	■ do they have an extended social network?
	■ what kind of social life would they prefer?
	■ impact of problem on these social networks
Recreation	■ way in which free time is used
	■ hobbies and preferred activities
	■ what changes might be desirable?
General health	■ states of health throughout the person's lifetime
	■ maintenance of health through diet, exercise, etc.
Drugs	■ use of drugs whether prescribed, over-the-counter, or illicit
	■ how does the person feel about drug taking?
	■ amount, route of administration, frequency and duration of any drug use
	■ is present problem and use of any drugs connected?
Past treatment	■ any past treatments for presenting problem
	■ effects of any treatments and preferences/feelings toward them
Coping	■ coping strategies employed to deal with life's problems
	■ successful strategies that have been employed previously
Outstanding problems	■ problems that the person perceives to be beyond help
	■ feelings towards them and likely reactions, including anger/attempting suicide

Table 10.6 Developing the history (After Barker 2004)

Subjective–self assessments require the use of open-ended questions and reflective listening skills to elaborate a person's description of their experience. We might ask:

■ What are your feelings about that experience?
■ What thoughts did you have at the time?
■ Could you say a little more about what that means for you?

It follows that the information we receive needs to be recorded in the person's own words, otherwise we are documenting our interpretations of what they say and are missing an opportunity to understand fully the person's *subjective–self*. Interpretations and judgements about their need for care will still be made, but in the case of the upper left quadrant these should be predicated on an individual's verbatim account of their inner world.

Frameworks

It is possible to bring order to the verbatim recording of a person's thoughts and feelings, though rarely are these separated from objective actions or behaviours. In Chapter 2 we introduced Ellis's (1962) ABC framework in which A stands for 'activating event', B stands for 'beliefs' about the event and C stands for the emotional (or behavioural) 'consequence' that follows. Barker (2004) offers a variation on this theme referring to 'actions', 'emotions' and 'thoughts'. Both frameworks provide a structure for eliciting and documenting aspects of a person's inner world, though each incorporates a behavioural component in its analysis.

Subjective–community

The lower left quadrant of Figure 10.1 represents the meaning, values and beliefs that a person holds regarding their sense of self in community. These include cultural identity and world-views. Allied to these are negative correlates including racism, social exclusion and stigma. In Chapter 1 when we demonstrated how stigma and social exclusion have a bearing on people's mental health. For example, the experiences of African-Caribbean communities in the UK, which include poorer housing, higher levels of unemployment and lower average incomes than the indigenous population are sufficient to engender mental health problems (Modood *et al.* 1998). In this particular quadrant it is not the quantifiable attributes themselves but the meaning they have for people that contributes to the formation of mental health problems.

As with the *subjective–self* (upper left) we can only comprehend the personal meaning of these aspects of a person by asking them directly through open-ended questions and reflective listening. For example, someone may appear socially isolated or excluded but we cannot fully comprehend such observations without understanding the meaning they hold for the person.

Of contemporary interest in this quadrant is the emergence of the recovery approach and the meaning it holds for service users (cf. Chapter 5). The Chief Nursing Officer's review of mental health nursing (DH 2006) recommends that the profession incorporates the broad principles of the recovery approach into every aspect of their practice, including assessment. This means understanding the goals that are important for service users, being positive about change and promoting social inclusion.

Objective–self

The upper right quadrant of Figure 10.1 represents external, measurable, quantifiable attributes of the person. This includes their physiological and biological self, and associated indices, as well as measurements of their functioning or mental state through the use of questionnaires and rating scales. Functioning is a broad term that incorporates thoughts, feelings and behaviours associated with self as well as those associated with self in community. The latter is often referred to as social functioning, which is examined in the next section (*objective–community*). A number of instruments incorporate both self and community measures of functioning, particularly global assessments of need such as the *Health of the Nation Outcome Scales* (*HoNOS*) (Wing *et al.* 1995) and the *Camberwell Assessment of Need* (*CAN*) (Phelan *et al.* 1995). Each taps into personal attributes such as physical health and symptom severity as well as measures of social functioning such as interpersonal behaviours and social engagement.

Gamble and Brennan (2006) provide a detailed account of questionnaires and rating scales that are designed to capture in quantifiable terms the experience of illness. Less evident are instruments that tap into the experience of health, although some are cited in

Barker's (2004) work. We draw on this literature to present a selected overview (in Table 10.7) of questionnaires and rating scales that are available for *objective–self* assessments. Readers may wish to review subsequent chapters for assessment instruments relevant to the specific problems/conditions that people experience.

Objective–community

The lower right quadrant of Figure 10.1 represents external, measurable, quantifiable attributes of the self in community. In the earlier section that described presenting problems and personal histories, the collection of information pertaining to these attributes was recommended. For example, in Table 10.6 Barker (2004) emphasizes the importance of enquiring about a person's occupation and social structures. These are examples of self in community data. In the *objective–community* quadrant these attributes are quantified according to questionnaires, rating scales and other objective data. However, we can also seek to understand a person's subjective experience of these phenomena (*subjective–community*).

Instrument	Commentary
Brief Psychiatric Rating Scale (BPRS) (Overall and Gorham 1962)	One of the oldest and most commonly used instruments for assessing the presence of various forms of mental illness including anxiety, depression and thought disturbance. All items are rated on a 7-point scale from 'not present' to 'extremely severe'. Administered through direct questioning but relies also on observations made at the time of administration.
Beck Depression Inventory (BDI) (Beck *et al.* 1961)	Another much used instrument designed to measure the severity of depressive states. Containing 21 items, each is rated on a 4-point scale and can be completed by the person in care directly or through interview technique.
Positive and Negative Syndrome Scale (PANSS) (Kay *et al.* 1987)	Designed to assess key symptom types associated with schizophrenia. The instrument contains 30 items a proportion of which are completed through interview and the remainder through observation. Each is rated on a 7-point scale.
Beliefs About Voices Questionnaire (BAVQ) (Chadwick and Birchwood 1995)	Designed to elicit the feelings a person has about hallucinatory voices. The questionnaire contains 30 items, all of which are answered with simple yes or no responses.
Self-Esteem Scale (Rosenberg 1965)	This brief 10-item instrument taps into a key component of health or well-being. It is easy to administer with each item rated on a 4-point scale.
Self-Efficacy Scale (Sherer *et al.* 1982)	A further instrument to gauge aspects of a person's health. Of the 30 items the majority tap into general self-efficacy and the remainder examine social self-efficacy (lower right quadrant). Each is rated on a 5-point scale.

Table 10.7 Instruments to assess illness and health in the individual

For objective measurement, instruments that tap a person's social functioning and to a lesser extent their quality of life are important. We include the latter, which often straddle both the *objective–self* and *objective–community* quadrants of Figure 10.1, but which typically measure an individual's quality of life in its broadest sense, and are, therefore, grounded in the self in community. Measures of social functioning are often concerned with problem areas and deficits while quality of life measures are more broadly focused and accommodate measurement of a person's sense of health. We would include also in this quadrant the objective views of carers and significant others involved in a person's care. Table 10.8 presents a selected overview of instruments that are available for *objective–community* assessments.

Instrument	Commentary
Social Functioning Scale (SFS) (Birchwood *et al.* 1990)	This instrument covers seven main areas of social functioning including independence in living skills and social engagement. All areas reflect aspects of day-to-day social functioning that can be adversely affected by mental health problems. The authors designed this instrument specifically for use in family intervention programmes.
Instrumental and Expressive Functions of Social Support (IEFSS) (Ensel and Woelfel 1986)	This instrument is designed to assess the function and emotional content of a person's social relationships. A 5-point scale is used to rate 28 problem areas, which cover demands, money, companionship, marital conflict and communication.
Quality of Life Scale (QLS) (Heinrichs *et al.* 1984)	This instrument has 21 items, each of which is rated on a 7-point scale. They cover three key areas deemed to be representative of a person's quality of life: interpersonal relations; occupational role; and richness of personal experience. The scale specifically taps into a person's capability to manage social roles and with this emphasis on capability is oriented towards health rather than illness.
Manchester Short Assessment of Quality of Life (MANSA) (Priebe *et al.* 2002)	In addition to gathering sociodemographic data this instrument asks 16 questions pertaining to employment, finance, friendships, leisure, accommodation, family, safety and health. Each is rated on a 7-point scale. As with the QLS the emphasis is upon health rather than illness.
Carers' Assessment of Managing Index (CAMI) (Nolan *et al.* 1995)	Designed to assess coping style and management of stress in the carers of people with mental health problems. Examples of coping strategies are given, which respondents report their use of and the degree to which they are effective.

Table 10.8 Instruments to assess illness and health of self in community

Conclusion

We have presented assessment as an ongoing continuous process, which in its many forms underpins all nursing activity. Its purpose incorporates both the collection of information and the use of that information to make judgements about a person's need for health care. Traditionally these judgements are based on a person's problems, deficits and abnormalities though we encourage a broader perspective that accommodates strengths, assets and skills.

We advocate the principle of holistic assessment and have presented a framework for that purpose, which takes account of a person's *subjective* and *objective* sense of *self* and their *subjective* and *objective* sense of *community*. In each respect consideration needs to be given to a person's problems (illness) and their strengths (health).

This holistic framework does not require mental health nurses to be skilled in all areas of assessment, but does require acknowledgement of its scope and thus the need to collaborate with others who have complementary assessment skills.

In summary, the main points of this chapter are:

- Assessment is an ongoing cycle of activity that all nurses perform in all nursing situations.
- Assessments can be more or less explicit and formal depending upon the person being assessed and their reason for assessment.
- The process of assessment involves decision-making, which requires the collection and interpretation of information to make judgements about a person's need for care.
- Holistic assessment requires information on a person's *subjective* and *objective* sense of *self* and their *subjective* and *objective* sense of *community* and, in each area, indicators of both health and illness should be explored.
- Mental health nurses need to develop an integrated understanding of the scope of assessment to be demonstrated in collaborative partnerships with service users and professional colleagues.

Questions for reflection and discussion

1   In relation to Figure 10.1 undertake an assessment of yourself, listing indicators for both health and illness in each of the four quadrants.
2   Reflect on the mental health care of someone you have nursed and consider whether their assessment and care incorporated an interest in their health. If not, what indicators of health are you able to recall and how might recognition of these have altered the care they received?
3   In a health care culture that deals primarily with the management of risk, deficits and problems, how feasible is it to redress this balance with health-oriented assessments? What factors might hinder such developments and how can these be overcome?
4   Reread Tom's case study in this chapter. How open you are to the possibility of health among people who experience mental illness, and, how willing are you to help people find a way to live in spite of their illness?

Annotated bibliography

- Barker, P. (2004) *Assessment in Psychiatric and Mental Health Nursing: In Search of the Whole Person* (2nd edn). Cheltenham: Stanley Thornes. This text provides a detailed contemporary account of theoretical principles, methodologies and instruments for conducting mental health nursing assessments. Practical examples of how to assess a range of disorders are provided, including anxiety states, psychotic experiences and human relations. The text includes an examination of the moral and ethical issues surrounding assessment, and provides a selected bibliography of assessment instruments.

- Gamble, C. and Brennan, G. (2006) Assessments: A rationale and glossary of tools, in C. Gamble and G. Brennan (eds) (2nd edn) *Working with Serious Mental Illness: A Manual for Clinical Practice*. London: Elsevier. A valuable chapter in which the authors provide a rationale for systematic assessments, describe the core elements of information to be collected and provide an extensive glossary of standardized assessment tools. The chapter provides also some practical strategies to aid the interpretation and effective implementation of assessment data.
- Bowling, A. (2004) *Measuring Health: A Review of Quality of Life Measurement Scales* (3rd edn). Milton Keynes: Open University Press. This text provides a comprehensive collection of quality of life measurement scales that have been selected for inclusion either because they have been well tested for reliability and validity or because considerable interest has been expressed in their content area. The author provides a useful discussion of the conceptualization of functioning, health and quality of life. The text includes instruments and methods to measure functional ability, health status, psychological well-being, social networks and support, and life satisfaction and morale.
- Bowling, A. (1995) *Measuring Disease: A Review of Disease-Specific Quality of Life Measurement Scales* (2nd edn). Buckingham: Open University Press. Though not specific to mental health this book complements Bowling's 1997 text. The strengths, weaknesses and coverage of a range of instruments designed to measure aspects of disease are reviewed.

References

Barker, P. (2004) *Assessment in Psychiatric and Mental Health Nursing: In Search of the Whole Person* (2nd edn). Cheltenham: Nelson Thornes Ltd.

Beck, A., Ward, C., Mendelson, M. *et al.* (1961) An inventory for measuring depression. *Archives of General Psychiatry* **4**: 561–71.

Birchwood, M., Smith, J. and Cochrane, R. (1990) The Social Functioning Scale: the development and validation of a new scale of social adjustment in use in family interventions programmes with schizophrenic patients. *British Journal of Psychiatry* **157**: 853–9.

Bradshaw, J. (1972) The concept of social need. *New Society* **21**: 640–3.

Chadwick, P. and Birchwood, M. (1995) The omnipotence of voices II: The beliefs about voices questionnaire. *British Journal of Psychiatry* **166**: 11–19.

Department of Health (1999) *A National Service Framework for Mental Health*. London: The Stationery Office.

Department of Health (2006) *From Values to Action: The Chief Nursing Officer's review of mental health nursing: Summary*. London: DH.

Egan, G. (1994) *The Skilled Helper* (4th edn). Monterey, CA: Brooks/Cole.

Ellis, A. (1962) *Reason and Emotion in Psychotherapy*. New York: Stuart.

Ensel, W. and Woelfel, J. (1986) Measuring the instrumental and expressive functions of social support, in N. Lin, A. Dean and W. Ensel (eds) *Social Support, Life Events and Depression*. New York: Academic Press.

Fox, J. and Conroy, P. (2000) Assessing client's needs: the semi-structured interview, in C. Gamble and G. Brennan (eds) *Working with Serious Mental Illness: A Manual for Clinical Practice*. London: Baillière Tindall.

Gamble, C. and Brennan, G. (2006) Assessments: a rationale for choosing and using, in C. Gamble and G. Brennan (eds) (2nd edn) *Working with Serious Mental Illness: A Manual for Clinical Practice.* London: Elsevier.

Heinrichs, D., Hanlon, T. and Carpenter, W. (1984) The quality of life scale: an instrument for rating the schizophrenic deficit syndrome. *Schizophrenia Bulletin* **10**: 388–98.

Kay, S., Fiszebein, A. and Opler, L. (1987) Positive and negative syndrome scale. *Schizophrenia Bulletin* **13**: 261–76.

McConnell, H. (1998) Psychological and behavioral correlates of blood and CSF laboratory tests, in P. Snyder and P. Nussbaum (eds) *Clinical Neuropsychology for House Staff.* Washington DC: American Psychological Press.

Modood, T., Berthoud, R., Lakey, J. *et al.* (1998) *Ethnic Minorities in Britain: Diversity and Disadvantage. The Fourth National Survey of Ethnic Minorities.* London: Policy Studies Institute.

Newell, R. (1994) *Interviewing Skills for Nurses and Other Health Care Professionals.* London: Routledge.

Nolan, M., Keady, J. and Grant, G. (1995) CAMI: a basis for assessment and support with family carers. *British Journal of Nursing Quarterly* **4**: 822–6.

Overall, J. and Gorham, D. (1962) Brief Psychiatric Rating Scale. *Psychological Reports* **10**: 799–812.

Phelan, M., Slade, M., Thornicroft, G. *et al.* (1995) The Camberwell Assessment of Need: the validity and reliability of an instrument to assess the needs of people with severe mental illness. *British Journal of Psychiatry* **167**: 589–95.

Pickin, C. and St. Leger, S. (1993) *Assessing Health Need Using the Life Cycle Framework.* Milton Keynes: Open University Press.

Plant, J. and Stephenson, J. (2008) *Beating Stress, Anxiety and Depression.* London: Piatkus Books.

Priebe, S., Huxley, P., Knight, S. and Evans, S. (2002) *Manchester Short Assessment of Quality of Life.* Manchester: The University of Manchester.

Repper, J. (2000) Adjusting the focus of mental health nursing: Incorporating service users' experiences of recovery. *Journal of Mental Health* **9**: 575–87.

Rollnick, S., Miller, W. and Butler, C. (2008) *Motivational Interviewing in Healthcare: Helping patients change behaviour.* New York: Guilford Press.

Rosenberg, M. (1965) *The Measurement of Self-esteem.* Princeton, NJ: Princeton University Press.

Savage, P. (1991) Patient assessment in psychiatric nursing. *Journal of Advanced Nursing* **16**: 311–16.

Sherer, M., Maddux, J., Mercandante, B. *et al.* (1982) The self-efficacy scale: construction and validation. *Psychological Reports* **51**: 663–71.

Ward, M. (1992) *The Nursing Process in Psychiatry* (2nd edn). Edinburgh: Churchill Livingstone.

Wilkinson, J. Bywaters, J. Chappel, D. and Glover, G. (2007) *Indicators of Public Health in the English Regions: Mental Health.* York: Association of Public Health Observatories.

Wing, J., Curtis, R. and Beevor, A. (1995) *Measurement of Mental Health: Health of the Nation Outcome Scales.* London: Royal College of Psychiatrists Research Unit.

CHAPTER 11

Working with risk

Steve Morgan and Andrew Wetherell

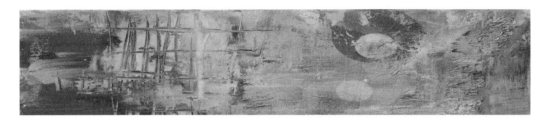

Chapter overview

In recent years the concept of risk has increasingly permeated the policy and practice agenda in mental health care. Legislative guidance and administrative documentation have introduced more bureaucracy, which can undermine confidence in practice and also promote a 'blame culture' where opportunities for positive risk-taking may be overlooked. This chapter unpacks the concept of risk and encourages the reader to look beyond its negative connotations to include the positive risks we must all take in the course of our lives. Types of risk and their associated factors are detailed and processes for assessing and managing risk are examined. The chapter places particular emphasis on the 'service-user perspective' and encourages the promotion of genuine involvement and collaboration with service users in the assessment and management of risk.

This chapter covers:

- An introduction to risk;
- Policy guidance and legislative context;
- The service-user experience;
- Positive risk-taking;
- Risk assessment and risk management;
- Risk categories;
- Paper institution or practical tools?
- Confidentiality.

An introduction to risk

Risk is enmeshed in all aspects of our daily functioning; it is essentially the art of living with uncertainty. For some, the emphasis is on the positive – a chance for gain; while for others, it takes on a more negative focus – the experience of pain. For many people, at least for some of the time, risk simply 'is', with little conscious acknowledgement of its influences. Whatever your personal standpoint, the passions for living or dying are sustained by the very existence and temptations of risk. A life devoid of risk is likely to have no challenge and very little real meaning.

In mental health, the term schizophrenia is broadly used as a diagnosis for conditions that are often represented by disjointed thinking and distorted perceptions. It may equally apply as a diagnosis of the diverse reactions observed in relation to the concept of risk in mental health. It becomes an emotive subject, generating conflicting priorities and agendas: a linked public safety and political policy agenda; an organizational bureaucratic and administrative agenda; and a clinical preventative and restrictive agenda. What these appear to have in common, when examined in some detail, is a 'cover-your-back' agenda. Seldom do we find a serious attempt to engage the service user's personal agenda!

The public safety agenda

One of the repeated inaccurate messages to emerge from years of homicide inquiries is the implication of danger in pursuing a policy of community care, which may be serving to release dangerously deranged individuals into the community. In defence of this position, there are detailed reports of inquiries which highlight the failure of treatment and care for individuals who did go on to commit horrendous and fatal acts of violence against family members or other members of the public (Ritchie *et al.* 1994; Sheppard 1996). The political policy reaction has carried implications of blame for those who provide mental health services, with accompanying government guidance and legislation focused specifically on those who present a high risk (NHS Executive 1994; DH 1995). The more general framework of managing care for the broader constituency of those diagnosed with mental health problems, the Care Programme Approach, is also taking on a stronger risk management focus (DH 1999a, DH 2008) and the intention is very much directed towards the need to ensure public safety. The underlining premise appears to be that people experiencing mental health problems are primarily a threat to others.

To counterbalance this prevailing argument, less well publicized but researched evidence suggests that we do live in a more violent society than a generation ago. However, the progressive policy of community care has contributed nothing to the increase in homicide statistics during the second half of the twentieth century (Taylor and Gunn 1999). Either by a consistently high dose of luck, or the unnoticed application of some good practice, many risks are being effectively identified and managed, with the immeasurable outcome of potential incidents being prevented.

Undoubtedly, some horrendous tragedies have occurred that could otherwise have been avoided with attention to important principles of practice and a major dose of hindsight. However, we seem to have fallen into the trap of losing sight of realistic expectations in the face of sensationalist media headlines and political sound bites. The implications that risk can be accurately assessed and managed appear to be linked to measures of success based on the notion of 'risk elimination'. The unpredictability of human behaviour dictates that 'risk minimization' or reduction is a more realistic outcome to expect.

An organizational agenda

This is where senior management frequently find themselves caught between the ideals of guiding and supporting front-line staff to provide high quality services for those who need them, and the need to be seen to respond to the powerful external pressures and demands of the imagination-capturing, vote-winning, paper-selling public safety ticket. In its simplest form, it suggests that the staff are the organization's most valuable resource, that good service-user-involving practice is paramount, and that a flexible and creative response to individually assessed need is the way to deliver a first-class service. On the other hand, completion of the Care Programme Approach (CPA), risk assessment, carers' assessment, audit tools, daily notes and monitoring forms should be done on everyone seen by the service, primarily to meet externally determined performance targets. An inevitable consequence is the pressure put on to staff to manage the higher caseloads and workloads that accompany increasing expectations.

When, in this conflicting scenario, something goes wrong, the initial organizational response, at least as perceived by the majority of practitioners, is a 'guilty until proven innocent' stance. There often appears to be a management assumption that people with serious mental health problems can be comprehensively assessed with rigorous research tools. On this basis they can either be given the necessary support to live in the community without posing threats or fears to those around them, or they can be provided with varying degrees of restriction to ensure that no harm comes to unsuspecting members of the public. The unrealistic external expectations of those who know no better appear to be assimilated by people higher up within the organization, who should know better.

The challenge to this way of thinking is not a call to condone poor or negligent practice. Staff work daily with difficult challenges, and need to feel supported rather than blamed the instant things go wrong. Instead, their more usual experience leaves them with little doubt that the organization focuses more on externally established targets and perceptions than the gritty reality of messages from practice.

The practitioner agenda

As the providers of direct treatment, support and care, most practitioners are fully aware of the place of risk and safety in their working lives. With few exceptions, their intentions are to provide a good quality of service that meets the needs of the people referred to them. They also expect reasonable resources, guidance and support in order to provide the necessary quality of care. Fears are that the role is gradually changing from primarily one of good nursing practice to a more generic notion of multi-disciplinary/multiagency workers; to the administrator of care coordination; to the specific role of social policing; and where to next?

Mental health practitioners fear that their work has recently become dominated by risk, and maybe they are not doing the caring and supporting functions they came into the job to do, and from which they derive so much of their job satisfaction. They fear that external forces have conspired to make the mental health business into a risk business (Rose 1998). Yet risk has always been there – in the asylums, the mini-institutions, the development of community mental health initiatives, every time people come into direct contact; and the times when they do not. Perhaps the problem is not so much that we have become the risk business, but rather that we have become the 'bureaucratic and administrative business' – a face of authority that it is easy to 'risk against'.

Many different and conflicting agendas have become established in relation to the conceptualization of risk in mental health. However, one significant question generally seems to be overlooked: Whatever happened to the notion that it could be the people experiencing the mental health problems who are the ones most at risk?

Definition of risk

❝   The likelihood of an event happening with potentially harmful or beneficial outcomes for self and/or others ... possible behaviours include suicide, self-harm, aggression and violence, and neglect; with an additional range of other positive or negative service user experiences.

(Morgan 2007a)   ❞

This is a helpful definition in that it does acknowledge risk as not totally negative by stating there can be beneficial outcomes for self and/or others. In addition, it registers that there are a whole range of additional service-user experiences, which need to be taken into account.

Policy guidance and legislative context

National Service Framework (NSF) for Mental Health (DH 1999b) and NHS Plan (DH 2000)

These documents set the scene as statements of intent and injections of resources, which imply that criticisms presented by repeated reports of inquiry are being dealt with. One positive development is the placing of a stronger emphasis on the category of suicide risk (NSF for Mental Health, Standard 7), thus recognizing the negative impact of circumstances on the service user, as opposed to solely being seen as the perpetrators of risk. The downside of this emphasis is a continued reliance on setting targets, in this instance the reduction of suicide rates by 20 per cent by 2010 (DH 1999c). Any appreciation of the complexities that underpin the individuality of the suicidal act is only reflected in the statements of how Standards 1–6 will contribute towards the achievement of this ambitious target. Once again, expectations are set up, with the inevitable sense that they will become benchmarks of future service failures.

Overall, the *NSF for Mental Health* represents a more balanced view of risk than some of the earlier examples of guidance and legislation in the 1990s. Only in Standards 4 and 5 (covering 'Effective Services for People with Severe Mental Illness') does a more specific emphasis on assessing and managing risk appear, with reference to 'risk to others'; but, this is also counterbalanced by an acknowledgement of service users' potential risks of vulnerability.

Review of the Mental Health Act 1983

Following their failure to implement their original Mental Health Bill the government has introduced revisions to the Mental Health Act 1983. The details of these revisions remain a cause for concern for all who have formed the Mental Health Alliance (service users, voluntary organizations, and representatives of all mental health professions). Some of the controversial aspects of the previous bill remain, particularly the implementation of compulsory treatment in the community, and an extension of the definition of mental illness to include personality disorder whether or not it responds to medical forms of treatment.

Madden (2006) reviews 25 homicide inquiries using the structured HCR20 forensic risk assessment tool and applying Root Cause Analysis and concludes that compulsory community treatment is the only means that would break the revolving door of hospital admissions. The Department of Health commissioned this report and promotes it as supportive evidence for its intended revisions of the Act, but it fails to make a convincing argument of how it extrapolates such wide-ranging repercussions from so few examples of extreme events. Service users fear further restrictions being placed on their liberties, and practitioners fear a further erosion of good practice weighed down by further bureaucracy and the unwarranted elevation of the public safety agenda.

Human Rights Act 1998

This legislation requires that all public authorities should act in a manner compatible with the European Convention of Human Rights (ECHR) (cf. Chapter 6). It will now be unlawful for them to act in a way that is incompatible with the ECHR, unless the specific requirements of other legislation appear to contradict the ECHR. How can the legislators marry together a promotion of human rights with a need for greater 'surveillance and supervision' of certain individuals, assumed to be required of mental health services charged with upholding public safety?

Briefing Paper 12 (Sainsbury Centre for Mental Health 2000) examines some of the potential impact of this legislation, highlighting:

Article 2:   the right to life.
Article 3:   prohibition of torture and inhuman and degrading treatment.
Article 5:   the right to liberty and security.
Article 8:   the right to respect for private and family life, home and correspondence.

The National Health Service Litigation Authority (NHSLA) provide regular emailed briefing papers to NHS Trusts and other bodies that reflect on the specific messages learned from the application of this legislation to specific legal cases across all sectors of the NHS, including mental health. Practitioners need to be aware of the likely wide-ranging impact of their work on the rights of service users and carers. They need to ensure that any perceived interference with individual rights needs to be clearly justified, reasoned and recorded. 'Risk' will be a significant area, as the issues of restriction and detention are generally closely aligned with the potential for risk.

Reviews of restriction at tribunal hearings may also pose a human rights minefield; both in terms of scrutinizing the validity of the act of restriction in some individual cases, but also through unreasonable delays in arranging review dates. However, there may also be future potential for this legislation to be considered in support of reasoned positive risk-taking in mental health services.

Social Care Risk Framework (DH 2007a) and Best Practice in Managing Risk (DH 2007b)

In May and June 2007 two new Department of Health risk frameworks have been published. The Social Care framework (DH 2007a) is a cross-disabilities publication that sets out the importance of the value-base that any individual brings to their work, and sets the context of supporting choice and personal decision-making within a person-centred approach. The Risk Tools framework (DH 2007b) is mental health specific, and focuses attention on the underlying principles of good practice, and evaluates a broad range of tools for the job.

Together they present a coherent message of what positive practice should and often does look like, quite different from the on-going rhetoric which has driven the changes to the Mental Health Act.

Refocusing the Care Programme Approach (DH 2008a)

Reinforces the need to see th CPA as service user-focused, underpinned by a clear set of values and principles, and integral to processes that underpin best practice in risk management. A specific set of CPA resources have been developed for service users and carers (DH 2008b), placing good practice in working with risk within the wider context of comprehensive assessment, care planing and review, and promoting the service users own reflections and identification of risks.

The service-user experience

Some areas of government policy have been extremely disappointing to many service users, not least of which is the *National Service Framework* (*NSF*) *for Mental Health* (DH 1999b). While this document is generally to be welcomed, the overwhelming view of many service users, and indeed practitioners, is that the standards it outlines should be regarded as minimums – not optimums. Therefore, the aim should be to try to build more effective and supportive services from those stated within the NSF.

It is important to note that a number of service-user participants on the government's External Reference Group, which helped to shape the *NSF for Mental Health* actually resigned from the group as they were unhappy not only with the process but also the general direction which was being taken. To highlight just one of the potentially serious areas in this context, it is worth considering the continuing proposals to implement Compulsory Treatment Orders in the community (CTOs). Most service users and practitioners which the authors of this chapter have spoken to around the UK feel that this type of approach to community mental health will be a retrograde step which will have real potential to increase risk. Service users may be driven away from services rather than being properly engaged in an effective and sensitive way as the vital therapeutic relationship between service user and practitioner is broken down by inappropriate and highly unhelpful policy.

While the government policy agenda of reducing stigma and promoting social inclusion is warmly welcomed by most service users, the public safety agenda creates something of a paradox in that it only helps to stigmatize mental health service users even further by adding to some highly inappropriate and inaccurate myths connected with mental distress.

Further, the whole 'protection of the public' approach fails to fully register the far higher risks of self-harm, serious self-neglect and suicide, as well as abuse, attack and exploitation from other members of the public, which face many service users each day. In other words, mental health service users are more often than not vulnerable human beings who are far more likely to be victims of violence rather than the perpetrators of it (Wetherell 2000).

Taylor and Gunn (1999) looked at the homicide figures for the period 1957–95 and, overall, they found there was a fivefold increase in homicides within the UK. However, they found a decline of 3 per cent per annum in contribution to these figures by people with mental illness. Therefore, it is important to note that while we are now living in a significantly more violent society, proportionally, homicides by people with mental health problems are reducing.

As stated at the beginning of this chapter, risk is enmeshed in all aspects of our daily functioning; it is essentially the art of living with uncertainty. Therefore, in reality there will always be tragedies whether we deliver mental health care in the community, within large institutions, on acute wards or from specialist units. Most service users accept the above and are willing to live with risk in their lives so long as they are provided with accessible, person-centred, effective services, which are sensitive to their needs.

Service users are sometimes put at risk because inflexible systems and services are unable to respond to individual clinical needs as they occur. As an example, although Care Programme Approach (CPA) can be of great assistance in managing risk, systems failures can cause people to fall through the safety net despite good service-user focused planning. Therefore, it is essential that services are able to respond to specific risk management and crisis plans in a swift and appropriate manner at all times and such an approach should include the following:

■ monitoring for early warning signs/relapse signatures;
■ agreed crisis and contingency plans;
■ proactive follow-up for service users who do not attend appointments;
■ a named care coordinator whose telephone number is available to all those in the network of care.

All of the above need to be supported with a thorough, detailed and up-to-date care plan which names the individual professionals responsible for each element of care, timescales and recommended responses, etc.

The service user's experience of risk in relation to acute care is another important area to consider. A survey of the quality of care in acute psychiatric wards (Sainsbury Centre for Mental Health 1998) highlighted that most acute ward environments have limited therapeutic input and can be dangerous places for both patients and staff. Service users commonly said that they felt unsafe on acute wards, and women in particular expressed concerns about their personal safety. In many areas, there is constant demand for beds that leads to inappropriate early discharge thereby putting service users at increased risk. Therefore, a comprehensive risk assessment needs to take place both for service users who are being discharged as well as for those being considered for leave. The serious difficulties identified in acute in-patient environments have at least sparked further attempts to develop initiatives as a response to the challenges (Sainsbury Centre for Mental Health 2005, 2006).

As stated within Standard 7 (Preventing Suicide) of the *NSF for Mental Health*, care plans for those with severe mental illness should include an urgent follow-up within one week of discharge from hospital as it is recognized that this period carries a significantly increased risk of suicide. Although the suicide rate has fallen by more than 12 per cent since 1982 (Kelly and Bunting 1998), some people remain at a relatively higher risk of death by suicide. The following statistics taken from the *NSF for Mental Health* (DH 1999b) help to highlight some of the higher risk areas:

■ Men are three times more likely than women to commit suicide. It is the leading cause of death among men aged 15–24 and the second most common cause of death among people aged under 35.
■ Men in unskilled occupations are four times more likely to commit suicide than are those in professional work.

- Among women living in England, those born in India and East Africa have a 40 per cent higher suicide rate than those born in England and Wales.
- Certain occupational groups are at higher risk, for example, doctors, nurses, pharmacists, vets and farmers, due to access to means.
- More than 1 in 10 people with severe mental illness kill themselves.
- Risk is raised further for those with depression and/or suffering major loss.
- Previous histories of self-harm, or drug and alcohol misuse are at relatively higher risk of suicide.
- There are high rates of suicide in prisons.

Positive risk-taking

Broadly speaking, individuals can only grow through measured and justifiable risk-taking. It would also be a rather dull world if it were devoid of all risks and associated choices. Life consists of exercising one choice over another, and this liberty should apply to service users as much as it does to other members of society. It is also important to remember that we all engage in risky behaviour to some degree as a normal part of daily living. Mental health managers, service commissioners, practitioners and service users alike all take some risks every day. It would be virtually impossible to actually live a normal life without some form of risk-taking.

Some obvious, common examples would include: smoking, drinking alcohol, poor diet, taking recreational drugs, driving while tired, breaking the speed limit, and crossing a busy road. Risk is often an important and positive element within our lives – people learn and grow through taking measured and justifiable risks, and so it is not all about danger and negativity, by any means.

While some would argue that positive risk-taking is a relatively new concept in risk management, it is true to say that many nurses and other practitioners have been working collaboratively with service users in this way for many years in their everyday working practice. The idea of positive risk-taking is usually most popular with service users and practitioners alike, as it takes a different approach by focusing on service users' strengths and positive attributes (Morgan 2004). This will be a different way of working to many practitioners as it is not problems oriented. However, it can be a useful, refreshing and empowering way to work collaboratively with service users (Morgan 2007a).

Any positive risks taken, together with the reasoning behind them, need to be clearly documented, and supported by a collaborative approach. To be 'defensible' in the face of opposition and scrutiny they need to be:

- justifiable;
- measured;
- intelligent;
- negotiated with the service user and carer(s) (Wetherell 2001b).

Some basic examples of what could be positive risk-taking are shown below and include some things which general members of the community would do as a matter of course in their daily lives:

- having a bank account;

- shopping;
- visiting family or friends;
- independent living;
- voluntary or paid work;
- going on holiday;
- 'controlled' self-harm;
- medication reduction or withdrawal.

Probably one of the most radical issues listed above is the 'controlled self-harm'. As a concept, self-harm needs to be more fully understood and accepted as a coping strategy that some people need to engage in order to prevent something even worse from happening. It should not simply be seen as behaviour associated with a suicide attempt. Therefore, if service users are going to engage in self-harm, from a risk perspective is it not better they do so with appropriate knowledge of harm minimization, which will help to reduce risk?

As an example, the National Self-Harm Network has produced some helpful literature in *The Hurt Yourself Less Workbook* (Dace *et al.* 1998) which is focused on harm reduction or minimization and includes information on informing service users of 'safer self-harm' approaches, effective first aid and wound dressing, etc.

When approaching the management of self-harm behaviours from a risk viewpoint, it is helpful to be aware of the following common inaccurate myths in this connection. Some people incorrectly believe that self-harm is:

- attention seeking;
- attempted suicide (although in some cases it has accidentally led to death);
- masochism;
- a form of manipulation;
- unworthy for treatment within hospital settings, particularly accident and emergency departments.

Understanding why people engage in self-harm behaviours may also be helpful in assessing and managing risk. Some possible reasons include:

- to feel alive;
- preventing something worse from happening (for example, a suicide attempt);
- to reduce or stop intrusive thoughts;
- self-hatred;
- self-punishment;
- to achieve relief/release of emotions;
- a distraction from 'intolerable reality'.

With a focus on effective management of self-harm behaviours, the following approaches may be of assistance within clinical practice:

- Encourage the individual to talk about how they are feeling.
- Show care and respect for the person behind the self-harm behaviour.
- Recognize that trying to extinguish self-harm behaviour can be unrealistic and can deprive the service user of a coping strategy. Working towards harm minimization or reduction may be a more realistic goal.
- Acknowledge the emotional distress and trauma that the person is experiencing.

■ Even if self-harm is considered to be part of a 'Personality Disorder' try to remember that behind every 'personality disorder' there is a personality and; behind every personality there is a person.

Clearly, contingency plans need to be formulated just in case any positive risk-taking begins to go wrong or if the service user reaches a crisis at any time. Additionally, there can be value in making contracts with service users so that everyone is clear of the boundaries and any appropriate action to be taken should risk increase to an unacceptable level. At all times of any positive risk-taking process, practitioners, carers and service users themselves need to be monitoring for any early warning signs of relapse or increased risk, and an agreed course of action can then be taken in line with the contingency plan and/or the contract with the service user.

While we need to work towards a culture which accepts and positively encourages positive risk-taking, we need at all times to remember that there may be team conflict in this connection. This, of course, needs to be managed and constructive, objective dialogue needs to take place between all practitioners concerned, wherever possible leading to a negotiated consensus within the team.

Case study: Kate – a study in positive risk-taking

Personal history

Kate is 35 years old, born in Dublin, but moved to Manchester with her family (parents, older sister, younger brother) when she was 14. She was married at 26 and divorced at 33. Her ex-husband was awarded custody of their two sons owing to her mental health problems. Her working life was mainly spent in accountancy, before her marriage and parenthood. During the last 18 months, Kate held a part-time job (usually two days per week) in a local shop, using her accountancy skills. The shop owner has taken a flexible and supportive approach to employing Kate, even through numerous spells of time spent in hospital.

Psychiatric history

Kate was sexually abused by an uncle, between the ages of 6 and 14. Any attempts by Kate to discuss the abuse with her parents were quickly dismissed or denied. First contact with child and adolescent psychiatric services was at the age of 8, experiencing depressive episodes and low levels of self-worth and confidence. When she was 10 the family GP prescribed Ativan, which Kate became addicted to, and was not properly supported to come off it until her late teenage years. Further developments in her teenage years included drug and alcohol misuse, and self-harm (cutting and burning).

A serious suicide attempt, through paracetamol overdose combined with vodka, followed her divorce. She was found by emergency services who were alerted by concerns of a close friend. Kate has had 11 hospital admissions during the last five years, most being short-term crisis admissions of up to three weeks' duration, with a couple of admissions extending up to six weeks. The longer-term diagnoses of depression and anxiety remain, but approximately four years ago Kate was diagnosed with borderline personality disorder, due to her chaotic lifestyle, self-harming behaviour and substance misuse becoming more pronounced features of her presentation.

Relationships

While the relationship with her parents is not very good, they are on speaking terms, and Kate usually sees them at least monthly. She maintains occasional contact and reasonably good relationships with her brother and sister. Weekly contact is maintained with two close friends from the local badminton club, and very good relationships are sustained with her two sons – they normally stay with her most Saturdays. Good relationships with mental health professionals are rare, and only established where she feels a strong sense of trust and safety; but on occasions she has become very attached to individual members of nursing staff, leading to unhealthy levels of dependency.

Current situation

Kate's ex-husband is due to remarry in the next few weeks. Concerns over her future contacts with her sons precipitated a series of arguments with him. She was admitted to the local psychiatric unit a few days ago following several days' drinking and drug use, leading to a serious incident of deep cutting, which damaged her arm. During the admission, a member of staff discovered Kate pushing paper tissue down her throat, in an attempt to asphyxiate herself. She was placed on one-to-one close observations. She has also attracted unwanted attention from young male patients on the unit, and feels a strong need for staff to ensure her safety over this issue.

Interests and aspirations

Maintaining the contact with her two sons is her main priority; and sustaining her part-time job in the local shop is something she feels respects her skills and abilities. Kate particularly values her few close friendships, and she has read some information on the psychiatric unit about the National Self-Harm Network. After discussions with another patient on the unit she is expressing a desire to contact the network, with the aim of meeting likeminded people and possibly taking some personal control and management of her self-harming behaviours.

Consideration of risk-taking

After a full multi-disciplinary discussion, with Kate proactively involved, a plan for early discharge was formulated based on:

1 a counselling and coordination role provided by the community psychiatric nurse based in the GP practice (no referral to the community mental health team);
2 establishing Kate's links with local people in the National Self-Harm Network;
3 Kate's self-monitoring of an early warning signs and relapse signature plan, developed with an inpatient nurse with whom she has a trusting relationship;
4 opportunities for Kate to occasionally initiate contact with the inpatient nurse to discuss her progress or concerns (the nurse will establish regular contact with the primary care CPN to coordinate such contacts);
5 discharge on no medication, but with progress reviews established with the GP, and 6-monthly outpatient appointments;
6 clear documentation of the reasoned decision-making: discussions, plans and contingencies for potential difficulties.

Risk assessment and risk management

For the purposes of a textbook or training event, the concepts of risk assessment and risk management can be analysed separately. However, in reality they are closely interlinked – risk cannot be effectively managed until it has been clearly identified and defined; and when a risk is identified we instantly respond with considerations of how it is best managed. In recent years, there has been a shift of conceptual thinking, from a singular and static determination of dangerousness, to a more dynamic and changeable concept of risk (Rose 1998). Risk assessment and management have become continuous elements of good clinical practice.

This development has coincided with some of the consistent requirements emerging from the homicide inquiry reports, namely that:

- high quality and up-to-date risk information is essential;
- information needs to be shared as widely as possible between agencies and individuals, as appropriate;
- collaborative working between all individuals and organizations is crucial.

Risk assessment

" A gathering of information through processes of communication, investigation, observation and persistence; and analysis of the potential outcomes of identified behaviours. Identifying specific risk factors of relevance to an individual and the circumstances in which they may occur. This process requires linking the context of historical information to current circumstances to anticipate possible future change.

(Morgan 2007a) "

Specific categories and risk factors will be discussed in detail in the next section; here we will focus consideration more on the skills and general areas of assessment. There is no mystique about risk assessment, as with all other types of assessment it depends on the accessibility and quality of information gathered. To this end, it requires persistence in pursuit of the relevant information held at multiple sources. The skill lies more in the delicate manner and approach to enquiring after appropriate information from the service user, and all others with relevant knowledge to contribute. The basic skills include active listening, empathic understanding and reflective communication, supplemented by alert observation of the non-verbal cues or signs of change.

Once information has been collected, the next skill required of the practitioner is that of reasoned analysis, towards the formulation of a plan of action. At this stage, accurate historical information needs to be evaluated against current patterns of behaviour. One previous incident, 20 years ago, does not necessarily indicate a high risk of reoccurrence; though such an eventuality should not be entirely ruled out. A repeated pattern of risk behaviours over time begins to present a stronger basis for predicting a reoccurrence. Never lose sight of the human potential to change behaviour patterns, even those that appear to be well established. The keys to a good assessment of risk are as follows.

Context

It is vitally important to look at any changing personal circumstances when assessing risk in relation to a particular individual. If someone is experiencing significant change within their life such as moving, the bereavement of someone close to them, or the allocation of a new care coordinator, there could well be increased risk present. An individual who may be at risk in one particular situation, or specific relationships, could actually be at little or no risk in another setting. For instance, the likelihood of self-injury or suicide may increase significantly in an individual faced with an inpatient admission, or in a specific relationship. On the other hand, inpatient admission could reduce risk for other individuals who feel safer within an acute hospital setting (Wetherell 2001a).

Environment

As well as assessing the individual, how well they are functioning, and their general behaviour, we need to look at the current environment, and the community in which the person lives (Morgan 2007a). Whether the person may be at risk from local people needs to be considered – some service users are highly vulnerable and are open to abuse and/or exploitation in many ways. Local hazards have to be appreciated and taken into account, for example, a drug culture or robberies on the street. It is crucial to remember that these potential risks are faced not only by the service user, but also by the practitioner who might go to particular known areas to carry out home visits (Wetherell 2001a).

Another area of consideration is the degree of emotional arousal dependent upon the setting. For instance, one person may become emotionally aroused within a formal setting, whereas another person may find such a setting to be calming and safe. There is also the issue of potential weapons to be considered in the rare circumstances where a service user may pose the threat of violence to others. Anything can be a weapon, and practitioners need to give due consideration to this, in relation to the potential emotional arousal, as well as to the physical layout of the environment in any given circumstance.

Research information

Research information is a key part of risk assessment, and it can assist in identifying potentially risky circumstances or individuals (DH 2001). For instance, men under 35 years of age are more likely to pose a risk of violence. If you then add the taking of drugs and/or alcohol, the risk increases further. Certain psychotic phenomenon, for example, persecutory delusions specifying an individual(s), or auditory command hallucinations then increase the risks even higher (Buchanan 1997). Risk factors are discussed in more detail in the next section.

Predictive ability

One expectation of risk assessment is that it enables predictive judgements on the probability of certain behavioural outcomes. Prediction is a very uncertain element, though its accuracy can be partly improved by shortening timescales. In this instance, risk has some parallels with trying to predict the weather (Monahan and Steadman 1996). A glance out of the window will tell you if you need to take an umbrella with you in ten minutes' time. Predicting whether you will need an umbrella at the same time a week later becomes a totally different, more complex and difficult to gauge scenario. Similarly with risk – events are generally easier to predict over the next few hours and days than the next few weeks and months.

Practitioner confidence in assessing risks grows with experience. However, the key to a good risk assessment process has to be a collaborative multi-disciplinary and multi-agency approach, where good quality information is shared as appropriate between all relevant parties, leading to shared decision-making for good risk management.

Risk management

66 A statement of plans and an allocation of individual responsibilities for translating collective decisions into real actions. It is the activity of exercising a duty of care where risks (positive and negative) are identified. It entails a broad range of responses linked closely to the wider process of care planning. The activities may involve preventative, responsive and supportive measures to diminish the potential negative consequences of risk and to promote potential benefits of taking appropriate risks. These will occasionally involve more restrictive measures and crisis responses where the identified risks have an increased potential for harmful outcomes. It should also identify a review date for the assessment and management plan.

(Morgan 2007a) 99

Risk management receives far less attention in the literature than risk assessment. For more than a decade we have seen an overall change of emphasis, not just for the concept of risk generally, but also risk management specifically. The latter has shifted from a means of trying to control the volume of medical negligence, to a clinical initiative for addressing potentially harmful outcomes for service users (Vincent 1997). Morgan (2007a) suggests that clinical risk management is focused on the interpretation and implementation of individualized care plans, through targeting treatment, care and support options to the issues identified in a comprehensive assessment (including risk assessment). In reality risk management is about actions, and the responsibilities for ensuring they are carried out and monitored as effectively as possible.

Morgan and Hemming (1999) outline a structure for procedural risk management that stresses three levels of intervention:

■ preventative risk management (including attention to the working relationship, education and early warning signs of relapse);
■ management of escalating situations (including de-escalation techniques, rapid responses and crisis intervention);
■ post-incident supportive management (including positive support for victims and a culture of learning rather than instant retribution through blaming).

The effectiveness of risk management will be determined by the local team operational policies and daily procedures of clinical practice. The context that holds the most influence in this respect is that of team resources, space for imagination, reflection through individual and peer supervision, and attending to the tensions between the need for safety and least restriction of all people engaged in the process, not least the service user (Morgan and Hemming 1999).

One of the key messages for all nursing staff and other mental health workers is the need to move away from an approach relying on the sole responsibility of individual practitioners.

The need for collaborative approaches and collective responsibility cannot be over-emphasized. It is recommended that this method of working is supported by organizational management, policies and procedures emphasizing the concept of collective responsibility. It is therefore vital that collaborative working takes place, where high quality information is shared and where colleagues use each other as sounding boards in order to check out thoughts, intuitive feelings, or concerns. In terms of good risk management practice, regular review at appropriate intervals is therefore required (DH 1999a).

'A collective approach should lead to collective responsibility in the event of "x"' (Wetherell 2001b: 15). We need to learn the valuable lessons from what has gone wrong in the past, and the 'near miss' situations, in order that similar risks can be minimized in the future. The current patterns of investigation immediately set up anxieties in practitioners, even before the full facts have been established. A sense of 'guilty until proven innocent' is established. It is highly unlikely that this approach generates the necessary confidence of practitioners, either in their own abilities or in the support of the organizations. This approach may also seriously contribute to a more fearful, and consequently closed attitude towards reporting events that nearly became incidents.

Therefore, we should welcome a culture that strives to encourage and support a 'blame-free, near-miss reporting' mechanism, in order to develop the confidence to learn. This may require a more confidential set of arrangements to be established within or across organizations, enabling people to pass on important messages to the people who can ensure they are heard without any attachment of blame to those doing the reporting (unless serious negligence has arisen). Similar arrangements currently exist in the aviation industry to learn about near misses without targeting blame to individuals.

Risk categories

Risk categories together with the various factors under each should assist nursing staff and other practitioners in their assessment and management of risk within their daily clinical practice. However, they should be used as a helpful aide-mémoire or as a tool to support professional judgement based on practical experience. This section is designed to help the reader examine the risk categories we are suggesting as well as the individual factors under each of the headings set out later on in this section.

Seven broad categories are considered:

- suicide;
- neglect;
- aggression/violence;
- risk associated with disability;
- physical/medical risks;
- self-harm;
- other risks.

Risk categories and their constituent factors can be used to develop tools that systematically gather these data in relation to individual service users. However, a few broad considerations will arise in practice:

- Provision for 'past' and 'current' (and possibly 'potential' in relation to the 'current' category). A frequent question raised by practitioners is, 'What constitutes "past" and what constitutes "present"?' One approach is to provide a cut-off date in the operational policy and on the risk documentation, for example, three months. However, this approach can lead to various problems including occurrences that are just a few days away from the cut-off point. Under which category should they be entered?

■ Documenting 'potential' risks under the 'current' section. Arguably anything could be described as 'potential'. Therefore, the preferred option is to rely upon good clinical judgement, based upon sound professional approaches and experience. As far as possible where areas of potential confusion occur, it is preferable for practitioners to check out thinking, ideas and concerns with colleagues with a view to arriving at some sort of consensus on the issue in question.

■ Inclusion of tick boxes for 'yes', 'no' and 'don't know' against each of the category factors (creating the opportunity for practitioners to highlight areas where more information or clarification is required by ticking the 'don't know' box). However, some documentation in use around the country only has provision for 'yes' or 'no', which can lead to people being forced to tick one of these when, in reality, it would be far more appropriate to be recording some items as 'don't know'.

Risk categories and associated factors

Tables 11.1–11.7 list the seven risk categories we are suggesting together with some of the associated risk factors for each. We pose a question to the reader regarding which categories they could come up with personally, and how they might re-arrange the individual factors, which are listed under each section.

	Examples (where appropriate)
Helplessness or hopelessness	Severe depression
Misuse of drugs and/or alcohol	
Family history of suicide	
Major psychiatric diagnoses	Manic depression, schizophrenia,
clinical depression	
Separated/widowed/divorced	
Expressing suicidal ideas	
Unemployed/retired	
Considered/planned intent	
Attempts on their life	Taking of overdoses/hanging
Expressing high levels of distress	Highly emotional, agitated
Use of violent methods	Cutting of wrists
Significant life events	Bereavement of close relative or friend
Believe no control over their life	
Other (to be specified)	

Table 11.1 Suicide risk factors

	Examples (*where appropriate*)
Periods of neglect	Neglect when abusing drugs
Lack of positive social contacts	Abusive peer contacts
Failing to drink properly	
Unable to shop for self	
Failing to eat properly	
Insufficient/inappropriate clothing	
Difficulty managing physical health	Ignoring dental needs
Difficulty maintaining hygiene	
Living in inadequate accommodation	
Experiencing financial difficulties	
Lacking basic amenities (water/heat/light)	
Difficulty in communicating needs	Client with psychosis
Pressure of eviction/repossession	
Denies problems perceived by others	Lack of insight/denial
Other (to be specified)	

Table 11.2 Risk factors for neglect

	Examples (*where appropriate*)
Incidents of violence	
Paranoid delusions about others	'They are poisoning me'
Use of weapons	
Violent command hallucinations	Voices say 'Hit that nurse'
Misuse of drugs and/or alcohol	
Signs of anger and/or frustration	Shouting/banging fists
Sexually inappropriate behaviour	Touching/stroking others
Known personal trigger factors	Visit from family
Preoccupation with violent fantasy	Rape/hostage taking
Expressing intent to harm others	
Admissions to secure settings	High, medium or low security provisions or use of seclusion
Dangerous impulsive acts	Deliberate fire setting
Denial of previous dangerous acts	
Other (to be specified)	

Table 11.3 Risk factors for aggression/violence

	Examples (where appropriate)
Sensory impairments	
Intellectual impairments	Poor social skills
Physical suitability of home	
Mobility inside the home	
Mobility outside the home	
Risk of falls	Frail/elderly person
Risk of wandering	Client with dementia
Risk of accidental injury	Learning disability client drinking a boiling hot drink
Communication difficulties	
Expressing sexuality	
Consequences of impulsivity	Assault on client
Challenges to services	Poor service resourcing
Risks associated with driving	Partial sighted or epilepsy
Other (to be specified)	

Table 11.4 Risk factors associated with disability

	Examples (where appropriate)
Physical impairments	Loss of limb(s)
Medical conditions	Asthma/epilepsy
Self-managing medication	
Monitoring medication side effects	
Risks of withdrawal	Relapse/fit/seizures
Risks from smoking	Health/fire
Manual handling risks	
Incontinence	
Other (to be specified)	

Table 11.5 Physical/medical risk factors

	Examples (where appropriate)
Cutting	Use of razor blades/glass
Burning	
Insertion of objects	Pushing items into veins
Overdosing	
Eating disorders	Bulimia/anorexia
Taking of laxatives	
Hair pulling	
Head banging	Striking head against wall
Striking self with objects	
Breaking of bones	
Other (to be specified)	

Table 11.6 Risk factors for self-harm

	Examples (where appropriate)
Exploitation by others	Finance issues
Exploitation of others	Manipulation
Stated abuse by others	Physical/sexual
Abuse of others	Verbal/physical/sexual
Harassment by others	Racial
Harassment of others	Verbal
Risks to child(ren)	
Living alone (with no support)	Isolation
Culturally isolated situation	
Religious or spiritual persecution	
Arson (deliberate fire-setting only)	
Staff conveying clients in own vehicles	Volatile behaviour of client
Other (to be specified)	

Table 11.7 Other risk factors

The following case study challenges you to consider risk categories and associated factors. The case study itself is a composite, for illustration purposes only, as it would be rare to find a service user who would exhibit major factors in all of the category areas.

Case study: Martha – a study to illustrate risk categories and factors

Personal history

Martha is 71 years of age, white British, and was born in Scotland. She experienced physical, sexual and emotional abuse from the age of 4 by her aunt who brought her up as her mother and father were unfit to look after her due to chronic alcoholism.

Martha did reasonably well at school despite the severe problems at home and subsequently obtained a job in a local bakery. She worked in various bakers' shops between 16 and 35 years of age. At 25, Martha married someone she met during one of her inpatient spells in hospital but unfortunately he was physically and emotionally abusive towards her and they eventually divorced when she was 36.

Approximately a year before the divorce, Martha was pushed down the stairs by her husband, through which she acquired a head injury leading to a mild learning disability. This incident also left her with epilepsy and she tends to get an attack every couple of months although she manages to cope with this quite well.

Residing in the Leeds area since the age of 23, Martha now lives alone in a 24-hour warden-assisted ground-floor flat where she normally copes reasonably well, receiving weekly support through her community psychiatric nurse (CPN) from the elderly service.

Psychiatric history and associated factors

Martha experienced her first episode of what is now known as bipolar disorder at the age of 19 and she had numerous hospital admissions up to 30 years of age. Fortunately, she was able to gain an immense degree of insight and applied herself to managing her illness and this led to dramatically reduced hospital admissions.

Following the head injury she sustained at the age of 35, Martha was admitted to Rampton High Security Hospital as she was considered too difficult to manage within her local hospital and, at that time, there were no other appropriate services to deliver her care. She was discharged from Rampton Hospital at the age of 40 to her local hospital in Leeds where she spent two months before being resettled into the community.

Three years ago, Martha had a major stroke that has left her right side very weak. Although she has responded well to physiotherapy, she still needs the aid of a stick when walking and she can be quite unsteady on her feet. In addition, it is impossible for her to climb stairs or walk much more than three-quarters of a mile without having to have a long rest. The following are some of the main risk factors that have been present at various times during the past ten years:

- *Self-harming behaviour*: Martha has been known to insert objects in her arm, swallow batteries and also cut herself when she is distressed.
- *Alcohol misuse*: She often drinks excessive amounts of gin when feeling depressed/not coping.
- *Exploitation*: Martha usually becomes very free and loose with her money when high and/or when she feels lonely and wants company.
- *Self-neglect*: When depressed and/or drinking heavily she usually does not wash or take a shower and fails to eat properly.
- *Aggression/violence*: During periods of psychosis, Martha has been known to lash out with her hands at various people who come into contact with her.

Martha has a standing agreement (by way of a 'contract' with her clinical team) to notify them when her clinical management requires inpatient care. This arrangement usually works well and short admissions of three weeks or so are usually sufficient to get her stabilized. She has the support of an advocate from the local advocacy service in relation to this set-up as well as for other issues which arise from time to time.

Relationships

She enjoys an excellent relationship with her CPN who previously worked in a challenging behaviour unit and is, therefore, well experienced in dealing with how she presents sometimes. As well as a good relationship with her advocate, Martha enjoys a close friendship with a fellow woman resident who lives upstairs – they usually have tea and biscuits with each other at least twice a week.

Current situation

Martha's cousin passed away three days ago and this has led to a difficult period for her. Since receiving the awful news, Martha has been drinking heavily in order to escape from the intolerable reality and this has led to the usual problems of self-neglect.

In addition, she has been cutting her arm again and inserting objects into it as part of her coping strategy. On today's visit of the CPN, there were signs of psychotic symptoms in that Martha was talking rapidly and not making much sense at times. In addition, she became quite distressed twice during the visit and shouted abusively at her CPN.

The environment of the flat appeared to be extremely untidy with cigarette ends, ash, empty bottles and other items scattered around. Martha was also dishevelled and has been ignoring personal hygiene. Finally, as the CPN left the flat, he thought he heard Martha mumbling something about 'bringing an end to it all'. However, when he asked her if she was suicidal she said 'no'.

Service user strengths/positive attributes:

- some insight when she is becoming unwell;
- excellent relationship with CPN;
- most of the time she manages to live relatively independently;
- sociable and reasonable communicator when well;
- normally requests support/assistance via her CPN when she needs it;
- good relationships with her advocate and fellow woman resident;
- normally does most of her own shopping as there is a helpful shopkeeper 300 yards from the flat.

Box 11.1 summarizes the risk categories and risk factors illustrated by the case of Martha, and associated risk management interventions.

Box 11.1 Martha: Risk categories and factors and risk

Risk categories	Risk factors	Risk management
Suicide	Manic depression diagnosis. Recent bereavement. Possibly expressing suicidal intent.	Increase CPN input to daily and encourage client to talk about how she feels.
Neglect	Failing to eat properly. Not shopping for self. Not maintaining personal hygiene.	As above, plus try to see if neighbour can assist by offering practical help. Also, consider meals-on-wheels.
Aggression/violence	Misuse of alcohol. Signs of distress and frustration. Previous admission to high security hospital.	CPN to closely monitor for early warning signs/relapse signature(s) and consider short-term hospitalization.
Risk associated with disability	Poor mobility and risk of falls. Poor communicator when unwell.	OT home assessment. Try to get warden and neighbour to monitor the flat between CPN visits.
Physical/medical risks	Risk of fire from smoking. Epilepsy condition. Frail following stroke.	Ensure smoke alarms are working. Arrange regular GP home visits.
Self-harm	Cutting arm and inserting objects.	CPN to monitor on a daily basis – check for new injuries/dress wounds.
Other risks	Possible verbal/physical abuse towards others. Exploitation by others.	CPN to monitor on a daily basis and to liaise with Martha's neighbour and warden.

Paper institution or practical tools?

One of the greatest fears currently has to be that the tools of bureaucracy are turning skilled clinicians into deskilled 'risk administrators'. The mechanisms for this change are the volumes of paperwork required in contemporary mental health practice, particularly in relation to risk. The need for the paper mountain (Morgan 2001) is driven by the culture of blame – something goes wrong and we all need to find a scapegoat.

The brick walls of the Victorian institutions were held together by mortar, but they seem to have been replaced by the paper walls of the modern institution held together by red tape (Rose 1998). However, is the issue of paperwork all seen as negative? Human services are essentially about the giving and receiving of information, and the paperwork and computer systems are the currency for these transactions. The dilemma is how to create the right balance of time for doing, and time for writing. At another level, whether communicating important information, sharing good practice, or facing the rigours of a serious incident inquiry, written documentation is vitally important. What you knew and what you thought is what you have written. Without such a system requirement, we would be open to many abuses, through bad practices easily defended by the 'but I thought ...' whim.

The types of paperwork currently in use are voluminous – referral forms, care programme approach documentation, comprehensive needs assessments, full risk assessments, supervised discharge documentation, Mental Health Act assessment forms, carers' assessments, detailed daily notes, copies to all, notes of all telephone conversations, letters of confirmation of all agreements, registers, lists, workload statistics, compatibility with team-organization-profession requirements, written requests on the relevant forms for the relevant organizations, incident report forms, and so on.

What is the purpose of all this documentation? For whose benefit is it? How much is necessary? Who has access to it? When do we arrive at the summit of this paper mountain? Who is involved or consulted in its design and implementation? What about the issues of duplication ... accessibility ... confidentiality? So many significant issues, yet often so little discussion at the local service level between all the relevant parties. Morgan (2001) suggests that one of the major challenges is that of shifting perceptions of paperwork, away from the negative demands of a remote bureaucracy, to one of a practical tool supporting good practice. However, this should not cloud the need to scrutinize the relevance of all the requirements, determining baseline minimum standards, involving practitioners and service users more in the design of relevant formats, and ensuring that there is a shared understanding of how these mechanisms are to operate.

One apparent answer would be to develop the technology by transferring all records to computer systems. The ideal situation would be a unified system of electronic patient record keeping. All practitioners would have access to desktops, laptops or palmtops as needed; so that relevant information could be entered or downloaded at the time of need. Records and assessments could be recalled and edited while in the review meetings. Duplication could be avoided, and new information could be shared with all relevant individuals as soon as it was available. People could search for key words or specific information without having to sift through what are often very bulky files, and different agencies would be using compatible systems that communicated with each other. At-risk individuals would be identified, and appropriate protocols implemented to ensure the risk information was passed to all people who need to know it.

In these days of information technology, this should be an achievable goal. However, the general experience in practice is that within individual organizations, even within the NHS, there are numerous different operating systems in place, which are not compatible with one another. The above scenario appears to remain a long way off, even with current attempts to develop an NHS system through 'Connecting for Health' by 2012, and is only partly the answer to the paperwork conundrum. While it may save 'some' time for some people, services may still be populated by technophobes who require training and technical support; sufficient capital investment has been made into the supply of accessible equipment; and it still does not address the validity of all that is required to be recorded, or sufficiently addresses the confidentiality and accessibility of information issue.

How to shift from 'disabling' to 'enabling' risk assessments and management plans

A number of important principles would need to be established:

- information efficiently communicated, through a more collaborative process;
- a transparent 'need-to-know basis' established;
- a sense of ownership of documentation, developed through practical processes of consultation and testing of ideas;
- eradication of duplication;
- an awareness of realistic expectations openly acknowledged by all parties, that risks can be minimized or reduced but not eliminated;
- a recognizable culture shift to a more open use of risk-assessment information for the purpose of meeting service-user needs rather than just as a way to find out what went wrong, and who made the mistakes.

This type of development could have significant benefits: for the service manager, the possibility of collaborative working towards recognized good practice, supported by relevant research and practical evidence; for the practitioner, an appreciation of the place and function of essential administrative needs, able to both support and reflect the reality of working relationships; for the service user, fears heard and listened to, through more open discussion of the needs for minimum standards of essential documentation. The gathering of information needs to respect individual circumstances – achievements, strengths and personal priorities, not just to detail problems and difficulties.

Whether we are aiming towards the more difficult task of national standards for documentation, or supporting local decisions, an agreed minimum standard of what is needed has to be achieved. The Department of Health have commissioned two National Risk Frameworks, one for mental health and the other for social care DH 2007a, 2007b, which will aim to re-establish the underlying values and principles of good practice. The mental health framework will also review the complex issue of evidence-based practice and available risk tools. Essentially, what most people will want is the maximum information with the minimum time and effort – the impossible tension between being brief and comprehensive at the same time. It has been said, by some practitioners, that the best format for documenting a risk assessment is a blank sheet. While this will allow for complete individuality of the assessment recording process, it does not guarantee good practice in recording information by all nurses, and other practitioners. Furthermore, it offers no guidance on what a risk assessment should cover, and may encourage some people to write in a style that becomes inaccessible or not read. For many people, the absence of a structure will result in their attempting to devise a structure to their method of recording. There are no great merits in a system where the structure of recording is completely ad hoc.

Getting down to the basics – it is not so much the form, more the quality of the information. But, designed properly, the form structures the thought processes and the resulting information in a meaningful way. It must be used with clear explanations to service users, about why, how and with whom it will be shared. Forms involving assessments of need and risks must incorporate equal attention to positive strengths, resources and opportunities for positive risk-taking (Morgan 2007a).

The vitally important point to stress in this connection is that good risk documentation should always be a supportive tool to good clinical practice and not a burdensome hindrance. In a blame culture, it is important to remember that 'paperwork protects practitioners and patients' (Wetherell 2001b: 15). Where vital information was not accessed, it is still important in these instances to document the need for additional information, and the attempts to gain it. At all times professional training, practical experience and multi-disciplinary approaches arriving at sound clinical judgement should be the focus, supported, of course, by effective processes of risk assessment and management.

What about scoring mechanisms and numerical scales?

Some of the existing risk assessments on the open market have devised their own numerical systems of quantifying the risks identified (Worthing Priority Care 1995; O'Rourke and Hammond 2000). In practice and in workshops, the responses to this format are mixed. They seem primarily to be meeting the audit and research agenda for numbers that can be more easily analysed and evaluated. For this reason, they have some merit in comparison of assessments across time.

However, in the particular instant where clinical decisions need to be made about how a risk assessment may inform a risk management plan, they can become more misrepresentative of circumstances, and more inclined to the quantitative rather than qualitative values. Numerical systems are generally poor at representing the thinking and communication that informed a risk decision (Stein 1998). They may also be cynically seen as a useful tool for rationing services at times of pressure, rather than focusing on the reality of risks being faced.

What about risk management plans?

Clinical practice is fraught with demands on the practitioner's time, and the emphasis of many clinical tools is on the assessment of need, with a commensurate neglect of the management of the risks identified. In many instances, the design of clinical tools stops short at simply offering a final box headed 'management plan', lacking the guidance previously afforded to the process of assessment. Morgan (2007a) presents one example of how more space and guidelines may be offered, to inform the discussions that direct a risk decision to be represented in a more formal plan. This plan may equally be located within the overall 'care plan', or stand as a specific risk management plan attachment to the care plan. Accessibility and utility of the plan are the important issues.

The subsequent management of a risk, including the taking of risks, should be afforded at least equal importance and attention as the initial identification of risk through assessment. Ultimately, a thoroughly assessed risk that was haphazardly managed is still likely to result in negative consequences.

Confidentiality

One of the great paradoxes facing mental health professionals today is the need for greater disclosure and for confidentiality (Cordess 2001) (cf. Chapter 6). In conjunction with the inquiry reports calling for more sharing of information, we struggle to square the circle in mental health services. Guidance, legislation and local policy statements often exist, but serve to cloud the issues in the reality of day-to-day practice. Maybe it is one of the issues that simply defies clarity.

On the one hand, confidentiality is a crucial part of the risk assessment and management process, an essential cornerstone of the trusting working relationship. On the other, it has the potential for abuse, where playing the confidentiality card for all of the wrong reasons acts as a defence. In the latter circumstances, confidentiality may prevent the passing of information that should be communicated for important safety reasons.

Service users may not always be the people who use 'confidentiality' as a blocking mechanism. However, they are well within their rights to use it as a demand for more transparency in the use and communication of sensitive information about their personal lives. The person who is not told where information will be shared, and for what purposes, is understandably going to raise concerns about its widespread broadcasting. Where there is more transparency on behalf of the service providers there is likely to be more understanding and acceptance from most service users.

In its simplest form, transparency may be linked to the CPA network of care: indicating that these are the people who the information will be shared with, as they are all working together to offer care and support. As with ripples in a pond, this picture may spread further as we explain how some of these individuals will be part of working supervision relationships, and team-working, requiring some disclosure to aid ideas and care planning. Even where the information appears to be seeping through more widely, we may still be able to define reasoned boundaries to its sharing. We need to clarify the 'need-to-know' test.

Mental health services introduce many complications to this simple picture. Health and social services are often likely to operate different policies and procedures for information sharing and accessibility. The statutory sector services may express concerns about widely differing practices across a diverse voluntary sector. Some services, for example advocates, may actively refuse to accept information passed on, preferring to take a blank slate approach to assessing individual needs (and taking their own precautions about the potential for risks as something you deal with if and when it arises).

A further complication arises when we are thinking about the mechanisms for recording information, their accessibility, and frequent incompatibility. Many practitioners experience that frequent heart-sinking feeling – so many different places to be recording so many types of data – that it becomes a challenge to determine where a specific piece of information should go; none of it is cross-referenced, and the thought of considering with whom it should be shared is a thought too far!

Some psychotherapeutic relationships are established on a strict basis of confidentiality. In this context, some disclosures may have been made on the premise that nothing is shared outside of the relationship. This approach is contra-indicated by the repeated reports of inquiries, which highlight a consistent factor of poor risk management, in the failure to pass on vitally important information to people who could have used it to possibly avoid a disaster. US and UK case law over the last 25 years has pointed towards the breaching of confidentiality, where information about a serious and imminent risk of harm to an identified individual is divulged (Monahan 1993).

There will be many 'what if' scenarios in relation to this issue, defying any attempts to secure an answer for all eventualities. What we do need, as a basic standard for practitioners, is guidance that indicates:

- service and team operational policy statements outlining the importance of confidentiality, and openly recognizing the dilemmas it throws up;
- development of leaflets/statements to present information about confidentiality and information-sharing to service users;

- the need for transparency with service users about how information is to be used;
- the setting of reasonable boundaries that recognize the rare circumstances where breaching confidentiality will be needed for personal safety of service user and/or others;
- clear documenting of the reasons for decisions to breach confidentiality;
- clear documenting of the reasons for decisions made not to share information with specific individuals;
- inter-agency agreements about issues of confidentiality and information sharing.

Conclusion

This chapter has examined the concept of risk and emphasized its importance in all our lives. Positive risk-taking can promote growth, while other types of risk can pose serious threats to the health and well-being of individuals and/or those around them. We summarize the main points of this chapter below:

- Risk cannot be eliminated. However, it can be reduced or minimized through good working practice and sound clinical approaches which, as far as possible are multi-disciplinary/multi-agency.
- Risk is dynamic and each case needs to be treated separately with due regard to its own particular elements.
- Risk assessment and risk management more often feel like 'done to' rather than 'collaborated with' processes for many service users. This promotes more stigma and hinders real recovery.
- Carefully considered positive risk-taking initiatives offer the most tangible form of defensible decisions.
- All people directly involved in mental health services need to collaborate in demonstrating the reality of everyday circumstances, and challenge the unrealistic expectations perpetuated by media misrepresentation, public perceptions and legislative bureaucracy.

Questions for reflection and discussion

1   Review the case study 'Kate – a study in positive risk-taking'. What are the potential outcomes of the stated plan, and what needs to be in place in your local services to make these types of decisions a reality?
2   What tensions exist between the roles of service documentation/paperwork tools and clinical judgement, in the routine assessment and management of risk?
3   Confidentiality of service-user information is of paramount importance, and good risk assessment and management plans require the sharing of accurate information. How do you square the circle?
4   What elements should be prioritized in 'training' and 'practice development' programmes, for supporting the implementation of good practice in assessing and managing risks in local mental health services?

Annotated bibliography

- University of Manchester (2006) *Avoidable death: five year report of the National Confidential Inquiry into Suicide and Homicide by People with Mental Illness.* Manchester University of Manchester. This provides the most comprehensive statistics on the suicides and homicides in England and Wales. It focuses specifically on the populations in contact with mental health services, but importantly places these within the context of the figures for the whole population. Significant recommendations are drawn out for the wide-ranging areas of the service, from inpatient care to community support, and the vital place of primary care.
- Langan, J. and Lindow, V. (2004) *Living with Risk: Mental health service user involvement in risk assessment and management.* Bristol: Joseph Rowntree Foundation/Policy Press. This report of interviews with service users, carers and practitioners indicated that the stigma associated with risk has caused service users distress in terms of their personal safety, and led occasionally to disengagement from services. Service users felt practice around risk assessment was inconsistent, and agreement between themselves and professionals regarding levels of risk was extremely variable.
- O'Rourke, M. and Bird, L. (2000) *Risk Management in Mental Health.* London: Mental Health Foundation. A short practical booklet setting out clear bullet-point lists of the key themes and messages about the context and practice of risk assessment and management. In RAMAS it outlines one specific example of a locally developed and nationally recognized systematic approach to documenting and auditing the identified research risk factors and management responses.
- Rose, N. (1998) Living dangerously: risk-thinking and risk management in mental health care. *Mental Health Care* **1**(8): 263–6. A thought-provoking challenge to the way risk assessment and management have come to dominate the thinking and working of mental health services. It argues that we have become the 'risk business', with a greater emphasis on the administration of risk, rather than on the care and support of people experiencing mental health problems.

References

Buchanan, A. (1997) The investigation of acting on delusions as a tool for risk assessment in the mentally disordered. *British Journal of Psychiatry* **170**(Suppl. 32): 12–16.

Cordess, C. (ed.) (2001) *Confidentiality and Mental Health.* London: Jessica Kingsley.

Dace, E., Faulkner, A., Frost, M. *et al.* (1998) *The Hurt Yourself Less Workbook.* London: National Self-Harm Network.

Department of Health (1995) Mental Health (Patients in the Community) Act. London: The Stationery Office.

Department of Health (1999a) *Effective Care Co-ordination in Mental Health Services: Modernising the Care Programme Approach.* London: The Stationery Office.

Department of Health (1999b) *A National Service Framework for Mental Health.* London: The Stationery Office.

Department of Health (1999c) *Saving Lives: Our Healthier Nation.* London: The Stationery Office.

Department of Health (2000) *The NHS Plan.* London: The Stationery Office.

Department of Health (2007a) *Independence, choice and risk: a guide to best practice in supported decision-making.* London: Department of Health (DH_074773)

Department of Health (2007b) *Best practice in managing risk: principles and guidance for best practice in the assessment and management of risk to self and others in mental health services.* London: Department of Health (DH_076511).

Department of Health (2008a) *Refocusing the Care Programme Approach: Policy and Positive Practice Guidance.* London: Department of Health.

Department of Health (2008b) *Service Users & Carers and the Care Programme Approach: Making the CPA Work for You.* Leaflet, Booklet & DVD. London: Department of Health.

Kelly, S. and Bunting, J. (1998) *Trends in Suicide in England and Wales 1982–1996.* London: Population Trends.

Madden, A. (2006) *Review of Homicides by Patients with Severe Mental Illness.* London: Department of Health and Imperial College.

Monahan, J. (1993) Limiting therapist exposure to Tarasoff liability: Guidelines for risk containment. *American Psychologist* **48**: 242–50.

Monahan, J. and Steadman, H.J. (1996) Violent storms and violent people. *American Psychologist* **51**(9): 931–8.

Morgan, S. (2001) Scaling paper mountains *Openmind* **107**: 20–1.

Morgan, S. (2004) www.practicebasedevidence.com

Morgan, S. (2007a) *Working with Risk: A Practitioner Manual.* Brighton: Pavilion.

Morgan, S. (2007b) CPA: process or event? *Openmind* **143**: 19–21.

Morgan, S. and Hemming, M. (1999) Balancing care and control: risk management and compulsory community treatment. *Mental Health and Learning Disabilities Care* **3**(1): 19–21.

NHS Executive (1994) *Introduction of Supervision Registers for Mentally Ill People.* HSG(94)5. Leeds: NHSE.

O'Rourke, M. and Hammond, S. (2000) *Risk Management: Towards Safe, Sound and Supportive Services.* Surrey Hampshire Borders NHS Trust and South Thames Research and Development Fund.

Ritchie, J.H., Dick, D. and Lingham, R. (1994) *The Report of the Inquiry into the Care and Treatment of Christopher Cluref.* London: The Stationery Office.

Rose, N. (1998) Living dangerously: risk-thinking and risk management in mental healthcare. *Mental Health Care* **1**(8): 263–6.

Sainsbury Centre for Mental Health (1998) *Acute Problems.* London: Sainsbury Centre for Mental Health.

Sainsbury Centre for Mental Health (2000) *An Executive Briefing on the Implications of the Human Rights Act 1998 for Mental Health Services* (Briefing Paper 12). London: Sainsbury Centre for Mental Health.

Sainsbury Centre for Mental Health (2005) *Acute Care 2004: A national survey of adult psychiatric wards in England.* London: Sainsbury Centre for Mental Health.

Sainsbury Centre for Mental Health (2006) *The Search for Acute Solutions: Improving the quality of care in acute psychiatric wards.* London: Sainsbury Centre for Mental Health.

Sheppard, D. (1996) *Learning the Lessons* (2nd edn). London: the Zito Trust.

Stein, W. (1998) The use of standardised scales and measures for identification, assessment and control of risk in mental health. Unpublished thesis. Glasgow Caledonian University.

Taylor, P.J. and Gunn, J. (1999) Homicides by people with mental illness: myth and reality. *British Journal of Psychiatry* **174**: 9–14.

Vincent, C. (1997) Risk, safety and the dark side of quality. *British Medical Journal* **314**: 1775–6.

Wetherell, A. (2000) Risk in mental health – Part 1. *Breakthrough* **6**(4): 22–3.

Wetherell, A. (2001a) Risk in mental health – Part 2. *Breakthrough* **7**(1): 17–18.

Wetherell, A. (2001b) Risk in mental health – Part 3. *Breakthrough* **7**(4): 15–16.

Worthing Priority Care (1995) The Worthing Weighted Risk Indicator. Unpublished. Available from the Nursing Directorate, Worthing Priority Care NHS Trust, Worthing, UK.

CHAPTER 12

Modern milieus: psychiatric inpatient treatment in the twenty-first century

Anne Aiyegbusi and Kingsley Norton

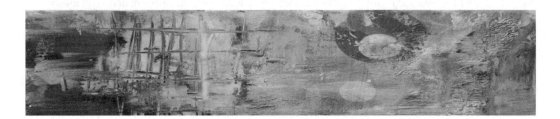

Introduction

Staff working on inpatient psychiatric wards report that it is hard to provide both safe custody as well as excellence in clinical care (Haigh 2002) and patients voice their dissatisfaction about the treatment received therein (Beadsmore *et al.* 1998; Ford *et al.* 1998). In one survey of ex-inpatients, over half had found their hospital admission to be un-therapeutic, with 45 per cent claiming that it was detrimental to their mental health, and 30 per cent experiencing it as unsafe (Baker 2000). Indeed, in a damning indictment of the UK services they commissioned, the Department of Health (England) (DH, formerly DoH) acknowledged that there was 'incontrovertible and compelling evidence' that mental health service users found hospital care to be 'neither safe nor therapeutic' (2002: 8).

Problems with delivering a high standard of care and treatment to mentally ill patients in hospital settings are not new. Over the years, many potential solutions have been conceived. The late eighteenth century, for example, saw a sea change in attitudes to mentally ill patients who were incarcerated, resulting in the so-called 'moral treatments'. This innovative and humane approach (developed by Tuke and others) was based on a concept of 'shared responsibility for the physical maintenance of the shared living space, participation and democratic decision-making in the governance of the project' (Whiteley 2004). Following on from this, although there have been many significant pharmacological and psychotherapeutic developments in treatment for mentally ill patients, the latter have not resulted simply in modern inpatient settings – 'milieus' – being therapeutic, as the surveys referred to above attest. It is therefore timely to consider what lessons from the past might be learned.

In this chapter, we illustrate the problems associated with providing a therapeutic environment for inpatients and summarize some of the relevant therapeutic milieu literature, with the aim of offering a practical guide to staff, particularly nursing staff. We put the latter centre stage and discuss a range of issues around the theme of what contributes to making an inpatient environment therapeutic. From a psychodynamic and systemic perspective, we also consider aspects that can undermine the therapeutic endeavour, again concentrating mainly on the nurses' perspective. Drawing on a growing academic literature, we try to shed light on the complexity of the nursing role, the difficulty of performing it effectively, and its central importance in optimizing the inpatient health care environment- realising the therapeutic potential of the milieu. Finally, we describe the application of some therapeutic milieu principles to working effectively within outpatient and community settings.

Therapeutic milieus

The 1960s and 1970s saw an upsurge of academic interest and clinical experimentation in inpatient settings, including the re-kindling of interest in some of the ideologies of previous generations of mental health care reformers and psychiatric clinicians (Whiteley 2004). The term 'therapeutic milieu' was coined to refer to 'a method of providing specific treatments in an effective manner' (Abroms 1969: 560). The main aims of the therapeutic milieu were defined:

- to control or set limits on pathological behaviour (such as destructiveness, disorganization, deviancy, dysphoria and dependency);
- to promote psychosocial skills (such as orientation, assertion, occupation and recreation).

Achieving these aims required the construction of a 'stable, coherent social organization, which provides an integrated, extensive treatment context' (Abroms 1969: 560). However, creating such an organization is problematic. In part this is because of the upsetting, anxiety-inducing and disturbing effects of psychiatric disorders, not only for patients but also for those around them, especially those who are emotionally close or otherwise attached to them. It is difficult to produce the necessary degree of organization and integration, relying as it ultimately does on the capacity of staff and patients to work together effectively. Delivering a 'therapeutic' outcome, within a given ward, is further complicated by the fact that what an individual patient might require, at a specific point in time, can differ markedly from what is appropriate for another patient at the same time, in the same ward. Yet, a single ward environment is required to cater, more or less equally, for all the patients who inhabit it – for the collective, as well as for the individual patient's needs.

In addressing the relevant issues, it has been found useful to consider the particular therapeutic functions that might need to be undertaken by an inpatient ward, in order for it to be able to maximize the chances of its being therapeutically effective (Gunderson 1978). Five functions were defined: containment; support; structure; involvement; and validation. These would be enacted according to the prevailing needs of the 'ward as a whole'. At times, the emphasis is on the requirement for the first aim – control – but, at other times, there is scope to promote patients' recovery by the provision of opportunities to acquire pertinent skills. With the high turnover of patients in many modern wards, and the associated short duration of many admissions, some of the functions concerned with the second aim of the therapeutic milieu – promoting psychosocial skills – are increasingly delivered in outpatient and community settings. Nonetheless, a consideration of the whole range of functions helps steer the professional in the direction of providing an integrated and coordinated treatment package, which remains patient-centred, across different settings – from inpatient unit to wider community.

Why inpatient settings are not simply therapeutic

Case vignette

Cecelia is a 25-year-old woman who has a primary (Axis I) diagnosis of bipolar disorder and a secondary (Axis II) diagnosis of borderline personality disorder. She has a long history of contact with mental health services, presenting as a 'revolving door' patient. She typically spends a few weeks in hospital followed by a short period of time in the community which precedes a further hospital stay. When in hospital, Cecelia poses mental health services with a number of challenging behaviours. She exhibits a range of self-harming behaviours, has engaged in violence as an inpatient and is extremely verbally abusive to staff, launching spiteful personal attacks on professionals. As an inpatient, Cecelia also regularly complains of physical health problems, which when investigated are usually found to have no organic basis.

Between hospital admissions, Cecelia takes occasional overdoses and consequently attends the local accident and emergency department. While there, she tends to be uncooperative and abusive to the medical and nursing staff. They feel confused and annoyed, failing to understand why Cecelia should self-harm rather than ask for help from a health service, and cannot understand why she behaves as though they have attacked her in some way, criticizing them and abusing them personally. Sometimes, Cecelia places herself in dangerous situations, such as threatening to throw herself from a motorway bridge while intoxicated, which require the intervention of the police. When the latter arrive on the scene, Cecelia is similarly abusive towards them, fighting with them and accusing them of manhandling her as they try to restrain her to safety.

There is a discernible pattern to Cecelia's admissions. Her behaviour challenges ward staff and taints their entire view of her. By most, although not all of the staff, she is seen as someone to be tolerated, more than treated. To ensure her safety, Cecelia is placed on increasingly high levels of 'observations'. She receives medication, against her will, as a response to her violent behaviour. Consequently, her challenging behaviour gradually lessens and finally stops. There is little time to reflect on what might lie behind her behavioural presentation. Attention focuses on discharge follow-up care and planning which team is best placed to provide – a matter that is not usually swiftly resolved. During this period she often takes her own discharge. Back in her flat, and complying poorly with taking her medication, Cecelia's social isolation also contributes to the cycle being continued, with Cecelia bringing herself to the attention of emergency services by putting herself at risk. Thereafter, almost inevitably, she is admitted compulsorily into hospital again. Worryingly, Cecelia's risk-taking behaviour appears to be increasing in seriousness. Staff fear that she could kill herself, probably without really intending to do so.

Commentary

The above case vignette of 'Cecelia' is a composite case, based on many actual examples of inpatients known to us, male as well as female. This case serves to paint a picture of a commonplace clinical situation, where a patient has more than one diagnosis and so-called 'complex needs'. Cecelia's case also illustrates the fact that such patients in acute psychiatric wards are not simply helped by their experience therein. This patient's diagnosis of borderline personality disorder suggests a pattern of unstable mood and associated impulsive behaviours, related to profound fears of abandonment, in the face of threatened or actual loss or separation. This forms the backdrop to and complicates the management of her bipolar disorder. This is especially so as her discharge date nears – the threat of separation. In her case, some symptoms are controllable with medication. However, Cecelia's erratic compliance with the relevant medications, as with other aspects of her care plan, means that it has not been clearly established how much she could be helped by it. Her isolation and lack of social support, between hospital admissions, represent other influences that impact negatively on her capacity for recovery. The clinical management of Cecelia is far from simple.

From the nursing staff's perspective, it feels as if they have no time to think or plan their patient's care. They find themselves 'fire-fighting', i.e. responding to the next acute and dramatic episode of Cecelia's dangerous or worrying behaviour. In doing so, they are adopting (and accepting) a stance which is essentially reactive. However, not all staff feel the same way about Cecelia and her care. Some feel defeated, despairing and frustrated, believing that she is beyond help and others that she does not merit it. Some believe that the system is failing their patient and that Cecelia might be helped if only others (within the health care, social or penal systems) worked differently or harder. Staff find themselves, at times, arguing strongly against or blaming one another. It is also very tempting for them to become critical of colleagues from other agencies who share Cecelia's case. Failures by the health care system to communicate effectively and work together, consistently and systematically, sometimes do result in their patient being admitted to hospital. Hospital admission may relieve those staff initiating it of some anxiety associated with Cecelia's self-injurious behaviour. The ward-based staff on the receiving end, however, often feel they have little or nothing to offer. Once Cecelia is in hospital, a familiar pattern becomes enacted, as if inevitably, even though none consciously wishes it to be so.

Controlling maladaptive behaviour and promoting psychosocial skills

Ideally, the inpatient ward provides patients like Cecelia with an interpersonal environment that provides not only a safe place but also avoids reinforcing maladaptive coping strategies, so that some learning of new coping strategies and skills might take place. This state of affairs has been aptly described as 'preventing "bad" things from happening and allowing "good" things to occur' (Gunderson 1978: 332). However, it is much simpler to describe than to deliver as Cecelia's case testifies. Modern wards may be better at achieving Abroms' first aim – controlling maladaptive behaviour – than his second – promoting psychosocial skills (Abroms 1969). In the following section, therefore, we outline therapeutic functions and processes of a therapeutic milieu, which represents a brief summary of Gunderson's pertinent concepts. He reasons that, in order to provide a therapeutic setting, inpatient ward staff need to understand the wide range of functions that they may be called upon to deliver. This is so that they can select and deploy relevant aspects of care and treatment, based on the changing needs of their patients, according to their mental state, risk status, the stage in their disorder and the phase of their recovery.

Containment

According to Gunderson (1978), the function of 'containment' is to sustain the physical well-being of patients and remove from them the burdens of self-control or feelings of omnipotence. It is effected through the provision of food, shelter and at least temporary removal from the stressors of the outside world. The aim of containment is to prevent assaults and to minimize physical deterioration and dangerousness in those who lack judgement, as was almost always the case with Cecelia's inpatient admissions. The effect of admission is to reinforce, at least temporarily, the patient's internal controls and to reality-test their omnipotent beliefs, concerning their destructiveness. Effective containment thus demonstrates to the patient that their violence can be stopped, i.e. they are *not* all-powerful.

There is a risk that a given inpatient ward could over-emphasize containment, thereby suppressing the patient's own initiative, reinforcing feelings of isolation in them and leading to an increased sense of hopelessness and despair. Cecelia appeared to suffer from an increase of such feelings, especially once a discharge date for her had been set. The staff caring for her also felt increasingly hopeless and despairing, as re-admission relentlessly followed admission. Even though she was not in a fit state to benefit from other functions, outlined below, Cecelia did at least experience some containment. Her physical well-being was sustained. Indeed, her life was almost certainly prolonged by the treatment she received.

Support

'Support' refers to deliberate efforts, effected through the social network of the inpatient environment, to help patients feel better about themselves (Gunderson 1978). There is an acceptance that patients have certain needs, which staff can fulfil, and also that they have limitations to which staff need to make accommodation. Relevant supportive activities include the provision of escorts and other behavioural provisions (such as advice and education) aimed at preserving and reinforcing the patient's existing ego functions. This may also include assisting patients to do things which they protest are impossible but under circumstances where success is almost certainly guaranteed. Those milieus that emphasize support are recognizable as retreats that provide nurturance and permit, encourage and direct patients to venture into other, more specific, therapies such as psychotherapy, rehabilitation or family therapy.

With the costs of health care being intensively scrutinized and carefully controlled, one consequence of shorter acute psychiatric admissions is that there is less time available for forming and strengthening a therapeutic alliance between patient and staff. A weaker alliance means that it is harder to form a secure platform, post-discharge from hospital, upon which to develop further therapeutic interventions that can promote the patients' fuller recovery. Certainly, the suddenness and speed with which Cecelia is usually discharged, means that there is little or no time to reflect on what has transpired or to engage actively and meaningfully in her care plan. Cecelia therefore is not in a position to benefit from the functions specified below, which previously were more often part of an inpatient stay, at least in some psychiatric inpatient settings.

Structure

'Structure' represents all aspects of an inpatient milieu that provide for a predictable organization in terms of time, place and person. It acts to make the environment less amorphous and to support the patient's reality-testing, by making the ward's treatment programme intelligible to patients (Gunderson 1978). Structure facilitates the safe attachment of patients to their environment (Haigh 1999). Ideally, the latter feel neither invaded nor detached and alone. Structure promotes changes in patients' symptoms and action patterns, especially where these are considered to be socially maladaptive, e.g. as with forensic patients. It can contribute to this outcome through helping them to consider consequences of their behaviour for both themselves and others. This can gradually help them deal differently with their emotions and impulses, delaying their acting upon depressive feelings or destructive impulses. The beneficial effect of structure, is mediated by, among others, hierarchical privilege systems and the use of treatment contracts (see Miller 1990). These draw on the patients' healthy capacities.

In practice, many inpatient staff are predominantly reacting to the prevailing crisis – part of the routine of fire-fighting, as in the case of Cecelia, and not concentrating on making the environment intelligible to the patients. This detracts from the setting's capacity to function predictably, with the result that the patient's sense of reality orientation may even be further impoverished, as inpatient surveys have shown (Baker 2000). With little or no negotiation or joint planning (given the short time available between the acute situation being managed and Cecelia's discharge from the ward), the potential for promoting more adaptive behaviour, on the basis of her greater insight, is seldom realized.

Involvement

'Involvement' refers to those processes that cause patients to attend actively to their social environment and to interact with it. The purpose of involvement is to utilize and strengthen a patient's ego and to modify aversive or destructive interpersonal patterns. In particular, it confronts patients' passivity, i.e. their wishes to have others do things to or for them. Means of facilitating involvement include 'open doors', patient-led groups, negotiation of therapeutic goals, mandatory participation in milieu groups, collective activities. Placing a high emphasis on the interpersonal meaning of symptomatic behaviours (such as deliberate self-harm) conveys to patients the belief that such aspects are within their control and thus their responsibility. Therefore, patients who talk about their 'needs' not being met may find these being re-framed (by staff or fellow patients) as unrealistic or inappropriate 'wants' (Gunderson 1978). The treatment aims to reinforce ego strengths by encouraging social skills and developing feelings of competence. Along with this, patients are expected to relinquish or subordinate private, anti-social or unrealistic wishes. Wards that emphasize involvement will have a distribution of power and decision-making, some blurring of traditional roles, and an emphasis on the group processes of cooperation, compromise, confrontation and conformity.

Cecelia's behaviour on the acute inpatient ward reveals that she does little that is constructive and staff have little time to confront, constructively, her lack of engagement. Her challenging behaviour elicits a predictable 'containing' response, which appears only to reinforce more such behaviour. For reasons that are not understood, her destructive behaviour ceases and discharge follows imminently. Cecelia does not appear to have a sense of herself as an effective 'agent', except in relation to her destructive and dangerous behaviour and the impulsive taking of her own discharge.

Validation

'Validation' refers to the processes and activities that occur in the hospital ward setting that affirm a patient's individuality. Patients are validated through the staff's attention to a range of aspects of individualized treatment programming: respect for a patient's right to some privacy, to be alone; frequent exploratory one-to-one talks; an emphasis on issues concerning separation and loss, and encouraging individuals to operate at the limits of their known capacities, including 'opportunities to fail'. This requires the staff's acceptance and understanding of the patients' incompetence, regressions or symptoms as meaningful personal expressions. They need to know that such aspects should not be ignored but nor do they necessarily have to be eradicated. Validation, which takes many forms, might include encouraging patients to talk about their hallucinations and to consider them as expressive of some unclear but important aspect of themselves. The patient who self-harms might be asked to recall a recent episode of the behaviour and explain why it had made sense to act in that way (Gunderson 1978). Unfortunately, this ideal is not achieved in respect of Cecelia. It appears to be only her negative self-image that is 'validated' by the vicious circle of re-admission.

Dynamic interactions between Cecelia and the healthcare system

In the context of an inpatient setting, by definition involving a number of patients and staff, the need to cater for the differing needs of individual patients is potentially problematic. In effect, giving to one can mean taking from another and, due to the priority that crises demand, time that might be spent in conversation with patients is easily eroded. However, even where time is available and patients are motivated, the latter may not be able to confide, for a wide variety of reasons, including high emotional arousal, fear of stigma, shame, humiliation, and feelings of vulnerability. Many patients, such as Cecelia, are unable to speak openly about themselves. Instead, they present themselves, as if as a puzzle for the professional to solve, without their own active participation.

Staff may experience this passivity, and lack of engagement, as exasperating. However, patients often have no concept of a shared enterprise of any kind. Their previous experience of the world and of other people has not exposed them to any such mutually respectful encounters. This situation may go unrecognized, with the staff member assuming a level of engagement which is actually missing. It may be only once the 'therapeutic' relationship has become seriously derailed or undermined (e.g. with some violation of the usual professional relationship boundary) that the professional discovers that something is, and has been, amiss. Often relevant training and supervision of complex cases and problematic encounters is not available to those in most need of it. Knowing something of Cecelia's early life history can shed some light on her presentation.

Cecelia is the eldest of nine children. Her mother also suffered from bipolar disorder and was frequently hospitalized during Cecelia's childhood. During those times, both her father and the other siblings expected Cecelia to stand in for her mother. This involved her in doing the bulk of the housework and shopping, with the result that her attendance at school was patchy and her academic achievement poor. However, she undertook the maternal role with energy and not without some success, albeit she was authoritarian, strict and occasionally violent to those in her charge. Partly on account of this, and deterioration in her behaviour at school, Cecelia was placed in care. While there she was subjected to physical, sexual and emotional abuse on various occasions and in various placements. When her mother was home from hospital, Cecelia was returned to the family setting, which was inevitably chaotic, with all the children (unsettled and insecure after yet another period of upheaval and on occasions, trauma) vying for their mother's attention. The mother was never able to meet the children's needs. Nevertheless, the only periods when Cecelia felt hopeful were when she was awaiting return home to her family having been in care. Once returned, however, she soon experienced the familiar feelings of insecurity, derived from being part of such a dysfunctional family. Parallels between this past scenario to that of the present, in the context of the acute ward admission, are plain to see.

The effects of Cecelia's past abuse and neglect have left her scarred emotionally (as well as physically) and with an extremely limited behavioural and psychological repertoire to deploy in relation to other people. Her style of asking for help is confusing and misleading. Her mode of interacting with authority figures, including ward staff and police, is (unconsciously) designed to keep them at bay – at a safe emotional distance. In doing so, Cecelia's inner self is kept private hence potentially safer. However, this does not allow her to become emotionally close to others, which she both longs for but also fears.

Establishing and maintaining therapeutic alliances in the ward setting

Case vignette

John was admitted to a medium secure mental health service in his thirties. He was suffering from severe depression and had been drinking heavily for a number of years and was in and out of prison, on account of offences involving petty theft and acts of minor violence. During the course of his imprisonment, the quality of relationship with his long-term female partner deteriorated, as John became convinced that she was being unfaithful to him. After a particularly large alcohol binge, shortly after having been released from prison, John carried out a frenzied knife attack on her, leaving her paralysed. He had no recollection of the assault.

In the medium secure ward setting, John was difficult to engage. He preferred a solitary existence. On the surface, he appeared to function well, being self-sufficient and having good personal care skills. However, he did not talk about how he felt. With his primary nurse, he spent most of the sessions looking down at the floor and did not make eye contact. He did not provide anything the nurse felt she could work with. She found the individual sessions with John excruciating and persecutory. The whole team treating John felt immense sympathy for his ex-partner, who was languishing in a long-term hospital bed, and a sense of grievance on her behalf, for the injury their (perpetrator) 'patient' had caused. John evoked little or no sympathy from them. Most believed that he should have been serving a prison sentence. All felt stuck, believing that treatment was achieving nothing.

Commentary

It was difficult for staff to make any empathic connection with John. However, they had not considered whether, unwittingly, they were playing a part in the therapeutic stalemate. It was only after a presentation of John's case, by a new and relatively junior member of the nursing staff, who had undertaken a particularly thorough summary of his copious case files, that the team began to think more deeply about what was going on, between him and them, and were able to take a step back.

The nurse's presentation revealed that John's mother had suffered from alcohol problems for many years before and after John was born. When he was young, his mother was unable to put his needs before her own need to drink. She managed to cut herself off from John's vulnerability and dependence on her, experiencing his cries for care as him being deliberately persecutory. This instilled in John an inappropriate degree of 'independence' (actually, withdrawal from meaningful emotional contact, from early on). Although John's father was kindly towards him, his father's priority was to pacify and placate his wife. When older, John was drawn into this placatory dynamic as a way of relating to others, not just his mother. He had internalized his mother's view that he was a nuisance and the cause of her 'bad moods'. John's basic sense of himself was that he was evil.

John believed that he would inevitably damage anybody with whom he tried to get close. Except when under the influence of alcohol, he was solitary and uncommunicative. This latter presentation was evident in the hospital setting. Despite the fact of his lonely, loveless life being documented in his case notes, John did not impress as a person who needed or merited care. This replicated his experience with his mother, who was not able to acknowledge the needs he had. It is possible that John's emotional inaccessibility was too much for the ward nurses to bear, especially his primary nurse. Rather than trying to understand what John's introversion and isolation might represent, it was as if John's nursing team set about simply confirming their own belief that there was nothing wrong with him but that he was 'bad'. Worse, their negative attitudes and avoidant behaviour confirmed his belief that he was too much trouble for others to bother with, reinforcing his existing impoverished self-image.

Recognizing and dealing with destructive processes

Developed in the context of psychoanalysis, 'therapeutic alliance' is a concept that recognizes that the quality of the professional–patient relationship should not be taken for granted (Greenson 1967). The concept refers to a more healthy, 'rational relationship' between patient and therapist (alongside a more 'neurotic', unhealthy one) which makes it possible for the patient to work purposefully in therapy (1967: 46). Within a psychiatric inpatient ward, this more rational relationship between staff and patient is often more of an aspiration than an expectation. However, attempting to enable patients to perform their role as patient 'rationally' is a relevant task. It can include information-sharing, for example, so that patients understand what is expected of them, for them to get the help they need to improve their health in the particular ward setting. This can foster the patient's active involvement in their treatment. However, many factors can interfere with the achievement of this apparently modest goal. Therefore it is prudent to identify them and consider how they conspire to make a therapeutic outcome less likely.

Identifying negative aspects and processes may not be easy. This is because they derive not only from the deliberate, conscious behaviour of people in the inpatient situation but also from influences that derive from the unconscious part of their minds. The following destructive processes and phenomena have been described as 'the destructiveness of the isolated individual; destructive group phenomena; the contribution of staff to destructiveness; and destructive structural manifestations' (Roberts 1980).

An individual patient may carry out actual acts of destruction, aimed at the fabric of the building or the individual's own body, rarely towards another member of the inpatient ward. Often this behaviour is considered to reflect alienation, which the patient experiences anew within the treatment setting. Certain patients may be especially at risk of isolation: the new patient, the scapegoat (perhaps a patient from a minority ethnic group), the psychotic patient, those with schizoid personality features, the borderline patient, those who repeatedly act out early rejection experiences, and those dependent on alcohol and drugs (Roberts 1980). Cecelia and John would both fall into a number of these categories. However, according to Roberts, their behaviour and that of their respective ward staff, should not be construed as being solely due to their conscious motivation but to unconscious factors.

Unconscious factors derive, in part, from the operation of defence mechanisms. Such are deployed involuntarily to do away with or minimize anxiety that would otherwise threaten the psychological integrity of the individual. The effect of the unconscious defensive operation is to distort the 'reality' of the situation, at least by degree. Certain defences, such as 'splitting', 'projection' and 'denial' exert a far-reaching and distorting effect (Kernberg 1984), which usually serves to simplify perceptions and beliefs. Denial, for example, can remove the anxiety associated with dealing with a painful dilemma. Such anxiety would have been present in staff, if they had acknowledged that John had emotional needs that they should have been meeting and had consciously struggled with their guilt at not feeling any compassion towards him. Defence mechanisms often function in concert. Denial, splitting and projection frequently act together. This combination can account for staff viewing John as being 'all bad', so allowing them to feel better about themselves, i.e. not defeated in their therapeutic endeavours in relation to him. In this way, they would not experience inadequacy and hence feel guilty. Rather, they would locate their inadequacy (and blame) elsewhere – in John and the wider criminal justice system that had placed him inappropriately in the health care system. Such perceptions and beliefs are over-simplifications, which do not do justice to the complex state of affairs.

In the multi-disciplinary staff team, the phenomenon of splitting can result in simple polarizations, often painful and marked by extreme animosity, around a particular contentious issue. Allies to the opposing factions may collect and lead to a paralysis of usual, more cohesive, team functioning – as with Cecelia's nursing team. According to Roberts (1980), other manifestations may follow in the wake of splitting, such as 'sub-culturing', 'idealization' and 'splits in leadership'. The last can be particularly destructive in its effect. The leaders' capacity for thinking, which might be directed at solving the difficulties within their team, is otherwise expended in a futile battle between themselves, for example, between the ward nurse manager and medical consultant or responsible clinician. As above, other staff may be drawn into the battle or elect to retreat as excited or helpless onlookers.

Roberts also considers the role of 'idealization' another important unconscious defence mechanism, the effect of which may be especially hard to recognize for people working in the caring professions. Its operation can cause staff to try to live up to unrealistic expectations placed on them by patients. They may believe that they have the authority or skills to achieve them. Consequently, they can overwork, becoming stressed and eventually even becoming mentally ill themselves. All of this can foster the development of further destructive splitting processes and so contribute to the breakdown of cooperative working among different members of the team, leading to an inconsistent delivery of the overall treatment programme for a given patient, hence a poorer prognosis for a given patient.

Roberts considers structural manifestations of destructive processes, identifying three main conditions: 'autolysis', 'crystallization' and 'encapsulation'. Autolysis represents the breaking down of internal structures, such as the dissolution of time boundaries for the treatment programme or a lack of clarity between the respective roles of staff and patients. Crystallization reflects an internal organization that has become so rigid and entangled that change is impossible. Flexible functioning suffers; for example, the ward is unable to adapt itself to move swiftly to containment mode, in the face of an emergency. Encapsulation is the situation where the institution has stopped interacting effectively with its environment – senior management, referrers or funders. All of these states can appear within a given part of an organization, for example a hospital ward. In the case of specialist or autonomous units, closure may be the consequence of encapsulation. In other situations, where closure is not so readily conceivable, the consequence is likely to be an increase in serious untoward incidents. The latter may be the first recognizable signs that destructive processes are operating at an unacceptable level. (For a fuller account of relevant aspects please see Campling *et al.* 2004.)

Unconscious roots of un-therapeutic practice

Like Roberts, others have argued that the problematic functioning of health care staff often results from 'unconscious processes' (see Hinshelwood 2002). Therefore, if meaningful behavioural change for the better is to be achieved, health care organizations must address these particular processes (Obholzer 1994). Obholzer advocates a psychoanalytic approach, in order to understand the difficulties experienced by health care workers in their interpersonal interactions with patients. As the group whose work takes place predominantly in the 'public' areas of the ward environment is nursing, this is the profession that has been the subject of (mainly psychoanalytic) observational studies (Sinanoglou 1987; Donati 1989; Chiesa 2000).

Nurses in mental health services have been found to experience difficulty sustaining interpersonal engagement with patients. In a seminal study, Menzies-Lyth developed the application of a psychoanalytic approach to the evaluation of a general nursing service within a large hospital. She described how many practices were determined not by the needs of patients but by their own unconscious needs. Unconsciously, nurses defended themselves against the emotional effects of close interpersonal proximity to human suffering and death by deploying a range of motor activities (Menzies-Lyth 1988). Such practices actually impeded the delivery of effective nursing care.

Chiesa conducted a series of psychoanalytic observations in an acute mental health admission ward and found that nurses tended to neutralize any potentially meaningful human interactions between themselves and the patients (Chiesa 2000). He observed that nurses employed continual motor activity as a 'manic' defence against anxiety provoked by their proximity to the psychological distress patients experienced. Sinanoglou (1987), studying nursing attitudes in a mental health unit, also concluded that excessive motor activity was employed by nurses to defend against anxieties provoked by making emotional and interpersonal contact with psychological distress associated with patients' psychotic states.

Other observational studies have utilized the perspective of unconscious processes of anxiety and defence to understand the phenomena of nurses' impoverished interpersonal interactions with patients. Donati undertook 12 one-hour psychoanalytic observations within a 'chronic psychiatric ward' and concluded that nurses made 'high use of inappropriate, defensive maneuvers' in response to anxiety associated with their therapeutic impotence in the face of patients' enduring conditions (Donati 1989: 42). Defensive nursing practices which were identified included the maintaining of superficial, ritualized interpersonal contacts with patients and ensuring that all feelings of failure and poor self-image remained located in the patients, to raise the nurses' own self-image – as was the case with John.

A number of researchers have observed that nurses are less likely to engage interpersonally with patients who present with certain types of behaviours: poor compliance with clinical programmes (Rosenthal *et al.* 1980); demandingness and complaining (Sarosi 1968; Stockwell 1972; Armitage 1980); over-dependence on nurses (Rosenthal *et al.* 1980); and rule breaking (Spitzer and Sobel 1962; Armitage 1980). Both Cecelia and John would certainly fit into the first behavioural category – poor compliance. Altschul (1972) employed a quantitative approach to examine nurse–patient relationships by observing interactions between patients and nurses in an acute mental health service and found that the patients who nurses engaged with most were more likely to enjoy a good treatment outcome. However, this study also noted that nurses lacked a theoretical framework for 'organizing' (i.e. understanding and interpreting) their relationships with patients and that they tended to have more contacts and to spend more time with non-neurotic patients (Altschul 1972). Interestingly, it has been shown that an increase in the quality of interpersonal care provided by nurses is associated with higher rates of recovery from illness (Stockwell 1972).

Overall, the (limited) literature paints a picture of impoverished interpersonal communications and interactions between patients and mental health nurses (Altschul 1972; Macilwaine 1983; Donati 1989; Chiesa 2000). This has been construed as reflecting unconscious defensive manoeuvres against anxiety which enable professional survival in the nursing role and the maintenance of self-esteem. The anxiety stems from a combination of the patients' disturbing presentations and the nurses' own (individual and collective) impotence. There is no reason to suppose that any other professional group exposed to the ward environment for such prolonged periods would fare better or operate differently than those in the nursing profession. However, it might be that the training, support and supervision of other professional groups allow them greater access to useful theoretical frameworks, with which to 'organize' their relationships with their patients.

Changing staff attitudes and practices

If nursing (and other) staff are to be facilitated to improve the quality of their demanding work, within the pressurized and stressful environment of the inpatient ward, they require appropriate training, support and supervision (see also Kurtz 2005). This will vary according to the nature and function of the particular ward. However, without such input, it is hard to imagine that staff could be in a state of mind to develop new perspectives on their work – to have new ways of 'organizing' their interactions with patients. They need this if they are to incorporate an understanding of the role of unconscious processes which influence the process of health care, and to be able to translate the new concepts into practical changes in their individual behaviour and the functioning of the teams of which they are a part.

In the case of John, the new nurse's presentation of his case appeared to be a watershed and 'wake up call' for many members of the multi-disciplinary team, even though, by the time of that presentation, they had known this patient for many months. The members had become accustomed to his negative attitudes and passive behaviour, believing that this was the whole picture. They saw no prospect of change. However, their collective belief was somewhat surprising, if John's frenzied, violent attack and forensic history is recalled and put alongside his passive demeanor within the ward. This disparity might have begged questions about how and why John's aggression seemed to be absent. It is interesting therefore to speculate what was going on to stifle the curiosity of the staff. The operation of unconscious defensive manoeuvres might have accounted for the staff's over-simplified perception of John (based on splitting etc.), simply seeing him as a perpetrator and his ex-partner as victim and meriting sympathy. Such a 'split' perspective probably served to save the team from feeling therapeutically impotent, through their not acknowledging any potential for therapeutic optimism.

Reflective practice

'Paralysis' was a theme that emerged in the context of weekly 'Reflective Practice' sessions that were started on John's ward, a few weeks after this case had been presented by the junior nurse. All multi-disciplinary staff working on the ward were expected to attend. The meeting lasted for one and a quarter hours and was facilitated by someone trained in a psychoanalytic understanding of institutions, who neither worked on the ward in question nor had managerial relationship to any of the staff who worked there. Staff brought various issues for discussion. Early on it was senior or the more extravert individuals who spoke and dominated the conversation with their preoccupations and concerns. Later, in the absence of some of the usual seniors, the nurse who had presented John's case ventured to say that there had been no observable change, either in the patient or in the team's approach to him, in spite of the apparent 'insight' that the presentation had helped to generate. This observation was greeted with a few affirmative nods but nobody actually said anything aloud, to confirm or refute what the nurse had said.

The male facilitator picked up on this non-verbal communication style within the Reflective Practice group, wondering aloud how the absence of verbal support might have left the outspoken nurse feeling. He wondered whether she might be left uncomfortable by the group's feeble response, being unsure whether she really had the agreement and support of her (still relatively new) colleagues or not. He thought that being thus unsupported it might be a disincentive to speak up in the future. He commented also that it was relatively unusual for a more junior member of the team to risk speaking. Following this comment, the meeting became energized. A deeper discussion of John's case – their prevailing feeling of impotence – ensued. Staff also spoke, with verbal support for one another, at the disgust they had felt on first hearing of the index offence. They spoke of their lack of sympathy, let alone empathy, for John. They were more preoccupied with his ex-partner and her immediate family, none of whom was actually known to any in the team. The facilitator was able to help the team to explore this over-simplified formulation, with the result that a more complicated picture of both parties emerged.

Over the next few weeks, the team returned to the topic of John and his treatment, within the Reflective Practice sessions and the facilitator commented that there appeared to be more energy and interest in identifying some of the complexities in his case and an atmosphere of greater optimism. As reported, John's own activity level on the ward had increased, although the team were surprised that he had been expressing quite depressive and, at times, suicidal thoughts. He had been observed to be in tears by a number of staff, whereas previously such behaviour had not been witnessed. He expressed ideas of guilt, not only for the injuries caused to his partner, but also for a catalogue of events from his childhood and other criminal acts, which he felt he had been responsible for. Gradually he was supported to talk about these with his primary nurse in their weekly individual sessions. Movement and feeling was entering the previously paralysed (and emotionally impoverished) interaction between patient and staff team.

Application of therapeutic milieu priniciples to outpatient/community settings

With the closure of many inpatient beds – acute, long-stay and rehabilitation – a much greater proportion of psychiatric patients is treated in outpatient or community settings. While outpatients whose needs are relatively straightforward probably get these met satisfactorily (and increasingly by primary care-based services), those with more complex needs fare less well. Among such patient populations are those with: severe personality disorder; substance misuse; serious eating disorders; learning disability and dual diagnosis. The list is a long one and, for these groups at least, there is a need to attempt to provide in a dispersed form something in the community that was previously available within the therapeutic milieu.

Managing therapeutic resources outside a hospital requires much planning – arguably more than to achieve the same aim within such an establishment. This is because there is still a need to provide an integrated package of care, involving a range of professionals and often a range of modalities, but with a team which is virtual, i.e. not literally meeting together on a regular basis. Indeed, the 'team' may not know or agree on its own membership! For most psychiatric patients with complex needs there is reason to believe that successful treatments (NIMHE 2003) have the following characteristics:

- set out clear aims;
- specify the treatment methods to achieve aims;
- have consistency during phases of transition from one (part of) a service to another;
- utilize skilled and motivated professionals;
- have good inter-communication among all those involved;
- are supported educationally and managerially;
- pay particular attention to the termination phase of treatment.

In practice, however, it is hard to achieve the above, given the geographical dispersal of human resources and the need for all those involved to collaborate, respecting and valuing one another's contributions to the shared therapeutic venture. Patients such as Cecelia, with complex needs, who might have been catered for previously as inpatients, sometimes over extended periods (months or years), now find themselves seeing a range of professionals, often in a range of different settings and locations. Like Cecelia and John, many patients are unable to articulate their needs, presenting themselves as a problem to be solved by the professional. Their oppositional or passive presentations may alienate them from professionals who are more comfortable with an insightful and compliant patient. Professionals working outside the hospital will thus also face their share of frustrations. Like their inpatient staff counterparts, they may not have ways of 'organizing' their transactions with their patients, so as to avoid some of the pitfalls associated with falling prey to the operation of defence mechanisms (e.g. splitting), which complicate management of the case and can also impair the necessary collaborative working. A crucial clinical task therefore is to identify when and how the clinical transaction with a given patient is going wrong – deviating from the straightforward path that was originally envisaged for it (Norton and McGauley 1998).

Case vignette

Cecelia's 'local' inpatient team found themselves at loggerheads with the 'crisis team', which functioned as a gateway (or, as the local team viewed it, a barrier) to inpatient wards. This was because the inpatient team also operated within the community but could not directly admit its patients to its ward! The latter had to be referred for an assessment by the crisis team. Sometimes all proceeded relatively smoothly, when the crisis team agreed with the local team's assessment, i.e. the need for Cecelia to be admitted. At other times, it worked out differently and there were more of the latter outcomes, when Cecelia was not admitted.

There had been sufficient of the 'disagreeable' outcomes between the two teams to produce a barely concealed hostility, which Cecelia would almost certainly have noticed. She certainly expressed confusion to her community psychiatric nurse about who was looking after her at any given time while out of hospital, stating that she did not know to whom to turn when she felt herself to be in a crisis. Wittingly or unwittingly (i.e. unconsciously), Cecelia added fuel to the fire of division that existed between the local and crisis teams. She would be praising of the staff member she was speaking to but scathing of the efforts of staff who were not present to contradict or otherwise defend their reputations! In her case, when it came to the point of giving a date for discharge from hospital, there was often disagreement over which team was better placed to deliver this. The plan to give a date would be thus postponed and Cecelia, as was her norm, would end up taking her own discharge, in the absence of agreement about the precise detail of follow-up. On one occasion, in this state of limbo, in the community, Cecelia took a substantial overdose, necessitating admission to a general hospital. She spent a number of weeks there, having almost died.

The senior clinicians involved with Cecelia's case felt guilty about the overdose. They thought, not altogether unreasonably, that their indecision and divisions could have exerted a negative influence on their mutual patient's mental state, increasing her suicidality. A psychodynamic psychotherapist was asked to provide a 'second opinion'. This was obtained by the calling of a meeting of senior staff from the two teams. The purpose was to learn about the patient and to see if the disharmonious working arrangements might reflect factors from the patient's past that were being rekindled and enacted in the current interactions within and between the two teams.

Both teams attended this extraordinary meeting, setting aside one hour for it. However, the presentation of their shared patient was dominated by descriptions of Cecelia's various behaviours – overdoses, self-harming, violence to staff – and the two teams' range of responses, their reactions – admit, discharge, crisis treatment, admit, discharge, crisis intervention etc. Forty-five minutes into the presentation only the most meagre of personal and family detail had been reported. This left the psychotherapist with no sense of the person who went by the name of Cecelia, family details having emerged almost incidentally, as it was mentioned that Cecelia had had visitors while in the general hospital. Otherwise it was as if the patient's personal distinguishing features had no bearing on the management of her complex clinical case – not a patient-centred approach!

A plan was hatched for the psychotherapist to interview the patient to provide a psychodynamic assessment that might inform the combined approach of the two teams. This was carried out and the formulation shared with the two teams. Discussion followed, as the formulation was more or less accepted as capturing the main elements. These included, in particular, how staff felt misled, manipulated and rendered ineffectual by the patient and how Cecelia was feeling rejected, confused and abandoned, believing that neither team actually had her interests at heart. A fuller meeting was arranged, to which the patient and her family doctor were invited. In this extended forum, the psychotherapist was invited to feedback her formulation and Cecelia and the family doctor were invited to respond.

Commentary

Further meetings in this format followed and at least some of the heat had been released from the problematic set of professional relationships, as the different 'sides' were enabled to see things from the other's perspective. At least for a period, Cecelia was more settled in the community, with a greater sense of working together with those professionals involved. The revised care plan, with her involvement, also included her referral to a creative therapy group in order to help her focus on some of her strengths ('validation') and also to be exposed to forming some more healthy social contacts ('involvement').

With patients such as Cecelia, there is a need to create and maintain a network of all the relevant individuals who are involved. Ideally, such coming together of relevant parties occurs before a crisis has occurred, although with her this occurred only after the particularly dangerous overdose. Optimally, the patient is aware and part of the meeting, which also includes key players in the patient's own family or social network. In this instance Cecelia had no significant people living local to her and her family had only been in intermittent contact. She had kept her condition and circumstances from them, a pattern of secrecy that had started in her childhood.

Information-sharing and clinical networking

Engagement

As with the inpatient therapeutic milieu, attention must be paid by staff to the securing of the patient's active engagement in their treatment – involvement. This is achieved through education, discussion and negotiation, when the patient is not highly anxious and the professional has adequate time at their disposal – they are not anxious nor too frustrated or angry with the patient. Education, part of Gunderson's 'structure', refers to information being imparted to enable the patient to understand what are their *responsibilities* – what they should and should not do and their *rights*, especially in terms of what they can expect of the professional(s) and what they cannot. It can be helpful to draw up a written contract, once the negotiations are complete. This can serve as a reminder, if (and when) things start to depart significantly from what was agreed at the outset. The contract thus forms part of the 'structure' of treatment. An effective treatment contract is usually characterized (after Miller 1990) by the following:

- being mutually agreed by all parties, including patient and/or carer(s);
- having clear specified responsibilities for all parties, as above;
- bearing a minimum of detail so that it can be readily recalled, when needed;
- providing for alternative strategies for the client to manage intolerable feelings;
- providing positive reinforcement for the client's adaptive change;
- being strictly enforced but allowing for reasonable negotiated modification;
- fostering a therapeutic alliance.

(NB A contract can fail for many reasons, including it being unduly restrictive of the patient, becoming a substitute for therapeutic activity, and being used by the professional as a punishment, even if only unconsciously so.)

Information

How relevant information is collected and disseminated varies according to the circumstances of the case but general principles remain the same (see Norton and Vince 2002). In each case the responsible senior professionals need to ask themselves if there is an adequate network, with rules governing the frequency of contact and what should be communicated to whom, if an emergency arises, whose nature could be predicted. Such a network is ideally in place as soon as it is clear that the case is complex. Otherwise it is likely that it will have to be hastily put together in the face of an unanticipated crisis. The latter is more difficult to do, as was the case with Cecelia. It also needs to be recognized that collaborative working can be undermined by a range of factors and influences, including the negative effects of unconscious defensive mechanisms.

Information about treatment and the importance of a therapeutic alliance will be imparted according to the patient's intellectual, psychological and social circumstances, as well as the overall complexity of the clinical task and treatment package. In Cecelia's case, additional time was set aside to go over with her what was discussed in the relevant meetings with the team, since it was anticipated that these might be anxiety inducing, which would make it harder for her to take in all that was being said. In addition to verbal discussion, therefore, written material may be particularly helpful since this can be consulted by the patient in his or her own time and when they may be more relaxed and better able to absorb its content. Cecelia was copied into the relevant correspondence that was sent as a summary to all the staff involved in the extraordinary meetings.

Information might usefully include facts about the patient's condition as well as what has been agreed about their treatment. Ideally, it conveys the logic of the latter, given the former. The patient's ambivalence to treatment and their difficulty with forming a trusting relationship (possibly on the basis of low self-esteem, fear of stigma and the rekindling of feelings of insecurity) might also be acknowledged, where this is considered to be helpful – a matter of judgement in the particular case. The patient should have been made aware of the limits of confidentiality, i.e. the conditions under which it will be broken, in what way, and to whom. This should happen at an early stage, before the necessity to do so has been encountered! There needs to be an ongoing monitoring of the relationship network to ascertain, as far as possible, the state of authenticity of the patient's engagement, which should not be seen as 'all or nothing' or 'once and for all'. The client can therefore be informed that there will be regular or periodic reviews of his or her care, in addition to any statutory requirements. Professionals need to be able to form a shared opinion about the quality of the engagement of their shared client. This usually requires at least some face-to-face meetings of the key personnel.

Regular communication

There needs to be regular communication among the relevant professionals, in addition to the monitoring of the therapeutic alliance, to judge if the relevant treatment goals are being achieved. This may not prove easy to do. First, the client may provide differing accounts to different 'points' in the network. Second, even if the same account is given to each part of the network, it may be that the professionals differ in how they construe it – progress, regress, status quo! Third, sometimes it appears, in relation to the client's gross behaviour that they are not changing. However, at such times, seemingly subtle signs, such as the quality of the therapeutic alliance, reflected by the level of the patient's factual disclosure or emotional candour, can be decisive.

Realizing that 'splits' can develop among those providing treatment in complex cases can also be revealing of the patient's internal world, and their appearance should not therefore be construed as simply negative (Gabbard 1986). Apparently disparate views can sometimes be imaginatively integrated when both 'sides' of the split can be held, with neither party battling to establish supremacy over the other – as if only one could be correct or have the whole truth. Such a mature state of affairs, however, is difficult to achieve, especially where there is high anxiety over a patient's violent potential or over the prospect of blame being apportioned to the professional in the event of an untoward incident (see Davies 1995). Good, as in mutually respectful, relationships between professionals can have a containing effect on the patient, who may be unused to having people working concertedly with their interests at heart. This became the situation with John and the two 'sides' of the staff team and also with Cecelia, as the 'local' and 'crisis' teams began to appreciate that the views that they held were only partial and they needed also the other team's perspective.

Terminating treatment

Endings of treatment are often extremely difficult where complex cases are concerned, as with Cecelia and John, where many professionals have been involved or where the treatment process has been particularly lengthy. Such situations require more than the usual attention to effective communication. Meetings among the professionals involved might need to be *increased* in frequency. It should also be expected that some patients might well regress, with a return of earlier symptoms, which those involved had thought to be a thing of the distant past. There might be disappointment expressed by the patient (or their carers or significant others) that they are 'back at square one'. However, where there has been a relatively sustained and identifiable therapeutic process, not too abrupt or magical changes for the better, and where there is no particular adverse recent circumstance to account for the apparent deterioration, the professionals should not simply agree/collude with the patient's apparently negative evaluation. Regression is a phenomenon that is frequently observable at the latter stages of lengthy treatments, particularly with non-psychotic patients. It may arise solely out of increasing anxiety about the uncertainty of the future, beyond therapy. It is important therefore, under the particular circumstances, that the patient is helped to sift the relevant evidence and be assisted to arrive at a balanced judgement about what has been achieved and what problem areas actually remain, which might require further attention in the future or might need to be endured.

Conclusion

Inpatient wards form only one part of the whole mental health care system. As the whole evolves and develops, for instance, in response to policy directives and resource re-allocation, so the parts are required to change and re-align. The process is dynamic and ongoing. A review of mental health nursing by the Chief Nursing Officer for England (CNO) identified the need for nurses to promote the empowerment of patients and their social inclusion through the development of positive therapeutic relationships (DH 2006). This report describes the set of values and principles that underpin the so-called 'recovery model' (see also Chapter 5). Recovery is not so much viewed as necessarily a return to life as it was before illness but to a life experienced as worthwhile which might depend upon the development of new expectations, skills and ways of living. To assist in this process, nurses and other professionals are required to approach their roles with hope and optimism regarding patients' capacities to make progress.

At present, in the UK (though the system differs in different locations), overall bed numbers within the inpatient system are much smaller than formerly. This is the consequence of developing more community-based services, with the corresponding transfer of financial and other resources to enable assertive outreach, crisis and home treatment and early intervention in psychosis services. The resulting increase in the proportion of ward patients compulsorily detained, with little scope to disperse them and rehouse them in wards that might represent a potentially therapeutic mix, has meant that it is difficult for staff to retain their therapeutic optimism. Staff are more taxed than formerly to provide a therapeutic, as well as a custodial, environment. There is often tension between 'therapists' who visit the ward (or are visited by patients from the ward in pursuit of their therapy) and those staff (mostly nurses and care assistants) who must remain anchored to the inpatient environment. The latter groups of staff are destined to spend the duration of their shift, at least potentially, in close proximity to very disabled, disturbed and socially deteriorated patients. Their personal and interpersonal coping strategies can be tested to the limit and their psychological functioning and mental health can be impaired in the process.

According to some researchers and other commentators, unconscious processes account for at least some of the failure of concerted and therapeutic action of staff, within inpatient settings. Some studies have found that nursing staff defend themselves against contact with their patients by a range of means, which are not usually deliberate – keeping on the move, blaming patients and falling out with colleagues, whether within their profession or outside. There is no reason to believe that nurses are essentially different from other health care professionals or that their responses are anything but natural human defences deployed in the face of overwhelming emotional difficulty. The fictitious case vignettes presented in this chapter illustrate the inability of many inpatient milieus to do more than contain their patients, with an inability to provide higher functions.

To effect change in ward environments requires training, support and supervision to enable ward staff to understand the processes that operate when extremely disturbed and disordered patients are housed with staff who are not necessarily appropriately trained or experienced (Kurtz 2005) and when their role responsibilities are not clear or clearly understood in relation to those of colleagues (Burns 2000). The consequences of this mismatch, of patient requirement and staff resource, can be damaging to all parties. This situation can be improved if staff, individually and collectively, are aided to stand back to reflect on their work. To effect this, protected time and space are required, so that staff's anxiety levels are low enough to enable learning to take place – to imbibe new concepts, such as the influence of unconscious defence mechanisms. Training is also needed to facilitate staff to embed new skills, through the provision of supervision, in order to change overall ward functioning. In this way, some of the 'higher functions' might be able to be reintroduced to the wards and integrated during the patient's stay in that environment.

By providing a safe transfer from the ward environment to the community, higher functions, required to support patients to 'recover', can be deployed there. However, even within the community, coordinated functioning between different health care disciplines and agencies is hard to achieve. Just like ward-based staff, community-based workers also fall prey to the stress of working with patients such as Cecelia and John, whose needs are complex and behaviours challenging. The source of anxiety may not be identical and the lone professional may feel they could be blamed more readily for a 'critical untoward incident', since their role and influence is more clearly identifiable than for inpatient staff. Splitting is prevalent as a defence. Consequently, there is a need for relevant staff training, support and supervision so that its destructive effect on 'team' functioning is recognized and dealt with creatively. Otherwise, the Cecelias and Johns of the psychiatric world will continue to find that they are little helped by the services offered to them and the staff working with them will have low job satisfaction and may even find their own mental health deteriorating.

Questions for reflection and discussion

1   Consider with colleagues the extent to which the ward in which you work, or to which you are connected, embodies the principles and practice of a therapeutic milieu. The following checklist might be helpful:

   ■   Do staff and patients in the ward know what the enterprise is trying to achieve?

   ■   Do patients know how the ward is organized and what ingredients or treatment sessions they might encounter in any given week?

   ■   Are staff clear and explicit with patients about the rules that apply, what is expected of them and what supports are available to help them flourish?

   ■   To what extent do staff from the same and different disciplines work collaboratively with each other and with patients?

   ■   Does the ward regime empower patients and provide them with sufficient opportunities to voice their concerns?

   ■   Is there an explicit statement about the values of the inpatient setting, such as abhorrence of racism and sexism?

   ■   Do staff have regular reflective practice or supervision sessions whereby the unconscious processes at work in the milieu are clarified?

■   What practical steps might be taken to increase the therapeutic potential of the inpatient environment? In collaboration with others, draw up an action plan for implementation.

2   Are there one or more patients on your ward who might be alienated from care and treatment? If so, consider with colleagues whether the patient(s) developmental history might make their social behaviour more understandable so that they might feel more socially included.

3   Can you identify 'recovery' values and principles in your practice, as identified in the report of the Chief Nursing Officer (DH 2006)?

Annotated bibliography

■   Campling, P., Davies, S. and Farquarson, G. (2004) *From Toxic Institutions to Therapeutic Environments.* London: Gaskell. A very useful text which describes the processes that support the development of effective therapeutic milieus and those which underpin anti-therapeutic in-patient services.

■   Hinshelwood, R. D. (2002) Abusive help – helping abuse: the psychodynamic impact of severe personality disorder on caring institutions. *Criminal Behaviour And Mental Health* **12**: 20–30. A paper which lucidly describes the interpersonal processes that lead to people becoming alienated from mental health care.

■   Kurtz, A. (2005) The needs of staff who care for people with a diagnosis of personality disorder who are considered to be a risk to others. *Journal of Forensic Psychiatry and Psychology* **16**(2): 399–422. A detailed, thorough account of what services require to have in place for staff, including nurses, if they are to work effectively with people who have a diagnosis of personality disorder and who present a risk to others.

■   Pflaffin, F. and Adshead, G. (2003) *A Matter of Security: The Application of Attachment Theory to Forensic Psychiatry and Psychotherapy.* London: JKP. A book of edited papers applying attachment theory to the forensic context. This is a very useful book and makes a lot of reference to the institutional setting.

Acknowledgements

We are grateful to Mr Mark Jenkinson, Service Manager, St. Bernard's Hospital, Middlesex, for his thoughtful comments on an early draft of this chapter.

References

Abroms, G.M. (1969) Defining milieu therapy. *Archives of General Psychiatry* **21**: 553–5.
Altschul, A. (1972) *Patient Nurse Interaction.* Edinburgh: Churchill Livingstone.
Armitage, S. (1980) Non Compliant Recipients of Health Care. *Nursing Times* **76**: 1–3.
Baker, S. (2000) *Environmentally Friendly?: Patients' Views of Conditions on Psychiatric Wards.* London: MIND.
Beadsmore, A., Moore, C., Muijen, M. *et al.* (1998) *Acute Problems: A Survey of the Quality of Care in Acute Psychiatric Wards.* London: Sainsbury Centre Mental Health Publications.

Burns, T. (2000) The legacy of the therapeutic community practice in modern community health services. *Therapeutic Communities* **21**(3): 165–74.

Campling, P., Davies, S. and Farquarson, G. (2004) *From Toxic Institutions to Therapeutic Environments.* London: Gaskell.

Chiesa, M. (2000) At a crossroad between institutional and community psychiatry: an acute admission ward, in R.D. Hinshelwood and W. Skogstad (eds) *Observing Organizations: Anxiety, Defence and Culture in Health Care.* London: Routledge, pp. 54–67.

Davies, R. (1995) The inter-disciplinary network and the internal world of the offender, in C. Cordess and M. Cox (eds) *Forensic Psychotherapy.* London: Jessica Kingsley.

Department of Health (2002) *Mental Health Policy Implementation Guide: Adult acute inpatient care provision.* London: DH.

Department of Health (2006) *From Values to Action: The Chief Nursing Officer's Review of Mental Health Nursing.* London: DH.

Donati, F. (1989) A psychodynamic observer in a chronic psychiatric ward. *British Journal of Psychotherapy* **5**: 317–29.

Ford, R., Durcan, G., Warner, L., Hardy, P. and Muijen, M. (1998) One day survey by the Mental Health Act Commission of acute adult psychiatric inpatient wards in England and Wales. *British Medical Journal* **317**: 1279–83.

Gabbard, G. (1986) The treatment of the 'special' patient in a psychoanalysis hospital. *International Review of Psychoanalysis* **13**: 333–47.

Greenson, R. (1967) *The Technique and Practice of Psychoanalysis: Vol 1.* New York: International Universities Press.

Gunderson, J.G. (1978) Defining the therapeutic processes in psychiatric milieus. *Psychiatry* **41**: 327–35.

Haigh, R. (1999) The quintessence of a therapeutic environment: five universal qualities, in P. Campling and R. Haigh (eds) *Therapeutic Communities Past, Present and Future*, vol. 2. London: Jessica Kingsley Publishers.

Haigh, R. (2002) Acute wards: problems and solutions. Modern Milieux: therapeutic community solutions to acute ward problems. *Psychiatric Bulletin* **26**(12): 380–2.

Hinshelwood, R.D. (2002) Abusive help – helping abuse: the psychodynamic impact of severe personality disorder on caring institutions. *Criminal Behaviour and Mental Health* **12**: 20–30.

Kernberg, O.F. (1984) *Severe Personality Disorders: psychotherapeutic strategies.* New York: Vail-Ballon Press.

Kurtz. A. (2005) The needs of staff who care for people with a diagnosis of personality disorder who are considered to be a risk to others. *Journal of Forensic Psychiatry and Psychology* **16**(2): 399–422.

Macilwaine, H. (1983) The communication patterns of female neurotic patients with nursing staff in psychiatric units of general hospitals, in J. Wilson-Barnett (ed.) *Nursing Research: Ten Studies in Patient Care.* Chichester: Wiley, pp. 1–24.

Menzies-Lyth, I. (1988) The functioning of social systems as a defence against anxiety: a report on a study of the nursing service of a general hospital, in *Containing Anxiety in Institutions. Selected Essays Volume 1.* London: Free Association Books.

Miller, L.J. (1990) The formal treatment contract in the inpatient management of borderline personality disorder. *Hospital and Community Psychiatry* **41**(9): 985–7.

NIMHE (2003) *Personality Disorder: no longer a diagnosis of exclusion.* Policy implementation guidance for the development of services for people with personality disorder. London: NIMHE.

Norton, K. and Vince, J. (2002) Out-patient psychotherapy and mentally disordered offenders, in A. Buchanan (ed.) *Care of the Mentally Disordered Offender in the Community.* Oxford: Oxford Medical Publications.

Norton, K.R.W. and McGauley, G. (1998) *Counselling Difficult Clients.* London: Sage.

Obholzer, A. (1994) Managing social anxieties in public sector organizations, in A. Obholzer and V.Z. Roberts (eds) *The Unconscious at Work: Individual and Organizational Stress in the Human Services.* London: Routledge, pp. 169–78.

Roberts, J.P. (1980) Destructive processes in a therapeutic community. *International Journal of Therapeutic Communities* **1**: 159–70.

Rosenthal, C.J., Marshall, V.W., MacPherson, A.S. and French, S.E. (1980) *Nurses, Patients and Families.* London: Croom Helm.

Sarosi, G.M. (1968) A critical theory: the nurse as a fully human being. *Nursing Forum* **7**: 349–64.

Sinanoglou, I. (1987) Basic anxieties affecting psychiatric staff and their attitudes to psychotic patients. *Psychoanalytic Psychotherapy* **3**: 27–37.

Spitzer, S. and Sobel, R. (1962) Preferences for patients and patient behaviour. *Nursing Research* **11**: 233–5.

Stockwell, F. (1972) *The Unpopular Patient.* Royal College of Nursing Research Project. Series 1. No. 2. London: RCN.

Whiteley, J.S. (2004) The evolution of the therapeutic community. *Psychiatric Quarterly* **75**(3): 233–48.

CHAPTER 13

Strategies for living and lifestyle options

Alison Faulkner and Iain Ryrie

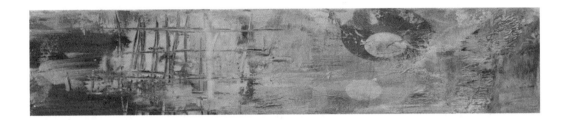

Introduction

This chapter explores strategies for living and lifestyle options from the perspective of people who have experienced mental health problems. In this respect the chapter concerns itself with the rest of our lives, on the principle that we are all more than the treatments and the services that we use. Starting with the service user-led research 'Strategies for Living', the chapter looks at the different strategies and supports that service users themselves have identified as helpful in managing and living with mental health problems. It then goes on to review a number of self-management approaches or programmes, many of which incorporate a variety of different strategies.

Traditionally these approaches have not attracted large-scale research funds or the interest of pharmaceutical companies, resulting in a relative paucity of research evidence, although this is now changing. Many of the strategies reported in this chapter rely on a different kind of evidence: the evidence of service users and carers (sometimes deemed 'anecdotal'), of dedicated practitioners and, often, the voluntary sector. This should not prevent us from living our lives as we want to or from trying out different things to help us in our own individual journeys. Furthermore, the first-person account and other forms of personal testimony are legitimate sources of evidence and are often corroborated by more objective scientific approaches as we demonstrate in this chapter. It is therefore important that we listen to service users about what works for them/for us, and take it seriously. This chapter covers:

- the service user/survivor movement;
- definitions;
- strategies for living;
- self-management approaches;
- common threads.

The service user/survivor movement

Much of the campaigning energy of the user/survivor movement in the UK has been directed towards existing psychiatric services and treatments, motivated by the desire to change and improve them, which is perhaps why 'user involvement' has become such a major development within UK mental health services. Evidence of dissatisfaction with mental health services can be traced back to the nineteenth century: individuals voicing dissatisfaction with the treatment given them in the name of psychiatry. In the mid-1980s the voices of protest became more recognizably organized as a user or survivor movement. Initially the formation of hospital-based Patients' Councils and a proliferation of user-led self-help and advocacy groups developed alongside the formation of more formally organized networks such as Survivors Speak Out, the Hearing Voices Network and the UK Advocacy Network. Other contemporaneous developments included campaigns for women-only services and advocacy, and the campaign against electroconvulsive therapy (ECT).

In the 1990s the user/survivor movement increasingly turned its attention towards the development of self-help or self-management strategies and user-led alternatives, with the aim of broadening the agenda beyond that of seeking change to existing services. A seminal publication is Viv Lindow's (1994) *Self-Help Alternatives to Mental Health Services*. In it, she stated that what is different about user-controlled alternatives is 'the existence of choice and freedom in meeting our needs'.

The strength in these developments lies not just in identifying the coping strategies themselves, but also in the development of alternative explanations for distress and the establishment of the concept of 'experts by experience'. They are motivated by both a desire to address the power imbalance of being treated by psychiatric services as a mental patient (particularly in the long term), and, for some people, the failure of those services to deal with many of the symptoms and problems associated with a mental illness diagnosis. In addition to this there is recognition of the power of self-help and mutual support, an approach often marginalized in the past by mental health services and professionals.

Some definitions

So, what are these alternatives? First of all it is important to draw a distinction between user-controlled alternative *services* and user-controlled alternative *strategies*. Viv Lindow's survey in the 1990s focused primarily on the former and found a range of housing support projects, clubhouses, employment training and support schemes, crisis houses and self-help groups around the world as well as a few in the UK. Our focus in this chapter is primarily on 'strategies', but we should not forget the parallel developments going on in the interests of developing user-controlled services, not least because they often become the location for the activity of many of these strategies.

Another important distinction is between *self-help* and *self-management*. Self-help is a term often coined to describe something that you do for yourself, often by yourself. There are self-help manuals and books, self-help groups and self-help computer software. Self-help tools are often developed around a particular issue, diagnosis or symptom, such as depression or anxiety, phobias or panic attacks (see Chapter 29). However, self-help within the voluntary sector and service user movement more often refers to mutual support among people who share similar experiences. Self-management refers to a more comprehensive approach to dealing with your life. It may also engage with a particular diagnosis, but it tends to take a whole-life approach towards managing your life with the diagnosis and to include reference to all of your strategies, services and treatments whether or not they are themselves self-help strategies. An example of this is the self-management programme developed by the Bipolar Organization (formerly the Manic Depression Fellowship).

Strategies for living

In 1997, the Mental Health Foundation launched the Strategies for Living Programme. Funded by the National Lottery, Strategies for Living sought to 'document and disseminate people's strategies for living with mental distress'. The programme was 'user-led' in that the staff team and the Advisory Group were predominantly people with experience of mental distress and/or of using mental health services. However, it took place within a conventional mental health voluntary organization which was not (and is not) user-controlled. The approach taken was in part modelled on the ethos adopted within the field of Aids and HIV: that we are people 'living with' a diagnosis and need to develop and share the things that we find helpful. In this sense it was closely aligned with the concept of recovery (see Chapter 5). The programme started with a large-scale piece of qualitative research and subsequently funded service users to carry out their own smaller research projects into subjects of interest to them.

The initial research (Faulkner and Layzell 2000) concerned itself simply with finding out what people find helpful in managing or living with mental health problems. For that reason it is a useful springboard for a chapter exploring lifestyle options and choices. The interviews covered different aspects of people's lives, from their use of medication, treatments and services to a wide range of lifestyle options, such as physical exercise, complementary therapies, religion and spirituality and creativity.

Table 13.1 gives an overall picture of the different strategies and supports people had found to be the 'most helpful' to them overall. Many people gave a combination of two or three supports, people or activities, while a few found that one factor alone – or one person – stood out for them.

The overwhelmingly predominant theme running through people's responses to what was 'most helpful' to them was the role and value of relationships with other people. While for some people, it was individuals, family or friends, for others it meant the company of people encountered through groups or local day centres. For other people, the most important people in their lives were mental health professionals: counsellors or community psychiatric nurses (CPNs), support workers or social workers. The interviews were testament to the value of peer support and friendship; many people talked about the importance of meeting other people with similar experiences or who shared a similar diagnosis.

One important issue to emerge from this research is the relative absence of mental health services and treatments from this list. Medication, when prescribed with information and choice, could relieve symptoms and improve mood, and there were a number of mental health professionals who received special mention for the support they provided. However, the 'most important' sources of help remained predominantly outside the statutory mental

Relationships with others	Medication
■ Friends, relatives	■ Physical exercise
■ Other service users/people with similar problems	■ Religious and spiritual beliefs
■ Mental health professionals	
■ Counsellors/therapists	
■ People encountered in day centres, drop-ins, voluntary sector projects	Money
Personal strategies	Other activities
■ Peace of mind	■ Hobbies and interests
■ Thinking positively, taking control	■ Creative expression
■ Home	■ Information

Table 13.1 Strategies and supports rated 'most helpful'

health services. Voluntary sector drop-ins and day centres, some of them provided by local mental health charities, and some of them addressing particular life experiences such as sexual abuse, received enormous and grateful praise.

At this level, the research gives us an idea of the different things that people find helpful, but perhaps of greater importance to our understanding are the underlying themes, or the meanings that people place on these strategies and supports. Table 13.2 lists the themes that emerged from a more in-depth analysis.

- ■ Acceptance
- ■ Shared experience... shared identity
- ■ Emotional support... 'being there'
- ■ A reason for living
- ■ Finding meaning... and purpose
- ■ Peace of mind... and relaxation
- ■ Taking control... having choices
- ■ Security... and safety
- ■ Pleasure

Table 13.2 Underlying themes

In some ways, these themes are so self-explanatory that they hardly need further comment. That people should need a sense of acceptance, of belonging, a reason for living and a sense of purpose, peace of mind and security, choices and pleasure, should not be any surprise to us. Perhaps, however, we are now influenced by the recovery approach to mental health which acknowledges many of these themes. At the time of the research, which was published in 2000, it was ground-breaking in its own way. It serves perhaps also to remind us that people with mental health problems are no different to the rest of society – are indeed a part of society – and consequently have the same, or similar, needs and preferences about our lives.

The research is also useful in pointing us towards some of the options that we might want to consider when thinking about what might be helpful to ourselves or when advising someone with mental health problems about what they might find helpful. There is not the space here to go through all of the possible strategies and supports included so we have selected three to explore in more detail: physical exercise, religion and spirituality, and peer support. To this we have added diet and nutrition, which although not a focus of the 'Strategies for Living' programme has gained increasing credibility as an approach to managing mental health problems and to promoting our sense of health and well-being.

Physical exercise

A review of research into exercise and mental health (Glenister 1996) suggested that regular aerobic exercise can bring about a reduction in depression. It also suggested that exercise is not enough in itself to improve depression, but that a personal or subjective perception of improvement is an important part of the whole. In 2001, a meta-analysis of studies examining the effectiveness of exercise as a treatment for depression, published in the *British Medical Journal*, found that exercise compared with no treatment showed a significant difference on the Beck Depression Inventory (Lawler and Hopker 2001). However, most such research studies have been conducted on 'healthy populations' although they do tend to show positive improvements in psychological health and stress reduction.

The 'Strategies for Living' research indicates that physical exercise might be beneficial for a range of mental health problems. Many people reported that some form of sport or physical exercise was a valuable part of their lives. They mentioned a wide variety of activities, such as walking, swimming, running, using the gym, cycling, dancing, badminton, gardening, and hard physical work. For some people, physical exercise was a way of maintaining physical health and weight control (weight gain being a side effect of many psychiatric medications). Others talked about exercise having a positive effect on their mental health, self-esteem and well-being, relieving stress or helping them to relax. Another important benefit from engaging in physical exercise was its ability to provide distraction from feelings, thoughts or from hearing voices.

There are at least three other important ways in which engaging in sport and physical exercise might help a person's mental health and well-being. One is the element of control that it gives over a person's life and well-being (see the Mental Health Foundation (2005) report *Up and Running*). The sense of actively engaging in one's own recovery, taking responsibility and doing something that does not rely on the role of patient or service user, can become empowering. The second way in which sports and physical activities can help is by providing an opportunity for taking part in a group activity, meeting people and 'fitting in' (as someone in the 'Strategies for Living' research described it). In other words, it can become a route towards social inclusion. Thirdly, exercise leads to an increased release of endorphins and enkephalins, chemicals in the brain that are known to promote feelings of well-being and pain relief.

The difficulty experienced by many people in relation to physical exercise lay in summoning the motivation to participate. Depression in itself can suppress the motivation to do many things, and the effort of getting out of the house to go to the gym or to walk or participate in a sport was often too much for people. Fortunately, there are now over 800 exercise referral schemes across the UK to support people take up regular exercise (Labour

Research Department 2004). These are often referred to as 'exercise on prescription' schemes and operate in a variety of forms, often involving a partnership between primary care trusts and local leisure services. Typically, GPs and other health professionals can refer patients including those with mental health problems, particularly anxiety and depression. Once referred, clients are seen by exercise professionals who have been trained specifically to work with exercise referral populations. Clients can draw on this support throughout their programme for motivation and technical advice, and this appears to be vital to the success of the schemes.

The Mental Health Foundation's research into exercise referral schemes (MHF 2005) revealed that 42 per cent of GPs are knowledgeable of these services and have access to them. However, none reported that they 'very frequently' referred patients with mild or moderate depression to these schemes and only 15 per cent referred patients 'fairly frequently'. In contrast, 92 per cent of GPs tend to use antidepressants as one of their three most common responses for treating depression. These findings are disappointing given the voices from the 'Strategies for Living' programme and are at odds with guidelines from the then National Institute for Health and Clinical Excellence (2004) for treating depression in primary and secondary care that state: 'Patients of all ages should be advised of the benefits of following a structured and supervised exercise programme of typically up to three session per week of moderate duration (45 minutes to one hour) for between 10 and 12 weeks.'

Religion and spirituality

Arguably, it was the role of the Mental Health Foundation's *Knowing our own Minds* report (Faulkner 1997) in highlighting the importance of religion and spirituality to mental health service users that has led to a growth in local and national initiatives, conferences and publications. Subsequent interest in the subject and a seminar resulted in another publication (MHF 1999) 'The Courage to Bare our Souls' in which a number of people wrote about their own personal experiences of religion, spirituality and mental distress. What became clear, both in 'Strategies for Living' and beyond, is that many people have experienced stigma and discrimination in their attempts to explore and express their spiritual or religious beliefs at times of mental distress. And yet, it is a valid and valuable strategy for managing, expressing and explaining mental distress.

Spirituality means different things to different people. They may interpret it as:

- their religion or faith;
- giving meaning and direction to their life, sometimes described as their 'journey';
- a way of understanding the world and their place in the world;
- belief in a higher being or a force greater than any individual;
- a core part of their identity and essential humanity;
- a feeling of belonging or connectedness;
- a quest for wholeness, hope or harmony;
- a sense that there is more to life than material things.

It is only possible to scratch the surface of this complex issue in one small section. However, service users in the 'Strategies for Living' research spoke of religion and spirituality as a source of hope and meaning, a reason for living. Some found peace and comfort through their religious beliefs and through prayer and feeling the presence of God; for others it was the support of other people they found through meeting in church and religious organizations. While many people mentioned the value of their beliefs or the support of their faith, there were some who talked of the potential for harm within religious organizations. They talked of the difficulties surrounding the interpretation of guilt and sin, and sometimes of a failure on the part of religious communities to understand or support people experiencing serious mental health problems.

A recent publication (Coyte *et al.* 2007) gathers together personal and professional contributions from mental health professionals, carers and mental health service users and survivors. It addresses the stigma that can surround both mental health and spirituality and explores the place of the spiritual in mental health care, and its implications for research, education, training and good practice. It is aimed at mental health practitioners, carers and service users, chaplains, faith leaders, faith communities, as well as students and professionals working in the field of spirituality and mental health.

In writing of the experiences of people in distress *et al.* (2007: chapter 16), Coyte suggests that spiritual practice can have a direct bearing on mental well-being and mental distress. She suggests that a purely clinical approach without a knowledge of spirituality can both 'define and foster' mental health problems.

> " We who experience mental distress are given models of belief by psychiatry and religion which often do not encompass our experience. We struggle at the edge trying to make sense of our situation. Where we have the ability and courage to frame our experience in our own spiritual terms we can find a way to a meaningful centre. "

More recently still, Plant and Stephenson (2008) have reviewed the contribution of spirituality and faith to the management of mental health problems and conclude:

> " There is no doubt that, whatever the illness, having a faith helps and all the scientific evidence supports this. "

Peer support and friendship

In the 'Strategies for Living' research, the role and value of relationships with other people was perhaps the strongest theme to emerge overall. For some people, it was individual family members or friends, while for others it was about the company of people they met in day centres and self-help groups. For still others, the significant people in their lives were mental health professionals: counsellors or CPNs, support workers or social workers.

The value of peer support and friendship lay in the emotional support, companionship, the sense of belonging, and practical support offered. In particular, people talked of acceptance; both from others and from within themselves. This sense of acceptance and belonging was strongest where people met others who had similar experiences to their own. They valued the sense that they did not need to explain or justify themselves, there was a mutual understanding that brought people together. Some people talked of this in contrast to the stigma and discrimination they experienced elsewhere in the community.

> ❝ [the drop-in] is like a safe haven really, from out there. Presumably there are some people a lot worse off than me – maybe mental health problems that will lead them to behave in very unusual, unacceptable ways which result in them receiving derisive comments and ridicule. They have to suffer all that outside and in here they don't – they are just accepted for the person they are, underneath the illness. That really is the key to it all here. ❞

Some people met each other in dedicated self-help groups, whether for a specific diagnosis or a particular life experience, such as child sexual abuse – as in the case of the following quotation. There were indications in many of the interviews that meeting other people who had similar experiences was a significant turning point or stepping stone in an individual's recovery.

> ❝ … it was quite fantastic to be with other women who had actually the same kind of experience … it was just this feeling that I wasn't this kind of monster who had this very sordid kind of life. ❞

Self-help groups have an increasingly strong role to play in people's lives and within the context of voluntary sector service provision; they can provide a context for support and mutual help, as well as for campaigning, empowerment and political action. There is relatively little research to support their effectiveness, but there is an increasing interest in such research – both from professionals and from service users (Lucock *et al.* 2007). A brief literature review (Nelson 2007) found the following benefits of self-help groups:

- feeling less isolated;
- accessing relevant information;
- sharing common experiences;
- gaining empowerment over one's own health;
- increasing self-esteem;
- finding inspiration from others;
- being able to help others;
- learning new skills.

Diet and nutrition

There is mounting evidence that nutrition is key to our mental health and well-being, and that the right kind of food can dramatically improve outcomes for people with mental health problems (Plant and Stephenson 2008). This work is predicated on the brain as the organ that determines our mental health, which is made up of essential fatty acids, water and other nutrients.

Just like the heart, stomach and liver, the brain is an organ that is acutely sensitive to what we eat and drink. To remain healthy, it needs different amounts of complex carbohydrates, essential fatty acids, amino acids, vitamins and minerals, and water. Anyone who has ever smoked, drank alcohol, tea or coffee, or eaten chocolate knows that such products can improve one's mood, at least a little and temporarily. What seems to be less well understood is that some foods can have a lasting influence on mood and mental well-being because of the impact they have on the structure and function of the brain.

It is beyond the scope of this section to give a detailed account of all the nutritional factors that are believed to influence our mental health and well-being. We have chosen to look specifically at the role of neurotransmitters, which pass messages between neurons in the brain. These include acetylcholine, serotonin, dopamine and GABA. We have chosen these because they are often the target of pharmacological interventions, e.g. selective serotonin reuptake inhibitors.

A balance of neurotransmitters is essential for good mental health, as they are influential in the feelings of contentment and anxiety, memory and cognitive function (Mental Health Foundation 2006). Some foods are perfect at temporarily promoting a neurotransmitter that we may lack and, as we crave and then consume them, they 'trick' us into feeling better, for a while.

By making the brain less sensitive to its own transmitters and less able to produce healthy patterns of brain activity, these substances encourage the brain to down-regulate. Down-regulation is the brain's instinctive mechanism for achieving homeostasis: when the brain is 'flooded' by an artificial influx of a neurotransmitter (for example, adrenaline triggered by strong coffee), the brain's receptors respond by 'closing down' until the excess is metabolized away. This can create a vicious cycle, where the brain down-regulates in response to certain substances, which in turn prompt the individual to increase their intake of those substances to get the release of the neurotransmitter that their brain is lacking. This is one reason why people sometimes crave certain products. Fortunately, there are many more nutrients that serve the brain without deception or damage, and can improve mood and well-being (Table 13.3).

The foods listed in Table 13.3 can help to release an efficient balance of neurotransmitters that will not lead to down-regulation. However, this is but one aspect of diet and its effects on our mental health and well-being. Other important considerations include our intake of essential fatty acids, complex carbohydrates, vitamins and minerals, and water. For a thorough review of these nutritional considerations see the Mental Health Foundation report 'Feeding Minds' (MHF 2006).

Sadly, the use of nutritional therapies within mainstream psychiatry is not common and more often service users need to turn to voluntary sector services (e.g. The Food and Mood Project www.foodandmood.org) or to private sector providers (e.g. Institute of Optimum Nutrition www.brainbiocentre.com). However, there are exceptions including the Rotherham Early Intervention Team for Psychosis in the UK. All new service users have a nutritional assessment and analysis. Nutritional deficiencies in the diet are initially increased by using supplements and service users who have an excess of poor nutrients are advised to reduce their intake of saturated fats and sugar. Continuing nutritional feedback is given with the aim of achieving optimum nutrition from a balanced diet, without the need for continuing supplements. More integrated services of this type are needed to equip service users with the necessary knowledge, skills and support to manage their own mental health.

Neurotransmitter	Effects of deficiency	Foods to avoid	Foods to consume
Acetylcholilne	Deterioration of memory and imagination Fewer dreams Increased confusion, forgetfulness and disorganization	Sugar Deep fried food Junk food Refined and processed foods Cigarettes Alcohol	Organic/free range eggs Organic or wild fish – especially salmon, mackerel, sardines and fresh tuna
Serotonin	Low mood Difficulty sleeping Feeling 'disconnected' Lacking joy	Alcohol	Fish Fruit Eggs Avocado Wheatgerm Low-fat cheese Lean, organic poultry
Dopamine	Lacking drive, motivation and/or enthusiasm Crave stimulants	Tea and coffee Caffeinated drinks and pills	Regular, balanced meals Fruit and vegetables high in vitamin C Wheatgerm Yeast spread
GABA	Hard to relax Can't switch off Anxious about things Irritable Self-critical	Sugar Alcohol Tea and coffee Caffeinated drinks	Dark green vegetables Seeds and nuts Potatoes Bananas Eggs

Table 13.3 Neurotransmitters and their effects
From Holford (2003)

Self-management

Self-management approaches to mental health have been expanding and proliferating in recent years; while they appear to come from a variety of sources and different countries, most tend to have originated with people who have experience of mental health problems. There are a number of 'condition-specific' approaches, such as self-management of bipolar disorder and of schizophrenia, and more generic approaches as promoted through the recovery approach and WRAP (Wellness Recovery Action Plan) which originated with Mary Ellen Copeland in the USA.

Some of these are more structured than others, as they have been designed as a programme for training people. Some UK mental health charities such as the Bipolar Organization (formerly the Manic Depression Fellowship), Depression Alliance, and No Panic have self-management programmes currently running or in development. The approach taken by these and other 'condition specific' organizations in the UK has been to design a self-management course which suits the particular needs of a group of people who share a similar experience. While they may be based within the personal experience of people who share that experience, they have in some cases drifted away from those origins in the context of seeking research evidence for their effectiveness and/or safety.

There are common themes across the different approaches and tools that have been developed, but perhaps the core of self-management lies within the need to regain or take control over one's life, distress, symptoms or illness. In all of these programmes and approaches there is a fundamental belief in the 'expert by experience'. Slightly different approaches have been taken by these different groups. Rethink's self-management programme (for people with a diagnosis of schizophrenia) identified the following themes through research working closely with service users:

- occupation, including education, voluntary work, work with the user movement, art and creative occupations, and paid employment;
- relationships with other people, including family and friends and other service users;
- personal qualities involved in maintaining morale;
- coping strategies for the experiences of schizophrenia;
- managing medication, including managing relationships with prescribers;
- exploring and understanding the experience labelled schizophrenia, including getting information;
- religion;
- counselling and psychotherapy;
- complementary therapies;
- healthy living, such as diet and exercise.

These themes are not dissimilar from those identified in the Strategies for Living research – which also took the approach that people with experience of mental health problems could take the lead in defining what is helpful to them.

In a rather different approach, WRAP (on which the Bipolar Organization's programme is based) takes people through the following:

1 increasing awareness at the day-to-day level of what triggers off small changes that can upset our equilibrium;
2 more general ways of ensuring our good health through our lifestyle;
3 signs that things are deteriorating;
4 letting others know what we want to happen and who we want involved if we are in crisis;
5 being quite specific about interventions and treatment;
6 semi-legal written advanced directives.

The programme offered by the Bipolar Organization aims 'to teach the individual with bipolar disorder how to recognize the triggers for, and warning signs of, an impending episode of illness. Participants learn to take action to prevent or reduce the severity of an episode.' The Bipolar Organization offers training in the following sessions:

1 describes the principles of self-management and the aims and objectives of the course;
2 discusses the personal expectations of the participants and the nature and impact of manic depression;

3   identification of triggers and warning signs;
4   coping strategies and self medication;
5   support networks and action plans;
6   strategies for maintaining a healthy lifestyle and drawing up an advance directive;
7   complementary therapies, coping strategies and finalizing action plans.

The Bipolar Organization works to constantly review and develop its programme and its training on the basis of feedback received from trainees. It also claims to be the first self-management programme to be written and run by an independent user-led mental health organization.

Two more approaches that fall within a broad definition of self-management deserve special mention. Both were developed and remain within service user control: these are the Hearing Voices Network and the National Self-Harm Network. These are in reality user-controlled organizations which have developed and disseminated strategies for managing their respective experiences. Both have worked to enable the experience of people who hear voices or who self-harm to be understood by others. They have in common the promotion of different ways of understanding these experiences, based on the views of service users and challenging the medical and psychiatric frameworks of understanding that tend to predominate.

Although the Hearing Voices Network was inspired by Professor Marius Romme and Sandra Escher (from the Netherlands) it developed as a user-controlled network of self-help groups around the UK, with the aim of helping people to develop their own self-help strategies for managing the experience of hearing voices. Once again the theme of power and control emerges. The aim of the self-help groups is to help people to accept and live with their voices 'in a way that gives some control and helps them to regain some power over their lives'.

In a similar way, the National Self-Harm Network (NSHN) has been a survivor-led organization since 1994. They are committed campaigners for the rights and understanding of people who self-harm. The aims and objectives of the National Self-Harm Network include the following:

■   to support and empower people who self-harm;
■   to provide information, contacts and workshops on matters relating to self-harm and to promote survivor written literature;
■   to challenge assumptions and demystify common misconceptions surrounding self-harm;
■   to promote and advocate for the interests, needs and aspirations of people who self-harm and to influence social and health care policies at a local and national level;
■   to raise awareness among the general public, health services, hospitals and their staff of the needs of people who self-harm.

The NSHN provides a number of resources, training packs and publications which aim to support people who self-harm and their friends and family, and to promote understanding of self-harm among health care professionals. One example is the *Hurt Yourself Less Workbook* which was written by people who self-injure and aims to provide people with ways of understanding their own self-injury and exercises to help reduce the harm.

Conclusion

By way of a conclusion we draw out some of the common threads from the evidence presented. There are probably as many ways of managing and coping with mental distress as there are people experiencing it. One of the conclusions of the 'Strategies for Living' research was simply that people are all individuals and have their own different ways of understanding and coping with their difficulties. It is worthwhile considering some of the common threads that run through these different approaches:

- power and control – a sense of 'agency';
- meaning and purpose;
- symptom management;
- acceptance – of self and by others;
- crisis management;
- relationships and peer support;
- peace of mind.

If we are fully informed and have the power and resources with which to make choices, we can choose the things that work for us. However, this is rarely the case. Information is often not widely available on how different lifestyle approaches – such as diet and exercise – might help with our mental health, or how adopting certain strategies to help manage voices or self-harm might be helpful to us. Similarly, many people are living on benefits and consequently may be less able to access some of the beneficial therapies or strategies.

It is also true that many professionals working in the mental health field are unfamiliar with the potential contribution lifestyle approaches can make to an individual's mental health and well-being. There is some evidence that this is beginning to change but not at a pace which we believe is adequate or optimum for the well-being of individuals, their families and communities.

The service user/survivor movement and innovative statutory developments such as exercise referral schemes and the use of nutritional therapy in the Rotherham early intervention service demonstrate what could be possible. We do not advocate the wholesale rejection of traditional methods in mainstream psychiatry but we do call for a better balance of options, many of which could and should aim to support service users to take greater control of their own mental health.

Questions for reflection and discussion

1   Reflect on your own mental health and make an inventory of the behaviours and activities that you feel support or deplete your sense of well-being.
2   Think about a patient or service user you have cared for and consider their circumstances against the inventory you have made and the content of this chapter. What advice and support could you offer to promote their mental health and well-being?
3   Think about the service you work in or a placement you have been on and consider how it could be developed to provide a more comprehensive range of service to support patients or service users through mental health difficulties.

4   How many exercise referral schemes are available to you in your locality? (You can use an internet search engine to check your knowledge or make enquiries through your local PCT.)

Annotated bibliography

- Mental Health Foundation (2000) *Strategies for Living Summary*. London: MHF. Available to download from http://www.mentalhealth.org.uk/publications/?EntryId5=43591. This report summarizes much of the evidence presented in this chapter. The research reported in the summary aimed to explore the expertise of mental health service users in depth and in detail, and to reach a better understanding of what it is like to live with and manage mental distress.
- Mental Health Foundation (2005) *Feeding Minds: The impact of food on mental health*. London: MHF. Available to download from http://www.mentalhealth.org.uk/publications/?EntryId5=38571. This report provides a comprehensive overview of the effects of diet and nutrition on our mental health and well-being. It includes an overview of the biology and neuroscience that underpins nutritional approaches as well as practical advice to improve our diet. It also includes six case studies of services across the statutory, voluntary and private sectors that use nutritional therapy.
- Plant, J. and Stephenson, J. (2008) *Beating Stress, Anxiety and Depression*. London: Piatkus Books. This textbook provides a refreshing alternative to traditional mainstream psychiatric approaches to treating anxiety and depression. It provides ten lifestyle factors and ten food factors that can reduce the risk of mental health problems and dramatically improve our sense of well-being.
- Servan-Schreiber, D. (2005) *Healing without Freud or Prozac*. London: Rodale International. This exciting textbook provides compelling alternatives to the treatment of mental health problems without recourse to the traditions of psychiatry. It describes seven highly effective treatments that work through the body to tap into the emotional brain's self-healing process. It does this by combining cutting edge science with alternative medicine and points the way for a psychiatry of the future.

References

Coyte, M., Gilbert, P. and Nicholls, V. (eds) (2007) *Spirituality, Values and Mental Health: Jewels for the Journey*. London: Jessica Kingsley.

Faulkner, A. (1997) *Knowing our own Minds*. London: Mental Health Foundation.

Faulkner, A. and Layzell, S. (2000). *Strategies for Living: A Report of user-led research into People's Strategies for Living with Mental Distress*. London: Mental Health Foundation.

Glenister, G. (1996) Exercise and mental health: A review. *Journal of the Royal Society for the Promotion of Health* **116**: 7–13.

Holford, P. (2003) *Optimum Nutrition for the Mind*. London: Piatkus.

Labour Research Department (2004) *Exercise on Prescription: A report for the Chartered Society of Physiotherapy*. London: Labour Research Department.

Lawler, D. and Hopker, S. (2001) The effectiveness of exercise as an intervention in the management of depression. *British Medical Journal* **322**: 1–8.

Lindow, V. (1994) *Self-Help Alternatives to Mental Health Services.* London: MIND Publications.

Lucock, M., Barber, R., Jones, A. and Lovell, J. (2007) Service users' views of self-help strategies and research in the UK. *Journal of Mental Health* **16**(6): 795–805.

Mental Health Foundation (1999) *The Courage to Bare our Souls: a collection of pieces written out of mental distress.* London: Mental Health Foundation (out of print).

Mental Health Foundation (2005) *Up and Running: Exercise therapy and the treatment of mild or moderate depression in primary care.* London: MHF.

Mental Health Foundation (2006) *Feeding Minds: The impact of food on mental health.* London: MHF.

National Institute for Health and Clinical Excellence (2004) *Depression: management of depression in primary and secondary care.* NICE guidance. London: NICE.

National Self-Harm Network (Undated) *The Hurt Yourself Less Workbook.* Available from the NSHN (address below).

Nelson, S. (2007) You need to have been there: do self-help groups help, and how? *Mental Health Today* July/August, 37–9.

Nicholls, V. (2002) *Taken Seriously: The Somerset Spirituality Project.* London: MHF.

Plant, J. and Stephenson, J. (2008) *Beating Stress, Anxiety and Depression.* London: Piatkus Books.

Useful organizations

- **Hearing Voices Network**, 79 Lever St., Manchester M1 1FL. 0845 1228641; info@hearing-voices.org
- **MDF The Bipolar Organization**, Castle Works, 21 St. George's Road, London SE1 6ES; 08456 340 540 (UK only)
- **The National Self Harm Network**, PO Box 7264, Nottingham NG1 6WJ; www.nshn.co.uk
- **The Food and Mood Project**, Box 2737, Lewes, East Sussex BN7 2GN; www.foodandmood.org
- **Institute of Optimum Nutrition – Brain Bio Centre**, 13 Blades Court, Deodar Road, London SW15 2NU; www.brainbiocentre.com

CHAPTER 14

Psychosocial interventions

Catherine Gamble and Iain Ryrie with Jacqueline Curthoys

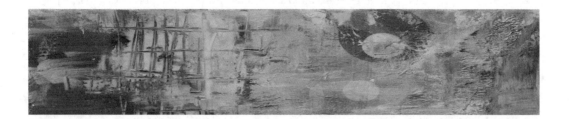

Chapter overview

The seminal work of Brown *et al.* (1972) and Zubin and Spring (1977) has been instrumental in the development of psychosocial interventions. Their work demonstrated the influence of life events and background stressors on the course of a serious mental illness. This understanding created the potential to develop interventions other than medication which would support people to manage life events and background stressors in ways that reduced their tendency to generate 'psychiatric symptomatology'. The effective delivery of psychosocial interventions necessitated a different type of relationship between staff and service users. By definition, collaborative relationships were required in which clients became active participants in the management of their symptoms.

This chapter begins with an overview of the theoretical rationale for psychosocial interventions and examines its implications for the relationship between service users and health care providers. Psychosocial interventions to support engagement, manage psychotic symptoms and involve families in care are described and their evidence base reviewed. Case studies illustrate use of the interventions and their value is appraised through the eyes of one client with first hand experience. The chapter provides a foundation for Chapters 30 and 31 in which Gega considers the practical application of behavioural and cognitive techniques when working with clients. This chapter covers:

- Rationale for psychosocial interventions;
- Developing a working alliance;
- Psychosocial interventions:
    - engagement and outcome-oriented assessment
    - individual psychosocial approaches
    - working with families;
- A personal experience of talking therapies.

Rationale for psychosocial interventions

There are a number of theoretically compelling explanations to support the efficacy of psychosocial interventions, the most widely reported of which has been Zubin and Spring's (1977) stress-vulnerability model. It proposes that psychotic illnesses arise from a combination of innate vulnerabilities and stress levels that exceed an individual's ability to cope with their present circumstances. Innate vulnerabilities include genetic predisposition and early life experiences while stress is classified as either ambient or discrete in the form of life events (Table 14.1). This separation of stress from innate vulnerabilities to explain the course of a psychotic illness provided the basis for psychosocial interventions including work with families and teaching social problem solving to individuals.

Type	Example
Ambient	Household/family dynamics
	Social expectations/barriers
	Work pressures
Life events	Loss of job
	Death of someone close
	Relationship break up

Table 14.1 Types of stress

A person's cognitive appraisal of ambient stress or life events is another important part of the Zubin and Spring model. A person might appraise a stressor as positive, negative or neutral, each with its own implications for their response. This is true of many of the symptoms of psychosis so that a person who experiences an auditory hallucination is either overwhelmed or able to rationalize it as an unreal if frustrating experience. This aspect of the model gradually led to the development of psychosocial interventions to include strategies for the psychological management of psychotic symptoms.

In contrast to the administration of medication, which is by and large a fairly passive act for service users, psychosocial interventions require active partnerships between those involved. The interventions aim to impart strategies that service users, their carers and families can use to better cope with the symptoms and course of serious mental illness. The therapeutic or working alliance is therefore key to the likely success of any intervention.

Developing a working alliance

Carl Rogers, the renowned psychotherapist, established principles for client-centred interactions, which are now considered fundamental to the development and sustainability of therapeutic relationships. The guiding principles include:

- accurate empathy, which is sensitive to others' feelings;
- genuineness, which is reflected in an open, honest approach;
- unconditional positive regard, which is achieved by accepting others as individuals who are entitled to respect and care.

Rogers (1983) believes that exposure to these qualities in another person supports learning and change in people. They are able to see themselves differently, accept their feelings more readily, become more accepting of others, and more self confident and self-directing. The promotion of these attributes provides common ground regardless of which treatment philosophy or affiliated school of thought is adopted. Indeed, at the core of any contemporary practice is the recognition that people are unique, that irrespective of their diagnosis they are able to collaborate, and that positive outcomes are unlikely if these principles are not adhered to and used by practitioners.

However, in today's busy clinical settings nurses and other health care professionals can become easily harassed resulting in any negative feelings they hold being expressed in their interactions with others. All too frequently professionals fail to apply Rogerian principles in their routine contact with clients (McQueen 2000). In this respect it may be salutary to ask 'How far do we always:

- act in ways that are trustworthy, dependable and consistent?
- communicate unambiguously?
- promote positive attitudes, such as warmth, caring, liking, respect?
- ensure that our personal feelings do not negatively influence our interactions?
- encourage clients to be individuals, rather than expect them to do as we say?
- understand and acknowledge clients' feelings and experiences, and respect their cultural and spiritual beliefs?
- act with sufficient sensitivity when presented with behaviours that seem threatening?

To some degree the quality of your answers will reflect the quality of your working alliance with clients, which is one marker for the effectiveness of any intervention you provide. That alliance can be enhanced in a number of ways in addition to the use of Rogerian principles including:

- challenging assumptions and reviewing attitudes;
- learning to listen;
- promoting collaboration;
- multi-disciplinary working.

Challenging assumptions and reviewing attitudes

Adverse views of people with serious mental illness stem from a number of assumptions including their perceived tendency to be violent, that they 'choose' to behave as they do, that they are unpredictable and difficult to treat (Haywood and Bright 1997). Promoting and sustaining positive working alliances involves challenging these negative beliefs and assumptions. Mental health professionals are part of a society that perpetuates these unconstructive suppositions and at one time or other, are likely to have shared all or some of them. Therefore, before entering into any relationship with a client, it is important to consider how to minimize these assumptions, so that a more optimistic outlook is created. Haywood and Bright's (1997) adapted model, shown in Table 14.2 provides some guidance.

Assumption	Methods
Mentally ill are violent and dangerous	360 homicides are committed each year in the UK, 10 per cent of this population are 'mentally ill'. Use of such statistics help to challenge the view that all those with severe mental health problems are violent and dangerous (James 2001).
They 'choose' to behave as they do	Utilize your educational role as a nurse. Challenge this view whenever it is expressed, strive to portray clients as rounded individuals – severe mental illness is not self-inflicted.
Prognosis is chronic	Many people go on to lead meaningful and successful lives – quote examples such as Ron Coleman (James 2001) and the work of Romme and Escher (1993). Moreover, it is possible to challenge this view when contemporary PSI, such as family work can produce significant benefits for clients long beyond the term of intervention (Sellwood *et al.* 2001)
Mentally ill are unpredictable and don't behave 'normally'	Does everyone always behave predictably and 'normally'? If we did wouldn't the world be full of robots? Challenge yourself to consider what is 'normal'. Review potential or actual 'strange' behaviours or ideas you have, such as, déjà vu, a belief in the occult, ghosts, reincarnation, aliens, astrology and tarot, etc.
Symptoms are difficult to treat	Incorporate cultural, psychological and biological models of health care, in doing so you will have a greater sense that there are self-management steps that can be used with symptoms that are perceived to be hard to treat (Kingdon and Turkington 1994)
This client group is hard to work with	Promote discussions with service users – learning to listen in this way you will be more likely to realize that working with this client group is a privileged lifelong learning experience.

Table 14.2 Methods to counterbalance maladaptive views

Learning to listen

Listening requires intelligent concentration to pay attention to context and content, and to paraphrase what is being said without changing the meaning of the words (Bostrom 1997). Skilled listeners are less likely to force-feed their own ideas onto clients or contaminate what they hear with their own thoughts and opinions. A key skill for all practitioners is to listen reflectively. This may be achieved by repeating single words that seem to be of importance, paraphrasing to elaborate a point or summarizing what has been said to check for understanding. Reflective listening develops empathy as the practitioner communicates their interest in and understanding of a person's experience. Accurate empathy is a Rogerian principle and a foundation stone for the working alliance. Table 14.3 lists a number of strategies that underpin the art of listening.

The art of listening involves four Cs:	Potential barriers include:	Methods to overcome involve:
Considering situations in which you may find it difficult to concentrate	Interruptions; noisy external exchanges; when there is more than one thing on the agenda, someone interrupting the session or going over the allocated time.	Planning for and reporting your unavailability. Put a 'do not disturb' sign up for the duration of the meeting; challenging interruptions if they are made. Setting an agenda, a realistic timeframe and adhering to it.
	Client's current symptoms may be too troublesome and distracting for them. TV and radio on.	Assess how the client feels, is this the right time and place to be meeting? Negotiate where and when would be more appropriate and/or turn off the TV or radio.
Collating methods to facilitate being a 'better listener'	Not planning for the interaction and missing valuable cues. Others not agreeing to formalized approach.	Discuss your interaction with another experienced member of the team. Plan how to structure and evaluate the session. Balancing note taking with personalized interaction.
	Tape recording and/or note taking perceived to be journalistic rather than therapeutic.	Adhering to trust and/or university guidelines, so it does not breach local confidentiality guidelines.
	Clients and/or carers will be suspicious, won't they?	Providing a rationale for note taking and/or audio-taping. No harm in just asking and gaining consent to audio-taping. Challenging own and others' assumptions.
Constructing a rationale for why you can't always listen	Being occupied by all the above and other clinical responsibilities.	Being honest. Acknowledging distractions and reporting other items on the agenda. Recognizing inability to time manage.
Consolidating what you will do with the information	Information obtained challenges others' perceptions.	Reflective listening; repeating, paraphrasing and summarizing. Encouraging others to listen to client's and/or carers' viewpoint.
	Unable to objectively document or report on what you had learnt.	Documenting what you have learnt in the case notes.
	Other members of the team don't want to acknowledge and there is no forum to feedback.	Disseminating to other 'listeners' such as the client, their carers and others on the team.
		Attending the next possible clinical review meeting to feedback.

Table 14.3 The art of listening

Promoting collaboration

Some clients may find psychosocial approaches overwhelming if they have been used to more traditional methods of care. Meaningful collaboration can only be realized if there is an appreciation of the degree to which clients want to participate in their care (Carhill 1998). Although this may fluctuate and be difficult to judge one approach is to consider a client's motivation to change. Prochaska and DiClemente (1986) have produced a trans-theoretical model of change that contains five stages. A person may be unaware of a need to change (pre-contemplation), aware of the need but not inclined to change (contemplation), aware and determined to change (determination), engaged in change behaviour (active change) or have successfully negotiated the change process (maintenance). Being aware of a client's readiness to change and providing interventions in line with that awareness are necessary parts of collaborative partnerships (cf. Chapter 22).

Multi-disciplinary working

Users and their carers often complain that despite every communication effort on their part they are at times confronted with an array of conflicting messages from different members of the team. Unless professionals are willing to communicate effectively, share working practices and value each other's contribution, it is unlikely that sustained working partnerships and positive outcomes for service users will be achieved. This is particularly true of psychosocial interventions which are dependent on high quality training and expert clinical supervision within broader operational strategies (Brooker 2001).

The quality of team functioning and collaboration between professionals are factors that influence the outcomes achieved by clients (Zwarenstein and Bryant 2002). Furthermore, reported barriers to implementing psychosocial interventions include the negative assumptions professionals hold about each other (Campbell 2000). Dennis (2000) has called for greater awareness and understanding of each other's roles and responsibilities and more negotiation between professionals. Thus team members would feel more valued, would identify and exhibit loyalty to the team rather than their own discipline alone and would be more likely to acknowledge and be more confident of each other's skills. Just as the working alliance requires accurate empathy between clients and staff this quality is also needed between members of the multi-disciplinary team.

Psychosocial interventions

Psychosocial interventions have been defined as formulation-driven interventions that ameliorate a user's or carer's problem associated with a psychosis, using an approach based on psychological principles or addressing a change in social circumstances. They include a range of evidence-based approaches that are typically grouped into two broad categories; individual approaches and working with families. All interventions are underpinned with a focus on engagement and are initiated by outcome-oriented assessments.

Engagement and outcome-orientated assessment

Outcome-orientated assessments provide a baseline to summarize the extent to which interventions do what they are intended to do for a particular client or population. Undertaking a thorough assessment of a client may be perceived by some practitioners to be too complex, drawn out and time consuming. Furthermore, some may consider form filling to be a barrier to engagement especially if the assessment requires that clients are confronted with lengthy assessment tools. People do not want to be overwhelmed so it is very important to be pragmatic and considerate when selecting assessment tools. However, due to the complex nature of the problems people experience, assessment does take multiple forms looking at symptoms, social functioning and needs assessment (Fleet 2004). The assumption that all clients and their carers will feel bombarded has also to be reviewed. Clinical experience suggests that many clients and carers perceive formal assessment approaches as a refreshing change. It can be reassuring when sound, practical interviewing and rating procedures are therapeutically utilized, since this process demonstrates that assumptions are not being made, that accurate observations are sought and that systematic procedures are being followed. Formulating a working hypothesis, through systematic assessment is an integral part of PSI implementation; the following case study of Claudette provides evidence of the therapeutic value of such an approach.

Case study: Claudette

Claudette is a 26-year-old African-Caribbean woman with a diagnosis of paranoid schizophrenia. She lives with her family and is currently unemployed. She was first admitted to hospital six years ago while she was studying hairdressing at the local college. She became concerned that another classmate was reading her thoughts and copying her ideas. Her coursework deteriorated and she became increasingly paranoid, irritable and secretive. She aggressively demanded screens to be erected in the classroom, lashed out at her tutors and despite every effort on their part her behaviour became so unmanageable she had to be asked to withdraw from the course. Her behaviour and symptoms worsened and she was eventually admitted to hospital. She made a satisfactory recovery and was in remission for nearly two years until she stopped taking her medication. She again became aggressive and paranoid, tried to strangle her mother and was re-admitted. Despite being compliant with treatment, Claudette failed to respond fully to anti-psychotic medication with hallucinations remaining the most prominent and distressing symptom. At this point Claudette expressed feeling overwhelmed by her incapacity to socialize, concentrate or motivate herself and she expressed 'this is ruining my life'.

The initial phase of the assessment process included conveying to Claudette that her current concerns and problems would be addressed and taken seriously. In doing so it was possible to describe the process of therapy and introduce the idea that a formal review of symptoms and the problems she was experiencing via systematic assessment was required. She readily agreed to participate in this approach, in part because the supporting explanation conveyed to her that 'talking therapy' could be formalized and that there was hope for the future. Over the next six weeks she participated in the following assessments:

Krawiecka, Goldberg and Vaughn, Manchester Symptom Severity Scale

The KGV (M) is a standardized global semi-structured instrument which measures the severity of symptoms. It comprises 14 items, which are rated on a 0–4 scale: 0 = no symptoms, 1 =

mild, 2 = moderate, 3 = marked and 4 = severe symptoms reported in the last month. The first six items are rated by the mental health professional on the basis of the client's verbal responses and next eight are rated on observations made during the interview (Krawiecka *et al.* 1977). Claudette's main symptoms produced the following ratings:

Anxiety	3
Depression	3
Suicidal thoughts and behaviour	1
Hallucinations	4
Delusions	2

This assessment showed that anxiety, depression and hallucinations were Claudette's most prevalent reported symptoms but, through observation, it was clear also that others were evident, these included:

Flattened affect	2
Psychomotor retardation	2
Poverty of speech	2

By reviewing these ratings, anxiety, depression and hallucinations appeared more prevalent than negative symptoms. At this stage it would have been easy to hypothesize about how to intervene, especially in relation to her reported anxiety. However, it is important not to rush in with a 'quick fix' anxiety-management programme; a fuller picture is always more preferable and further detail was recognized to be required. For instance, from this assessment it was not possible to measure the impact that some symptoms were having on Claudette's life and it was important to draw upon the initial concerns about her socializing, concentration and motivation capabilities.

Four further assessments were therefore undertaken, as follows:

Hospital Anxiety and Depression Scale (HAD)

This validated self-report questionnaire assesses anxiety and depression. It comprises 14 items; half of these assess anxiety and the other half assess depression. Items are rated on a 0–3 scale. Thus, the highest possible score for each symptom is 21. The client is asked to report how they have felt during the past 1–2 days (Snaith 1993). The HAD was used in Claudette's case because it is more sensitive than the KGV (M) at measuring the current impact anxiety and depressive symptoms and it assesses depressive–negative symptoms. It thus complements the third assessment tool selected – the Schedule for the Assessment of Negative Symptoms (Hogg 1996).

Schedule for the Assessment of Negative Symptoms (SANS)

This scale assesses symptoms such as affective flattening (decreased range in emotional responses), alogia (poverty of thought), avolition (loss of motivation or drive), apathy, anhedonia (diminished capacity to experience pleasure), asociality and attention. All symptoms are rated on a 0–5 scale of increasing severity (Andreasen 1982).

In Claudette's case the HAD and SANS assessments produced the following scores:

Anxiety	9
Depression	4
Affective flattening or blunting	2

Alogia	2
Avolition–apathy	3
Anhendonia–asociality	4
Attention	1

The results from the HAD were illuminating. The score of 9 for anxiety was borderline, which contradicted the results of the KGV (M) which had rated her anxiety as 'marked'. Social anxiety and deficits in social functioning are viewed generally as core problems for individuals with psychotic disorders (Birchwood *et al*. 1990) and these results demonstrate why it had been essential to listen to Claudette's own appraisal of her problems, use more than one assessment tool and not to rush in with solutions.

Impaired social functioning is a recognized hallmark of schizophrenia either as an early sign or as residual symptoms. Therefore, before commencing any intervention a baseline of Claudette's abilities in this area was undertaken, using the Social Functioning Scale.

The Social Functioning Scale

Birchwood *et al*. (1990) designed this instrument to cover seven main areas of social functioning including: social engagement, relationships, independence in living skills (competence and performance) and employment. All seven categories are rated independently, high scores indicating higher social functioning. From Claudette's results (Table 14.4) it was possible to conclude that she seemed to be doing quite well in all aspects of social functioning since all scores exceeded 100 (the population mean), with the exception of social activities, which scored 98. The scores in this case, however, were not accurate or sensitive to her level of functioning with respect to 'relationships'. Claudette, since leaving college, had lost contact with many of her peers, had no 'real' friends and only socialized with her parents. In spite of this her 'relationships' score was 145, which is well above the population mean of 100.

Categories	Raw score	Transformed score
Social withdrawal	12	110.0
Relationships	17	145.0
Social activities	10	98.0
Recreational activities	21	113.0
Independence (c)	39	123.0
Independence (p)	37	124.0
Employment	4	103.0
TOTAL SCORE	140	816.0

Table 14.4 Social Functioning Scale data

Beliefs about voices questionnaire

By administering the beliefs about voices questionnaire time was spent reviewing Claudette's beliefs about her voice hearing experiences (Chadwick and Birchwood 1994). From this is was possible to conclude that in the past week, her voices had caused her to feel anxious, but she had been telling them to leave her alone and she felt confident in being able to control them.

As previously mentioned, Claudette's assessment took six weeks. Throughout this period mental health professionals adopted a quizzical non-threatening approach and the rationale for going slowly trying to achieve a clear picture of Claudette was reiterated. Furthermore, as each assessment was completed Claudette was provided with feedback. It was imperative that this feedback was coherent and informative because Claudette's previous experience of her 'case' being reviewed had not produced the results she had been promised and much of the information obtained had not been used by the multi-disciplinary team. Claudette clearly appreciated the time that had been spent gathering this information; she described the experience as 'the detective period' and often questioned why she had never had the opportunity to do this following previous admissions.

The results of these assessments were drawn on to formulate a programme of care for Claudette, which could be monitored over time. Members of the mental health team discussed ideas for future interventions with her and with each other. These interventions included:

- activity scheduling and problem solving to increase Claudette's motivation, activity levels, social and independent living skills;
- cognitive therapy for voice hearing, utilizing, for example, coping strategy enhancement techniques;
- reviewing Claudette's medication, the side effects she was experiencing and examining her motivation to continue to take what she had been prescribed (via motivational interviewing);
- monitoring progress by revisiting the previous assessments and continuing to gather further details from other reliable sources, such as her family;
- collaborating and working with her family.

Individual psychosocial approaches

Individual psychosocial interventions described in this section include coping strategy enhancement, relapse prevention and problem solving.

Coping strategy enhancement

Coping strategy enhancement (CSE) is one of a number of psychosocial approaches that use cognitive behavioural therapy (CBT) techniques. CBT for people who experience psychosis aims to help clients gain knowledge about schizophrenia and its symptoms, overcome helplessness, reduce distress from symptoms, reduce dysfunctional emotions and behaviour, and help them analyse and modify beliefs and assumptions (Haddock and Slade 1996). It focuses on the cognitive appraisals clients make of psychotic symptoms and employs the ABC model in assessments. Thus, by examining Activating events, such as stresses that trigger or exacerbate delusions or voice hearing, and the Beliefs held about those ideas or thoughts, it is possible to understand the emotional or behavioural Consequences that the Belief invokes.

Through structured psychotherapeutic processes clients are invited to consider and question their cognitive appraisals with reference to the ABC framework. Possible biases in reasoning processes and errors in thinking are explored, alternative hypotheses are established and coping responses identified. CBT strengthens the rational part of the person enabling them to control the influence of their intuitive self. Fleet (2004) refers to this as encouraging a split between the 'feeling' and 'knowing' self. CBT therefore focuses on altering the thoughts, emotions and behaviours of people by teaching them skills to challenge and modify beliefs about their delusions and hallucinations (Healy *et al.* 2006).

Coping strategy enhancement (CSE) involves undertaking a detailed assessment of a client's psychotic experiences, then constructing highly individualized coping methods to deal with each distressing symptom when they occur (Tarrier 1992). Many clients have developed and learned to use a labyrinth of strategies that are designed to cope with problems and emotions. A selection is presented in Table 14.5.

Type	Examples
Behaviour control	Passive distraction, e.g. listening to music Active distraction, e.g. writing a diary
Cognitive control	Suppression of unwanted thoughts or perceptions Redirecting attention Active problem solving
Distraction	Listening to music, reading aloud, watching TV Counting backwards from 100 Describing an object in detail
Interacting	Telling the voices to go away Agreeing to listen to the voices at particular times
Activity	Walking Going to the gym Having a relaxing bath
Social	Talking to a trusted friend Phoning a helpline Visiting a favourite place

Table 14.5 Coping strategies
(After Fleet 2004)

Introducing CSE techniques involves a great deal of diplomacy, expertise and support. It takes time for clients to talk about their experiences, especially if their symptoms are pervading and intrusive. Furthermore, it is important to review a client's overall motivation and be aware of the sort of terminology you are using when introducing the idea and rationale for using CSE. Romme and Escher (2000) recommend adhering to the following principles:

■ Be willing and able to focus on the client's experiences, remembering that it is they who are the experts, but some may find it difficult to talk about strange and intangible influences in an open way – it requires lots of practice.

■ Take a journalistic approach to asking questions – use open questions until the picture is complete – try not to preempt what the client is trying to say and refrain from interpreting material too early. Practise introductions and interviewing – there are pitfalls which only experience can help you negotiate. A story may seem complete – but afterwards it may become clear that something is missing – this is not a disaster and can always be revisited. It will become less of a problem with time; you soon learn to get a sense of what is too vague and needs clarification.

These approaches have been studied in some detail over the last two decades in Great Britain with encouraging results. Kuipers *et al.*'s (1997) randomized controlled study allocated 60 outpatient clients with medication-resistant symptoms of psychosis to either CBT or standard care. CBT was individualized and lasted for nine months. Improvements were found only in the CBT group, in which there was a 25 per cent reduction in symptoms. It was concluded that CBT could facilitate clients with long histories to talk about the meaning of their psychotic symptoms, which helped to improve their coping strategies and decrease their symptoms.

Turkington *et al.* (2002) demonstrated the benefits that can accrue for patients when CBT is administered by community psychiatric nurses who receive weekly supervision. Individual trials (Garety *et al.* 2000) and reviews of randomized controlled trials (Cormac *et al.* 2001; Gould *et al.* 2001) all indicate that cognitive behavioural interventions offer a promising approach for targeting the positive symptoms of persistent delusions and hallucinations in people with a diagnosis of schizophrenia. Overall, however, the evidence base is only beginning to emerge and Healy *et al.* (2006) have argued that the case for wider use of CBT is far from conclusive (Cormac *et al.* 2001). CBT for psychosis appears to work for some of the people some of the time (Paley and Shapiro 2002). Nevertheless, work to date has challenged the widely held view that people with severe and enduring mental health problems cannot learn strategies to cope with their symptoms and gain positive clinical outcomes (Gamble and Brennan 2006).

Self-monitoring approaches: relapse prevention

The success of CBT in reducing positive symptoms led to a belief that self-monitoring could be used to help prevent relapse. The early work of Herz and Melville (1980) stimulated this interest as their study showed that by observing changes in thoughts, feelings or behaviours 70 per cent of clients and 93 per cent of families could predict when they, or their relative, were becoming unwell. There are four general categories of the early signs of relapse as presented in Table 14.6.

Type	Example
Anxiety and agitation	Irritability
	Sleep problems
	Tensions
	Fear
Depression or withdrawal	Quiet
	Low mood
	Loss of appetite
Disinhibition	Restlessness
	Stubbornness
	Aggression
Incipient psychosis	Persecutory feelings
	Odd behaviours

Table 14.6 Early signs of relapse
After Fleet (2004)

As self-monitoring involves identifying signs of psychosis, it seemed logical to develop a structured way to help clients identify and manage their individual relapse signatures and offer interventions to prevent florid psychosis (Spencer *et al.* 2000). This work may be undertaken on a one-to-one basis but a valuable strategy is to incorporate as many key stakeholders as possible. The approach involves five steps:

1   engagement and education;
2   identification of the relapse signatures, such as the signs noted above;
3   development of a relapse drill and a clear framework within which clients and/or their carers can voice their concerns: that is who will do what, when and how if particular signs or symptoms occur;
4   rehearsal and monitoring;
5   clarification of the relapse signature and drill, which involves ensuring that all concerned are aware of and willing to act if the drill is required (Spencer *et al.* 2000).

The first step is to provide education as this offers one way to engage service users in the development of a collaborative management plan. Furthermore, it provides an ideal way to share goals and establish common ground with staff and services. One approach is to inform the client and his or her carers about the stress vulnerability model by relating stressful events such as, siblings moving away from home, parents divorcing, losing a job, moving house, etc. to particular personal experiences of increased psychosis. Clinical experience shows that clients and carers can learn how to anticipate and manage potentially stressful experiences.

Information regarding an individual's relapse signature can be placed on a chart which incorporates the progression of symptoms, from minor to extreme and outlines what actions can be taken, by whom, and when to prevent escalation. With the client's consent, this chart can be circulated to all the key stakeholders involved in the client's care, and can act as a valuable aide-mémoire for them. Sharing information in this way generates an open approach by all those most closely involved in the client's care, and if further potential relapse behaviours emerge, such as the client becoming isolative or withdrawing from usual activities, they can be addressed using a predetermined problem-solving strategy. An example of a self-monitoring and relapse chart is shown in Table 14.7.

Stage	Signs noted by client (C)	Signs noted by family (F)	Signs noted by staff (S)	Actions to be taken
3 = Extreme	Become obsessed with my mum. Not wanting her to go out. Not sleeping at all.	Won't leave mum alone. More arguments in the house.	Very irritable, increasingly suspicious and paces.	C = try to listen to the advice I am given!!! Don't panic. F = arrange a meeting with doctor, encourage to take increase in medication. S = monitor, take to clinic if family not able, increase contact to at least daily; liaise with doctor to review medication.
2 = Moderate	Sleep is disturbed.	Slightly clinging to mum, suspicious of other family members.	Becoming unkempt – less likely to go out.	C = talk to sister about feelings, ignore voices. F = be available to listen. S = encourage to go out with me. Feedback observations – encourage doing the actions outlined below.
1 = Mild	Feeling stressed, get cross with my mum.	Has a slightly odd look about the eyes.	Slightly irritable, not as interested in appearance.	C = go to bed earlier, take a break, visit mates. F = give space, encourage to do slightly less. S = reinforce the above, reflect on this in sessions.

Table 14.7 Example of a self-monitoring and relapse prevention chart

Problem solving

Problem solving is an integral part of a cognitive behavioural approach and a common element in successful PSI programmes for individuals and families (Mari *et al.* 1996; Falloon *et al.* 2007). Based on structured and comprehensive assessment, problem solving aims to elicit detailed information concerning the nature of the client's and/or carer's difficulties and thus generate specific goals, which can be formulated and tested. By identifying the problem or issues that are causing dissatisfaction it is possible to learn systematic methods to solve them and thus instil a sense of control. Ultimately this helps to tackle problems if and when they occur in the future (Hawton *et al.* 1989).

The first step in teaching clients and carers effective problem solving involves promoting effective communication styles. Falloon and Graham-Hole (1994) advocate teaching these skills through specific behavioural tasks, which incorporate learning how to listen, praise, be assertive and make positive requests. Once these have been put into practice effectively, the likelihood of arguments occurring reduces and it becomes possible to amicably discuss previous coping strategies in response to problems, review past experiences and then move on to formulating a brief description or statement of the current difficulty, as the target for future work. This statement can incorporate behaviours, thoughts, feelings, material circumstances or individuals that the problem is affecting, such as the client, family, nurse, psychiatrist or neighbours.

Overall, the problem statement should indicate clearly who is involved in the problem, and describe specific thoughts, feelings or behaviours that constitute the problem. Those problems judged as having a reasonable chance of achieving improvement in a short time (weeks or perhaps months) should be targeted first, and progress measured.

The second step in a problem-solving approach is to develop a brief description of an agreed goal which the client, carers or practitioners have to pursue. For example:

> Problem: John lies in bed all day, he is missing the work scheme he is supposed to attend which causes him to argue with his mother.
> Goal: For John to get up every weekday morning by 11.00 a.m., attend the work scheme twice a week for the next month, and avoid arguments with his mother.
> Step three is to generate a list of possible solutions, to the aforementioned problem statement and goal. The skill, at this stage is to merely devise solutions; not to discuss their pros and cons.

Step four involves identifying advantages and disadvantages of the possible solutions. It is not uncommon for some aspects of the different possible solutions to be incorporated together and it is important to be flexible enough to allow an eclectic solution to develop. Figure 14.1 provides some examples of potential solutions to John's problem, and Table 14.8 lists the pros and cons of each.

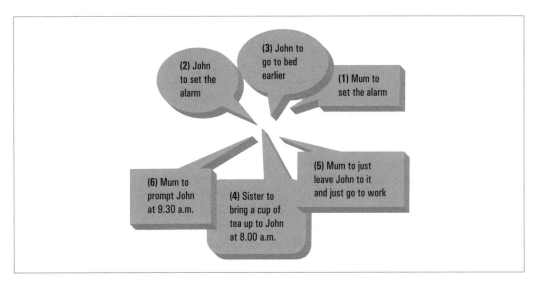

Figure 14.1 Potential solutions

Solutions	Advantages	Disadvantages
Mum to set the alarm	Mum would know it would have been set.	Places all the responsibility on Mum.
John to set the alarm	Places responsibility on John.	Might forget. Once it's switched off there will be nothing to wake him again.
John to go to bed earlier	Wouldn't be so tired in the morning. The house will be quieter.	Difficult to change routine. Miss late-night TV.
Sister to bring a cup of tea.	Nice thing to do. Good to see John before I leave for work.	
Mum to just leave.	Go to work and be there on time.	Would worry that nothing will change. More arguments.
Mum to prompt John at 9.30 a.m.	Would see him awake.	Might cause argument.

Table 14.8 Advantages and disadvantages of potential solutions

Through the above process it is possible to choose the best solution which should be valued by all involved, i.e. they should understand the anticipated benefits and agree to its implementation. Furthermore, everyone should be clear about what to do if the best solution generated does not work. Indeed, specific cognitive or behavioural steps should be described and clearly stipulated so the people involved know exactly what part they will play. For example:

■ John's sister will wake him up with a cup of tea at 8.00 a.m.
■ Mum will prompt John at 9.30 a.m., set the alarm and go to work.
■ John will get up at 11.00 a.m. and make his own way to the work centre.

■   The solution's effectiveness will be reviewed at the next session and in the meantime no one will blame each other if it does not appear to work immediately.

At their next meeting the mental health worker and client, together with others involved, will review progress, identify potential barriers to further progress, and address how these may be overcome by, for example, either redefining the problem or reducing the goal into smaller, more easily accomplished components. When one target problem has been solved, the next is identified by mutual agreement.

It is important for mental health care staff to recognize that it takes time for people to change and take on new principles. This highlights the importance of the worker developing therapeutic collaborative relationships with the client and his or her carers. The preferred approach is to regard problem solving as 'team work' which involves identifying and working with the client's and their carer's personal strengths, resources and the supportive/confiding relationships they have and utilize. Problem solving should also include considering how other professionals might be involved to help clients reduce sources of external stresses, such as poor housing, inadequate finance and unemployment.

Working with families

Seminal work by Brown and Rutter (1966) was influential in developing psychosocial family interventions. These authors developed the concept of 'expressed emotion' (EE) suggesting that stressful factors in a person's home environment and particularly in their family were associated with higher levels of relapse. People with a diagnosis of schizophrenia who experienced high levels of negative EE in their families have a significantly higher relapse rate than clients living in low negative EE families (Fleet 2004). Following Pharoah *et al.* (2002) psychosocial interventions with families include family engagement, education, communication training, goal setting, problem solving, cognitive behavioural self-management, increasing family well-being and maintenance of skills.

Family work for psychosis is now one of the most efficacious of all the PSIs. Over the past 20 years its effectiveness has been intensively evaluated in a number of different settings and cultures. Individual studies and systematic reviews have concluded that family work reduces relapse beyond the protection of medication, produces substantial long-term benefits for clients and provides families with the skills to cope more effectively with their relative's illness (Sellwood *et al.* 2001; Pharoah *et al.* 2002).

In spite of its strong evidence base, family work continues to be difficult to integrate into routine clinical practice. Faddon and Birchwood (2002) identify a number of reasons for this. The first appears to be directly related to service provision. Rigid service styles prevent integrating family work into existing caseload demands and practitioners are not routinely given time off in lieu for work undertaken in the evenings (which is when most family members are more likely to be able to participate). Second, there is a general lack of confidence and skill-experience in cognitive behavioural techniques, thus some practitioners feel ill-prepared to keep family sessions on track or tailor the approach to meet the family's needs. Third, professionals may feel themselves unable to deal with the maelstrom of problems professionals think they will encounter if they get involved with families, or they may fear breaching confidentiality or an escalating and unmanageable workload as further problems are unearthed (Leff and Gamble 1995; Furlong and Leggatt 1996; Faddon and Birchwood 2002).

What is clear, however, from clinical experience and the case studies presented in this chapter is that even if clients do not appear to be members of stereotypical families, it is rare to find them completely isolated. We know that family and friends are important in promoting recovery (cf. Chapter 5) and in helping clients find ways of coping (Baker and Strong 2001). Thus, it is essential that professionals overcome rigid working methods, revise their negative fears about undertaking family work, find practical solutions to overcome the risk of breaching confidentiality and embrace clients' families and friends as valued members of the care team.

The following case study of Sophie provides some ideas as to how the issues described may be addressed in order to work with carers more effectively.

Case study: Sophie and her son, Charlie

A referral for family intervention was received via a telephone call from a team who described themselves as 'desperate'. The mother of one of their clients was a 'terrifying, over-protective, management problem' and they needed help! It was agreed that the family workers should visit her to objectively assess her needs. On arriving outside the family home, thoughts of being lynched by an ogre were invoked by the image portrayed by the team. Then an ordinary woman (Sophie) in her late sixties walked up the road and went into the house. She was not 14 feet high and she definitely did not look like she could say boo to a goose. She was affable, welcoming and delighted when the idea of undertaking a comprehensive needs-led assessment was introduced.

The Knowledge about Schizophrenia Interview, which assesses a carer's knowledge about six broad aspects of schizophrenia was completed (Barrowclough and Tarrier 1992). From this it was possible to ascertain that she understood the diagnosis, recognized the positive symptoms and knew what her son was being treated for. She was also aware that its cause was stress related and knew his medication regime, the names of his drugs, the times they should be taken and was clearly worried that he would have problems again. She reported that 'services don't tell me anything and do nothing for him. I can't stop caring – I'm his mother and if I don't look out for him, who will?'

From her responses to the Relatives' Assessment Interview (Barrowclough and Tarrier 1992) it emerged that she was a lone carer who, after immigrating to England 20 years ago, was left to bring up seven children on her own. One of her daughters, who still lived with her, had severe hearing problems and she had chronic arthritis. When her son Charlie became ill, she was the only one from whom he would accept medication, therefore the psychiatrist asked for her help. This was one of the main reasons why she now reported walking across town every day to ensure he took his medication. Following discharge, Charlie also experienced housing problems; the ceiling of his council flat fell in and he was without gas or electricity. Despite his mum asking – nothing was done about this for four months. Sophie had to start shouting at service personnel, and when she still wasn't heard she involved a solicitor.

The assessent process had elicited that Sophie was a great advocate, a deeply religious person who provided support not only for her immediate family – but also to her elderly neighbour. She endeavoured to maintain a life of her own; she was undertaking a creative writing course. Furthermore, it was clear that she had a clear set of realistic goals for Charlie – she stipulated that it was essential that he started to be more responsible, learn to take his own medication, take care of his cat and that she would like him to achieve this over the next year. But despite all this, the care team had 'pathologized' her behaviour and she had been labelled as demanding and over protective!

The sessions that followed involved reiterating that, from henceforth, rigid boundaries that had hitherto prevented Charlie's family from being fully involved in his care and care planning would be dismantled. Charlie welcomed this and described how he had previously felt like a 'pig in the middle!' The sessions also involved feeding back and reinforcing the family's strengths and providing all family members, including Charlie, with more information about Charlie's illness, especially with regard to negative symptoms (cf. Chapter 18), which family members reported never having heard of previously. It was clear that Charlie was experiencing some severe negative symptoms, which resulted in him being unable to motivate himself. Thus he had become increasingly socially withdrawn from his supportive family.

Charlie's family were keen to help him overcome these symptoms and were genuinely pleased when intervention ideas were proposed, as this provided them and Charlie with optimism for the future. Hogg (1996) suggests that activity scheduling is one of the simplest and most useful techniques to help clients overcome their negative symptoms. Initially Charlie and his family were encouraged to note down what he did throughout the day. By obtaining this baseline it was possible to monitor change in his activities and his progress. Engaging Charlie in activities that would give him the greatest sense of achievement is key to this work. Therefore, he and his family were asked to brainstorm all the activities he would like to undertake and Charlie was asked to rate on a 0–10 scale how pleasurable he would find them. Going to the gym, going back to college and visiting his mum emerged as Charlie's most pleasurable activities. It was clear that realizing some of these activities would be easier than others. In the short term, it was decided to focus on attending the local gym and visiting his mum. Ways to achieve these were problem solved, using the strategy outlined earlier in the chapter, and various members of his family volunteered to help Charlie to achieve these goals. Charlie's mum was clearly delighted, because increasing Charlie's ability to visit her meant that she would not need to travel across town as frequently as before to ensure that he took his medication.

Mum's dissatisfaction with mental health and other services was also addressed. The family's workers alleviated her concerns by liaising with Charlie's care team, which helped to defuse some of the myths that had been generated about this family previously. In turn, by observing the results that family interventions brought about, the whole multi-disciplinary team began to embrace the philosophy of family work and sought to implement Standard 6 of the *National Service Framework for Mental Health* (Department of Health 1999) (assessing the needs of carers – cf. Chapter 4) and thus integrate it into every client's treatment package.

A personal experience of 'talking therapies': Jacqueline's story

Hitherto this chapter has described the range of psychosocial interventions available, and their application by health professionals to the care of particular clients. The following section considers psychosocial interventions, not from the viewpoint of the professional, but as experienced by a client. There follows a personal account of the experiences of one client who has experienced 'talking therapies' within the context of mental health services:

My experiences as a user of mental health services have been somewhat unexpected. About five years ago, I was a happily married successful professional planning to start a family. I was in good physical and mental health. Friends, if asked, would probably have described me as a lively outgoing individual who enjoyed socializing and liked to have a laugh and a drink in a variety of social circumstances. I enjoyed my job, and took an especial interest in the mental health list I was developing at the time, through which I was meeting a number of leading authors and practitioners.

The company I was working for was going through a sustained period of change involving major takeovers and changes in personnel. I was fortunate enough to be promoted to a job which involved a great deal of travelling and considerable extra responsibilities. Within a matter of months, I started to feel the strain; suddenly it seemed as if I would arrive at my desk in the morning, turn on the PC and within an hour was sobbing uncontrollably behind the office door. I couldn't cope and the less I tried, the more insurmountable the workload became. Eventually, I went to my general practitioner, desperate. I had no idea what could possibly be done, but had no idea what else to do. The GP signed me off with 'work-related stress', told me I was depressed (how could I be – I thought that meant staring at the walls?) and put me on Prozac. Bang, problem solved.

For a while, it was a miracle drug. I was back at my desk within a fortnight and felt like a new woman, completely back to my old self – in fact even better. I was the life and soul, confidence brimming, and could have become a passable stand-up comic.

If this sounds too good to be true, it indeed was. A few months later, I found my elation was getting to be a problem in itself. I started to wonder if Prozac might not be contributing to the over-excitement I experienced. I was not feeling depressed any more, so I weaned myself off it.

One of the 'problems' my over-confidence had caused was that I was now engaged in an affair, which my husband had discovered, and we were experiencing considerable marital difficulties as a result. Over the next 12 months, I went into another period of depression, deeper this time and my marriage began to break down irretrievably. During this period I went back on Prozac and was referred by my GP for six counselling sessions with the practice-based counsellor.

My initial reaction to this referral was one of suspicion. I had little belief that counselling would help. Frankly I felt my problems were of my own making and that my depression was my fault. Moreover, it would be 'cured' by Prozac, not talking, although that seemed to be taking longer to work this time. My professional background made me quite curious about the approach that would be taken, but almost cynical about the efficacy. As it was, these suspicions appeared to be borne out by the experience.

The counselling itself took place in a room above the GP's, and the counsellor seemed young and inexperienced. My initial assessment of her was 'stereotypical'. I believed her to be some kind of 'hello trees, hello flowers, hello sky' hippy chick in Laura Ashley, who clearly had no life experience to speak of. Unfortunately, she couldn't explain or justify the 'approach' she was taking although she described it as Rogerian and told me that this meant she would be positive about anything I said. We spent sessions mostly in uncomfortable silence as most of her questions seemed unworthy of response. Any response I gave would generally be repeated back to me parrot fashion in the form of a question. I could see little or no reason to trust her sufficiently to tell her personal or intimate details of my life as to me she lacked credibility, intelligence, or any ability to provide me with any of the 'answers' I so desperately sought. I now see that I was expecting advice, which she of course diligently withheld, and perversely I would never have taken from her anyway. It may seem immaterial, but I was never going to respect anyone who simply couldn't spell, which was clear from the notes she showed me. She came across as pleasant, well-intentioned, but ultimately useless. We parted after the six free sessions came to an end.

Despite this experience, after a further year of coping with both the highs and lows, I became intensely depressed once more and had to take several weeks off work. The thought of returning filled me with fear and anxiety and in desperation I began to see another counsellor who I subsequently saw regularly for nearly a year.

From the beginning our relationship was helpful. The counsellor was considerably older than I was and her experience seemed to me to provide a secure environment of trust. She was open and explicit about the aims of counselling and the approach she was taking which she described as 'Rogerian with common sense'. The actual environment was very comforting; a large quiet slightly darkened room, where we both sat. She listened attentively and her questions always seemed pertinent and thought-provoking. She expressed herself well and helped me to do so, often prompting me to explain thoughts in ways I had not previously considered, to see them in new contexts. I was impressed by her apparent ability to recall details from previous sessions, which made the process seem very personal. She was non-judgemental and empathetic, yet did not avoid speaking herself or giving me advice, sometimes of a psychological nature, sometimes very practical. My only criticism, if I have one, is that as the agenda for each meeting was purely mine, the process lacked a certain structure and we would weave seemingly aimlessly across time periods and incidents. However, as I explained earlier, her skill lay in apparently extracting the themes which emerged and attempting to make me see a larger pattern to my thinking. Ultimately though, I was left feeling that we were looking for long-term solutions; for answers that were buried in some distant past that we might never find, while meanwhile my immediate problems in the form of deepening depression re-emerged. The counsellor did provide me with one hugely useful insight into my problems when she suggested that there was a bipolar element to my moods and in her opinion I ought to be seeking more expert psychiatric help than she was able to give.

Fortunately, shortly after this time I was referred to the local hospital and I began to attend a local clinic, seeing a psychiatrist there primarily for depression, which this time was crippling, and I was unable to work for three months. As the depression began to lift, I was naturally keen to return to work, and anxious that although my employers had been supportive, this was not an open-ended arrangement. Work also meant to me self-esteem and returning to 'normality'. I cannot overstate at this time how important it was to me not to feel as if I had a long-term problem or was in any way 'mad'. One condition of my return was that I had to attend several private sessions with a consultant psychiatrist.

I find it difficult to discuss this experience. I was clearly quite ill and the antidepressants I had been taking all winter were now swinging me into mania. I did not feel comfortable speaking honestly to someone I perceived to be in the pay of my employers. The formal setting which was intimidating compounded this and the manner of the psychiatrist was patronizing and distant. I was told I was fine and my company was being over-cautious as I was clearly no longer depressed. Just in case, the dose of antidepressants I was taking was doubled. Striving to keep my job I tried to buy into the relationship. I was grateful to have access to some kind of support at this time, but I had no idea what purpose the sessions served. The relationship did not work, I was made to feel that I was a neurotic malingerer. In turn the psychiatrist often seemed distracted and bored and allowed long periods of silence to develop which I had no idea how to fill. I was galloping towards a major breakdown, he recommended inpatient treatment for what was described as 'treatment resistant alcoholism'. I was naturally terrified and summoned every remaining outward appearance of sanity I had in order to remain in control and to leave the premises.

One aspect I have not included in this account has been the often crucial role of family and friends. This is partly because of the selfish nature of depression which by its very nature turns you completely inwards and away from believing that help is available to you in any form. Compounding this is the fear that it often induces in those close to you who do not know as my mother succinctly put it 'where the old Jackie has gone', and fear the unknown country which mental illness often appears to be. I had some enormously supportive experiences of friendship during this period; people who were prepared to simply be there for me and tolerate having a miserable boring self-obsessed person in their homes through long winter evenings. Conversely, I also discovered that 'advice' from people perceived previously as friends, can be patronizing and destructive, simply confirming and compounding your own sense of worthlessness and inadequacy. Often these are the same people who enjoy the grandeur of your manic self-delusion as they confirm to you that all is well when in fact you are at your most unwell.

Ultimately, however, the important thing for health professionals to be aware of is that mental illness in any individual has a huge impact on their family and social networks, an impact which is often misunderstood or overlooked. There remains an almost Victorian sense that ultimately families provide the safety net for sufferers of mental illness, which in most cases is simply not practical in today's fractured society. How many of you reading this live within an hour's drive of your parents? How many of you come from nuclear families? Most of the time when I have been ill, I have spent alone, partly through choice but mainly through circumstance. Yet paradoxically there has been little or no attempt to involve family or friends in the treatment I have received or to acknowledge their role.

One illustrative example that is worth giving in brief concerns the manic breakdown I experienced. My account of this episode is by definition patchy. I have little recollection of much of the time that had elapsed – it is like a dream, leaving strong impressions which remain intensely vivid now at the time of writing almost exactly a year after the events.

As far as I know I spent a 48-hour period alone in a completely euphoric state experiencing intense delusions and hearing voices. During this period, I was convinced that my friends had planned a huge surprise party for me which was due to begin at any time. A CPN who was scheduled to visit me during this period arrived to assess me. I had been told I should not leave the house in case she arrived, so clearly she was simply a decoy, in fact some kind of minor celebrity brought in to launch the party. Hordes of friends were in hiding around my house, monitoring my every move via the use of Big Brother-type hidden cameras. When she finally arrived, three or four hours after the scheduled appointment time, I delighted in 'playing her game' and teasing her about the true nature of her visit. I was so excited about the party, and very pleased with myself that I had been clever enough to discover their plans. When she left, I felt as if I had been extremely cunning.

I had already spent the morning calling loads of friends, including my ex-husband, none of whom had any idea who to call or how they could help. Luckily a friend who is a senior mental health nurse had been contacted by one of my other friends and she came round to find me now intensely paranoid, cowering in my front room, terrified, knowing above all that

I had gone completely mad. The counselling in crisis I received from her at that point was life-saving, literally and metaphorically. My friend spent several patient hours talking me back into something approaching normality and was able to liaise with the mental health services. It is unlikely that most people are as fortunate in their choice of friends as I was in this instance. She talked to me with patience, reassurance, and above all humour which promoted my sense of normality and trust in her and more importantly in myself. It still frightens me to realize now that under other circumstances I would have had to endure this alone.

I had been referred to the clinical psychology team via my psychiatrist at my local hospital in the previous January, but it took until December for this referral to come through. I was depressed following the mania of the summer recounted above (I had also lost my job), and I was as ever cynical about whether anyone could help me. Initially, a clinical psychologist and a student assessed me, and it was explained to me that a cognitive behavioural approach would be used. I knew something of CBT from my work and had heard that it had very positive results for depression in combination with antidepressant drugs which I was taking once more.

The initial assessment was very reassuring. Both clinicians were open and explicit about the aims of the session and about the therapeutic approach. They explained themselves well and equally listened carefully to my answers to their questions. The session ended with a number of questionnaires which I recognized as depression and hopelessness inventories, and I was then reassured that they would be able to help me. Their confidence astounded me at the time: they even put a limit on it – in 8–16 weeks I'd be better!

The therapy itself commenced after the Christmas break. From the outset, I appreciated the structured nature of the sessions and the fact that the agenda was explicit and clear. Instead of feeling that I had to fill up the sessions, the therapist would provide a structure and guidance to which I contributed where I felt I could. I didn't feel at this stage able to contribute much at all, but I was pleased that we were going to focus on specific problems I was presently experiencing and how to alleviate them rather than dwelling on past problems, or far distant roots of psychological stress. The approach seemed refreshingly practical and grounded. A lot of time was spent in the initial sessions explaining the approach and encouraging me to 'buy into' each stage through understanding how it might work, even if results might take a little longer. The process was broken into manageable, and, above all, negotiated steps, addressing both mental and physical needs, and I was always given handouts to read as well as homework to complete, mostly diaries of my empty days. At each session the therapist was open and encouraging, and explicit in the aims and agenda of each session and what we wished to achieve in the following week. Terminology was explained and supported by reading matter and handouts. I felt supported while in some limited way able to take some charge of my own treatment in a way I hadn't been able to before. Even in a small way I was being encouraged to contribute to and take control of my own well-being. From time to time, I completed further mood inventories and these were used to show me how I was progressing. The benefits of monitoring my own mood changes and their triggers soon became clear and by working through these each week with the therapist, I was able to tackle some immediate negative thought barriers which I had thought not so much impassable as simply an intrinsic part of my life.

So is CBT the ultimate answer? I remain a partial convert. It is by far the most effective talking therapy I have encountered while in deep depression, but it has many downsides. It is intellectually demanding and jargon ridden. I am not a stupid person, but hypothesis testing as a concept is not a simple one, and one of the things you feel when you are depressed is stupid and unable to take on abstract ideas. The book from which my handouts were taken was a US text, no doubt seminal but the examples did not always seem really relevant to my experiences. Over-reliance on the agenda in a session can make the experience seem as if you are both simply working through a checklist and the sessions can seem limited and over-prescribed. Most importantly, when you feel the therapy isn't working for you, it is easy to feel that you are simply too dumb to apply it properly and if you were less lazy and worked harder you'd be better. I felt guilty for leaving the homework to the last possible moment, yet that's hardly atypical of my character all my life! And thought records are really hard. Writing and thinking has been part of my professional life for almost 20 years and I found them and still find them a struggle.

My particular circumstances also taint my response to CBT. I was depressed and as ever the depression lifted. As I entered the inevitable following period of mania, the direction of the sessions became less focused. Two things have contributed to this: a lack of apparent understanding on the part of the therapist as to how CBT could be adapted from addressing the problems of depression to those of mania; and my own self-confidence, which in a manic state naturally leads me to assume that I don't need help anyway and that I am suddenly infinitely more intelligent than any therapist. I remain to an extent nervous of how CBT will be able to help me as I inevitably encounter depressive episodes in the future, as it requires self-confidence and analytical abilities that seem to desert me utterly when I'm depressed.

I'd also like to make the point that throughout this period I have also been seeing various psychiatrists to monitor the mood stabilizing medications I am on. Our sessions also involve communication though it is mainly restricted to discussion of the efficacy of medication. However, there is seemingly little or no cooperation or communication between the different personnel involved in my treatment, a situation which is not helped by the fact that both are on six-month rotations. It is left to me to try and keep the other informed of any significant goings on; they don't even share a single file for me. And of course each change in personnel involves a new period of attempting to establish a relationship, which each time feels like a potentially retrograde step.

I have reread what I have written above and would like to try and draw some conclusions. Although my experiences are as for any individual unique, I suspect they are not particularly unusual, and I have in fact been fortunate in the access to talking therapies I have had. However, the most important aspect is not the specific approach taken but the relationship of trust and security and mutual respect established. Acknowledging the reality and validity of the clients' experiences and life-situation, their key social and family relationships is crucial. What having a specific approach then contributes is that the therapist can provide an explicit framework of aims and outcomes, which the client can understand and hopefully buy into, thereby gaining joint ownership of the therapeutic relationship.

Conclusion

This chapter has described a range of psychosocial interventions and the requirements of the therapeutic relationship between staff and clients for these interventions to be effective. Case studies and a personal account of the experiences of receiving talking therapies have been used to illustrate psychosocial interventions in practice. The evidence base for these interventions is growing though it is clear that these interventions will not work equally effectively for everybody. It is also clear that the implementation of these complex, resource intensive interventions within routine practice remains an ongoing challenge. High quality training and expert clinical supervision within broader operational strategies that support psychosocial interventions are minimum requirements. The main points of the chapter are summarized below:

- A working alliance with a client is a prerequisite to the sensitive and effective application of evidence-based psychosocial interventions in clinical practice.
- The skills required by nurses to develop a working alliance with their patients can be learned and require practice.
- Rogerian principles are widely recognized as fundamental to the development of therapeutic relationships with clients. The challenge for nurses working in stressful health care settings is to demonstrate these principles in their everyday interactions with clients.
- Psychosocial interventions have been defined as formulation-driven interventions that ameliorate a user's or carer's problem associated with a psychosis, using an approach based on psychological principles or addressing a change in social circumstances.
- Formal assessment tools carefully selected and administered sensitively as part of assessment can be reassuring to clients because they demonstrate that mental health staff are seeking to identify and measure their problems accurately as a basis for care planning.
- Coping-strategy enhancement, self-monitoring and problem solving are psychological management approaches for psychosis, which draw upon techniques from educational interventions and cognitive behaviour therapy. They all assume that ambient stress, together with life events may trigger onset or relapse in some people.
- Current research evidence suggests that cognitive behaviour therapy approaches are a very promising intervention for those who experience psychosis, however, their efficacy has not yet been conclusively demonstrated.
- Research findings show conclusively that family work for psychosis can reduce relapse beyond the protection of medication, produces substantial long-term benefits for clients and provides families with skills to cope more effectively with their relative's illness.

Acknowledgements

The authors are indebted to all the users, carers and those whose reported experiences have helped shape this chapter, especially Jacqueline Curthoys for her sincere, humbling contribution.

Questions for reflection and discussion

Read Jacqueline's personal account of her experiences of talking therapies, together with the case studies in this chapter and take time to self-reflect and consider the following questions.

1   Am I willing to take time to listen, learn and communicate unambiguously with users, their significant others and my colleagues?

2   Do I promote positive attitudes, such as trustworthiness, warmth, caring, liking and respect in my interactions with clients?

3   Do I understand and encourage people to express their feelings and experiences?

4   Am I able to utilize the skills and the interventions described in this chapter? If not what attributes, support and guidance do I require to be able to do this?

Annotated bibliography

■ Rollnick, S., Miller, W. and Butler, C. (2008) *Motivational Interviewing in Healthcare: helping patients change behaviour.* New York: Guilford Press. This textbook translates complex psychological concepts into easy-to-understand terms that will support and guide health care practitioners in improving their consultations with patients. Practical examples and exercises make this book a powerful tool for use by health care practitioners and moves motivational interviewing (MI) into the realm of everyday health care practice. Though not focused solely on mental health problems this book provides a good generic introduction to motivational interviewing.

■ Gamble, C. and Brennan, G. (2006) *Working with Serious Mental Illness: A Manual for Clinical Practice* (2nd edn). London: Elsevier. Now in its second edition this popular textbook reflects the changing nature and evolution of health care. It provides a comprehensive overview of the basis for psychosocial interventions and includes chapters that deal in detail with cognitive behavioural approaches and family interventions. The book seeks to guide, plan and suggest down-to-earth ideas for individuals working with clients on a day-to-day basis.

■ Romme, M. and Escher, S. (2000) *Making Sense of Voices: A guide for mental health professionals working with voice hearers.* London: MIND Publications. This three-part easy to follow manual complements the discussion surrounding many of the interventions referred to in this chapter. The first coherently explains why it is necessary for mental health practitioners to develop new approaches to working with those who hear voices. The second provides step-by-step guidance as to how to interview clients and third, it describes the interventions that can help voice hearers learn how to deal with their experiences, in the short, medium and long term. Finally the appendices contain numerous user-friendly assessment tools.

■ Birchwood, M., Fowler, D. and Jackson, C. (2000) *Early Intervention in Psychosis: A guide to concepts, evidence and interventions.* London: Wiley. This book helps to challenge the belief that early onset schizophrenia is hard to treat. It contains three parts, which cover the concept of early intervention, related strategies and their implementation.

References

Andreasen, N. (1982) Negative symptoms in schizophrenia: definition and reliability. *Archives of General Psychiatry* **39**: 784–8.

Baker, S. and Strong, S. (2001) *Roads to Recovery: How People with Mental Health Problems Recover and Find Ways of Coping.* London: MIND Publications.

Barrowclough, C. and Tarrier, N. (1992) *Families of Schizophrenic Patients: Cognitive Behavioural Intervention.* London: Chapman & Hall.

Birchwood, M., Smith, J. and Cochrane, R. (1990) The Social Functioning Scale: the development and validation of a new scale of social adjustment for use in family interventions programmes with schizophrenic patients. *British Journal of Psychiatry* **157**: 853–9.

Bostrom, R.N. (1997) The process of listening, in O. Hargie (ed.) *The Handbook of Communication Skills,* 2nd edn. London: Routledge.

Brooker, C. (2001) A decade of evidence-based training for work with people with serious mental health problems: Progress in the development of psychosocial interventions. *Journal of Mental Health* **10**: 17–31.

Brown, G. and Rutter, M. (1966) The measurement of family activities and relationships: a methodological study. *Human Relations* **19**: 241–63.

Brown, G., Birley, J. and Wing, J. (1972) Influence of family life on the course of schizophrenic disorder. *British Journal of Psychiatry* **121**: 241–58.

Campbell, A. (2000) Evaluation of the West Midlands family intervention programme. Working with Families – Making it a Reality Conference. Stratford-upon-Avon, 20/21 March.

Carhill, J. (1998) Patient participation: a concept analysis. *Journal of Advanced Nursing* **24**(3): 119–28.

Chadwick, P. and Birchwood, M. (1994) The omnipotence of voices; a cognitive approach to auditory hallucinations. *British Journal of Psychiatry* **164**: 190–201.

Cormac, I., Jones, C. and Campbell, C. (2001) Cognitive behaviour therapy for schizophrenia (Cochrane Review), in *The Cochrane Library,* Issue 2, 2002. Oxford: Update Software.

Dennis, S. (2000) Professional considerations, in C. Gamble and G. Brennan (eds) *Working with Serious Mental Illness: A Manual for Clinical Practice.* London: Baillière Tindall.

Department of Health (1999) *A National Service Framework for Mental Health.* London: The Stationery Office.

Faddon, G. and Birchwood, M. (2002) British models for expanding family psychosocial education in routine practice, in H.P. Lefley and D.L. Johnson (eds) *Family Interventions in Mental Illness – International Perspectives.* Connecticut: Praeger Publishers.

Falloon, I.R.H. and Graham-Hole, V. (1994) *Comprehensive Management of Mental Disorders.* Buckingham Mental Health Service.

Falloon, I., Barbieri, L., Boggian, I. and Lamonaca, D. (2007) Problem solving training for schizophrenia: Rationale and review. *Journal of Mental Health* **16**: 553–68.

Fleet, M. (2004) Psychosocial interventions for people with serious mental illness, in S. Kirby *et al.* (eds) *Mental Health Nursing: Competencies for Practice.* Basingstoke: Palgrave Macmillan.

Furlong, M. and Leggatt, M. (1996) Reconciling the patient's right to confidentially and the families need to know. *Australian and New Zealand Journal of Psychiatry* **30**: 614–22.

Gamble, C. and Brennan, G. (2006) *Working with Serious Mental Illness: A Manual for Clinical Practice* (2nd edn). London: Elsevier.

Gould, R.A., Mueser, K.T., Bolton, E., Mays, V. and Go, D. (2001) Cognitive therapy for psychosis in schizophrenia: an effect size analysis. *Schizophrenia Research* **48**: 335–42.

Haddock, G. and Slade, P. (eds) (1996) *Cognitive Behavioural Interventions with Psychotic Disorders.* London: Routledge.

Hawton, K., Salkovskis, P.M., Kirk, L. and Clark, D. (1989) *Cognitive Behaviour Therapy for Psychiatric Problems.* Oxford: Oxford Medical Publications.

Haywood, P. and Bright, J.A. (1997) Stigma and mental illness: a review and critique. *Journal of Mental Health* **6**(4): 345–54.

Healy, H., Reader, D. and Midence, K. (2006) An introduction to and rationale for psychosocial interventions, in C. Gamble and G. Brennan (eds) *Working with Serious Mental Illness: A Manual for Clinical Practice.* London: Elsevier.

Herz, M. and Melville, C. (1980) Relapse in schizophrenia. *American Journal of Psychiatry* **137**: 801–12.

Hogg, L. (1996) Psychological treatment for negative symptoms, in G. Haddock and P. Slade (eds) *Cognitive Behavioural Interventions with Psychotic Disorders.* London: Routledge.

James, A. (2001) *Raising our Voices: An Account of the Hearing Voices Movement.* Gloucester: Handsell Publishing.

Kingdon, D.G. and Turkington, D. (1994) *Cognitive Behavioural Therapy for Schizophrenia.* Hove: Lawrence Erlbaum Associates.

Krawiecka, M., Goldberg, D. and Vaughn, M. (1977) A standardised psychiatric assessment scale for rating chronic psychotic patients. *Acta Psychiatrica Scandinavica* **55**: 299–308.

Kuipers, E., Garety, P., Fowler, D. *et al.* (1997) London-East Anglia randomised controlled trial of cognitive behavioural therapy for psychosis. I: effects of the treatment phase. *British Journal of Psychiatry* **171**: 319–27.

Leff, J. and Gamble, C. (1995) Developing a training for schizophrenia family work: Implications for its implementation into clinical practice, *International Journal of Mental Health* **24**(3): 76–88.

Mari, J.J., Adams, C.E. and Streiner, D. (1996) Family intervention for those with schizophrenia, in C. Adams, J. De Jesus Mari and P. White (eds) *Schizophrenia Module of the Cochrane Database of Systematic Reviews*, Issue 3. Oxford: The Cochrane Collaboration.

McQueen, A. (2000) Nurse-patient relationships and partnership in hospital care. *Journal of Clinical Nursing* **9**: 723–31.

Paley, G. and Shapiro, D. (2002) Lessons from psychotherapy research for psychological interventions for people with schizophrenia. *Psychology and Psychotherapy: Theory, Research and Practice* **75**: 5–17.

Pharoah, F., Mari, J. and Steiner, D. (2002) Family intervention. *Cochrane Database Systematic Review* (4).

Prochaska, J. and DiClemente, C. (1986) Toward a comprehensive model of change, in W. Miller and N. Heather (eds) *Treating addictive behaviours: processes of change*. New York: Plenum, pp. 3–27.

Rogers, C. (1983) *Freedom to Learn for the 80s*. Columbus: Merrill.

Romme, M. and Escher, S. (1993) *Accepting Voices*. London: MIND Publications.

Romme, M. and Escher, S. (2000) *Making Sense of Voices: A Guide for Mental Health Professionals Working with Voice Hearers*. London: MIND Publications.

Sellwood, W., Barrowclough, C., Tarrier, N. *et al.* (2001) Needs based cognitive behavioural family intervention for carers for patients suffering from schizophrenia: 12 month follow up. *Acta Psychiatrica Scandinavica* **104**: 346–55.

Snaith, P. (1993) Measuring anxiety and depression. *The Practitioner* **237**: 554–9.

Spencer, E., Murray, E. and Plaistow, J. (2000) Relapse prevention in early psychosis, in M. Birchwood, D. Fowler and C. Jackson (eds) *Early Intervention in Psychosis: A Guide to Concepts, Evidence and Interventions*. London: Wiley.

Tarrier, N. (1992) Management and modification of residual positive symptoms, in M. Birchwood and N. Tarrier (eds) *Innovations in the Psychological Management of Schizophrenia*. Chichester: Wiley.

Turkington, D., Kingdon, D. and Turner, T. (2002) Effectiveness of a brief cognitive behavioural therapy intervention in the treatment of schizophrenia. *British Journal of Psychiatry* **180**: 523–7.

Zwarenstein, M. and Bryant, W. (2002) Interventions to promote collaboration between nurses and doctors (Cochrane Review), in *The Cochrane Library*, Issue 2. Oxford: Update Software.

Zubin, J. and Spring, B. (1977) Vulnerability: a new view of schizophrenia. *Journal of Abnormal Psychology* **86**: 260–6.

CHAPTER 15

Physical health care and serious mental illness

Debbie Robson and Richard Gray

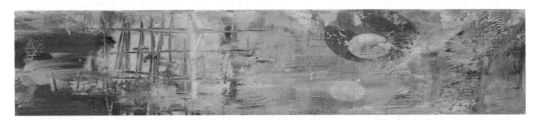

Chapter overview

- People with severe mental illness such as schizophrenia and bipolar disorder die at an early age due to poor physical health.
- Reasons for poor physical health in people with a severe mental illness include a complex interaction of health service related factors, health behaviours such as smoking and physical inactivity and the effects of psychotropic medication.
- We need to give equal priority to the risk assessment of physical health as we do to suicide and violence.
- Mental health workers can acquire the knowledge and skills to work collaboratively with service users to empower them to prevent and manage their own health.
- Interventions at the onset of people's illness could improve their physical health.
- Poor physical health is not inevitable.

Introduction

It has been estimated that the life expectancy of people with schizophrenia is reduced by 10 years (Newman and Bland 1991), although recent research suggests that this figure may have increased to 25 years (Parks *et al.* 2006). Suicide and accidents account for approximately 40 per cent of premature deaths in people with schizophrenia, whereas 60 per cent of premature deaths are as a result of physical health problems such as cardiovascular disease and diabetes (Brown 1997). These higher rates of morbidity and mortality do however need to be viewed within the context of a global increase in the rates of chronic diseases (Robson and Gray 2007).

Despite efforts over the past two decades to provide holistic and integrated health services for people with severe mental illness (SMI), the physical health care needs of this population have continued to be overlooked by both primary care and mental health practitioners in secondary care (Cohen and Hove 2001; Phelan *et al.* 2001). Mental health practitioners face the challenge of meeting service users mental health needs alongside their physical health needs.

To do this nurses need to understand the causes of physical health problems as well as feel confident in preventing, assessing, monitoring and managing potential and existing physical health conditions. The chapter begins by highlighting recent UK policy guidance about meeting the physical health care needs of people with SMI. We then discuss the physical health problems people with SMI experience and the reasons for this. Finally, we provide suggestions for risk assessment and management of physical health problems.

Policy

Recent health policy in the UK has included recommendations for the physical health care of people with SMI (DH 2005, 2006a). Guidelines from the National Institute for Health and Clinical Excellence for the treatment of schizophrenia in primary and secondary care (NICE 2002a) recommend that routine physical health checks should be carried out in primary care services. Where this is not possible either through service user choice or where the user has no general practitioner (GP), the responsibility for physical health monitoring must be taken up by secondary services. People admitted to psychiatric wards should also have physical health checks.

The Chief Nursing Officer for England's (CNO) review of mental health nursing (DH 2006a) emphasizes that mental health nurses must have the necessary skills to assess the physical health of service users and ensure that any identified needs are met. Following the CNO's review there is now guidance of the core competencies expected of mental health nurses at the point of registration (DH 2006b). Underpinning this focus on the physical assessment and intervention skills of the mental health nurse is the aspiration that service users should be viewed holistically rather than being seen fundamentally as recipients of treatment for a mental health problem (DH 2006a). This refocusing towards holistic health care delivery is central to the UK Government's drive to reduce health inequalities, support people to make informed healthy choices and improve partnership working across services (DH 2005). National guidelines exist for the management of diabetes (DH 2001), hypertension (NICE 2006) and coronary heart disease (DH 2000). Stakeholders need to think more broadly about the health of people with mental health disorders to ensure the rhetoric of holistic care becomes a reality.

What physical health conditions do people with SMI experience?

People with SMI have higher rates of cardiovascular disease than the general population; they also have higher than expected rates of infectious diseases, non-insulin dependant diabetes, respiratory diseases and some forms of cancers (Hippisley-Cox et al. 2007).

Cardiovascular disease

People with schizophrenia have rates of cardiovascular disease (CVD) two to three times higher than the general population (Brown et al. 2000; Osby et al. 2000). CVD includes conditions such as coronary heart disease, hypertension and high cholesterol and is caused by obesity, smoking, diabetes, lack of exercise and poor diet. These are all conditions and behaviours seen more commonly in people with SMI (Brown *et al.* 2000).

Respiratory disease

Up until 50 years ago respiratory diseases such as pneumonia and tuberculosis accounted for the majority of deaths among people with SMI who lived in institutions (Brown 1997). Respiratory diseases are still more prevalent in people with SMI, which are thought to result from high rates of smoking or passive smoking. People with SMI are more likely than the general population to suffer from asthma, chronic bronchitis and emphysema (Sokal *et al.* 2004).

Cancers

Researchers have consistently reported higher rates of digestive and breast cancer in people with schizophrenia. In a matched case control study of over 4 million patients registered with 454 general practices in the UK, patients with schizophrenia had a 42 per cent increased risk of breast cancer, and a 90 per cent increased risk of colorectal cancer (Hippisley-Cox *et al.* 2006). However, rates of lung cancer in people with schizophrenia are contradictory. The same study found a 46 per cent decreased risk of lung cancer (Hippisley-Cox *et al.* 2006). In a Danish sample of 9156 patients with schizophrenia, Mortensen (1994) found similar or lower rates compared with the general population, whereas Brown *et al.* (2000) and Lichtermann *et al.* (2001) both found mortality rates for lung cancer twice as high in people with schizophrenia than one would expect in the general population. Tobacco use is the single largest causative factor for lung cancer, followed by poor diet and physical inactivity.

Diabetes

Diabetes occurs in approximately 15 per cent of people with schizophrenia (Holt and Peveler 2006) and possibly even higher in people with mood disorders compared to approximately 5 per cent in the general population. It is influenced by a family history of diabetes, physical inactivity, poor diet, smoking and the metabolic effects of antipsychotic medication (Gough and Peveler 2004). The relationship between diabetes and schizophrenia has been discussed and investigated more than any other co-occurring physical and mental health problem. Controversy exists about how common diabetes is and its causes in people with SMI (Holt and Peveler 2006).

The association between schizophrenia and diabetes was first observed in the 1800s by the famous British psychiatrist Henry Maudsley (1897 cited by Koren 2004) who noted that 'diabetes is a disease which often shows itself in families in which insanity prevails'. Insulin resistance and glucose dysregulation have been observed in psychiatric patients since the 1920s (Koren 2004). We have therefore known that diabetes occurs independently of antipsychotic medication for over a century.

Reasons for poor physical health in people with SMI

There are many reasons why people with SMI have high rates of morbidity and mortality compared to the general population (Table 15.1).

Health behaviours	Smoking
	Diet
	Physical activity
	Alcohol and substance misuse
	Sexual behaviour
Illness	Positive symptoms
	Negative symptoms
	Cognitive and mood symptoms
	Poor spontaneous reporting of physical health problems
Health service	Lack of knowledge of mental health workforce
	Lack of training attitudes and confidence of mental health staff
	Attitudes of primary care staff
	Lack of integrated care
Adverse effects of medication	Extrapyramidal side effects
	Weight gain
	Glucose intolerance and diabetes
	Cardiovascular effects
	Sexual dysfunction
	Neuroleptic malignant syndrome
Environment	Poverty
	Poor housing
	Social exclusion

Table 15.1 Reasons for poor physical health in people with SMI
Source: Robson and Bragg, 2008

Health behaviours of people with SMI

The most commonly cited reasons for the increased rates of disease and death and in people with SMI are their high rates of smoking, poor diet, lack of exercise, co-morbid substance use and unsafe sexual practices (Lambert *et al.* 2003). In a survey of 102 service users with schizophrenia, McCreadie (2003) identified that 70 per cent were smokers, 86 per cent of women and 70 per cent of men were overweight, and 53 per cent had raised cholesterol, all significantly higher rates than in the general population. These behaviours are often referred in the literature as 'lifestyle choices'. Services users, however, would probably argue that these are not choices at all, but the physical, psychological, social and environmental consequences of having a severe mental illness and the treatments prescribed for them (Robson and Gray 2007).

Smoking

People with schizophrenia and bipolar disorder smoke up to three times more than the general population (Hughes *et al.* 1986; de Leon *et al.* 2002). They are heavier smokers, smoking, on average, more than 25 cigarettes a day (Kelly and McCreadie 2000) and are more likely to smoke high tar cigarettes. This population also experiences increased psychotic symptoms, more hospital admissions and higher doses of medication compared to service uses with schizophrenia who do not smoke. The reasons why people with SMI may have such high rates of smoking are well researched and include neurobiological, psychological, behavioural and social reasons. An increase in dopamine through inhaling nicotine has been shown to alleviate certain psychiatric symptoms (e.g. negative symptoms, cognitive dysfunction, side effects of antipsychotic medication) and therefore smoking has been viewed as a means of self-medication (Dalack *et al.* 1998). Smoking may also improve the attention and selective processing of information that is normally impaired in people with schizophrenia (Adler *et al.* 1998). Qualitative studies have found that people with schizophrenia smoke out of habit and routine, for relaxation purposes, as a way of making social contact, for pleasure and as a way of gaining control in their lives (Lawn *et al.* 2002). Smoking is ingrained in the culture of psychiatry. Health professionals often doubt this client group's motivation to stop smoking and promote smoking by using cigarettes to manage service users' behaviour (McNeill 2001).

Diet

Although the overall diet of the British public has improved in the past ten years, the consumption of fruit, vegetables, oily fish, wholegrain products and fibre are still below the recommended intake levels (Marriot and Buttris 2003). In a survey of the dietary habits of 102 people with SMI by McCreadie (2003), the average fruit and vegetable intake for these people was 16 portions a week, compared with recommended intake of 35 per week (DH 2004). In an American study of 146 outpatients with schizophrenia and schizoaffective disorder it was observed that service users ate a similar diet to the general population, but consumed significantly more calories (Strassnig *et al.* 2003). The physical health consequences of a poor diet include coronary heart disease, high blood pressure, diabetes, obesity, some cancers, osteoporosis and dental caries. Poor mental health outcomes in schizophrenia are associated with a diet high in saturated fat and unrefined sugar, whereas consumption of fish and sea food, particularly omega 3 fatty acids are associated with better outcomes (Peet 2004).

Physical activity

The World Health Organization (WHO) identifies physical inactivity as one of the leading causes of death in developed countries (2003). People with schizophrenia and bipolar disorder are less physically active than the general population (McCreadie 2003; Kilbourne *et al.* 2007) and are less likely to be encouraged to exercise by health workers (Kilbourne *et al.* 2007). In a cross-sectional survey of 120 service users with a mental illness, fatigue, mental health symptoms and lack of confidence were reported as the main barriers to regular exercise. Over half the respondents were positive about the benefits of exercise and said they were motivated to be more active (Ussher *et al.* 2007).

Health service factors

The physical health care needs of this population have long been overlooked by both primary care and mental health practitioners in secondary care (Phelan *et al.* 2001). This may be due to lack of clarity and guidance about whose role it is to assess and manage the physical health care of people with SMI. It may also be due to lack of training and the attitudes and confidence of the mental health workforce.

A retrospective case note review of 195 patients with schizophrenia, 390 matched controls with asthma and 390 matched general controls observed that service users with schizophrenia received less physical health checks from their primary care team than the matched controls (Roberts *et al.* 2006). The lack of assessment, monitoring and recording of the physical health status of people with SMI is also poor in mental health settings. Paton *et al.* (2004) reviewed case notes of 606 inpatients with SMI to determine if weight, cholesterol and triglycerides had been assessed during admission. Only 18 per cent (n=113) of patients had their weight recorded and 3.5 per cent (n =21) had their lipids monitored during their admission. In a survey of case notes of 63 patients in a community mental health service, 24 per cent (n=16) had their blood pressure (BP) recorded in the previous five years and 16 per cent (n=10) had their weight recorded (Greening 2005).

Nash's (2005) training needs analysis of 168 qualified mental health nurses in UK mental health trust found that 45 per cent (n=168) of mental health nurses had no formal training in physical health care, though 96 per cent (n=161) said they would be willing to attend a physical health training course. These nurses also reported lack of managerial support, staff shortages and lack of resources as potential barriers to attending training. Hyland *et al.* (2003) examined the attitudes and practice of 27 case managers working in Melbourne, Australia. Although 90 per cent of the sample believed that they had responsibility to improve the physical health care of people with SMI on their caseloads, a third of the sample believed that physical health needs were of secondary importance to mental health needs. Hyland *et al.* (2003) also reported that case managers did not systematically review health behaviours of the people on their caseloads, with preventative health checks receiving less attention.

Illness-related factors

In addition to health behaviours and the limitations of health services, we need to take into account the effect of severe mental illness on help seeking behaviour. It has been suggested that people with schizophrenia are less likely to report physical symptoms spontaneously (Jeste *et al.* 1996). They may be unaware of physical problems because of the cognitive deficits associated with the schizophrenia (Phelan *et al.* 2001), because of a high pain tolerance (Dworkin 1994) or due to reduced pain sensitivity associated with antipsychotic medication (Jeste *et al.* 1996).

Treatment-related factors

Effective treatment of mental illness relies upon a clearly thought-out package of multi-disciplinary care involving pharmacological and psychosocial interventions. Psychotropic medication is vital and necessary for the acute management of psychosis, mania and severe depression. It also plays an essential role in promoting recovery. Mental health professionals need to share information with service users and their carers about the benefits and risks of medication. Psychotropic medication is associated with weight gain, glucose dysregulation, sexual dysfunction and many other adverse effects. Antipsychotics, mood stabilizers and antidepressants have all been linked with weight gain. Clozapine has the greatest potential to cause weight gain followed by olanzapine, then quetiapine and risperidone (Taylor *et al.* 2007). Haloperidol and amisulpride are associated with a low risk of weight gain and aripiprazole may be weight neutral (Taylor *et al.* 2007).

Typical antipsychotics, in particular the low potency ones such as chlorpromazine, may induce or make existing diabetes worse (Newcomer *et al.* 2002). With regard to the atypical antipsychotics, clozapine and olanzapine have been most frequently associated with new onset or exacerbating type 2 diabetes, not just through their propensity to cause greater weight gain than other newer agents but because of their effects on glucose regulation (Newcomer *et al.* 2002). There are case reports linking respiridone and quetiapine to impaired glucose intolerance, diabetes and ketoacidosis (Taylor *et al.* 2007). Although research on the use of antipsychotics and its association with diabetes is copious, some argue that the quality of the research is methodologically weak and at this point in time more controlled prospective studies are needed before a definite causal link between antipsychotics and diabetes is confirmed (Holt and Peveler 2006).

The adrenergic and anticholinergic effects of antipsychotic medication affect sexual functioning and the antagonism of dopamine caused by antipsychotics in the tuberinfundibular part of the brain leads to hyperprolactinaemia (raised levels of the hormone prolactin). A consequence of raised prolactin levels is a decrease in testosterone in both men and women leading to sexual dysfunction and a decrease in oestrogen in women. Most studies have shown that the older antipsychotics are associated with a two- to tenfold increase in prolactin levels and usually develop over the first week of treatment and remain high throughout the period of use. Once treatment stops, prolactin levels return to normal within two to three weeks (Hummer and Huber 2004). The atypicals that have been associated with increased levels are amisulpride and risperidone (Halbreich and Kahn 2003). There are numerous clinical effects of hyperprolactinaemia seen in people with SMI who are taking antipsychotic medication. Women experience amenorrhea, disturbed menstrual cycle and anovulation. Both men and women experience galactorrhoea (leaking milk from the breasts) and gynaecomastia (painful and swollen breasts and sexual dysfunction (Dickson and Glazer 1999; Halbreich and Kahn 2003). There is contradictory evidence that the reduction in oestrogen caused by raised prolactin levels are associated with increased rates of breast cancer (Halbreich *et al.* 1996) and osteoporosis (Halbreich and Palter 1996).

Table 15.2 summarizes some of the common side effects of antipsychotic medication and gives some suggestions of how to assess and manage them.

Medication related side effect	Presentation	Assessment	Management (treatment options include)
Pseudo-parkinsonism	Tremor, rigidity, slow thinking, slow movements, stumbling gait, mask like expression.	Liverpool University Neuroleptic Rating Scale (LUNSERS) (Day et al. 1995). Simpson and Angus Scale (Simpson and Angus 1970)	Reduce dose. If patient is taking a typical antipsychotic, change to a atypical. Prescribe an anticholinergic and review regularly. Repeat measures following a change in medication or every 6 months (Taylor et al. 2007)
Acute or tardive dystonia	Muscle spasm in any part of the body (e.g. head and neck twisted, eyes rolling backwards, forceful rapid blinking. Laryngeal and pharyngeal muscles may go into spasm leading to difficulty in swallowing and speaking.	Acute: Observation and patient self report Tardive: Dystonia Movement Scale (Simpson et al. 1979)	Administer oral, intramuscular or intra venous anticholinergic medication, depending on the severity of symptoms (Taylor et al 2007).
Acute or tardive akathisia	Subjective: patient reports they feel an inner sense of restlessness, mental unease, an irresistible urge to move, tension and discomfort in the limbs. Objective: lower limb movements, e.g. rocking from foot to foot, walking on the spot, pacing up and down.	Rating Scale for Drug Induced Akathisia (Barnes 1989)	Reduce antipsychotic dose. Change to an atypical. Anticholinergic medication is not recommended. Repeat Rating Scale for Drug Induced Akathisia following change in medication regime (Taylor et al. 2007).

⇨

Medication related side effect	Presentation	Assessment	Management (treatment options include)
Tardive dyskinesia	A wide range of abnormal movements, e.g. tongue protrusion, lip smacking, chewing, choreiform hand movements, pelvic movements, patient may have problems eating and breathing (Gray *et al.* 2005).	Abnormal Involuntary Movement Scale (AIMS) (Guy 1976)	Stop anticholinergic if prescribed. Reduce dose of antipsychotic. Change to an atypical drug. Prescribe tetrabenazine (only licensed treatment for tardive dyskinesia in the UK). Repeat AIMS following change in medication regime (Taylor *et al.* 2007).
Changes in blood pressure Postural hypotension Hypertension	Optimal blood pressure (BP) is <120/80 mmHg. A fall in BP of 20 mmHg or more from a sitting to standing position (NICE 2006). Patient may complain of a headache, feeling faint, light headed. Persistent or repeated BP of >140/90 mmHg. Patient will often have no subjective symptoms though may experience headache and dizziness.	Patient interview of subjective symptoms. Take BP lying/sitting and standing. Patient interview of subjective symptoms. Take BP sitting.	Measure blood pressure before medication is prescribed. Ensure the patient is well hydrated. Educate patient about minimizing symptoms, e.g. avoiding alcohol, heavy meals, prolonged periods of lying down, long periods of standing still, hot showers. Switch to an atypical with low propensity to cause postural hypotension. Monitor BP regularly. Lifestyle interventions: Regular physical activity can reduce BP by 2–3 mmHg. Healthy, low calorie and low sodium diets can reduce BP by 3–6 mmHg. Help the patient to reduce any excessive alcohol and caffeine use. If BP is persistently high, the patient may need antihypertensive drug treatment. Medical care and the choice of medication for newly diagnosed hypertension should be informed by the NICE guideline for the management of hypertension (NICE 2006). ⇨

Medication related side effect	Presentation	Assessment	Management (treatment options include)
Sedation	Drowsiness, somnolence	Before prescribing medication assess sleep history and current sleep pattern.	Reassure that some sedation in the first couple of weeks of treatment may be expected and tolerance may develop. If sedation persists consider giving medication in divided doses/smaller doses in the morning or before bedtime. If the patient does not need the sedative effects of the medication consider switching to a less sedative drug.
Anticholinergic effects	Dry mouth, blurred vision, constipation	LUNSERS (Day *et al.* 1995) Patient self report Ensure that patients have regular dental check ups.	High fibre diet, plenty of fluids, sugar free gum. Good oral hygiene.
Weight gain	Significant weight gain from medication is defined as ≥7 per cent of baseline weight.	Prior to prescribing medication weigh patient calculate body mass index (weight in kg ÷ height in m²) BMI over 25 kg/m² = overweight BMI over 30 kg/m² = obese measure waist circumference (place the tape measure around the waist at the navel level). The waist circumference measurement at which there is an increased risk is defined as ≥94 cm for men and	Take a proactive approach to prevent weight gain through lifestyle advice. Educate patients about food labelling and how to plan meals. Consider switching to a drug that may cause less weight gain. Weigh monthly for the first 6 months of treatment, then every 3 months. Monitor BMI and waist circumference at the same time. Encourage patients to monitor their own weight and waist circumference in between appointments.

⇨

Medication related side effect	Presentation	Assessment	Management (treatment options include)
		≥80 cm for women (Lean *et al.* 1995). Food diaries are helpful to assess the type and amount of food the patient is eating.	
Glucose intolerance/ insulin resistance/ diabetes	Increased thirst, increased hunger (especially after meals) frequent urination, dry mouth, blurred vision, fatigue, slow healing wounds, repeated yeast infections, tingling in hands and feet.	Prior to prescribing medication carry out an assessment of known risk factors, i.e. family history of diabetes, obesity, sedentary lifestyle, hypertension; ethnic risk factors also include people from Asian and African-Caribbean origins. Patient's prescribed antipsychotic medication should have their plasma glucose levels monitored at baseline, every three months and then every 6 months if stable (Taylor *et al.* 2007).	Proactive approach is needed. Educate patient and carers about preventative strategies (e.g. dietary and lifestyle advice). Educate patients and carers in high risk groups about signs of diabetes and ketoacidosis (rapid onset of increased thirst, increased hunger, frequent urination, vomiting, abdominal pain, dehydration). Encourage patients and carers to report symptoms.

Medication related side effect	Presentation	Assessment	Management (treatment options include)
Hyperprolactinea-mia (raised prolactin levels)	Sexual dysfunction in men and women (e.g. reduced libido, ejaculatory and orgasmic dysfunction). Amenorrhea, lactation and painful swollen breasts (men and women).	Prior to prescribing medication -Take a sexual history and a menstrual history for women. - Rule out physiological causes. - During treatment assess for emerging symptoms of sexual dysfunction. - Useful validated questionnaires include the Psychotropic Related Sexual Dysfunction Questionnaire (Montejo & Rico-Villademoros, 2008). Serum prolactin levels can be taken if symptoms evident.	Reduce dose of antipsychotic. Switch to a prolactin sparing antipsychotic. Health promotion advice, e.g. the benefits of breast self examination, contraceptive advice. Regular monitoring for emerging or ongoing signs of sexual dysfunction using assessment tools.
Neuroleptic malignant syndrome	Rigidity, fever, sweating, fluctuating blood pressure, tachycardia, confusion	Take temperature, pulse, BP. Bloods to be taken for creatine kinase and liver function.	Stop antipsychotic – Monitor temperature, pulse, BP. Rehydrate the patient. Liaise with medical colleagues. Closely monitor patients temperature, pulse and BP when antipsychotic is re reintroduced. ⇨

Table 15.2 Medication side-effect assessment and management

> ## What can nurses and other mental health practitioners do to improve the physical health of people with serious mental illness?

Risk assessment

Risk assessment of suicide and violence has, quite rightly, dominated mental health care for the past two decades. However, one could argue that the increased focus of assessing and managing suicide and violence has contributed to the lack of focus on physical health risk. People with SMI are more likely to die at an earlier age than the general population from a physical illness than they are from suicide (Hansen *et al.* 2001). We need to give equal priority to the risk assessment of physical health as we do to suicide and violence.

Cardiovascular risk

The main non-modifiable risk factors are older age, gender and family history (Table 15.3). Over 83 per cent of people who die of coronary heart disease are 65 or older (American Heart Association (AHA) 2007). Men have a greater risk of heart attack than women, and they have attacks earlier in life. Even after the menopause, when women's death rate from heart disease increases, it is not as great as men's (AHA 2007). Modifiable risk factors are prevalent in people with schizophrenia. Mental health workers, service users and carers can share the responsibility and work in partnership to address these.

Cardiovascular risk factors		
	Modifiable	Non-modifiable
■ Tobacco smoke	■ Diabetes	■ Older age
■ Obesity	■ Dyslipidaemia	■ Gender (male)
■ Physical inactivity	■ Hypertension	■ Family history

Table 15.3 Risk factors for developing cardiovascular disease (adapted from AHA, 2008)

Assessing risk from tobacco smoke

Ask all service users about their smoking status and assess their level of dependence. The Fagerstrom Test for Nicotine Dependence (Table 15.4) (Heatherton *et al.* 1991) is a quick and reliable way of measuring levels of tobacco dependence. It comprises six questions which take just a few minutes to answer. Scores, which range from 0–10, identify varying levels of nicotine dependence, and feedback linked to the respondent's score (shown in Table 15.4). Assessing nicotine dependence is particularly important since tobacco smoke interacts with psychotropic medication.

When the service user is not acutely ill, or in a state of relapse, their readiness to quit can be assessed. Simply ask how ready the person is to quit: i.e. not ready, unsure or ready. Some service users will not be interested in stopping, others will be ambivalent and some people will be keen. Interventions can then be tailored to the person's stage of readiness.

Fagerstrom Test for Nicotine Dependence *

Is smoking 'just a habit' or are you addicted? Take this test and find out your level of dependence on nicotine.

1. How soon after you wake up do you smoke your first cigarette?

◆ After 60 minutes	(0)
◆ 31–60 minutes	(1)
◆ 6–30 minutes	(2)
◆ Within 5 minutes	(3)

2. Do you find it difficult to refrain from smoking in places where it is forbidden?

| ◆ No | (0) |
| ◆ Yes | (1) |

3. Which cigarette would you hate most to give up?

| ◆ The first in the morning | (1) |
| ◆ Any other | (0) |

4. How many cigarettes per day do you smoke?

◆ 10 or less	(0)
◆ 11–20	(1)
◆ 21–30	(2)
◆ 31 or more	(3)

5. Do you smoke more frequently during the first hours after awakening than during the rest of the day?

| ◆ No | (0) |
| ◆ Yes | (1) |

6. Do you smoke even if you are so ill that you are in bed most of the day?

| ◆ No | (0) |
| ◆ Yes | (1) |

* Heatherton, T.F., Kozlowski, L.T., Frecker, R.C. and Fagerstrom, K.O. (1991) The Fagerstrom Test for Nictoine Dependence: A revision of the Fagerstrom Tolerance Questionnaire. *British Journal of Addictions* **86**: 1119–27.

Click for score:

Your score was: . Your level of dependence on nicotine is: .

0–2 Very low dependence	6–7 High dependence
3–4 Low dependence	8–10 Very high dependence
5 Medium dependence	

[Scores under 5: 'Your level of nicotine dependence is still low. You should act now before your level of dependence increases.'
[Score of 5: 'Your level of nicotine dependence is moderate. If you don't quit soon, your level of dependence on nicotine will increase until you may be seriously addicted. Act now to end your dependence on nicotine.'
[Score over 7: 'Your level of dependence is high. You aren't in control of your smoking – it is in control of you! When you make the decision to quit, you may want to talk with your doctor about nicotine replacement therapy or other medications to help you break your addiction.'

Table 15.4 Fagerstrom test for nicotine dependence

Assessing risk of obesity

Body mass index (BMI) indicates if a person is a healthy weight in relation to their height. It is calculated by dividing a person's weight (in kilograms (kg) by their height (in metres squared). The healthy range is 18.5–24. People who have a BMI of 25 and over are considered to be overweight and those with a BMI of 30 and over are considered to be obese (World Health Organization 2003). There is contradictory evidence about whether people with SMI have higher rates of obesity than the general population (Wirshing and Meyer 2003). However, it is also recognized increasingly that people with SMI have higher rates of upper body obesity (i.e. visceral fat), which is more of a risk factor for developing metabolic complications than overall body fat (Ryan and Thakore 2001). Waist measurement can help to identify people at high risk of developing CVD and diabetes. Waist circumference should be measured at the level of the umbilicus. A waist circumference of more than 40 inches in men and 35 inches in women is thought to indicate a greater risk (Lean *et al.* 1995).

Assessing risk of diabetes

There are two main types of diabetes, type 1 and type 2. In type 1 the pancreas can no longer produce insulin because the insulin producing cells have usually been destroyed by the body's immune system. Type 1 has a rapid onset, usually days or weeks. In type 2 the insulin cells are not able to produce sufficient insulin or the body does not use it properly. Type 2 diabetes has a much slower onset. It often goes undiagnosed for 9–12 years (DH 2001). In the meantime prolonged exposure to raised blood glucose causes visual impairment and blindness, damage to kidneys, which can lead to renal failure, damage to nerves which can lead to loss of sensation in feet, foot or leg ulcers and finally amputation (DH 2001).

There is no clear consensus on testing for diabetes in patients with SMI. Initial testing should be carried out when service users first come in to contact with mental health services regardless of risk factors and presentation. Fasting plasma glucose (FPG) level is considered the optimum test, though this might be impractical for some service users. A random plasma glucose would be the best option in this case. This should be followed up by an oral glucose tolerance test if the FPG is ≥6.9mmol/L (≥126mg/dL) or the random plasma glucose is between 7.0mmol/L (126mg/dL) – 11mmol/L (200mg/dL) (Barnett *et al.* 2007). Fasting plasma glucose levels should be checked every six months or more frequently in service users if patients are gaining weight (Barnett *et al.* 2007). Service users should be asked about and observed for symptoms of diabetes, i.e. excessive thirst (polydipsia), frequent urination (polyuria), constant eating (polyphagia), fatigue and dizziness.

Assessing risk of dyslipidaemia

Too much cholesterol and triglycerides in the blood is one of the many risk factors for CVD and is influenced by health behaviours such as diet and smoking. Elevated levels of total cholesterol and low density lipoprotein (LDL) cholesterol and triglyceride and low levels of high density lipoprotein (HDL) cholesterol are independent risk factors for developing coronary heart disease. Both typical and atypical antipsychotics have been shown to have an effect on triglyceride and cholesterol levels with olanzapine and clozapine appearing to have the most impact (Taylor *et al.* 2007).

All service users should have their lipid levels measured before they are started on medication. Service users prescribed clozapine, olanzapine, quetiapine or phenothiazines should have their lipids measured every three months for the first year of treatment (Taylor *et al.* 2007). Those prescribed other antipsychotics should have them measured after three months and then annually (Taylor *et al.* 2007). Fasting lipid profiles will give the most accurate and reliable measurement, however, random levels are better than no levels from service users who may be too mentally unwell to comply with fasting requirements.

Assessing risk of hypertension

Blood pressure (BP) should be monitored routinely with all service users. Clozapine is associated with a sharp rise in BP when it is initiated and occasionally throughout treatment. Optimum blood pressure is <120/< 80 mmHg (NICE 2006). NICE guidelines on the management of hypertension in adults (NICE 2006) recommend the following when measuring blood pressure:

■ Where possible, standardize the environment, which should be warm, quiet and relaxed. The patient should be seated with their arm outstretched and supported.
■ Measure BP on both the patient's arms and use the arm with the higher value as the reference arm for future measurements.
■ If the first measurement exceeds 140/90 mmHg a second reading should be taken.
■ To identify hypertension (a persistent raised BP of above 140/90 mmHg) – check the BP on two more separate occasions (and twice on each occasion).
■ Devices for measuring BP should regularly maintained and calibrated.

Antihypertensive treatment is recommended for patients who have a persistent systolic BP of ≥160 mmHg and/or a persistent diastolic BP of ≥100 mmHg. If service users have other cardiovascular risk factors such as diabetes, treatment should be offered if they have a systolic BP of ≥140 mmHg and/or a diastolic BP of ≥90 mmHg (NICE 2006).

Assessing cancer risk

Screening programmes may be effective in detecting cancer early but the uptake of these programmes by patients with SMI is lower than in the general population. For example, in an American study of 46 women with schizophrenia aged 44–72, less than half of the women reported receiving one or more gender-specific preventive screenings within the past year: pelvic examination (45.7 per cent), pap test (43.5 per cent), or mammogram (41.3 per cent), and just over one third received none of the screenings. This was despite the majority being in receipt of regular medical and mental health care (Lindamer *et al.* 2006). The NHS Breast Screening Programme in the UK provides free breast screening every three years for all women aged 50 to 70 years of age. Also women between the ages of 25 and 64 are eligible for a free cervical screening test every three to five years. In July 2006 the NHS Bowel Cancer Screening Programme was introduced in England. This offers screening every two years to all men and women aged 60 to 69. Nurses and other mental health workers should ask service users if they have received routine screening to which they are entitled. If service users are reluctant to attend for screening appointments, it may be helpful to explore why. It may be they are unaware of the necessity or have fears about the examinations. Mental health workers can then help to facilitate attendance at screening appointments.

Interventions

Service users can adopt healthier lifestyles when interventions are tailored specifically to meet the complex needs associated with having a mental illness. Lifestyle interventions to improve overall health should be integrated into routine mental health care and should begin when the service user first comes into contact with mental health services (Robson and Gray 2007). Most mental health services have access to dieticians, physiotherapists and smoking cessation specialists. Mental health practitioners could actively collaborate with these professionals to design specialist health promotion programmes for people with SMI. There are also many simple interventions that mental health workers can incorporate into routine practice.

Healthy eating

We probably know from our own diets that simply giving people information about the type of foods to eat and avoid has little impact on sustained change. Food choices for people with SMI are influenced not only by individual choice but also by: the cost and affordability of food; access to kitchen equipment and storage; skills and confidence in budgeting, shopping and cooking; and knowledge of nutrition. It makes sense to start by helping service users sort out practical problems they may have with kitchen equipment, storage and accessibility of food. Clinical experience suggests it is not uncommon to visit a new service user at home to discover they do not have a fridge or cooker. Acquiring skills and confidence in budgeting, shopping and cooking could be done in partnership with other members of the multi-disciplinary team, such as occupational therapists and support workers. Educational information about nutrition and portion sizes can be shared with people in a way that is understandable and meaningful to people with SMI. There are many readable and easy to follow educational leaflets (for example, those produced by the British Heart Foundation) that are freely available to members of the public. Diets that are low in sugar, simple carbohydrates and saturated fat and high in whole grain products, complex carbohydrates, fibre, fruit, vegetables and omega 3 fatty acids should be encouraged. Some people may need practical help with how to modify eating habits, for example suggesting recipes and menu plans and how to read food labels. Clinical experience also suggests that creative solutions need to be found for service users on inpatient units who order in extra food from local take-aways to meet their increased appetite and compensate for lack of alternative food options.

There is increasing evidence that suggest both simple and more long-term interventions can have a positive impact on service users' health outcomes. A study by Wirshing et al. (2006) demonstrated increased knowledge about nutrition and healthy lifestyles following a single 30-minute education programme for inpatients with schizophrenia. In a nurse-led study by Vreeland et al. (2003) a 12-week programme that incorporated nutritional education, motivational counselling, cognitive, behavioural and exercise interventions, clients lost 2.7 kg in weight compared to a matched control group who put on weight.

Regular physical activity

Historically exercise and physical activity were integral to mental health institutional care and given the same priority as the relief of psychiatric symptoms. A number of studies have demonstrated the positive benefits of exercise on mental health. Faulkner and Sparkes (1999) conducted an ethnographic study that examined the influence of exercise as a therapy for schizophrenia. They reported that a ten week exercise programme of twice-weekly sessions appeared to help reduce participants' perceptions of auditory hallucinations, raise self-esteem, improve sleep patterns and general behaviour.

For general health benefits, adults need to achieve at least 30 minutes of moderately intense activity on at least five days per week (DH 2004). Service users may need an explanation of what is meant by moderate intensity (i.e. working hard enough to be breathing more heavily than normal, becoming slightly warmer but still able to talk). People also may need explanations of the different types of exercise available to improve and maintain overall health. For example, endurance or aerobic activities that improve cardiovascular health could include brisk walking, cycling, jogging, swimming and dancing. Activities for improving flexibility and mobility could include gardening, housework and walking. Strengthening exercises can improve balance, muscle tone, bone health and increase the rate at which the body burns calories, and can be achieved by climbing stairs, carrying shopping or walking uphill. Most inpatient mental health services have access to gyms and physical training instructors, and mental health workers can act as a link between such services. Building confidence in a hospital gym may help people feel more at ease with accessing public gyms once discharged, while acquiring tailored information about the best way to exercise. For those people who lack the confidence, motivation and finances to attend public gyms there are still many ways of increasing one's activity that can be incorporated into people's lives without any disruption or much more organization or effort. For example, breaking up the period of exercise into three ten-minute bouts of brisk walking throughout the day is initially more appealing than 30 minutes all at once and more manageable for inpatient staff trying to promote healthy behaviours on busy acute wards. Mental health workers can help people with SMI explore their beliefs about exercise and help people problem solve barriers to increasing activity.

Smoking cessation

Nicotine replacement therapy (NRT) is the most widely used drug to aid smoking cessation. There are many products to choose from including skin patches, chewing gum, lozenges, sublingual microtablets, nasal spray and inhalators. As all NRT products have similar success rates (NICE 2002b) the choice between them is a practical and personal one. Two drugs that do not replace nicotine but help the smoker by other mechanisms are buproprion and verenicline. Bupropion is an antidepressant and a nicotine antagonist. It is thought to act via doperminergic and noradrenergic pathways. Buprorion is known to lower the seizure threshold and induce mania so needs to be used with caution in service users with a history of seizures or mood disorder and also with medication that lowers the seizure threshold (NICE 2002b). Verenicline is the newest drug to be licensed specifically for smoking cessation and reduces the strength of the urge to smoke and the satisfaction from smoking, as well as withdrawal symptoms. There is currently no published evidence of the use of verenicline in patients with serious mental illness. NICE (2002b, 2007) have published guidelines on the use of NRT, buproprion and verenicline, which are estimated to double the chance of people in the general population quitting smoking. Access to support from a smoking cessation specialist further increases people's chances of successfully quitting (West *et al.* 2000).

A ban on smoking in public places including hospital and health care facilities is being introduced across Europe and America as a public health strategy to encourage people to stop smoking. The implementation of this ban in mental health facilitates has been contentious (Campion *et al.* 2006) and there appears to be a significant amount of resistance and scepticism, particularly from nurses about implementing the ban (Dickens *et al.* 2004). However, there is growing evidence that people with schizophrenia are able to stop smoking when given the opportunity to participate in smoking cessation programmes that are tailored specifically to meet the biological, cognitive, affective and social challenges this raises. A number of controlled and uncontrolled trials have evaluated the impact of smoking cessation packages for people with schizophrenia (e.g. George *et al.* 2002; Baker *et al.* 2006). Successful interventions combine atypical antipsychotic medication with either nicotine replacement therapy (NRT) or bupropion, in addition to psychological interventions, e.g. cognitive behaviour therapy or motivational interviewing. Quit rates at six months were 11–18.8 per cent for buproprion and psychological support, and 10–16 per cent for NRT and psychological support. These trials found no evidence of an increase in positive symptoms or extrapyramidal side effects. Although these interventions are more complex than those offered by mainstream smoking cessation clinics and do not reach the same quit rates as those in the general population, these results offer hope to people with schizophrenia who wish to stop smoking.

Service users who are prescribed certain psychotropic medicines need to be made aware of the effect smoking and smoking cessation has on the metabolism of their prescribed medication and the potential clinical effects of this. Some antipsychotics drugs (e.g. chlorpromazine, haloperidol, clozapine and olanzapine) are metabolized primarily by a liver enzyme (cytochrome P-450 1A2). Cigarette smoke increases the activity of this particular enzyme. This results in reduced plasma levels of these medicines in patients who smoke compared to non-smokers (Desai *et al.* 2001). There is evidence that smokers compared to non-smokers are prescribed higher doses of clozapine and olanzapine (Rostami-Hodjegan *et al.* 2004) perhaps as a way of compensating for this clinical effect. When a service user prescribed chlorpromazine, haloperidol, clozapine and olanzapine stops smoking, the activity of the liver enzyme (cytochrome P-450 1A2) slows down. Plasma levels of these drugs will rise quite rapidly and have the potential to cause toxicity. Meyer (2001) retrospectively analysed changes in clozapine levels in 11 patients who were receiving stable clozapine doses before and after the implementation of a no smoking policy in a large psychiatric hospital. Following implementation of the policy a mean increase in clozapine plasma levels of 71 per cent was reported. Skogh *et al.* (1999) describe a case study of a 35-year-old man with schizophrenia who was treated successfully with 700 mg of clozapine for over seven years. Two weeks after abrupt smoking cessation he developed tonic-clonic seizures, stupor and coma, thought to be attributed to increased plasma levels of clozapine. Serious adverse events can be avoided by collaborative medication management with pharmacists and medical colleagues.

Conclusion

It is well established that people with SMI have higher rates of death and physical illness compared to the general population (Harris and Barrowclough 1998) and die at a younger age (Newman and Bland 1991; Parks *et al.* 2006). The causes of poor physical health in people with an SMI are complex and interactive. Not only has the physical health care of people with SMI been neglected in the past, the training health professionals receive to assess, monitor and manage physical health care in people with SMI has also been lacking. Mental health practitioners have an opportunity to improve the physical and mental health of people with SMI through risk assessment and collaborative health promotion interventions initiated at the onset of people's illness. Poor physical health in people with SMI does not have to be inevitable.

Questions for reflection and discussion

1   Make a list of physical health checks you routinely carry out with clients you work with. Reflect on whether you think this is comprehensive enough. Do you think there are any health checks that are missing from your routine practice? What do you think you can do to address this?
2   Find out what resources are available in your work place or local area that can help service users who want to lose weight, increase their level of activity or stop smoking. Are these services specifically tailored for people with mental health problems? How can you work alongside service users and their families to help them access these services? If there are not any services available how can you collaborate with specialist health practitioners to meet this need?
3   Identify areas of your physical health care practice that you feel confident about and the areas you feel less confident about. Can you identify any personal training needs around physical health care that you need to address? (Find out what is available locally and nationally to meet your training needs.)

Annotated bibliography

■   Barnett, A., Mackin, P., Chaudhry, I. *et al.* (2007) Minimizing metabolic and cardiovascular risk in schizophenia: diabetes, obesity and dyslipedaemia. *Journal of*

Psychopharmacology **21**(4): 357–73. This comprehensive review provides a framework for the assessment, monitoring and management of metabolic and cardiovascular risk factors for service users with schizophrenia in UK clinical settings.

- Meyer, J.M. and Nasrallah, H.A. (2003) *Medical Illness and Schizophrenia*. London: American Psychiatric Publishing. Written by the world's leading experts in physical health and schizophrenia, this book provides an evidence-based account of the causes and treatment of a range of physical health problems experienced by service users. It argues for the provision of integrated medical and mental health care as a way of meeting the longstanding unmet needs of people with schizophrenia.

- Phelan, M., Stradins, L., Amin, D. *et al.* (2004) The Physical Health Check: a tool for mental health workers. *Journal of Mental Health* **13**(3): 277–84. This article describes the development and evaluation of a brief checklist to assess the physical health needs of mental health service users. The tool was piloted with 60 mental health service users and detected a high level of unmet need. The authors report a favourable evaluation of the tool and continue to work on its further development.

References

Adler, L.E., Olincy, A., Waldo *et al.* (1998) Schizophrenia, sensory gating and nicotinic receptors. *Schizophrenia Bulletin* **24**(2): 189–202.

American Heart Association (2007) *Heart Disease and Stroke Statistics*. Dallas: Texas, AHA.

Baker, A., Richmond, R., Haile, M. *et al.* (2006) A randomised controlled trial of a smoking cessation intervention among people with a psychotic disorder. *American Journal of Psychiatry* **163**: 1934–42.

Barnes, T.R.E. (1989) A rating scale for drug induced akathisia. *British Journal of Psychiatry* **154**: 672–676.

Barnett, A., Mackin, P., Chaudhry, I. *et al.* (2007) Minimising metabolic and cardiovascular risk in schizophenia: diabetes, obesity and dyslipedaemia. *Journal of Psychopharmacology* **21**(4): 357–73.

Brown, S. (1997) Excess mortality of schizophrenia: a meta analysis. *British Journal of Psychiatry* **171**: 502–8.

Brown, S., Inskipp, H. and Barraclough, B. (2000) Causes of excess mortality of schizophrenia. *British Journal of Psychiatry* **177**: 212–17.

Campion, J., McNeill, A. and Checkinski, K. (2006) Exempting mental health units from smoke free laws. *British Medical Journal* **333**: 407–8.

Cohen, A. and Hove, M. (2001) Physical health of the severe and enduring mentally ill. London: Sainsbury Centre.

Dalack, G.W., Healy, D.J. and Meador-Woodruff, J.H. (1998) Nicotine dependence in schizophrenia: clinical phenomena and laboratory findings. *American Journal of Psychiatry* **155**: 1490–501.

Day, J.C., Wood, G., Dewey, M. and Bentall, R.P. (1995) A self rating scale for measuring neuroleptic side effects. Validation in a group of schizophrenia patients. *British Journal of Psychiatry* **166**(5): 650–3.

de Leon, J., Becona, E., Gurpegui, M., Gonzalez-Pinto, A. and Diaz, F.J. (2002) The association between high nicotine dependence and severe mental illness may be consistent across countries. *Journal of Clinical Psychiatry* **63**(9): 812–16.

Department of Health (2000) *Coronary Heart Disease: National Service Framework for Coronary Heart Disease – modern standards and service models*. London: HMSO.

Department of Health (2001) *Diabetes National Service Framework*. London: HMSO.

Department of Health (2004) *At Least 5 a Week*. London: HMSO.

Department of Health (2005) *Choosing Health: Making healthy choices easier*. London: DH.

Department of Health (2006a) *From Values to Action: The Chief Nursing Officer's Review of Mental Health Nursing*. London: DH.

Department of Health (2006b) *Best Practice Competencies and Capabilities for Pre-registration Mental Health Nurses in England: The Chief Nursing Officer's review of mental health nursing.* London: DH.

Desai, H.D., Seabolt, J. and Jann, M.W. (2001) Smoking in patients receiving psychotropic medications: a pharmacokinetic perspective. *CNS Drugs* **15**(6): 469–94.

Dickens, G.L., Stubbs, J.H. and Haw, C.M. (2004) Smoking and mental health nurses: a survey of clinical staff in a psychiatric hospital. *Journal of Psychiatric and Mental Health Nursing* **11**: 445–51.

Dickson, R.A. and Glazer, W.M. (1999) Neuroleptic-induced hyperprolactinaemia. *Schizophrenia Research* **35**: s75–s86.

Dworkin, R.H. (1994) Pain insensitivity in schizophrenia: neglected phenomena and some implications. *Schizophrenia Bulletin* **20**: 235–48.

Faulkner, G. and Sparkes, A. (1999) Exercise therapy for schizophrenia: An ethnographic study. *Journal of Sport and Exercise* **21**: 39–51.

George, T.P., Vessichio, J.C. and Tremine, A. (2002) A placebo controlled trial of buproprion for smoking cessation in schizophrenia. *Biological Psychiatry* 52: 53–61.

Gough, S. and Peveler, R. (2004) Diabetes and its prevention: pragmatic solutions for people with schizophrenia. *British Journal of Psychiatry* **184**(suppl 47): s106–s111.

Gray, R., Parr, A.M. and Robson, D. (2005) Has tardive dyskinesia disappeared? *Mental Health Practice* **8**(10): 20–2.

Greening, J. (2005) Physical health of patients in rehabilitation and recovery: a survey of case note records. *Psychiatric Bulletin* 29: 210–12.

Guy, W. (1976) ECDEU Assessment manual for psychopharmacology. Washington: Department of Health and Welfare.

Halbreich, U. and Kahn, L.S. (2003) Hyperprolactinemia and schizophrenia: mechanisms and clinical aspects. *Journal of Psychiatric Practice* **9**(5): 344–51.

Halbreich, U., Shen, J. and Panaro, V. (1996) Are chronic psychiatric patients at an increased risk for developing breast cancer? *American Journal of Psychiatry* **153**: 559–60.

Hansen, V., Jacobson, B.K. and Arnesen, E. (2001) Cause specific mortality in psychiatric patients after deinstitutionalisation. *British Journal of Psychiatry* **179**: 438–43.

Harris, E.C. and Barrowclough, B. (1998) Excess mortality of mental disorder. *British Journal of Psychiatry* **173**: 11–53.

Heatherton, T.F., Kozlowski, L.T., Frecker, R.C. and Fagerstrom, K.O. (1991) The Fagerstrom Test for Nicotine Dependence: a revision of the Fagerstrom Tolerance Questionnaire. *British Journal of Addiction* **86**: 1119–27.

Hippisley-Cox, J., Vinogradova, Y., Coupland, C. and Parker, C. (2006) Risk of malignancy in patients with mental health problems. London: Disability Rights Commission.

Hippisley-Cox, J., Parker, C., Coupland, C. and Vinogradova, Y. (2007) Inequalities in the primary care of patients with coronary heart disease and serious mental health problems: a cross-sectional study. *Heart* **93**(10): 1256–62.

Holt, R.I.G. and Peveler, R.C. (2006) Association between antipsychotic drugs and diabetes. *Diabetes, Obesity and Metabolism* **8**: 125–35.

Hughes, J.R., Hatsukami, D.K., Mitchell, J.E. *et al.* (1986) Prevalence of smoking among psychiatric outpatients. *American Journal of Psychiatry* **143**: 993–7.

Hummer, M. and Huber, J. (2004) Hyperprolactinaemia and antipsychotic therapy in schizophrenia. *Current Medical Research Opinion* **20**(2): 189–97.

Hyland, B., Judd, F., Davidson, S., Jolly, D. and Hocking, B. (2003) Case managers attitudes to the physical health of their patients. *Australian and New Zealand Journal of Psychiatry* **37**(6): 710–14.

Jeste, D., Gladsjo, J., Lindmayer, L. and Lacro, J. (1996) Medical co morbidity in schizophrenia. *Schizophrenia Bulletin* **22**(3): 413–30.

Kelly, C. and McCreadie, R. (2000) Cigarette smoking and schizophrenia. *Advances in Psychiatric Treatment* **6**: 327–32.

Kilbourne, A.M., Rofey, D.L., McCarthy, J.F., Post, E.P., Welsh, D. and Blow, F.C. (2007) Nutrition and exercise behavior among patients with bipolar disorder. *Bipolar Disorder* **9**: 443–52.

Koren, D. (2004) Diabetes mellitus and schizophrenia: historical perspective. *British Journal of Psychiatry* **184**(suppl 47): s64–s66.

Lambert, T.J.R., Velakoulis, D. and Pantelis, C. (2003) Medical co morbidity in schizophrenia. *Medical Journal of Australia* **178**: S67–S70.

Lawn, S.J., Pols, R.G. and Barber, J.G. (2002) Smoking and quitting: a qualitative study with community-living psychiatric clients. *Social Science and Medicine* **54**: 93–104.

Lean, M.E.J., Han, T.S. and Morrison, C.E. (1995) Waist circumference as a measure for indicating need for weight management. *British Medical Journal* **311**(6998): 158–61.

Lichtermann, D., Ekelund. J., Pukkala, E. *et al.* (2001) Incidence of cancer among persons with schizophrenia and their relatives. *Archives of General Psychiatry* **58**(6): 573–8.

Marriot, H. and Buttris, J. (2003) Key points from the National Diet and Nutrition Survey of adults aged 16–64 years. *Nutrition Bulletin* **28**: 355–63.

McCreadie, R. (2003) Diet, smoking and cardiovascular risk in people with schizophrenia. *British Journal of Psychiatry* **183**: 534–9.

McNeill, A. (2001) *Smoking and Mental Health: a review of the literature.* London: ASH.

Meyer, J.M. (2001) Individual changes in clozapine levels after smoking cessation. *Journal of Clinical Psychopharmacology* **21**(6): 569–74.

Montejo A.L. & Rico-Villademoros F (2008) Psychometric properties of the Psychotropic-related Sexual Dysfunction Questionnaire in patients with schizophrenia and other psychotic disorders. T Sex Marital Ther 34(3): 227–239.

Mortensen, P.B. (1994) The occurrence of cancer in first admitted schizophrenic patients. *Schizophrenia Research* **12**: 185–94.

Nash, M. (2005) Physical care skills: a training needs analysis of inpatient and community mental health nurses. *Mental Health Practice* **9**(4): 20–3.

National Institute for Health and Clinical Excellence (2002a) *Schizophrenia: Core Interventions in the Treatment and Management of Schizophrenia in Primary and Secondary Care.* London: NICE.

National Institute for Health and Clinical Excellence (2002b) *Nicotine Replacement and Buproprion for Smoking Cessation.* Technical Appraisal. London: NICE.

National Institute for Health and Clinical Excellence (2006) *Management of Hypertension in Adults in Primary Care.* London: NICE.

National Institute for Health and Clinical Excellence (2007) *Final Appraisal Determination for Varenicline for Smoking Cessation.* NICE: London.

Newcomer, J., Haupt, D.W. and Fucetola, R. (2002) Abnormalities in glucose regulation during antipsychotic treatment of schizophrenia. *Archives of General Psychiatry* **59**: 337–45.

Newman, S.C. and Bland, R.C. (1991) Mortality in a cohort of patients with schizophrenia: a record linage study. *Canadian Journal of Psychiatry* **36**: 293–45.

Osby, U., Correia. N., Brant, L., Ekbom, A. and Sparen, P. (2000) Mortality and causes of death in schizophrenia in Stockholm County, Sweden. *Schizophrenia Research* **45**: 21–8.

Parks, J., Svensden, D., Singer, P. and Foti, M.E. (2006) *Morbidity and Mortality in People with Serious Mental Illness.* Virginia, USA: National Association of State Mental Health Program Directors.

Paton, C., Esop, R., Young, C. and Taylor, D. (2004) Obesity, dyslipedaemias and smoking in an inpatient population treated with antipsychotic drugs. *Acta Psychiatrica Scandinavica* **110**(4): 299–305.

Peet, M. (2004) Diet, diabetes and schizophrenia: review and hypothesis. *British Journal of Psychiatry* **184**(suppl 47): s102–s105.

Phelan, M., Stradins, L. and Morrison, S. (2001) Physical health of people with severe mental illness. *British Medical Journal* **322**: 443–4.

Roberts, L., Roalfe, A., Wilson, S. and Lester, H. (2006) Physical health care of patients with schizophrenia in primary care: a comparative study. *Family Practice* 24(1): 34–40.

Robson, D. and Gray, R. (2007) Serious mental illness and physical health problems: a discussion paper. *International Journal of Nursing Studies* **44**: 457–66.

Robson D & Bragg M (2008) Physical health and serious mental illness: promoting good health. In Hall A, Wren M, Kirbys Care Planning in Mental Health: promoting recovery. 199–222. Blackwell, Oxford.

Rostami-Hodjegan, A., Spencer, E.P., Lennard, M.S., Tucker, G.T. and Flanagan, R. (2004) *Journal Clinical Psychpharmacology* 24(1): 70–8.

Ryan, M.C. and Thakore, J.H. (2001) Physical consequences of schizophrenia and its treatment: the metabolic syndrome. *Life Sciences* **71**(3): 239–57.

Skogh, E., Bengtsson, F. and Nordin, C. (1999) Could discontinuing smoking be hazardous for patients administered clozapine? *Therapeutic Drugs Monitor* **21**(5): 580–2.

Simpson, G.M. and Angus, J.W.S. (1970) A rating scale for extrapyramidal side effects. *Acta Psychiatrica Scandinavica* **45**:(Suppl 212): 11–19.

Simpson GM, Lee J.H., Zoubok B. Gardos G (1979) A rating scale for tardive dyskinesia. Psychopharmacology 64: 171–179.

Sokal, J., Messias, E. and Dickerson, F.B. (2004) Comorbidity of medical illnesses among adults with serious mental illness who are receiving community psychiatric services. *Journal of Nervous and Mental Disease* **192**(6): 421–7.

Strassnig, M., Singh Brar, J. and Ganguli, R. (2003) Nutritional assessment of patients in schizophrenia. *Schizophrenia Bulletin* **29**(2): 393–7.

Taylor, D., Patton, C. and Kerwin, R. (2007) *The Maudsley Prescribing Guidelines* (9th edn). London: Informa Healthcare.

Ussher, M., Stanbury, L., Cheeseman, V. and Faulkner, G. (2007) Physical activity preferences and perceived barriers to activity among persons with severe mental illness in the United Kingdom. *Psychiatric Services* **58**: 405–8.

Vreeland, B., Minsky, S. and Menza , M. (2003) Program for managing weight gain associated with atypical antipsychotics. *Psychiatric Services* 54: 1155–7.

West, R., McNeill, A. and Raw, M. (2000) Smoking cessation guidelines for health professionals. *Thorax* **55**: 987–99.

Wirshing, D.A. and Meyer, J.M. (2003) Obesity in patients with schizophrenia, In J.M. Meyer and H.A. Nasrallah (eds) *Medical Illness and Schizophrenia*. Vancouver: American Psychiatric Publishing.

Wirshing, D., Smith, R.A., Erickson, Z., Mena, S.J. and Wirshing, W. (2006) A wellness class for inpatients with psychotic disorders. *Journal of Psychiatric Practice* **12**(1): 24–9.

World Health Organization (2003) *Global Strategy on Diet, Physical Activity and Health*. Geneva: WHO.

CHAPTER 16

Psychopharmacology

Richard Gray, Daniel Bressington and Howard Chadwick

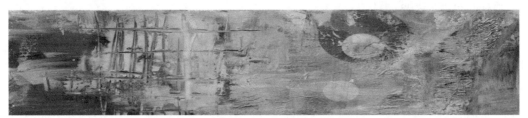

Introduction

The introduction of psychopharmacological treatments in the late 1940s revolutionized the treatment of psychosis, depression and other mental health problems. As in many other areas of health care pharmacotherapy often requires long-term maintenance treatment to maintain health and prevent relapse. Mental health nurses have always had an important role to play in medication management; working with service users to help them manage their treatment so that it fits in with their lifestyle and maximizes their health. This chapter will discuss pharmacological treatments for mental health problems and consider best practice in light of current evidence.

This chapter addresses the following:

- The brain;
- Pharmacology of antipsychotics:
  - typical antipsychotics
  - atypical antipsychotics
  - antipsychotic prescribing issues and clinical guidelines;
- Antidepressants;
- Mood stabilizers;
- Anxiolytics;
- Medicines against dementia;
- Rapid tranquillization;
- Chapter summary.

The brain

The human brain is a bit like a computer, it has an input (the sensory nervous system) and an output (the motor nervous system). Between these two systems the brain carries out mental processing such as thought, memory and interpretation of the world. When the brain goes wrong it causes neurological or psychiatric disturbances. It is helpful to consider the functions of different parts of the brain. The brain can be divided into a number of developmental and functional areas (Figure 16.1). The cerebral cortex at the top is the largest and most advanced region of the brain, responsible for our cognitive and conscious process.

Below this is the limbic system, made up of: the thalamus, hypothalamus, pituitary, amygdala and hippocampus. It is associated with preservation and emotions (such as fear) and behavioural patterns (such as eating). Next is the basal ganglia and cerebellum involved in the control of movement at an autonomic level. The brain stem is the most primitive part of the brain and is made up of three parts the pons; the reticular formation and the medulla, and is continuous with the spinal cord. The brain stem is involved with keeping the person alive at a physiological level, controlling the heart, blood pressure and lungs and other essential functions.

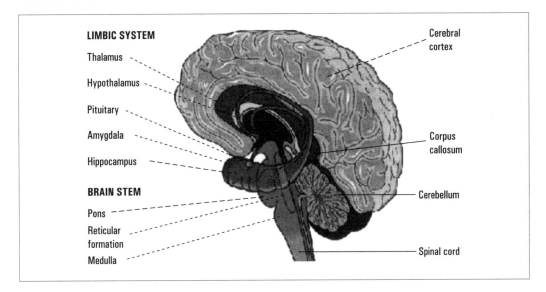

Figure 16.1 Areas of the human brain

The brain is made from grey and white matter. Grey matter is made from the cell bodies of brain cells or neurones. White matter is made from the axons of neurones. The brain and the spinal cord are covered by three layers – pia mater, arachnoid mater and dura mater – of membrane called the meninges. The subarachnoid space between two of these layers, the arachnoid and pia mater, contains cerebrospinal fluid (CSF) a watery fluid formed from blood plasma inside the brain that protects the central nervous system.

Blows (2003) has described the pathways between the different parts of the brain that are associated with mental health problems, psychotropic drug activity and medicine side effects. These are shown in Table 16.1.

Neural communication

Neurones are the functional unit of the nervous system. They have a cell body bearing dendrites and an axon (Figure 16.2). All nerve impulses (or action potentials) originate in neurones. Nerve cells communicate with each other via these electrical impulses. An impulse travels along the nerve axon and stimulates the release of chemical messengers known as neurotransmitters. They are released from storage vesicles in the pre-synaptic nerve and released into the synapse. The synapse is the gap between the pre-synaptic cell and the post-synaptic cell at a transmission site.

Pathway	From	To	Importance
Mesolimbic	Brain stem	Limbic system	Psychosis – positive symptoms (hallucinations and delusions)
Mesocorticol	Brain stem	Cerebral cortex	Psychosis – negative symptoms (isolation and withdrawal)
Nigostriatal	Substantia nigra	Corpus striatum	Extrapyramidal side effects
Diffuse modulatory systems	Brain stem	Limbic area and cerebral cortex	Depression and eating disorders
Median forebrain bundle	Brain stem	Frontal lobe of cerebrum	Reward pathways implicated in drugs of addiction
Dorsolateral prefrontal circuit	Frontal lobe	Basal ganglia	Deficits of frontal lobe executive functions
Lateral orbitofrontal circuit	Prefrontal cortex	Caudate nucleus	Involved in mood and personality changes

Table 16.1: Key brain pathways involved in mental health

The neurotransmitter travels across the synapse and binds with the appropriate receptor on the post-synaptic cell membrane. Receptors are selective cellular recognition sites for neurotransmitters, hormones and many drugs. This usually sets up an electrical impulse (an excitatory effect) in the post-synaptic nerve cell and so the message is passed on. Sometimes neurotransmitters have an inhibitory effect and stop further transmission of the message. After transmission, the neurotransmitter usually leaves the receptor and is taken back up into the pre-synaptic cell (reuptake) or destroyed by enzymes such as monoamine oxidase (MAO) at the synapse. Some of the most important neurotransmitters in mental health are dopamine, serotonin (5-hydroxytryptamine or 5-HT), noradrenaline and gamma-aminobutyric acid (GABA).

It has been hypothesized that over- or under-response within neurotransmission may be linked with some mental health problems. For example, psychosis may involve excessive dopamine neurotransmission (especially in the mesolimbic pathway) while depression and mania may involve disruption in the normal patterns of neurotransmission of noradrenaline and serotonin. This thinking about neurotransmission has led to the development of a range of pharmacological strategies to treat mental health problems. For example, antipsychotic drugs stop the neurotransmitter dopamine from binding to the post-synaptic receptor site by blocking – but not activating – receptors in the mesolimbic dopamine pathway. This reduces neurotransmission in that structure of the brain (Figure 16.3).

Some antidepressants such as SSRIs (selective serotonin reuptake inhibitors) stop the reuptake of the neurotransmitters noradrenaline and/or serotonin and regulate areas of the brain that produce them. Others such as monoamine oxidase inhibitors (MAOIs) prevent enzymatic metabolism of noradrenaline and serotonin. Both these actions result in increasing levels available at the synapse, increasing neuronal activity. The clinical effects of medicines

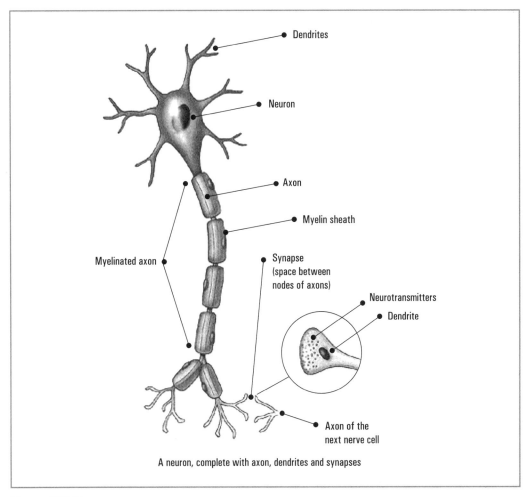

Dendrites

Neuron

Axon

Myelin sheath

Myelinated axon

Synapse
(space between
nodes of axons)

Neurotransmitters

Dendrite

Axon of the
next nerve cell

A neuron, complete with axon, dendrites and synapses

Figure 16.2 The neurone

used in psychiatry do not, however, confine themselves to the specific areas of the brain associated with mental health problems. Medicines will often interact with many other receptors causing unwanted symptoms or side effects and potential drug interactions during concomitant drug therapy.

It is important for mental health nurses to have an understanding of the effect of medicines on the body (this is called pharmacodynamics), the effects of the body on the drug over time (this is called pharmacokinetics) and the cross-ethnic, cross-racial profiles (this is called pharmacogenetics).

Antipsychotics

Antipsychotic medication has been the mainstay of treatment for schizophrenia since the 1950s when it was discovered that the dopamine antagonists, such as chlorpromazine, exert antipsychotic effects.

Pharmacology of antipsychotics

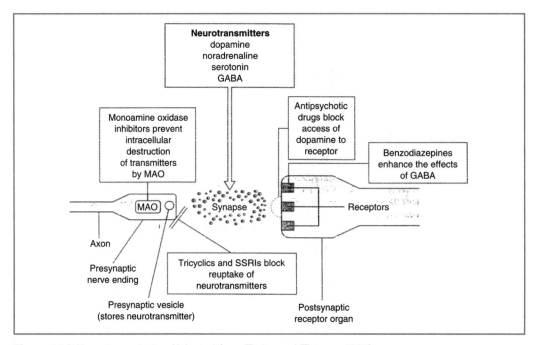

Figure 16.3 Neurotransmission (Adapted from Taylor and Thomas 1997)

Dopamine is a neurotransmitter mainly associated with reward and control of movement. Psychotic symptoms can be induced in healthy subjects by the administration of dopamine agonists, such as amphetamines or L-Dopa, the precursor molecule of dopamine. This, combined with knowledge of the action of antipsychotics in blockading dopamine receptors, led to the original dopamine hypothesis of psychosis. It was suggested that increased dopaminergic activity was associated with the symptoms of psychosis. Decades of research have demonstrated that this simple dopamine hypothesis is untenable and the pathological picture is highly complex. From a pharmacological perspective, much research attention has focused the role, function and distribution of dopamine receptors (see Figure 16.4).

Some authors suggest that a high affinity for D_2 receptors may not be the only basis for efficacy in antipsychotic agents. Although antipsychotics occupy receptors within a few hours of administration, there is often a one to three week delay before therapeutic benefits are reported. This suggests that these drugs act via a series of secondary, and as yet unknown, processes that evolve over days to weeks. There are suggestions that a number of other neuroreceptors, peptides and amino acid systems may be involved. This is further supported by the fact that changes in systems other than dopamine have been implicated in the aetiology of schizophrenia. For example, it has been proposed that the mediation of the sensory–motor gating function of the thalamus by the striatal complexes, which is in turn regulated by an inter-play of dopaminergic, GABAergic and glutamatergic systems, may be a key process in psychosis (Carlsson et al. 1999).

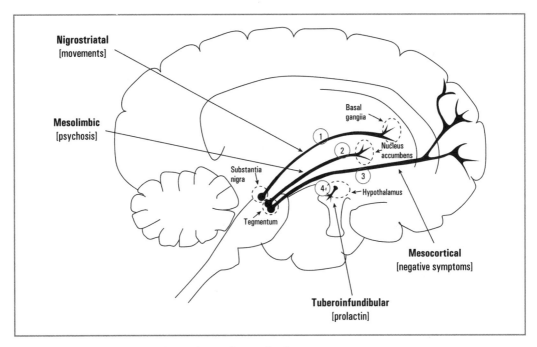

Figure 16.4 Important dopamine pathways in psychosis

Typical antipsychotics

Chlorpromazine, the first effective antipsychotic, was introduced during the 1950s. Subsequent research and development led to the introduction of a group of related drugs, the phenothiazines, and other drugs which acted in similar ways but were chemically distinct, such as the butyrephenones, haloperidol and droperidol, or thioxanthenes like zuclopenthixol. Collectively these may be considered the typical or first generation antipsychotics. Clinical trials have repeatedly shown that these drugs are effective in reducing the positive symptoms of schizophrenia such as hallucinations and delusions. About eight out of ten patients can expect to get some benefit from treatment, typically about a 50 per cent reduction in positive symptoms. Antipsychotic medicines exert the effect by blocking dopamine receptors in the mesolimbic pathway. However this serves merely to ameliorate the positive symptoms of psychosis, which often persist at a residual, albeit more tolerable, level.

Typical antipsychotic medicines are probably equally effective against the positive symptoms of schizophrenia. Their side-effect profile can differ dramatically and this can have important implication for patient treatment preference. Antipsychotic side effects are largely dependent on the drugs' effect on a range of neurotransmitter systems.

Dopamine system effects

Three key dopamine pathways, the mesocortical, nigrostriatal and tuberoinfundibular, are associated with important side effects associate with antipsychotic medication. Mesocortical blockade, for example has been implicated in the exacerbation of cognitive impairment and negative symptoms. It is thought that the mesocortical pathway may already have lowered dopaminergic activity in those suffering from schizophrenia and the antagonist effect of antipsychotics serves to compound this problem.

Nigrostriatal blockade causes predictable movement disorders that include dystonia and pseudo-Parkinsonism. Collectively these are referred to as extrapyramidal side effects or EPSE and are often distressing to people taking antipsychotics and may cause people to stop taking them. Acute dystonic reactions such as an oculogyric crisis where the eyes roll back in the head or torticollis where there is contraction of the neck muscles, are due to muscle constriction. Younger, treatment naive people are more likely to get these side effects. Anticholinergic medicines are often used to treat EPSE and exert their effect because of the reciprocal nature of dopamine and acetylcholine transmission in the nigrostriatal pathway. Dopamine antagonism produces a relative excess of cholinergic activity. By inhibiting the cholinergic activity the ratio between dopaminergic and cholinergic activity is restored to some extent, thus reducing the EPSE.

Akathisia is often considered an extrapyramidal side effect but in truth its cause is complex and poorly understood. What is known, though, is that akathisia causes considerable distress, aggression and even suicide in those that develop it. There is considerable debate regarding the treatment of akathisia. A systematic review (Rathbone and Soares-Weiser 2006) found there was no reliable evidence either for or against the use of antimuscarinic medicines or beta blockers, that are the most frequently prescribed treatments.

A particularly debilitating movement disorder associated with long-term treatment is tardive dyskinesia (TD). It is characterized by facial contortions, particularly of the mouth and tongue, and uncontrolled limb movements. Its cause remains rather unclear but appears to be a response to prolonged D2 antagonism in the nigrostriatal pathway whereby the receptors up-regulate or become supersensitive to combat blockade by the antipsychotic drug. In turn this leads to dopamine hyperactivity that may affect neurotransmission in other parts of the motor control system. Approximately 5 per cent of patients treated with typical antipsychotics will develop TD (Stahl 2000). According to Gray *et al.* (2005) risk factors that increase the likelihood of developing TD include:

- age, older adults are six times more likely to develop TD;
- female gender;
- smoking;
- a dual diagnosis of diabetes;
- the presence of negative symptoms;
- a previous history of EPSE;
- a concurrent mood disorder or dementia.

The blockade of dopamine receptors in the tuberoinfundibular pathway causes an increase in the level of the hormone prolactin. The pathway inhibits the release of prolactin. Dopamine antagonism therefore allows release leading to hyperprolactinaemia. There are a range of side effects associated with raised prolactin levels which include galactorrhea or the production of breast secretions, gynaecomastia, the production of breast tissue in men, amenorrhea, irregularity or absence of the menstrual cycle, and sexual dysfunction.

- **Side effects mediated by alpha 1 adrenergic receptors:** Alpha 1 adrenaline antagonism leads to cardiovascular side effects such as orthostatic hypotension and drowsiness;

- **Side effects mediated by H1 histaminergic receptors:** H1 histamine antagonism is responsible for drowsiness and weight gain;
- **Side effects mediated by M1 muscarinic receptors:** The blockade of acetylcholine at M1 muscarinic receptors produces a range of side effects such as dry mouth, blurred vision, constipation and cognitive impairment. However, drugs with a strong anticholinergic profile have a lower propensity to induce EPSE due to self regulating the dopamine–acetylcholine activity ratio in the nigrostriatal pathway.

Side effect groups

The varying propensity of phenothiazines to induce these side effects led them to be classified in three groups:

- Group 1 (e.g. chlorpromazine): highly sedating, moderate anticholinergic and moderate extrapyramidal side effects;
- Group 2 (e.g. pericyazine): highly anticholinergic, moderate sedating and moderate extrapyramidal side effects;
- Group 3 (e.g. trifuoperazine): highly extrapyramidal inducing, moderate sedating and moderate anticholinergic side effects.

All other typical antipsychotics, such as haloperidol and the typical depot preparations, have a profile similar to Group 3 in that they have a strong propensity to induce extrapyramidal side effects and are less problematic regarding sedation and anticholinergic activity.

Unpredictable side effects

Just as pharmacogenetics makes it difficult to predict an individual's response to a particular drug, there are side effects which it is not possible to predict from a drugs receptor binding profile. Most notable and serious is the condition known as neuroleptic malignant syndrome or NMS. This is characterized by pyrexia, muscle rigidity, confusion and labile blood pressure (Caroff and Mann 1993). Two indicative pathology results are a raised creatine phosphokinase (CPK) level and leukocytosis. Early recognition of the condition is important as it is potentially fatal and requires specialized intervention. All antipsychotics may induce it although trifluoperazine and haloperidol seem to present a higher risk and it is most likely to occur in the first two weeks of treatment. Estimates of incidence vary from 0.5 per cent to 2.2 per cent of cases. There is evidence to suggest that a diagnosis of bipolar affective disorder and administration by injection significantly increases the risk (Hermesh *et al.* 1992).

A further serious side effect is delay of cardiac repolarization measured by a prolonged QTc interval on electrocardiograph (ECG) recordings. This is caused by the blocking of the HERG I kr potassium channel. This may induce arrhythmias and can lead to a condition called torsades de pointes or 'twisted points' – a graphic description of the ECG trace appearance (Calderone *et al.* 2005). This in turn may lead to sudden death (Stollberger *et al.* 2005). A QT interval that is longer than 500 milliseconds is considered dangerous and is associated with life-threatening arrhythmias and sudden death (Gray 2001).

A variety of antipsychotics have been shown to cause this as well as other types of drugs such as tricyclic antidepressants, although some have a higher propensity than others to do so. Group 2 phenothiazines, particularly thioridazine, and higher doses generally (Warner *et al.* 1996), are prone to inducing this problem and it has been a cause of concern for a number of the atypical antipsychotics such as sertindole.

They may also cause a range of other side effects which are less common such as blood dyscrasias, including agranulocytosis and leucopenia, rashes, jaundice and photosensitization, for example.

While typical antipsychotics are undoubtedly effective at ameliorating positive symptoms of psychosis there is no doubt that they have many drawbacks. The search for more effective drugs with less disabling side effects led to the development of a second generation of antipsychotics.

Atypical antipsychotics

The term 'atypical' is applied to the second generation of antipsychotics due to their considerably reduced propensity to cause extrapyramidal side effects which distinguishes them from the 'typical' drugs. Clozapine was the original atypical antipsychotic which was first marketed in the 1970s to great excitement. It was said to avoid many of the drawbacks of conventional medicines. It reduced both positive and negative symptoms, was associated with few EPSEs and was effective for people who had not responded to other medicines.

Unfortunately in 1975, 21 out of 6100 people treated with clozapine in north Europe developed agranulocytosis (a blood dyscrasia), and clozapine was voluntarily withdrawn from the market. Nonetheless, the advent of clozapine marked an important advance in the treatment of schizophrenia, and introduced to psychiatry the term 'atypical' to describe a new class of antipsychotic medicine. In 1988 a pivotal multi-centre trial demonstrated that clozapine was far more effective than conventional antipsychotics for people with so-called treatment resistant schizophrenia (Kane *et al.* 1988). Subsequent studies have confirmed clozapine's efficacy in treating the positive and negative symptoms of schizophrenia with few EPSEs. In 1990 it was introduced to the UK, with strict guidelines for haematological monitoring. It was joined by a range of other drugs which, while chemically distinct, demonstrated a similarly low propensity to induce EPSE.

Like the typical antipsychotics, atypicals reduce positive symptoms through dopamine D2 antagonism in the meso-limbic pathway. In doing this they are equally as effective as typical antipsychotics with the possible exception of clozapine which is a fairly weak D2 antagonist. As a group they may be viewed as dopamine D2 and serotonin 5-HT2A antagonists but in other respects they are quite individual. Clozapine is the most complex, acting as an antagonist at seven serotonin and four dopamine receptor subtypes. How these actions combine remains unclear although evidence shows that it is superior in efficacy to typical antipsychotics (Wahlbeck *et al.* 1999) and helps a proportion of those resistant to conventional treatment (Lewis *et al.* 2006). Clinical experience has shown that treatment resistant people who respond to clozapine fall into two groups: rapid responders who demonstrate a notable improvement over a period of weeks; and slow responders who show an incremental improvement over a much longer period, in some cases years.

It is suggested that other atypicals may have some beneficial effect on negative symptoms but the evidence remains rather equivocal (Gardner *et al.* 2005). The hypothesis regarding both efficacy for negative symptoms and the low incidence of EPSEs concerns the atypicals serotonin 5-HT2A receptor antagonism. Serotonin has extensive influence on dopamine activity but this is not consistent between the dopamine pathways. In the meso-cortical pathway where dopaminergic deficiency is thought to relate to negative symptoms, 5-HT2A antagonism causes an increase in dopamine activity. In the nigrostriatal pathway serotonin inhibits dopamine release. 5-HT2A antagonism here enhances dopamine release allowing for greater competition at D2 receptor sites between the drug and dopamine and so reducing the proportion of D2 antagonized receptors and the consequent side effects (Stahl 2000).

Unsurprisingly there has been considerable research comparing not only the atypicals with typical antipsychotics but with each other. Overall it appears that there is little difference in symptom response between the atypicals and typicals or between them with the exception of clozapine (Gardner *et al.* 2005). Clozapine has been shown to help somewhere between 40 per cent and 70 per cent of people deemed treatment resistant. For those who have a poor response to clozapine various augmentation strategies have been tried but evidence concerning their efficacy remains equivocal (Kontaxakis *et al.* 2005; Remington *et al.* 2005).

Atypicals are far from side-effect free but they produce unwanted effects that differ from typicals. While the side-effect profile alters both from patient to patient and drug to drug, there are some characteristic unwanted results of treatment with this group.

Due to their 5-HT2A antagonism, atypical antipsychotics have a low propensity to induce EPSE but this does not mean to say that they never cause them (Margolese *et al.* 2005; Mendhekar 2005; Ghaemi *et al.* 2006). Risperidone is the most likely to induce movement disorders and this is dose related.

Weight gain causes considerable problems, being both a health risk, which may be associated with the onset of diabetes (Newcomer 2005) and also a major concordance issue. This is variable across the group with clozapine and olanzapine producing the greatest weight gain while having a higher incidence of diabetes (Mir and Taylor 2001) and ziprasidone the least (Gardner *et al.* 2005). Individual drugs have particular problems.

Probably the most serious side effect is the risk of agranulocytosis with clozapine. A potentially fatal condition, it affects the production of white cells thereby compromising the immune system, hence the need for regular blood tests. Clozapine may also cause hypersalivation which, although not dangerous, is highly debilitating socially. Clozapine can also be highly sedating to the point where it affects an individual's quality of life.

Similarly, amisulpiride which has a moderately low side-effect profile overall, is more likely to cause raised prolactin levels than other atypicals. There have also been concerns about some atypicals inducing prolonged QTc intervals. This caused sertindole to be withdrawn from the market although it is now undergoing further clinical trials.

Third generation antipsychotics

Typical and atypical (or first and second generation) antipsychotics bind to and block dopamine receptors in the mesolimbic and other dopamine pathways to exert their effects. It has long been considered that a drug that stabilizes rather than blocks dopamine activity may have great clinical benefit in reducing dopamine activity in the desired pathways rather than unintentionally disrupting dopamine transmission in other pathways causing adverse effects. Aripiprazole is a partial dopamine agonist that achieves this stabilizing effect by binding to dopamine receptors and partially activating them. Medicines that work to alleviate psychosis in this way are called third generation antipsychotics.

In addition to stabilizing dopamine D2 in the mesolimbic pathway aripiprazole has partial agonist activity at serotonin 5-HT1a receptors and antagonist activity at 5-HT2a receptors. Aripiprazole has a weak affinity for cholinergic, histaminergic and adrenergic receptors which results in a low incidence of adverse effects related to these neurotransmitters. Theoretically aripiprazole should alleviate the positive symptoms of psychosis without causing secondary negative symptoms.

The different receptor binding profile can make switching from first/second generation antipsychotics to aripiprazole complex. When the receptors previously blocked are unblocked there is a possibility of rebound receptor effects. These effects are clinically important and need to managed carefully; for example, a lack of sedation when switching to aripiprazole is due to increased histaminergic activity and may require short-term pharmacological and/or behavioural intervention.

A systematic review of clinical trials (El-Sayeh *et al.* 2006) has demonstrated that the efficacy of aripiprazole is similar to other atypical antipsychotics. At present there is little evidence available to demonstrate that it has superior treatment response or tolerability but there has been relatively little research hitherto.

Issues in the prescribing of antipsychotics

Decades of research have demonstrated the efficacy of both typical and atypical antipsychotic medication through the use of randomized controlled trials. However the results from these carefully controlled studies are rarely replicated under normal clinical conditions. Why then do antipsychotics not achieve their full therapeutic potential? The main reason appears to be that about 50 per cent of people do not take their medication as prescribed. This figure remains constant across all chronic illnesses.

The expectation that a reduction of the occurrence of EPSEs would improve the tolerability of atypicals over typicals led to the NICE guidelines recommending the use of atypicals as first line treatment (NICE 2002). This view has been challenged in the past few years by extensive research projects undertaken in both the UK (the CUtLASS trial, Jones *et al.* 2006) and the USA (the CATIE trial, Lieberman *et al.* 2005) where effectiveness and quality of life have been studied extensively in real life clinical situations. These studies suggest that there is no difference between typicals and atypicals when effectiveness and quality of life are compared, with the exception of clozapine, which continues to demonstrate a significant advantage compared to other drugs (Davis *et al.* 2003; McEvoy *et al.* 2006) but remains licensed only for those who do not respond to other drugs. A recent Health Technology Assessment based on randomized controlled trials in the UK (Lewis *et al.* 2006) concluded that, for people who were intolerant of current medication or had an inadequate response, there were advantages in utility, cost and quality adjusted life years in switching to a typical antipsychotic. For those with narrowly defined treatment resistance a significant advantage was shown in switching to clozapine in terms of symptoms.

While the CUtLASS and CATIE studies show no particular advantage to atypicals over typicals in the real world, there is evidence that consistently taken atypicals may have distinct advantages over typicals for long-term outcomes. It has been shown that atypicals have a neuroprotective capacity and induce higher levels of nerve growth factor than typical antipsychotics (Parik *et al.* 2004). It has been suggested that this may facilitate the cessation or even reverse the neuronal loss in frontotemporal cortical grey matter which is a common feature in schizophrenia (Nasrallah 2007). It has been argued that greater use of long-acting preparations in maintenance therapy would prove beneficial due to increased consistency of treatment which would result in better outcomes (Nasrallah 2007). At present, risperidone and olanzapine are available as long-acting formulations.

In today's health economy it is not possible to consider treatment without reference to the cost. In 2002, with reference to available evidence, NICE recommended atypicals as first line treatment. Atypicals are notably more expensive than typicals. For example a four-week supply of a maintenance dose of aripiprazole would cost £101.63, of risperidone £94.28 and of haloperidol £4.19 (Mehta 2007). In the light of the results being reported by the CATIE and CUtLASS studies, together with financial pressures, an increase in the prescribing of typical antipsychotics seems likely. While these cost disparities seem obvious, what remains less clear is the overall cost when aspects such as bed occupancy, social care and psychological support are included. It is also difficult to put a price on quality of life.

Ultimately the key to successful prescribing and effective treatment is a cost/benefit analysis between efficacy in symptom reduction and tolerability. This balance constitutes an idiosyncratic expression of the interaction of the person and the particular drug. Identifying the most effective treatment regime for a particular individual is often a matter of trial and error. Furthermore, it can be suggested that greater emphasis should be placed on medication concordance with professionals working alongside clients to maximize therapeutic benefit thereby improving outcomes (Gray *et al.* 2004).

It should be borne in mind however that antipsychotics do not constitute a cure. They do reduce symptoms and as such are a crucial part of a person's recovery process but need to be combined with an individualized package of psychosocial care to maximize their quality of life. Hogarty and Ulrich (1998) reviewed literature on relapse rates of people with psychosis to provide an estimate of how effective antipsychotic monotherapy is at preventing relapse. They estimate that relapse rate one year post hospitalization was 40 per cent if people were taking medication as prescribed and these rates were reduced by as much as 50 per cent when psychosocial care was included in the treatment package.

NICE guidance on atypical antipsychotics is that:

- the choice of drug should be made jointly between the individual and the clinician involving the carer if appropriate;
- atypical antipsychotics are the first line treatment for schizophrenia;
- individuals on typical antipsychotics should be considered for atypical drugs if they experience unpleasant side effects;
- clozapine is the treatment of choice for treatment resistant schizophrenia;
- clinicians should undertake a concordance assessment. If there is a risk of non-concordance a long-acting formulation may be indicated;
- the atypical antipsychotic with the lowest purchase price should be used if there is a choice;
- antipsychotic medication is part of a comprehensive package of care;
- atypical and typical antipsychotics should not be prescribed concurrently.

Antidepressants

Depression is one of the most common of all mental health problems and as a result antidepressants are prescribed widely both in primary and secondary care. Making the decision about whether to prescribe or not can be a difficult one, particularly as any class of antidepressant has a delayed onset of therapeutic action and can take upwards of several weeks to work. According to NICE guidelines (NICE 2004a) if a decision is made to prescribe medication for a depressive illness it should be a selective serotonin reuptake inhibitor (SSRI) and should be part of a package of care including psychosocial interventions such as cognitive behaviour therapy (CBT), problem solving and self-help techniques. Antidepressants are of little value (and therefore should not be prescribed) for people experiencing mild depression which appears to respond better to a psychosocial approach.

It has been proposed that depression is caused by a reduction in either serotonin or noradrenaline and mania by an excess of noradrenaline. MAOIs (monoamine oxidase inhibitors) effectively inhibit the destruction of these neurotransmitters while tricyclic antidepressants and SSRIs (selective serotonin reuptake inhibitors) prevent their reuptake at the pre-synaptic neurone. Both these mechanisms increase the amount of neurotransmitter at the synapse. Although this theory is widely taught to mental health nurses there are a number of substantial problems with it. Perhaps most importantly is the observation that 20–30 per cent of depressed people do not derive any benefit from the medicines. Although mainly used in the treatment of depression and related mental health problems there is evidence that they may be useful also for treating other illnesses such as obsessive compulsive disorder. It is important to remember that all antidepressant medicines may take four to six weeks to begin to work and service users cannot expect to realize a quick response to treatment.

Tricyclic antidepressants (TCAs) have been the mainstay for the treatment of depression for many years. Although very effective in the treatment of depressions it has long been known that they are poorly tolerated (common side effects include sedation, weight gain and anticholinergic symptoms) and, because of cardiotoxicity, are potentially fatal in overdose. Perhaps because of tolerability problems psychiatrists and general practitioners have tended to prescribe doses of TCAs that are known to be sub-therapeutic. Over the past decade their use in both primary and secondary care settings has reduced dramatically.

TCAs have now been largely replaced by SSRIs (such as citalopram, fluoxetine and sertraline) a group of drugs that inhibit the reuptake of serotonin at the pre-synaptic membrane promoting the neurotransmission of serotonin in the brain. Because they have specific affinity for serotonin receptors they have little effect at the transmission sites for other receptors and consequently are as effective as TCA but have fewer side effects. Venlafaxine is another newer antidepressant and is a SNRI (selective noradrenaline reuptake inhibitor). It increases levels of both serotonin and noradrenaline although claims of increased efficacy have been made for this medicine in practice it appears to be equally as effective as SSRIs and TCAs. SSRIs do not cause many of the side effects associated with traditional TCAs and they are much safer in overdose. The main side effects associated with SSRIs are nausea and agitation; they have also been associated with sexual dysfunction in both men and women and less commonly dry mouth and sedation.

The final group of antidepressant drugs to consider are monoamine oxidase inhibitors (MAOIs), for example, phenelzine and tranylcypromine. Although available for many years, and generally well tolerated, they have not been widely prescribed because clinicians are worried about the hypertensive crisis when tyramine-containing foods and some other medicines are taken with these drugs. More recently moclobemide, a new MAOI, has been marketed. Unlike previous MAOIs it only temporarily inhibits monoamine oxidase and consequently the tyramine reaction is substantially reduced and there are no dietary restrictions.

St John's wort (discussed also in Chapter 15) may have some effect in mild depression but due to a lack of empirical evidence it should not be prescribed or recommended. The known common adverse effects of St John's wort include: dry mouth, nausea, constipation, fatigue, headache and restlessness. Due to possible drug–drug interactions service users should always be asked if they are taking St John's wort (or any other non-prescribed treatment). St John's wort increases the action of P450 liver enzymes and this can result in a lowering of plasma levels of some concurrently prescribed drugs. Due to its action on serotonin it may cause serotonin syndrome if taken with some other prescribed antidepressants. The seriousness of possible interactions should be reinforced to patients who may view herbal remedies and over-the-counter medicines as being inherently harmless (NICE 2004a; Taylor *et al.* 2005).

NICE (2004a) strongly suggest that people about to be prescribed any class of antidepressant should be given clear information about the possibility of discontinuation syndrome. Discontinuation symptoms can occur if the drug is stopped abruptly, if doses are missed, and sometimes when the dose is reduced. The mechanism of action of discontinuation syndrome is thought to be related to a rebound effect of action at receptors that were previously blocked. The resulting symptoms are usually mild but can on occasion be quite severe. Severe symptoms are more likely if the medication is stopped abruptly and if the antidepressant has a short half life. Some of the symptoms experienced can be similar to the symptoms of depression and understandably service users who are not informed may feel that their illness is relapsing. All classes of antidepressants can cause discontinuation symptoms although there may be slight differences in symptoms between classes of drugs. TCAs and SSRIs cause very similar discontinuation symptoms such as flu-like symptoms, insomnia, vivid dreams, irritability and occasionally movement disorders. MAOIs do not appear to cause flu-like symptoms but they can cause other effects similar to SSRIs/TCAs, and, in addition, agitation, speech problems and occasionally hallucinations/delusions (Taylor *et al.* 2005).

Implications for clinical practice
- Antidepressants are effective in the treatment of depression.
- SSRIs are safer and better tolerated than TCAs.
- It takes several weeks for antidepressants to begin to ameliorate depressive symptoms.
- Service users need to be made aware of how to avoid and manage discontinuation syndrome.

Mood stabilizers

Mood stabilizers are the most widely used drugs to treat bipolar affective disorder and other related conditions such as unipolar depression and schizoaffective disorder. There is also evidence that lithium is effective in treating some non-affective mental health problems such as borderline personality disorder. Lithium has been the front-line drug for bipolar disorder for many years although increasingly carbamazepine and sodium valproate are becoming more popular. There is also emerging evidence that some other drugs – most notably the atypical antipsychotics clozapine, olanzapine and risperidone – may also be effective in the treatment of bipolar disorder.

Lithium has been used as a mood stabilizer since the late 1940s when it was first recognized to have anti-manic properties. However, the exact mechanism of action is poorly understood. It has been proposed that lithium corrects an ion exchange abnormality, alters sodium transport in nerves and muscle cells, normalizes synaptic neurotransmission of noradrenaline and changes receptor sensitivity. Lithium can be a complex drug to use. In high doses it can cause renal damage and reduce renal function. Hypothyroidism is also seen in service users taking lithium even at therapeutic doses. The maintenance dose for lithium must be individually tailored and carefully monitored and adjusted over time. Lithium is associated with a range of acute (such as tremor and fatigue) and long-term (such as thyroid dysfunction) side effects as well as the potential for toxicity (a clinical emergency).

Typically lithium is a first line treatment; however, two anticonvulsants, carbamazepine and sodium valproate, have been shown to be effective mood stabilizers. Typically these drugs are used only if service users have not responded to lithium therapy or if it is contraindicated.

Implications for clinical practice

- Lithium is an effective mood stabilizer but requires close monitoring.
- Lithium toxicity is an emergency situation.
- Carbamazepine and sodium valproate are also well-tolerated and effective mood stabilizers.

Anti-anxiety and sedative-hypnotic drugs

Benzodiazepines are the most widely prescribed group of drugs in the world although in recent years their popularity has waned because of their potential to cause tolerance and dependence. Benzodiazepines have a wide range of uses including anxiety, anxiety-related phobias, alcohol withdrawal, and sleep disorders. They are also used widely in the treatment of acute agitation and aggression in service users with psychosis.

NICE guidelines for the treatment of anxiety (NICE 2004b) recommend that the most effective and long-lasting treatment for anxiety is a psychosocial treatment or self-help approach based on CBT principles. However, access to such treatments is not always readily available in all areas and some patients will prefer drug treatment; this results in a variety of medicines being used to manage anxiety in clinical practice. NICE recommends that if a drug treatment is to be given it should be an SSRI antidepressant and if benzodiazepines are used they should be only prescribed for a short period (two to four weeks) and that they should be used for emergency management only (not for obsessive compulsive disorder or post-traumatic stress disorder).

Benzodiazepines (for example, diazepam, lorazepam and temazepam) reduce anxiety by potentiating the inhibitory neurotransmitter GABA. There are few clinical differences between the different types of benzodiazepines except for different half lives (the time for the plasma level of drug to reduce to half of peak level). Overdoses of benzodiazepines are almost never fatal (unless taken in conjunction with other central nervous system depressants such as alcohol and opiates) and the effect can be reversed by the specific antagonist, flumazenil. Side effects are rare and tend to be dose related. When used regularly tolerance increases therefore people need higher doses to obtain the same level of symptomatic relief. Prolonged use can result in physical dependency. Withdrawal symptoms range from insomnia and anxiety, to extreme agitation and convulsions. It may be fatal if not treated appropriately. However, if prescribed over a short term (around two weeks) dependence should not be an issue, especially if treatment is stopped gradually. It is also useful to advise service users to use benzodiazepines intermittently rather than regularly to reduce the risk of tolerance and dependence.

The use of barbiturates has been largely replaced by benzodiazepines as anti-anxiety and sedative-hypnotic drugs because of tolerability and safety issues (the range between therapeutic and toxic dose, leading to coma and respiratory arrest, is very narrow). Two drugs that are not structurally related to benzodiazepines and are licensed for the treatment of insomnia are zopiclone and zolpidem.

Another treatment for anxiety that is becoming more popular is buspirone. Buspirone is a non-benzodiazepine anxiolytic. Its mechanism of action has yet to be firmly established but is different to that of benzodiazepines as it does not act on GABA. It appears that its therapeutic effects are related to its action on the neurotransmitters dopamine, serotonin, noradrenaline and acetylcholine. It takes around three to six weeks to work and therefore has no place in the emergency management of anxiety. Buspirone does not appear to cause dependence and has no clinical sedative or anticonvulsant properties. Its common side effects include: dizziness, drowsiness, headache, fatigue, insomnia, nausea, dry mouth and palpitations. Rarely people may experience excitement, anger, hostility and nightmares. Buspirone should not be taken with MAOIs as this can cause hypertensive crisis. Serum levels of buspirone can be increased to toxic levels if taken with some drugs that inhibit some P450 liver enzymes (for example erythromycin and nefazadone).

Medicines for dementia

There are a wide range of drugs used to treat the variety of symptoms which can present with dementia. For example psychotic symptoms may develop and be treated with antipsychotics although olanzapine and risperidone should be avoided as they have an increased risk of stroke in the elderly with dementia (Ballard and Waite 2006). Antipsychotics should not be routinely prescribed solely for sedation or the management of challenging behaviours except in instances of severe distress or immediate risk of harm (NICE 2006a) due to increased risk mortality. It should be noted that dosing should generally be lower than normal due to lower metabolic rates in the elderly who make up the majority of dementia sufferers. This section examines those drugs designed to treat the cognitive impairment – largely memory deficits, which are characteristic of dementia.

Memory and learning is a highly complex function involving a multitude of pathways and a variety of neurotransmitters. As yet there is only an incomplete understanding of the processes involved. However, research has implicated the degeneration of cholinergic neurons originating in part of the amygdala called the nucleus basalis of Meynert as a major factor in the impairment of short-term memory and there seems an overall reduction in acetylcholine activity (Herholz *et al.* 2000). This led to the development of drugs designed to boost cholinergic activity in order to enhance cognitive function and memory impairment. These drugs are termed cholinesterase inhibitors.

Cholinesterase inhibitors

Three cholinesterase inhibitors are currently licensed for use in mild to moderate dementia in Alzheimer's disease: donepezil, galantamine and rivastigmine. One further drug, memantine, is licensed for use in moderate to severe dementia in Alzheimer's disease but it is not a cholinesterase inhibitor.

Cholinesterase inhibitors work in a similar way to the antidepressant monoamine oxidase inhibitors in that they inhibit the enzyme that breaks down the neurotransmitter. In this case the enzyme is acetylcholinesterase (AChE). By doing this there is an increase in the amount of acetylcholine available. The three drugs, although achieving the same therapeutic goal, are different from one another. Donepezil is a long-acting, reversible AChE inhibitor, rivastigmine is intermediate acting and pseudo-irreversible and galantamine may have a dual action in not only inhibiting acetylcholine breakdown in a similar way, but through its agonist activity at nicotinic receptors may induce acetylcholine release (Birks 2006).

A systematic review of studies of cholinesterase inhibitors used to treat mild to moderate dementia shows that there is no notable variation between the three drugs. Small benefits were noted in activities of daily living and behaviour as well as assessment scales. Similar benefits were also noted in cases of severe dementia but there are too few studies from which to draw conclusions (Loy and Schneider 2006). However small the benefits may appear, it can be argued that small or indeed no improvement over a period of six months, the timescale of a number of trials, constitutes a therapeutic success in what is a progressively degenerative disease.

Memantine has a different action altogether. It is thought that a mechanism responsible for neuronal injury or death is over exposure to the excitatory neurotransmitter glutamate. This is termed excitotoxicity. One receptor involved in this process is the glutamate N-methyl-d-aspartate (NMDA) receptor. Memantine is a non-competitive, low affinity, NMDA antagonist, allowing normal activity but having the ability to regulate excess $Ca2+$ ion influx under conditions of over-activation (Lipton 2005). This impedes the progression of symptoms.

The most common side effects encountered with cholinesterase inhibitors are gastrointestinal. These include nausea, vomiting and diarrhoea. Others such as headaches, insomnia, dizziness and psychiatric disturbances may also occur. Memantine can cause constipation, headaches, drowsiness and dizziness. Less commonly it can induce vomiting, confusion, hallucinations and fatigue. Seizures have also been reported but very rarely. The drugs for dementia have few strong interactions. Memantine has an increased risk of causing CNS toxicity when given with amantadine, ketamine or dextromethorphan and it is recommended that they are not used together. Galantamine may have its plasma concentration levels increased by a number of drugs, notably paroxetine and erythromycin.

The prescribing of these drugs has been the subject of considerable public debate. At the moment a revised technology appraisal by NICE recommends that they are made available only for moderate Alzheimer's disease sufferers as long as certain criteria are met (NICE 2006b). However, this recommendation has been questioned by a number of bodies including the Royal College of Nursing, the Royal College of Psychiatry, Age Concern and the Alzheimer's Society. It is of interest that a cost-effectiveness study of memantine in Finland concluded that the extended independence and delay of institutionalization more than offset the cost of treatment (Francois *et al.* 2004).

Rapid tranquillization

Rapid tranquillization (RT), the use of drugs to control acutely disturbed behaviour, is a high risk and anxiety provoking procedure for both service users and professionals. It is a treatment of last resort when all other attempts to de-escalate disturbed behaviour have either been ineffective or are inappropriate. Each time RT is used, the risk of the service user harming himself/herself or others must be balanced against the potential side effects of drug interventions. Decisions may need to be taken rapidly as a situation evolves. Surveys of RT have consistently found practice to be idiosyncratic and sub-optimal. A wide range of drugs and doses are used and polypharmacy is common, as is high dose prescribing (Mannion *et al.* 1997). There is also confusion regarding the desired outcome from RT and the time frame over which it is expected that this will be achieved.

The aim of RT is to calm the service user so that a comprehensive assessment of mental state can be undertaken; it is not to anaesthetize. Service users can slip into a deep sleep after RT and in these cases pulse-oximeters and other observations should be used to ensure their safety. Maintaining the airway is paramount.

Oral medication should be offered before using parenteral (IM/IV) in an emergency. The decision to use RT should be taken by a senior medical member of staff, where possible. If RT is considered necessary, and there is any uncertainty about previous medical history lorazepam should be considered as the first-line treatment. In cases where the client has previously responded to antipsychotics, haloperidol and lorazepam are sometimes used (NICE 2005; Taylor *et al.*).

Zuclopenthixol acetate (Acuphase) injection is not recommended for rapid tranquillization as it has a long onset and duration of action. However, it may be considered for use if: it is expected that the service user will be violent over a long period of time; the user has previously responded well to zuclopenthixol acetate; and the service user has a history of and is likely to need repeated short-acting injections. Zuclopenthixol acetate should never be administered to those without any previous exposure to antipsychotic medication (NICE 2005; Talor *et al.* 2005).

Conclusion

In this chapter we have considered that currently medication is the mainstay of mental health treatment. Modern medicines can offer safe and effective symptom reduction and relief for service users suffering from a range of mental health problems. Mental health nurses have a vital role to play in working in a collaborative partnership with service users in exploring and working through the multifaceted concept and process of medication concordance.

Questions for reflection and discussion

1 The UK Nursing and Midwifery Council indicates that practising mental health nurses who help clients manage their medication should assess and evaluate four areas of medication outcomes: safety, symptoms, side effects and client satisfaction. Consider how and why these four areas may differ between typical (1st generation) and atypical (2nd generation) antipsychotic medications.

2 Clients, relatives and carers often enquire about the most efficacious medication when making a decision about what to take. Given the content of this chapter what information would you give a client who was considering medication for a bipolar affective disorder?

3 Put yourself in the position of someone who is taking a medication that makes them feel nauseous, lethargic and forgetful. What practical strategies would you employ to counter the associated distress and who would you approach to help you?

4 Reflect on each of the following and consider what elements of each may influence adherence with medication:
   - the person
   - the illness/condition
   - the medication(s)

Annotated bibliography

- Bressington, D., Gray, R., Lathlean, J. and Mills, A. (2008) Antipsychotic medications in prisons: satisfaction and adherence to treatment. *Mental Health Practice* **11**(1): 18–21. This journal article explores and summarizes the influences on satisfaction with and adherence to antipsychotic medication in prisoners. Although the article relates to a specialist clinical setting the suggested interventions may be of use to anyone who is taking medication.

- Grant, A., Mills, J., Mulhern, R. and Short, N. (2004) *Cognitive Behavioural Therapy in Mental Health Care.* London: Sage Publications. Medication is only part of a package of care and clinical guidelines recommend the use of psychosocial approaches in conjunction with medicines. This book is an easy-to-read text that outlines the use of cognitive behavioural interventions with a range of disorders, it uses case examples in an extremely effective manner to illustrate how psychosocial approaches can be used to help people with a variety of problems.

- Turkington, D., Kingdon, D., Rathod, S. *et al.* (2009) *Back to Life, Back to Normality: Cognitive therapy, recovery and psychosis.* Cambridge: Cambridge University Press. This self-help book provides an excellent resource for mental health nurses to use to enable people with schizophrenia and their carers to manage their illness.

References

Ballard, C. and Waite, J. (2006) The effectiveness of atypical antipsychotics for the treatment of aggression and psychosis in Alzheimer's disease. *Cochrane Database of Systematic Reviews* 1: CD003476.

Birks, J. (2006) Cholinesterase inhibitors for Alzheimer's disease. *Cochrane Database of Systematic Reviews* 1: 10.1002./14651858.CD005593.

Blows, W.T. (2003) *The Biological Basis of Nursing: Mental Health.* London: Routledge.

Calderone, V., Testai, L., Martinotti, E., Del, T.M. and Breschi, M.C. (2005) Drug-induced block of cardiac HERG potassium channels and development of torsade de pointes arrhythmias: the case of antipsychotics. *Journal of Pharmacy and Pharmacology* **57**(2): 151–61.

Carlsson, A., Hansson, L.O., Waters, N. and Carlsson, M.L. (1999) A glutamatergic deficiency model of schizophrenia. *British Journal of Psychiatry* **174**(Suppl. 37): 2–6.

Caroff, S.N. and Mann, S.C. (1993) Neuroleptic malignant syndrome. *Medical Clinics of North America* **77**(1): 185–202.

Davis, J., Chen, N., Ira, S. and Glick, D. (2003) A meta-analysis of the efficacy of second-generation antipsychotics. *Archives of General Psychiatry* **60**: 553–64.

El-Sayeh, H.G., Morganti, C. and Adams, C.E. (2006) Aripiprazole for schizophrenia: Systematic review. *British Journal of Psychiatry* **189**: 102–8.

Francois, C., Sintonen, H., Sulkava, R. and Rive, B. (2004) Cost effectiveness of memantine in moderately severe to severe Alzheimer's disease: a Markov model in Finland. *Clinical Drug Investigation* **24**(7): 373–84.

Gardner, D.M., Baldessarini, R.J. and Waraich, P. (2005) Modern antipsychotic drugs: a critical overview. *Canadian Medical Association Journal* **172**(13): 1703–11.

Ghaemi, S.N., Hsu, D.J., Rosenquist, K.J., Pardo, T.B. and Goodwin, F.K. (2006) Extrapyramidal side effects with atypical neuroleptics in bipolar disorder. *Progress in Neuro-Psychopharmacology and Biological Psychiatry* **30**(2): 209–13.

Gray, R. (2001) Medication related cardiac risks and sudden deaths among people receiving antipsychotics for schizophrenia. *Mental Health Care* **4**(9): 302–4.

Gray, R., Wykes, T., Edmonds, M., Leese, M. and Gournay, K. (2004) Effect of medication management training package for nurses on clinical outcomes for patients with schizophrenia. *British Journal of Psychiatry* **185**: 157–62.

Gray, R., Parr, A.M. and Robson, D. (2005) Has tardive dyskinesia disappeared? *Mental Health Practice* **8**(10): 20–2.

Herholz, K., Bauer, B., Wienhard, K. *et al.* (2000) In-vivo measurements of regional acetylcholine esterase activity in degenerative dementia: comparison with blood flow and glucose metabolism. *Journal of Neural Transmission* **107**(12): 1457–68.

Hermesh, H., Aizenberg, D., Weizman, A., Lapidot, M., Mayor, C. and Munitz, H. (1992) Risk for definite neuroleptic malignant syndrome. A prospective study in 223 consecutive in-patients. *British Journal of Psychiatry* **161**: 254–7.

Hogarty, G.E. and Ulrich, R.F. (1998) The limitations of antipsychotic medications on schizophrenia. Relapse and adjustment and the contributions of psychosocial treatment. *Journal of Psychiatric Research* **32**: 243–50.

Kane, G., Honigfeld, J., Singer, J. and Meltzer, H. (1988) Clozapine for the treatment-resistant schizophrenia: a double-blind comparison with chlorpromazine. *Archives of General Psychiatry* **45**: 789–96.

Kontaxakis, V.P., Ferentinos, P.P., Havaki-Kontaxaki, B.J. and Roukas, D.K. (2005) Randomized controlled augmentation trials in clozapine-resistant schizophrenic patients: a critical review. *European Psychiatry: the Journal of the Association of European Psychiatrists* **20**(5–6): 409–15.

Lewis, S., Barnes, T. and Davies, L. (2006) Randomized controlled trial of effect of prescription of clozapine versus other second-generation antipsychotic drugs in resistant schizophrenia. *Schizophrenia Bulletin* **32**(4): 715–23.

Lieberman, J., Stroup, T., McEvoy, J. *et al.* (2005) Effectiveness of antipsychotic drugs in patients with chronic schizophrenia. *New England Journal of Medicine* **353**: 1209–23.

Lipton, S.A. (2005) The molecular basis of memantine action in Alzheimer's disease and other neurologic disorders: low-affinity, uncompetitive antagonism. *Current Alzheimer Research* **2**(2): 155–65.

Loy, C. and Schneider, L. (2006) Galantamine for Alzheimer's disease and mild cognitive impairment. *Cochrane Database of Systematic Reviews: Reviews 2006.* Issue. 1 DOI.: 10.1002./14651858.CD001747.pub3.

McEvoy, J.P., Lieberman, J.A., Stroup, T.S. *et al.* (2006) CATIE Investigators: Effectiveness of clozapine versus olanzapine, quetiapine, and risperidone in patients with chronic schizophrenia who did not respond to prior atypical antipsychotic treatment. *American Journal of Psychiatry* **163**: 600–10.

Mannion, L., Sloan, D. and Connolly, L. (1997) Rapid tranquillisation: are we getting it right? *Psychiatric Bulletin* **21**: 411–13.

Margolese, H.C., Chouinard, G., Kolivakis, T.T., Beauclair, L., Miller, R., and Annable, L. (2005) Tardive dyskinesia in the era of typical and atypical antipsychotics. Part 2: Incidence and management strategies in patients with schizophrenia. *Canadian Journal of Psychiatry – Revue Canadienne de Psychiatrie* **50**(11): 703–14.

Mehta, D. (ed.) (2007) *British National Formulary.* 53. London: BMJ Publishing Ltd.

Mendhekar, D.N. (2005) Ziprasidone-induced tardive dyskinesia. *Canadian Journal of Psychiatry – Revue Canadienne de Psychiatrie* **50**(9): 567–8.

Mir, S. and Taylor, D. (2001) Atypical antipsychotics and hyperglycaemia. *International Clinical Psychopharmacology* **16**(2): 63–73.

National Institute for Clinical Excellence (2002) *Guidance on the Use of Newer (Atypical) Antipsychotic Drugs for the Treatment of Schizophrenia*. London: NICE.

National Institute for Health and Clinical Excellence (2004a) *Depression: Management of Depression in Primary and Secondary Care. Clinical Guideline 23*. London: NICE.

National Institute for Health and Clinical Excellence (2004b) *Anxiety (Amended) Management of Anxiety (Panic Disorder with or without Agoraphobia and GAD) in Adults. NICE Clinical Guideline 22*. London: NICE.

National Institute for Health and Clinical Excellence (2005) *The Short-term Management of Disturbed/Violent Behaviour in In-patient Psychiatric Settings and Emergency Departments. NICE Clinical Guideline 25*. London: NICE.

National Institute for Health and Clinical Excellence (2006a) *Dementia: Supporting people with dementia and their carers in health and social care. NICE Clinical Guideline 42*. London: NICE.

National Institute for Health and Clinical Excellence (2006b) *Donepezil, galantamine, rivastigimine (review) and memantine for the treatment of Alzheimer's disease (amended). NICE technology appraisal guidance 111 (amended)* London: NICE.

Nasrallah, H.A. (2007) The case for long-acting antipsychotic agents in the post-CATIE era. *Acta Psychiatrica Scandanavica* **115**: 260–7.

Newcomer, J.W. (2005) Second-generation (atypical) antipsychotics and metabolic effects: a comprehensive literature review. *CNS Drugs* **19**(Suppl. 1): 1–93.

Parik, V., Khan, M.M., Terry, A. and Mahadik, S.P. (2004) Differential effects of typicaland atypical antipsychotics on nerve growth factor and acetylcholinesterase expression in the cortex and nucleus basalis of rats. *Journal of Psychiatric Research* **38**: 521–9.

Rathbone, J. and Soares-Weiser, K. (2006) Anticholinergics for neuroleptic-induced acute akathisia. *Cochrane Database of Systematic Reviews* **4**: CD003727. DOI: 10.1002/14651858. CD003727.pub3.

Remington, G., Saha, A., Chong, S.A. and Shammi, C. (2005) Augmentation strategies in clozapine-resistant schizophrenia. *CNS Drugs* **19**(10): 843–72.

Stahl, S.M. (2000) *Essential Psychopharmacology: Neuroscientific Basis and Practical Applications* (2nd edn). Cambridge: Cambridge University Press.

Stollberger, C., Huber, J.O. and Finsterer, J. (2005) Antipsychotic drugs and QT prolongation. *International Clinical Psychopharmacology* **20**(5): 243–51.

Taylor, D., Paton, C. and Kerwin, R. (2005) *The Maudsley Prescribing Guidelines* (8th edn). London: Taylor and Francis.

Wahlbeck, K., Cheine, M.V. and Essali, A. (1999) Clozapine versus typical neuroleptic medication for schizophrenia. *Cochrane Database of Systematic Reviews* **4** DOI.: 10.1002./14651858.CD000059.

Warner, J.P., Barnes, T.R. and Henry, J.A. (1996) Electrocardiographic changes in patients receiving neuroleptic medication. *Acta Psychiatrica Scandinavica* **93**: 311–13.

CHAPTER 17

Complementary and alternative therapies

Hagen Rampes and Karen Pilkington

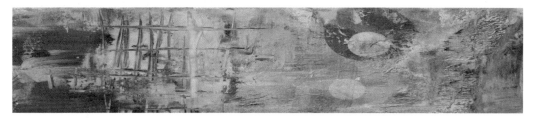

Chapter overview

This chapter describes the contribution of complementary and alternative therapies to the treatment and care of people who experience mental health problems. It is written from the perspective of a psychiatrist in the National Health Service who is trained in a number of complementary and alternative therapies and a clinical researcher with experience in assessing the research on complementary and alternative therapies in mental health. The chapter covers the following:

- What are complementary and alternative therapies?
- How many people use complementary and alternative therapies?
- Why do people use complementary and alternative therapies?
- Use of complementary and alternative therapies by people with mental health problems;
- Research on complementary and alternative therapies
  - Challenges in research
  - The contribution of qualitative studies;
- Specific complementary and alternative therapies
  - Acupuncture and related therapies
  - Aromatherapy, massage and reflexology
  - Herbal medicine
  - Homeopathy
  - Meditation, yoga and related therapies
  - Other therapies;
- The placebo effect – is it important?
- Conclusions and summary;
- Sources of information.

What are complementary and alternative therapies?

The term *alternative medicine* was originally introduced to refer to whole medical systems that did not fit with conventional medicine and which had different ideas on causes of disease, methods of diagnosis and approaches to treatment. *Complementary medicine* or *therapies* refers to those methods which can be used alongside or to 'complement' conventional medicine. There is considerable overlap between the two areas and what is considered to be complementary or alternative in one country may be considered conventional in another. *Complementary and alternative therapies* is often used to include both approaches and refers to any therapies, practices or approaches to health care outside mainstream conventional medicine. The Prince's Foundation for Integrated Health defines *integrated health care* as the best of all health care for the whole person.

Several organizations have developed definitions or categories of complementary and alternative therapies. The Cochrane Complementary Medicine Field defines complementary medicine as

> all such practices and ideas which are outside the domain of conventional medicine in several countries and defined by its users as preventing or treating illness, or promoting health and well being. These practices complement mainstream medicine by 1) contributing to a common whole, 2) satisfying a demand not met by conventional practices, and 3) diversifying the conceptual framework of medicine.
>
> (Manheimer and Berman 2006)

The National Center for Complementary and Alternative Medicine, which is a department of the National Institutes of Health established by the Congress of the United States of America, classifies complementary and alternative therapies into five categories or domains:

- ■ *Whole medical systems*
  Whole medical systems are built upon complete systems of theory and practice. Often, these systems have evolved apart from and earlier than conventional medicine in the West. Examples of whole medical systems that have developed in Western cultures include homeopathic medicine and naturopathic medicine. Examples of systems that have developed in non-western cultures include Ayurveda and traditional Chinese medicine.

- ■ *Mind–body medicine*
  Mind–body medicine uses a variety of techniques designed to enhance the mind's capacity to affect bodily function and symptoms. These techniques include meditation, prayer, mental healing and therapies that use creative outlets such as art, music or dance.

- ■ *Biologically based practices*
  Biologically based therapies in complementary and alternative therapy use substances found in nature, such as herbs, foods and vitamins. Some examples include dietary supplements or herbal products.

- ■ *Manipulative and body-based practices*
  Manipulative and body-based methods in complementary and alternative therapy are

based on manipulation and/or movement of one or more parts of the body. Some examples include chiropractic or osteopathic manipulation and massage.

■ *Energy medicine*
    Energy therapies involve the use of energy fields. Biofield therapies are intended to affect the energy fields that surround and penetrate the human body. The existence of such fields has not been scientifically proven. Some forms of energy therapy manipulate biofields by placing the hands in or through these fields. Pressure or manipulation may be applied to the body. Examples include qi gong, reiki and therapeutic touch. Bioelectromagnetic-based therapies involve the unconventional use of electromagnetic fields, such as pulsed fields, magnetic fields, alternating current fields or direct current fields.

Complementary and alternative therapies are then categorized by method of access or administration as listed in Box 17.1.

The boundaries between complementary and conventional medicine change over time as certain complementary practices become accepted and new approaches emerge. Several discussion papers on this topic may be of interest (Kaptchuk and Eisenberg 2001; Caspi *et al.* 2003; Wootton 2005).

How many people use complementary and alternative therapies?

Survey data suggest that complementary and alternative therapies are used by a sizeable proportion of the population in a number of countries: figures reported for some European countries in the early 1990s were between 20 and 50 per cent. A study from Germany reported an overall prevalence rate of 65 per cent in 1996, compared to a corresponding figure of 52 per cent in 1970 (Haussermann 1997). These figures are the highest reported anywhere. However, therapies such as herbal medicine, hydrotherapy and massage are firmly established in conventional medicine in many European countries.

Use of complementary and alternative therapies by US adults increased substantially between 1990 and 1997 (Eisenberg *et al.* 1998) but appeared to remain stable from 1997 to 2002 (Tindle *et al.* 2005). Overall, use of 15 therapies was similar between 1997 and 2002 (36.5%, vs. 35.0%, respectively, each representing about 72 million US adults). The most commonly used modalities in 2002 were herbal therapy, relaxation techniques and chiropractic and the greatest relative increase in use was seen for herbal medicine and yoga while the largest relative decrease occurred for chiropractic. A further survey in the US indicated that complementary and alternative therapies were most often used to treat back pain or back problems, head or chest colds, neck pain or neck problems, joint pain or stiffness, and anxiety or depression (Barnes *et al.* 2004).

It was estimated that in 1993, 8.5 per cent of the adult population in England visited at least one complementary and alternative therapy provider of acupuncture, chiropractic, homeopathy, hypnotherapy, herbal medicine or osteopathy during the past 12 months (Thomas *et al.* 1993). This figure increased to 10.6 per cent in 1998 using similar methodology, suggesting a slower growth than that reported by Eisenberg *et al.* in the USA over a similar time period (Thomas *et al.* 2001). However, if data for reflexology,

Box 17.1   Examples of complementary and alternative therapies

Treatments a person largely administers to himself or herself
Botanicals
Nutritional supplements
Health food
Meditation
Magnetic therapy

Treatments providers administer
Acupuncture
Massage therapy
Reflexology
Laser therapy
Balneotherapy
Chiropractic
Osteopathy
Psychological counselling certain types
Naturopathy

Treatments a person administers to himself or herself under the periodic observation of a provider
Yoga
Biofeedback
Tai chi
Homeopathy
Hydrotherapy
Alexander therapy
Nutritional therapy
Ayurveda

Other interventions
Qi gong
Anthroposophical medicines
Unani medicine
Traditional African medicine
Bach flower remedies
Clinical ecology
Colon cleansing or irrigation
Music or sound therapy

Diagnostic techniques
Iridology
Kinesiology
Vega testing
Biofunctional diagnostic testing
Electroacupuncture by Voll
Hair analysis

aromatherapy and remedies purchased over the counter were included in the analysis then the estimated one-year prevalence increased to 28.3 per cent. Over 4 million adults made 18 million visits to practitioners of one of six therapies: acupuncture, chiropractic, homeopathy, hypnotherapy, herbal medicine or osteopathy in England in 1998. The National Health Service provided about 10 per cent of these contacts. The majority of non-National Health Service visits represented direct out-of-pocket expenditures (Thomas *et al.* 2001). Frequency of use was greatest for osteopathy (4.3 per cent) and chiropractic (3.6 per cent). Other popular therapies included aromatherapy (3.5 per cent), reflexology (2.4 per cent), acupuncture (1.6 per cent) and herbal medicine (0.9 per cent). An estimated 10.0 per cent of the population had received any complementary and alternative therapy from a practitioner in the past year (Thomas and Coleman 2004).

Why do people use complementary and alternative therapies?

Furnham (1996) has summarized the main hypotheses relating to why people use complementary and alternative therapies. Some he described as 'push' factors. These include dissatisfaction with or outright rejection of conventional medicine through prior negative experiences or a general anti-establishment attitude. For these reasons, patients are pushed away from conventional treatment in search of alternatives. Other factors pull or attract patients towards complementary and alternative therapy. These include compatibility between the philosophy of certain therapies and patients' own beliefs and a greater sense of control over one's own treatment.

Kaptchuk and Eisenberg (1998) suggest that there are fundamental premises of most forms of complementary and alternative therapy, which contribute to its persuasive appeal. One of these is the perceived association of complementary and alternative therapy with nature. Complementary and alternative therapy is natural, pure and organic, whereas conventional medicine is artificial, synthetic and processed. Another fundamental component of complementary and alternative therapy is vitalism. The enhancement or balancing of 'life forces' known as *qi*, *prana* or *psychic energy* is central to many forms of complementary and alternative therapy. Another factor is spirituality. This bridges the gap between the domain of medical science with its search for causality and the domain of religion with its morals and values. Complementary and alternative therapy thus offers a satisfying unification of the physical and spiritual.

Another proposed explanation is that patients using complementary and alternative therapy are essentially neurotic and are drawn towards the touching or talking approach of many therapies. While levels of psychiatric disorder are reported to be high in patients visiting complementary and alternative therapists, and higher than those visiting a general practitioner (GP), this may simply be a reflection of the nature of the conditions being treated.

Several studies (Finnigan 1991; Resch *et al.* 1997) have compared patients' views of consultations with practitioners of conventional medicine and complementary and alternative therapy. Most studies have found complementary therapy practitioners to be perceived by patients as more friendly and personal, to have treated patients more like partners in care, and provided more time for the consultation. Patients were also more satisfied with the therapeutic encounter. The duration of consultation for complementary and alternative therapy is invariably longer than with conventional medicine; in Finnigan's (1991) study 68 per cent of patients reported a better relationship with the complementary and alternative practitioner than with their own GP. The hard-pressed GP can offer only a ten minute consultation. Complementary and alternative therapy consultations involve more discussion and explanation than that offered by conventional medical practitioners in the NHS.

In general, complementary and alternative therapy does not replace conventional medicine (Druss and Rosenheck 1999). Rather it serves as a substitute in some situations and as an adjunct in others, while being disregarded when not considered appropriate for the condition in question. This has been described as 'shopping for health'. Patients simply perceive complementary and alternative therapy as one of a range of treatment options available to them and exercise their freedom of choice and discriminating power accordingly. The desire to try all available options may be for some an attempt to leave no stone unturned as they become increasingly desperate for an effective treatment.

Astin's (1998) survey of 1500 North Americans found a number of predictors of complementary and alternative therapy use. Complementary and alternative therapy users were more likely than non-users to be better educated, have a holistic orientation to health and report current poor health status. Their main complaints were anxiety, back problems, chronic pain and urinary tract infections. They had often had an experience that had changed their world-view. They were also more likely to be committed to environmentalism, feminism, spirituality and personal growth.

Astin found that dissatisfaction with conventional medicine was not predictive of use of complementary and alternative therapy. However, in addition to being more educated and reporting poorer health status, most complementary and alternative therapy users find these health care approaches more congruent with their own values, beliefs and philosophical orientations towards health and life than conventional medicine.

Use of complementary and alternative therapies by people with mental health problems

A survey of over 16,000 people in the USA revealed that 9.8 per cent of those reporting a mental condition made a complementary visit, and about half of these (4.5%) made a visit to treat the mental condition. Persons reporting transient stress or adjustment disorders were most likely, and those with psychotic and affective conditions least likely, to use complementary therapies to treat their mental condition (Druss and Rosenheck 2000). A further study revealed that individuals with panic disorder and major depression were significantly more likely to use complementary and alternative therapies than those without those disorders (Unützer et al. 2000).

Davidson et al. (1998) conducted a study to determine the frequency of psychiatric disorders in a sample of patients receiving complementary medical care in the UK and the USA. Patients were randomly recruited from two sites. The UK study was conducted at the Royal London Homoeopathic Hospital. The North American component was conducted at a private complementary and alternative therapy practice in Durham, North Carolina. Patients were interviewed for demographic information and lifetime and current psychiatric disorders using a structured clinical interview.

Fifty patients (mean age 52.5, 79.6% female) were interviewed in London and 33 (mean age 46.9, 78.8% female) in North Carolina. Only 35.7 per cent of the patients in the British sample were married, whereas 66.7 per cent of the patients in the American sample were married. Of the British patients 78.3 per cent were white (13% were Asian and 8.7% were black) whereas 100 per cent of American patients were white. Fifty-six per cent of the British patients had graduated from sixth form whereas 100 per cent of the American patients had graduated from high school.

Rates of lifetime psychiatric diagnoses revealed a total of 74 per cent of the British patients and 60.6 per cent of the American patients having a diagnosis. Major depression (52% of UK and 33.3% of USA) and any anxiety disorders (50% of UK and 33.3% of USA) were the commonest lifetime diagnoses. Only post-traumatic stress disorder was significantly different (UK was 10% and the USA was 33.3%). Rates of current psychiatric disorder revealed 46 per cent of the UK patients and 30.3 per cent of the US patients having a diagnosis. Six per cent of the total suffered from a major depression and 25.3 per cent of the total met the criteria for at least one anxiety disorder, with social phobia and generalized anxiety being the commonest. Social phobia was significantly more common in the US patients. While generalized anxiety disorder, simple phobia and major depression occurred more often in the UK patients, these were not significantly different from the US patients. The demographic differences of ethnic, marital and education status may have been due to the sources of recruitment. The authors found that psychiatric disorders were not rare among patients who sought complementary medical care and that anxiety disorders were particularly represented.

A large study conducted between 2001 and 2003 of over 9000 people with 12-month DSM-IV anxiety, mood, impulse control, and substance disorders provided further insight into where they received treatment. In the 12 months before the interview, 41.1 per cent had received some form of treatment: 12.3 per cent were treated by a psychiatrist, 16.0 per cent by a non-psychiatrist mental health specialist, 22.8 per cent by a general medical provider, 8.1 per cent by a human services provider, and 6.8 per cent by a complementary and alternative medical provider (Wang *et al.* 2005).

The Mental Health Foundation's *Knowing Our Own Minds* survey (1997) of mental health service users' views on complementary and alternative therapy found that of the 401 users who participated, 37 per cent had received osteopathy, acupuncture, massage, aromatherapy or reflexology. Of these, 85 per cent had found the therapies helpful. Thirty-one per cent had experienced exercise, yoga or movement therapy, of whom 85 per cent had found it helpful. Twenty-seven per cent had received nutritional therapy, homeopathy, naturopathy or herbal medicine; 63 per cent of whom found it helpful. In each of these groups 2–5 per cent found the therapies unhelpful and 1 per cent found them harmful. What respondents valued most about complementary and alternative therapies was their relaxing and holistic nature. Some respondents found that the most helpful approach was to combine a number of different therapies and activities. In summary the survey found that mental health service users experienced complementary and alternative therapy as helpful in providing symptom relief and improving general health.

Several studies have investigated which therapies are used specifically for depression. Those most frequently sought in the USA included relaxation techniques, herbal medicine, imagery and spiritual healing (Kessler *et al.* 2001). A study in Australia revealed that massage and meditation is used for mild depression, aromatherapy, St John's wort, yoga and nutritional supplements for moderate depression and relaxation therapy for moderate to severe episodes (Jorm *et al.* 2004). No complementary therapies were reported to be used for severe depression.

Research on complementary and alternative therapies

Challenges in research

A wide range of different types of research has been conducted on complementary and alternative therapies but in comparison with conventional treatments, the actual numbers of studies are still very small. Surveys of use, outcome (uncontrolled) studies, non-randomized and randomized trials, systematic reviews and meta-analyses and qualitative studies have all been conducted. The Cochrane Library is an important resource for critically appraised research evidence on complementary and alternative therapies. The Cochrane Collaboration is collating all randomized controlled trials (RCTs) and the Complementary Medicine Field within the collaboration is compiling those pertinent to complementary and alternative therapies.

However, a number of problems have discouraged the use of RCTs in the complementary medicine field. Firstly, much treatment by complementary and alternative practitioners is individualized and involves combinations of different therapies, for example individualized acupuncture may be combined with dietary advice, massage and herbal treatment. This approach is difficult to accommodate in the design of RCTs where the main aim is to remove or reduce any variation in treatment. There are also difficulties in finding appropriate control or placebo treatments and blinding of patients and care givers is impossible for many therapies. Most therapies involve considerable interaction with a practitioner and RCTs do not always take account of this. Finally, there have been problems with recruiting sufficient numbers of people in trials where there is a possibility that they will not receive their chosen therapy.

For each complementary and alternative therapy, there are differing levels of evidence. Studies other than RCTs also have a role in assessment but more research, particularly large well-designed studies, needs to be conducted. There has been a lack of significant funding for research on complementary and alternative therapies in the UK. Several initiatives are underway to establish a research infrastructure and the number of trials conducted has increased. Nevertheless, systematic reviews which comprehensively identify, assess and summarize all the research on a specific topic, often conclude that there is a lack of good evidence on complementary and alternative therapies.

The contribution of qualitative studies

Nathan (2001) conducted a study of patients' perceptions and views on spiritual care in mental health practice in West London Mental Health NHS Trust. This study is an example of a qualitative study conducted by a nurse. This type of study is important since it raises interesting questions on how mental health professionals relate to patients.

The aim of the study was to establish patients' perceptions and views on spiritual care and to elicit whether or not mental health service users are of the opinion that spiritual care has any positive effects or benefits in mental health practice. A convenience sample of 13 patients from varied cultural and ethnic backgrounds was interviewed. Interviews were audiotaped and transcribed and the data were subjected to content analysis.

Four main themes that emerged were: religion, relationship, meaning making and work. Though all participants associated spiritual care with religion, none of them described spiritual care strictly as only religion. Patients described spiritual care as having to do with their relationship with others, daily activities that help them make meaning of life experiences and worship. Participants acknowledged that spiritual care is as important as all other aspects of care and its provision can contribute to their recovery and quality of life.

Patients were of the opinion that when spiritual care is appropriately provided it can enhance the effectiveness of other aspects of care (for example, social, physical and psychological). Elements of spiritual care were described as the quality that permeates all aspects of care and influences how each person provides or receives care.

One patient stated: 'My religious belief is very important to me, without my faith in God I would not have been alive today.' Some patients described spiritual care as providing opportunities to participate in creative activities.

> Art or music acts as a door or window into an imaginary world, which provides meaning and understanding to things that one cannot explain in words. Spiritual world is very personal and each person's world is different and depends on one's needs.

> Spiritual care is staff giving you time to talk through your problems ... it is helping you to deal with your inner feelings ... spiritual care is to do with your inner need, that which keeps you alive.

> Spiritual care is nothing more than the attitudes of staff to patients ... it is when you are made to feel valued ... it helps to bring dignity back to your life.

Qualitative research studies such as that by Nathan can make an important contribution to our understanding of the motivation and experience of users of complementary and alternative therapies. Qualitative studies can also provide the users' perspective on effectiveness and acceptability of therapies (e.g. Finucane and Mercer 2006). Practising nurses are well placed to contribute to this body of knowledge.

Specific complementary and alternative therapies

Acupuncture and related therapies

What is acupuncture?

Acupuncture encompasses differing philosophies and techniques. Acupuncture is the stimulation of special points on the body, usually by insertion of fine needles. How the points to be treated are selected depends on the teaching and background of the practitioner. At one end of the spectrum is the Traditional Chinese Medicine acupuncturist, who operates from a theoretical paradigm different from that of Western conventional medicine. Traditional Chinese Medicine includes the use of acupuncture, herbs, massage and dietary approaches. It has a belief in a vital force or 'Chi'. Disease results from imbalance of this 'energy'. The body has a number of 'energy' channels or meridians on which lie the acupuncture points. Traditional acupuncture theory sees illness in terms of excess or deficiencies in various exogenous and endogenous factors and treatment is aimed at restoring balance.

At the other end of the spectrum is the 'Scientific' or Western acupuncturist, who has divorced the Chinese theoretical basis of acupuncture and instead uses a set of acupuncture points to treat a variety of conditions empirically. Auriculo-acupuncture, i.e. acupuncture of the ears, although known to the Chinese, is a relatively new development advanced by Western doctors.

Following insertion of needles at acupuncture points, further stimulation of the points can be achieved by manual stimulation of the needle by rotation, application of heat to the needle by burning the herb *artemisia vulgaris* over the needle (moxibustion) or by applying an electric current to a pair of needles (electro-acupuncture). Electro-acupuncture is a modern development, which the Chinese also use. Other developments include the use of lasers to stimulate acupuncture points.

What is the evidence on acupuncture in mental illness?

Alcohol and substance misuse

Acupuncture has been used in the management of addiction. An early systematic review found encouraging evidence for efficacy of acupuncture in drug addiction and proposed that since acupuncture is quick, inexpensive and relatively safe, it may prove to be an important component of treatment (Moner 1996). Systematic reviews since then have not found sufficient evidence to confirm efficacy (Kunz et al. 2004; Gates et al. 2006). One review included seven studies with a total of 1433 participants but all were of generally low quality. It has also been suggested that some of the current supportive evidence for efficacy came from Chinese journals that have not yet been translated into English (Jordan 2006).

Smoking cessation

A review in 1997 concluded that acupuncture appeared promising although there was insufficient evidence to recommend it as an effective form of therapy (Ashenden et al. 1997). A 2006 Cochrane review still found no consistent evidence that acupuncture, acupressure, laser therapy or electrostimulation are effective for smoking cessation, but methodological problems meant that no firm conclusions could be drawn (White et al. 2006). Some researchers suggest that auricular (ear) acupuncture appears to be effective for smoking cessation, but the effect may not depend on point location (White & Moody 2006).

Anxiety

A systematic review of acupuncture in anxiety included ten RCTs: four focused on generalized anxiety disorder or anxiety neurosis and six on anxiety in the perioperative period (Pilkington et al. 2007). There were no studies on panic disorder, phobias or obsessive compulsive disorder. It was difficult to interpret the findings because of the range of interventions against which acupuncture was compared. All trials in generalized anxiety disorder/anxiety neurosis reported positive findings but lacked many basic methodological details. The perioperative anxiety trials were better and indicated that auricular acupuncture is more effective than acupuncture at sham points and may be as effective as drug therapy in this situation. The results were, however, based on subjective measures and blinding could not be guaranteed. Thus, there is some limited evidence in favour of auricular acupuncture in short-term anxiety suggesting that further research may prove valuable.

Dementia

No RCTs and only a few high quality trials were found on acupuncture in dementia and so the effectiveness is uncertain (Peng *et al.* 2007).

Depression

Research interest in acupuncture in depression followed animal experiments suggesting that it increased the synthesis and release of serotonin and noradrenaline in the central nervous system. One meta-analysis reviewed RCTs of acupuncture, electroacupuncture and laser acupuncture (Smith and Hay 2005). Seven trials of 517 subjects with generally mild to moderate depression met the inclusion criteria. The authors concluded that there was insufficient evidence to determine the efficacy of acupuncture compared to medication, wait list control or sham acupuncture. The second systematic review also included seven studies (Mukaino *et al.* 2005). The results of this review suggested that the effect of electroacupuncture may not be significantly different from that of antidepressants but it was unclear whether acupuncture has an additive effect when given with antidepressants. Both reviews concluded that, as the studies were generally small and poorly designed, further research is needed.

Schizophrenia

Five trials of acupuncture in schizophrenia provided insufficient evidence to recommend the use of acupuncture for people with schizophrenia because of inadequate numbers of participants and other problems (Rathbone and Xia 2005). Again, more well-designed studies are recommended.

Is acupuncture safe?

A review by Rampes and James (1995) revealed that serious adverse effects of acupuncture had been reported ranging from trauma to underlying organs (for example pneumothorax: puncture of the lung cavity) to infections (hepatitis B). Most serious adverse effects are preventable by appropriate practitioner training. In the past, practitioners used reusable needles, which required careful sterilization. Unfortunately, poor sterilization resulted in several outbreaks of hepatitis B worldwide. Overall, the conclusion of the review was that acupuncture is relatively safe. This has been confirmed by subsequent studies. The rate of adverse events reported by practitioners was investigated in two prospective surveys of a total of over 60,000 consultations (Macpherson *et al.* 2001; White *et al.* 2001). Eighty-six non-serious adverse events were reported, the most frequent being nausea, fainting and dizziness. In another study, patients reported a higher rate of adverse events (10.7%), most commonly severe tiredness, pain at the needling site and headache (Macpherson *et al.* 2004). However, the results of this study reinforced the perception that acupuncture is relatively safe in 'competent hands', that is those of regulated practitioners.

Who practises acupuncture?

The British Medical Acupuncture Society trains doctors and health care professionals. The British Academy of Western Acupuncture trains health care professionals. Physiotherapists and osteopaths have their own acupuncture training. The British Acupuncture Council represents non-medically qualified practitioners trained by several training colleges. Such practitioners are trained in traditional acupuncture. Currently acupuncture can be performed in the UK by practitioners who are either subject to statutory regulation (doctors, physiotherapists, nurses and other health professionals), voluntary self-regulation (members of the British Acupuncture Council), or by unregulated lay practitioners. A process is currently under way to organize statutory regulation of acupuncture in England.

Aromatherapy, massage and reflexology

What are aromatherapy, massage and reflexology?

Aromatherapy involves the use of essential oils from plants, which are considered to have a range of therapeutic properties. Oils may be inhaled or added to baths but are most frequently used in combination with massage. The aim of massage is to promote the circulation of blood and lymph, and relaxation of muscles, providing both physical and mental benefits. Reflexology is a method of massage in which pressure is applied to 'reflex' zones on the feet (or hands) thought to correspond to parts of the body including the major organs and glands and so connected with a range of health problems. The mechanism of action of reflexology is thought to be by stimulating the release of endorphins and encephalins in the same way as generalized massage. Other theories on action relate more closely to those of traditional Chinese medicine (Tiran 2002).

What is the evidence on aromatherapy, massage and reflexology in mental illness?

Anxiety and depression

It has been suggested that improvement of depression and trait anxiety are the largest effects of massage therapy and that a course of treatment provides benefits similar to psychotherapy (Moyer *et al.* 2004). A series of RCTs of massage therapy have been conducted in a range of groups including hospitalized children and adolescents with depression, adolescent mothers with depressive symptoms and women with postnatal depression (Pilkington *et al.* 2006a). Massage therapy (regular 30–60-minute sessions) compared favourably with relaxing activities such as viewing a videotape, yoga plus progressive muscular relaxation or no treatment. Similarly, massage appeared superior to no treatment or relaxation-based control treatment based on self-assessment of anxiety in range of situations (anxious elderly, post-traumatic stress disorder in children, premenstrual dysphoria disorder and preoperatively) (Pilkington *et al.* 2006b). There is currently insufficient research evidence on any single intervention or patient group for firm conclusions on effectiveness, role or long-term outcomes to be drawn. Aromatherapy massage was compared with massage alone in a small study in elderly patients with anxiety and/or depression. Promising results were reported for the combined intervention. It is difficult to assess the effects of aromatherapy alone as the studies were of insufficient quality. Several studies were found on the effects of reflexology on mood or depression in patients with conditions such as cancer but no published clinical trials specifically on anxiety disorders or depressive disorders (Pilkington *et al.* 2006c, 2006d).

Dementia

Aromatherapy showed benefit on measures of agitation and neuropsychiatric symptoms in people with dementia in the only trial of sufficient quality for analysis (Thorgrimsen *et al.*

2003). However, participants were taking a range of medication which may have affected the results and there was some concern over how treatment was randomized so further confirmation of the results is required.

Are aromatherapy, massage and reflexology safe?

Essential oils are potent chemicals virtually all of which require dilution before use. Several oils cannot be used due to potential toxicity and many are avoided during pregnancy due to lack of information on the possible risks. Problems with safety are most often due to inappropriate or excessive use, accidental ingestion and lack of patch testing in the allergy-prone (Buckle 2003). The purity and constituents of essential oils vary so their actions and potential for interaction with other therapies are not totally understood (Basch and Ulbricht 2005). While massage is not entirely risk free, serious adverse events are probably rare and qualified massage therapists were rarely implicated in the reported problems (Ernst 2003).

Who practises aromatherapy, massage and reflexology?

A number of organizations offer training and qualifications in these therapies and details can be found by following the link to 'CAM organizations' on the National Library for Health CAM Specialist Library website (http://www.library.nhs.uk/cam).

Herbal medicine

What is herbal medicine?

Herbal medicine utilizes the healing properties of plant substances to restore health. Since antiquity, mankind has used plants for healing. In fact, most of our modern drugs are originally derived from plant substances but are generally administered as the pure chemical. In earlier times, plants were venerated because they were known to have valuable properties. During medieval times, the use of herbs was laden with superstition, incantation and ritual.

Modern science has analysed and studied the therapeutic effects of plants. This has led to the identification, comparison and classification of the various properties so that plants with similar effects may be grouped together, and the most effective selected for further investigation. Medicinal plants are defined as those which produce one or more active constituents capable of preventing or curing an illness.

Many products are advertised with claims that they are effective in insomnia, stress, anxiety and even depression. Some of these have very seductive and inviting names such as 'Serenity'. People do find some of these preparations helpful. The risk and benefits of such preparations need to be compared with extant prescribed hypnotic medication. For example, the propensity for benzodiazepines to cause addiction is well recognized. Assessing effectiveness and safety of herbal medicines is difficult because they contain mixtures of constituents which vary considerably. Nevertheless, there has been considerable research and clinical interest in their use, particularly in anxiety and depression.

Is there a role for herbal medicine in mental illness?

Hypericum in depression

St John's wort (*Hypericum perforatum*) is a flowering plant that is widely used as a herbal remedy particularly for self-treatment for depression. The extract appears to increase serotonin, noradrenaline and dopamine content in the brain but the mechanism of action is not fully understood (Mennini and Gobbi 2004).

A series of systematic reviews have been published and in most cases findings have been positive when compared with placebo for mild to moderate depression. Recent larger trials have, however, been less positive and the current situation is probably best summed up in the 2005 Cochrane review:

> Current evidence regarding hypericum extracts is inconsistent and confusing. In patients who meet criteria for major depression, several recent placebo-controlled trials suggest that the tested hypericum extracts have minimal beneficial effects while other trials suggest that hypericum and standard antidepressants have similar beneficial effects ... several specific extracts of St. John's wort may be effective for treating mild to moderate depression, although the data are not fully convincing.
>
> (Linde *et al.* 2005)

Other herbal medicines of interest in mental illness

Ginko in dementia

A Cochrane review concluded that *Ginkgo biloba* appears to be safe with no excess side effects compared with placebo but evidence of predictable and clinically significant effects was not convincing as many of the early trials used unsatisfactory methods or were small (Birks and Grimley Evans 2007). There may also have been a tendency to over-report positive findings and two recent larger and better trials found no difference between placebo and ginkgo.

Kava for anxiety

A systematic review suggested that, compared with placebo, kava extract may be an effective symptomatic treatment for anxiety although the effect size was small (Pittler and Ernst 2003). Subsequently, concerns about suspected liver toxicity caused kava to be withdrawn from the UK market in 2003, a ban that remains in place (MHRA 2006).

Passiflora in anxiety

The findings from one study suggested an improvement in job performance in favour of passiflora and one study showed a lower rate of drowsiness as a side effect compared with mexazolam (Miyasaka *et al.* 2007). However, the trials were too few in number to permit any conclusions to be drawn.

Valerian in anxiety and insomnia

Only one small study on valerian in anxiety was located providing insufficient evidence to draw any conclusions about the efficacy or safety compared with placebo or diazepam for anxiety disorders (Miyasaka *et al.* 2006). The evidence for valerian in insomnia was promising but not conclusive as not all of the trials reported positive findings (Bent et al 2006).

Traditional Chinese herbs in schizophrenia

Traditional Chinese medicine (TCM) has been used to treat mental health disorders, including schizophrenia, for more than 2000 years. The use of Chinese herbs in a Western medicine context, without incorporating TCM methodology, has been evaluated in six trials (Rathbone *et al.* 2005). The results suggest that using Chinese herbs in conjunction with Western antipsychotic drugs may be beneficial in terms of mental state, global functioning and decrease of adverse effects. However, because study size and length were limited, further trials are needed before the effects of TCM for people with schizophrenia can be evaluated with any real confidence.

Is herbal medicine safe?

Drugs can be measured with reliability and are tested out on animals and humans before they are allowed to be prescribed. Herbal medicines are not subject to similar scientific scrutiny. Many plants are toxic and can be fatal. The National Poisons Unit at Guy's Hospital collects information on overdoses and poisoning with plant materials.

One widely used herb, kava has been shown to have serious toxicity problems as described above. Conversely, the available data suggest that hypericum is well tolerated and has an incidence of adverse effects similar to that of placebo. The most commonly reported adverse effects are gastrointestinal symptoms, dizziness and sedation. The only potentially serious adverse effects are photosensitization, which is extremely rare, and precipitation of manic symptoms in predisposed patients. However, problems may arise when patients take hypericum with other medications as it induces a hepatic enzyme through activation of the cytochrome P450 system. Thus hypericum can decrease the plasma level of a large range of prescribed drugs including anticoagulants, oral contraceptives and antiviral agents with possible clinically serious consequences. Some evidence also indicates that combining hypericum with selective serotonin inhibitors can lead to the serotonin syndrome, particularly in elderly patients. Hypericum can be easily purchased over the counter and, clearly, will appeal to some patients simply because it is a herbal antidepressant. Many different preparations are available and this raises questions of quality assurance in the manufacture of these preparations. The amount of active ingredient present also varies between preparations and this may affect effectiveness and the extent of interaction with other drugs.

There is a growing market in the over-the-counter herbal medicine field. This trend may not be in the best interests of patients, some of who may be misguided and desperately seeking help and self-medication inappropriately. There is also concern over the safety of constituents of some Chinese and other traditional herbal mixtures. Potential interactions with existing medication and possible contraindications of all herbal medicines should be thoroughly checked. Patient preference is important in terms of treatment adherence but it would be preferable for patients to be supervised by their general practitioner or psychiatrist. Thus, the patient's primary care giver(s) should be informed about any decision to take herbal medicines and health professionals should routinely enquire about possible use of these products. Suspected adverse effects should also be reported appropriately.

Who practises herbal medicine?

There are professional medical herbalists who belong to the National Institute of Medical Herbalists. They have good training in this discipline and often work in a private setting. However, the majority are not medically qualified.

Homeopathy

What is homeopathy?

Homeopathy is a school of medicine founded by Dr Samuel Hahnemann (1755–1843). The term homeopathy is derived from the Greek for 'like suffering'. It is based on the principle of 'let likes be treated with likes' or *similia similibus curentur*. This principle was known to Hippocrates but it was Hahnemann who coined the term 'homeopathy' and worked relentlessly in establishing it against much hostility from his contemporaries. Contemporary medical practice in Hahnemann's day consisted of techniques such as bloodletting, purging and prescribing toxic drugs. It was amid this background that Hahnemann developed his ideas on homeopathy. Homeopathy is used to treat a wide range of acute and chronic illness. Where a condition is beyond the scope of the body's normal self-repair mechanism, treatment is less likely to be curative, but may be palliative.

Homeopathic medicines are prepared from minerals, plant and animal substances. There are over 3000 medicines available. For example, a commonly prescribed medicine is lycopodium, which is derived from the plant club moss. The plant is macerated in 95 per cent alcohol and then this is filtered. This juice forms the basis of medicine preparation. A typical prescription would be lycopodium 30C. The number and letter refer to the degree of dilution of the original substance. One drop of the original substance is added to 99 drops of water and is then shaken vigorously. Then one drop of that is added to 99 drops of water and shaken vigorously. This is done 30 times! In fact by the laws of chemistry, lycopodium 30C is so dilute (ultramolecular) that not one atom of the original substance may be present in it. This is one of the most controversial aspects of homeopathy, which results in most people not being able to understand how homeopathic medicines may work.

Hahnemann hit upon the process of succussion or shaking by chance. This is said to potentize the medicine. It is important to understand that homeopathic medicines do not necessarily have to be very dilute. A substance can be prescribed homeopathically in its natural form. However, this would mean many toxic substances cannot be given for example, Arsenicum Album. Such toxic substances when used homeopathically are always prescribed very dilute to reduce or even abolish toxicity.

Is there a role for homeopathy in mental illness?

Anxiety

A systematic review located eight RCTs addressing test anxiety, generalized anxiety disorder and anxiety related to medical or physical conditions (Pilkington *et al.* 2006e). The trials reported contradictory results, were underpowered or provided insufficient details of methodology. Some used a single homeopathic remedy while others assessed a full homeopathy consultation with individualized prescribing of remedies. Several uncontrolled and observational studies reported positive results including high levels of patient satisfaction but because of the lack of a control group, it was difficult to assess the extent to which any response is due to homeopathy. Adverse effects reported appear limited to 'remedy reactions' and included temporary worsening of symptoms and reappearance of old symptoms. It was not possible to draw firm conclusions on the effectiveness of homeopathy for anxiety. However, homeopathy is quite frequently used by people suffering from anxiety and if proven to be effective, it would have benefits in terms of adverse effects and acceptability to patients.

Dementia

No trials were considered suitable for inclusion in a Cochrane review of homeopathy in dementia (Mccarney *et al.* 2003). The authors suggested that extent of homeopathic prescribing for people with dementia is not clear and so the importance of conducting trials in this area is uncertain.

Depression

A systematic review found only two RCTs of homeopathy in depression and one of these demonstrated problems with recruitment of patients in primary care (Pilkington *et al.* 2005a). Positive results and high levels of patient satisfaction were reported in uncontrolled and observational studies with adverse effects limited to 'remedy reactions' ('aggravations'). Exploratory qualitative studies to investigate how to overcome recruitment and other methodological problems are needed.

Is homeopathy safe?

Dantas and Rampes (2000) conducted a systematic review to evaluate the safety of homeopathic medicines by critically appraising reports of adverse effects published in English from 1970 to 1995. A comprehensive literature search was conducted by using electronic databases, by hand searching, by searching reference lists, by reviewing the bibliography of trials and other relevant articles, by contacting homeopathic pharmaceutical companies and drug regulatory agencies in the UK and the USA, and by communicating with experts in homeopathy.

The authors found that the overall incidence of adverse effects of homeopathic medicines was superior to placebo in controlled clinical trials but effects were minor, transient and comparable. There was a large incidence of pathogenetic effects in healthy volunteers taking homeopathic medicines but the methodological quality of these studies was generally low. Anecdotal reports of adverse effects in homeopathic publications were not well documented and mainly reported aggravation of current symptoms. Case reports in conventional medical journals pointed more to adverse effects of mislabelled 'homeopathic products' than to pure homeopathic medicines. The authors concluded that pure homeopathic medicines in high dilutions, prescribed by trained professionals, are probably safe and unlikely to provoke severe adverse reactions.

Who practises homeopathy?

Homeopathy has spread from Germany to all over the world. At the start of the twentieth century it flourished in America, where there were homeopathic medical schools, hospitals and even asylums. The Faculty of Homeopathy trains health professionals. There are four main homeopathic hospitals in the UK: in London, Glasgow, Bristol and Liverpool. These have been part of the NHS from the beginning in 1949. The Royal London Homoeopathic Hospital has provided homeopathic treatment since 1840. The Society of Homeopaths, which represents non-medically trained practitioners, is the largest organization. Homeopathy is not a statutorily regulated profession in the UK, so there is no legal definition of who can call themselves a homeopath. There are however National Occupational Standards for Homeopathy.

Meditation, yoga and related therapies

What are meditation and yoga?

The main types of meditation used in therapy are concentrative methods, transcendental meditation and insight forms such as mindfulness techniques although there is some overlap between these. Transcendental meditation was introduced to the West in the 1960s and involves use of a mantra (a repeated phrase, word or sound). The aim is to 'focus attention on an object and sustain attention until the mind achieves stillness' (Krisanaprakornkit *et al.* 2006). Mindfulness meditation emphasizes an awareness of any thoughts or feelings that enter the mind or anything that arises within the field of awareness.

Yoga originated in Indian culture and consists of a system of spiritual, moral and physical practices aimed at attaining 'self-awareness'. Hatha yoga, the system on which much of Western yoga is based, has three basic components: asanas (postures), pranayama (breathing exercises) and dhyana (meditation). Postures involving standing, bending, twisting and balancing the body to improve flexibility and strength, the controlled breathing helps to focus the mind and achieve relaxation while meditation aims to calm the mind. Several explanations have been proposed to account for the effects of yoga including an effect on autonomic nervous tone and an increase in the relaxation response in the neuromuscular system (Riley 2004).

Anxiety

One review located 12 controlled studies of meditation in people who had an anxiety disorder, were complaining of anxiety related symptoms, had raised anxiety levels or were being treated for anxiety related to a performance or test (Kirkwood *et al.* 2005a). Various styles of meditation were used although transcendental meditation was most frequently encountered. Most of the trials found no difference between meditation and other relaxation techniques. This could be because the interventions are equally effective or due to poor methodology or a small sample size.

A subsequent Cochrane review focused only on diagnosed anxiety disorders and concluded that the small number of studies located did not permit any firm conclusions to be drawn (Krisanaprakornkit *et al.* 2006). Transcendental meditation was found to be comparable with other kinds of relaxation therapies in reducing anxiety. Adverse effects of meditation were not reported but drop out rates were high so further investigation is required.

It was not possible to say whether yoga is effective in treating anxiety or anxiety disorders because of the range of anxiety-related conditions treated and the poor quality of the majority of studies (Kirkwood *et al.* 2005b). However, there are encouraging results, particularly in obsessive compulsive disorder.

Depression

A review of meditation in depression found that there is a general lack of research in this area and so it was impossible to draw any conclusions on either the effectiveness of meditation in easing depression or on its potential to exacerbate depression (Kirkwood *et al.* 2005c). Five trials of yoga interventions in depression were identified (Pilkington *et al.* 2005b). Different forms of yoga were used with twice weekly or daily practice for 20 to 60 minutes and rhythmic breathing was an important component in four trials. All trials reported positive findings. No adverse effects were reported with the exception of fatigue and breathlessness in participants in one study but participants in all the trials were under 50 years. Potentially beneficial effects of yoga interventions on depressive disorders were indicated although several of the interventions may not be feasible in those with reduced or impaired mobility. The findings should be interpreted with caution because of the variation in interventions and depression severity and the lack of some methodological details. Further investigation of which intervention is most effective, levels of severity of depression likely to respond and the effectiveness of anaerobic exercise (such as yoga) against aerobic exercise is needed.

Mindfulness-based stress reduction includes meditation and yoga components and promising results in depression have been reported (Grossman *et al.* 2004). Mindfulness-based cognitive therapy, based on aspects of cognitive behavioural therapy and of mindfulness-based stress reduction programmes may be useful in preventing relapse among people who have recovered from depression and is mentioned in current guidance (NICE 2004).

Are yoga and meditation safe?

A small number of cases of adverse psychological effects have been reported although these appear to be related specifically to meditation. A limited number of individual case reports of other serious adverse events have also been reported but these problems are likely to be rare and often linked to the more strenuous forms of yoga. As with other exercise programmes, yoga, particularly the more energetic forms, should only be undertaken on the advice of a health professional and practised under the supervision of skilled therapists. People with mental illness considering meditation should also consult their primary care giver.

Who practises meditation and yoga?

The British Wheel of Yoga, the largest organization in the UK can provide information and lists of accredited teachers (http://www.bwy.org.uk/).

Other therapies

Dietary supplements

A range of dietary supplements have been investigated in mental health conditions, with the majority of studies focused on dementia and depression. Melatonin, folic acid, lecithin and omega 3 fatty acids have all been assessed for their value in dementia. In each case, there was found to be insufficient evidence from good quality trials. The reviews of the evidence can be found on the Cochrane Library (http://www.cochrane.org/). Similarly, folate, inositol, tryptophan and 5-hydroxytryptophan, omega- 3 fatty acids (O3FA) and S-adenosyl-L-methionine (SAMe) have all been assessed as potential treatments in depression. These substances or their metabolites are often found to be depleted in depressed patients while low folate levels may cause a poor response to drug therapy. Cochrane reviews revealed potential of folate as a supplement to other treatment and for tryptophan and 5-hydroxytryptophan compared with placebo but a lack of evidence for inositol. Supplemental treatment with omega 3 fatty acids also appears promising (Schachter et al. 2005). However, the evidence was not conclusive and in each case, more investigations of safety are needed. Treatment with SAMe was found to be associated with an improvement of approximately six points (95% CI 2.2–9.0) on the Hamilton Rating Scale for Depression after three weeks, a statistically and clinically significant degree of improvement compared with placebo (Hardy et al. 2003). Outcomes from treatment with SAMe were not significantly different from those with conventional antidepressants. An overview concluded there was a 'favourable and significant' effect but all the studies were short term and the mechanism of action is still unclear (Williams et al. 2005).

A range of other therapies have been the focus as potential treatments for mental illness: art therapy in serious mental illness, autogenic training and guided imagery in depression, hypnosis for smoking cessation and schizophrenia, music therapy in dementia and schizophrenia and light therapy in non-seasonal depression. Systematic reviews of the research on these topics can be found on the Cochrane Library (http://www.cochrane.org/).

Ecotherapy

One therapy that has been the focus of attention recently is ecotherapy. Ecotherapy or 'green exercise' is a term used to refer to country walks, paying attention to seasonal changes or working in the countryside. Its effects were investigated in a group of 20 members of local MIND groups. After a 30-minute country walk, 71 per cent reported decreased levels of depression and feeling less tense while 90 per cent reported increased self-esteem. After participating in an equivalent length shopping centre walk, only 45 per cent experienced a decrease in depression, 50 per cent felt more tense and 22 per cent were more depressed. Over a hundred people with various mental health problems were also questioned about their experiences of ecotherapy. Over 90 per cent said green activities had benefited their mental health and lifted depression, the combination of nature and exercise having the greatest effect (full details are available at http://www.mind.org.uk/mindweek2007/report/, accessed July 2007).

The placebo effect – is it important?

No complementary therapy has an evidence base which compares with those of the antidepressants or cognitive behaviour therapy. RCTs do, however, focus on specific effects of treatment and the role of non-specific therapeutic or placebo effects also needs to be considered. Non-specific effects are related to the interpersonal aspects of the consultation and treatment and involve expectations, beliefs and behavioural factors of patients and health care providers (Kirsch 2002). Clinicians can have potent placebo effects, which could be judiciously harnessed and exploited in clinical interactions. A clinician's bedside manner, his or her empathy, eye contact and smile in greeting patients have healing effects that are hard to quantify and measure. Many of the therapies described above involve significant interaction between the patient and practitioner which may itself contribute to any measured response to treatment. This aspect is relevant regardless of the condition being treated but may be particularly important in patients with mental illness where significant non-specific effects are also seen with conventional treatment. Such non-specific effects of treatment are taken for granted and have been under-researched.

In complementary and alternative therapy, the main question is whether a given therapy has more than a placebo effect. Just as conventional medicine ignores the clinical significance of its own placebo effect, the placebo effect of complementary and alternative medicine is often ignored by its practitioners. The magic and ritual of medicine has ancient traditions. Perhaps complementary and alternative therapies have been better able to capture this magic for patients.

Conclusion

- Complementary and alternative therapies include a broad domain of 'practices and ideas which are outside the domain of conventional medicine in several countries and defined by its users as preventing or treating illness or promoting health and well-being' (Manheimer and Berman 2006).
- Survey data suggest that complementary and alternative therapy is used by a sizeable proportion of the population in a number of countries and that this proportion is increasing. One survey of a random sample of patients receiving complementary medical care in the UK and the USA found that almost three-quarters of the British patients, and just over three-fifths of the American patients had been diagnosed with a mental disorder; major depression and anxiety were most common. Over 4 million adults made 18 million visits to practitioners of one of six therapies in the UK in 1998.
- Currently there is some provision of complementary and alternative therapy in the NHS, but this is not readily available to people with mental health problems. These patients are often not aware of the services and lack the finances to access them.
- Patients use complementary and alternative therapy for different reasons. The majority of people who use complementary and alternative therapies do so in addition to conventional medicine, rather than as an alternative. Complementary and alternative therapy users tend to be better educated and have a holistic orientation to health.
- Explanations for the increasing use of complementary or alternative therapy can be classified as 'push factors' – such as dissatisfaction with conventional medicine through previous negative experiences or anti-establishment attitudes – or 'pull factors' – such as

compatibility between the philosophy of certain therapies and patients' beliefs, longer consultations and a greater sense of control over one's own treatment.

- There is a growing database of research evidence for complementary therapies; it is no longer true to say that there is no evidence. For the therapies reviewed in this chapter the evidence base would suggest that:
    - Acupuncture may have a role in the anxiety, depression and smoking cessation.
    - The evidence base for homeopathy is currently too poor to reach firm conclusions.
    - The evidence base for herbal medicines is variable but hypericum (St John's wort) appears to be more effective than placebo for the short-term treatment of mild to moderate depression.
    - There is some evidence that aromatherapy and massage reduces anxiety in the short term. It might be particularly useful as an intervention with people who are confused, have little or no preserved language, for whom verbal interaction is difficult and conventional medicine is seen as of only marginal benefit; for example for dementia sufferers.
    - Massage-related interventions can be delivered in a number of settings and may also have a potential role in, for example, mild depression where use of antidepressants as first-line treatment is discouraged (NICE 2004) particularly when use of antidepressants is problematic (elderly, depressed mothers, hospitalized children). The added benefits of incorporating essential oils into the massage treatment, the selection of appropriate massage techniques and safety of essential oils do, however, require further evaluation.
    - Various forms of yoga may be helpful in anxiety and mild depression while meditation may be as helpful as relaxation in anxiety and obsessive compulsive disorder.
    - Several dietary supplements may be helpful in patients with depleted levels but effectiveness and safety need further assessment.
- The question of combining therapies, i.e. what combinations of complementary and alternative therapy plus conventional might be most beneficial is one that deserves investigation. Compliance with medication is universally poor in medicine. The use of complementary and alternative therapy may improve compliance with medications.
- Many nurses are very interested in complementary and alternative therapies, and a number have been trained as practitioners in aromatherapy, in particular. Clinical experience suggests that there has been a move away from hands-on patient contact in nursing; complementary and alternative therapy has perhaps filled a lacuna in nurses' professional work. There is an important potential role for nurses as providers of some complementary therapies. As researchers, nurses are particularly well placed to conduct studies to contribute to our understanding of the motivation and experiences of users of complementary and alternative therapies.
- Mental health professionals need to be aware that their patients may be attending a complementary and alternative therapy provider and should enquire routinely about patients' use of complementary and alternative therapy.

Questions for reflection and discussion

1   Enquire about complementary and alternative therapy use by the patients with whom you work.
    (a)   What are their perceived benefits?
    (b)   How much do they cost?
    (c)   Are there any safety concerns?
2   Assess the evidence base of the therapies you encounter in daily practice.
3   Examine the patient–clinician encounter for non-specific effects of treatment.

Annotated bibliography

- Ernst, E., Pittler, M.H. and Wider B. (2006) *The Desktop Guide to Complementary and Alternative Medicine: An Evidence-based Approach* (2nd edn). London: Harcourt Publishers. Edzard Ernst has a chair in complementary medicine at the University of Exeter. With his team, he has made a significant scientific contribution to the critical appraisal of research into complementary and alternative medicine and has published many articles. This book has summarized the extant research in each field of complementary and alternative medicine.
- Boyd, H. (2000) *Banishing the Blues: Inspirational Ways to Improve Your Mood.* London: Mitchell Beazley. Hilary Boyd is a qualified nurse, journalist and author. This well-presented book has a section on depression and a section on use of complementary and alternative medicine in depression. It is aimed at patients but would be of interest to health care professionals in training as it gives pragmatic examples of how patients can help themselves. Dr Hagen Rampes was consultant editor for this book.
- Scott, S. (ed.) (2002) *Handbook of Complementary and Alternative Therapies in Mental Health.* London: Academic Press. A guide which addresses topics of relevance to practise, for example, integration of complementary therapy services into mental health care.

Useful websites

- *BluePages Depression Information.* The Centre for Mental Health Research, The Australian National University. Available at http://bluepages.anu.edu.au/
- *CAMEOL (Complementary and Alternative Medicine Evidence OnLine) database.* Research Council for Complementary Medicine/University of Westminster. Available at http://www.rccm.org.uk/cameol
- *National Centre for Complementary and Alternative Medicine* (NCCAM) National Institutes of Health. Available at http://www.nccam.nih.gov
- *National Library for Health Complementary and Alternative Medicine Specialist Library.* Available at http://www.library.nhs.uk/cam

References

Ashenden, R., Silagy, C.A., Lodge, M. and Fowler, G. (1997) A meta-analysis of the effectiveness of acupuncture in smoking cessation. *Drug and Alcohol Review* **16**: 33–40.

Astin, J. (1998) Why patients use alternative medicine. Results of a national survey. *Journal of the American Medical Association* **279**: 1548–53.

Barnes, P.M., Powell-Griner, E., McFann, K. and Nahin, R.L. (2004) Complementary and alternative medicine use among adults: United States, 2002. *Advance Data* **343**: 1–19.

Basch, E.M. and Ulbricht, C.E. (eds) (2005) *Natural Standard Herb and supplement Handbook: the clinical bottom line.* St Louis, Missouri: Mosby.

Bent, S., Padula, A., Moore, D., Patterson, M., Mehling, W. (2006) Valerian for sleep: a systematic review and meta-analysis. *American Journal of Medicine* **119**(12): 1005–12.

Birks, J. and Grimley Evans, J. (2007) Gingko biloba for cognitive impairment and dementia. *Cochrane Database of Systematic Reviews* Issue 2. Art. No.: CD003120. DOI: 0.1002/14651858.CD003120.pub2.

Buckle, J. (2003) *Clinical Aromatherapy: essential oils in practice* (2nd edn). London: Churchill Livingstone.

Caspi, O., Sechrest, L., Pitluk, H.C. *et al.* (2003). On the definition of complementary, alternative, and integrative medicine: societal mega-stereotypes vs. the patients' perspectives. *Alternative Therapies in Health and Medicine* **9**(6): 58–62.

Dantas, F. and Rampes, H. (2000) Do homeopathic medicines provoke adverse effects? A systematic review. *British Homeopathic Journal* **89**: S35–S38.

Davidson, J., Rampes, H., Eizen, M. *et al.* (1998) Psychiatric disorders in primary care patients receiving complementary medicine. *Comprehensive Psychiatry* **39**: 16–20.

Druss, B.G. and Rosenheck, R.A. (1999) Association between use of unconventional therapies and conventional medical services. *Journal of the American Medical Association* **282**: 651–6.

Druss, B.G. and Rosenheck, R.A. (2000) Use of practitioner-based complementary therapies by persons reporting mental conditions in the United States. *Archives of General Psychiatry* **57**(7): 708–14.

Eisenberg, D.M., Davis, R.B., Ettner, S.L. *et al.* (1998) Trends in alternative medicine use in the United States, 1990–1997: results of a follow-up national survey. *Journal of the American Medical Association* **280**: 1569–75.

Ernst, E. (2003) The safety of massage therapy. *Rheumatology* **42**(9): 1101–6.

Finnigan, M.D. (1991) The centre for the study of complementary medicine: an attempt to understand its popularity through psychological, demographic and operational criteria. *Complementary Medicine Research* **5**: 83–8.

Finucane, A. and Mercer, S.W. (2006) An exploratory mixed methods study of the acceptability and effectiveness of mindfulness-based cognitive therapy for patients with active depression and anxiety in primary care. *BMC Psychiatry* **6**: 14.

Furnham, A. (1996) Why do people choose and use complementary therapies? in E. Ernst (ed.) *Complementary Medicine: an objective appraisal.* Oxford: Butterworth Heinemann.

Gates, S., Smith, L.A. and Foxcroft, D.R. (2006) Auricular acupuncture for cocaine dependence. *Cochrane Database of Systematic Reviews* Issue 1. Art. No.: CD005192. DOI: 10.1002/14651858.CD005192.pub2.

Grossman, P., Niemann, L., Schmidt, S. and Walach, H. (2004) Mindfulness-based stress reduction and health benefits. A meta-analysis. *Journal of Psychosomatic Research* **57**(1): 35–43.

Hardy, M.L., Coulter, I., Morton, S.C. *et al.* (2003) S-adenosyl-L-methionine for treatment of depression, osteoarthritis, and liver disease. *Evidence Report/Technology Assessment* (Summary) **64**: 1–3.

Haussermann, D. (1997) Wachsendes Vertrauen in Naturheilmittel, *Deutsches Arzteblatt* **94**: 1857–8.

Jordan, J.B. (2006) Acupuncture treatment for opiate addiction: a systematic review. *Journal of Substance Abuse Treatment* **30**(4): 309–14.

Jorm, A.F., Griffiths, K.M., Christensen, H., Parslow, R.A. and Rogers, B. (2004) Actions taken to cope with depression at different levels of severity: a community survey. *Psychological Medicine* **34**: 293–9.

Kaptchuk, T.J. and Eisenberg, D.M. (1998) The persuasive appeal of alternative medicine. *Annals of Internal Medicine* **129**: 1061–5.

Kaptchuk, T.J. and Eisenberg, D.M. (2001) Varieties of healing. 2: a taxonomy of unconventional healing practices. *Annals of Internal Medicine* **135**(3): 196–204.

Kessler, R.C., Soukup, J., Davis, R.B. *et al.* (2001) The use of complementary and alternative therapies to treat anxiety and depression in the United States. *American Journal of Psychiatry* **158**: 289–94.

Kirkwood, G., Pilkington, K., Rampes, H. and Richardson, J. (2005a) Meditation for anxiety: a systematic review. *Complementary and Alternative Medicine Evidence Online (CAMEOL) Database.* Available at: http://www.rccm.org.uk/cameol/Default.aspx (accessed July 2007).

Kirkwood, G., Rampes, H., Tuffrey, V., Richardson, J. and Pilkington, K. (2005b) Yoga for anxiety: a systematic review of the research evidence. *British Journal of Sports Medicine* **39**(12): 884–91.

Kirkwood, G., Pilkington, K., Rampes, H. and Richardson, J. (2005c) Meditation for depression: a systematic review. *Complementary and Alternative Medicine Evidence Online (CAMEOL) Database.* Available at: http://www.rccm.org.uk/cameol/Default.aspx (accessed July 2007).

Kirsch, I. (2002) The placebo effect in complementary medicine, in G. Lewith, W. Jonas and H. Walach (eds) *Clinical Research in Complementary Therapies.* Edinburgh: Churchill Livingstone.

Krisanaprakornkit, T., Krisanaprakornkit, W., Piyavhatkul, N. and Laopaiboon, M. (2006) Meditation therapy for anxiety disorders. *Cochrane Database of Systematic Reviews* Issue 1. Art. No.: CD004998. DOI: 10.1002/14651858.CD004998.pub2.

Kunz, S., Schulz, M., Syrbe, G. and Driessen, M. (2004) Ohrakupunktur in der Therapie alkohol und substanzbezogener Störungen: eine Übersicht [Acupuncture of the ear as therapeutic approach in the treatment of alcohol and substance abuse: a systematic review]. *SUCHT* **50**(3): 196–203.

Linde, K., Mulrow, C.D., Berner, M. and Egger, M. (2005) St John's Wort for depression. *Cochrane Database of Systematic Reviews* Issue 3. Art. No.: CD000448. DOI: 10.1002/14651858.CD000448.pub2.

MacPherson, H., Thomas, K., Walters, S. *et al.* (2001) The York acupuncture safety study: prospective survey of 34,000 treatments by traditional acupuncturists. *British Medical Journal* **323**: 486–7.

MacPherson, H., Scullion, A., Thomas, K. and Walters, S. (2004) Patient reports of adverse events associated with acupuncture treatment: a prospective national survey. *Quality and Safety in Health Care* **13**: 349–55.

Manheimer, E. and Berman, B. (2006) Cochrane Complementary Medicine Field. *About The Cochrane Collaboration (Fields)* Issue 1. Art. No.: CE000052.

Mccarney, R., Warner, J., Fisher, P. and Van Haselen, R. (2003) Homeopathy for dementia. *Cochrane Database of Systematic Reviews* Issue 1. Art. No.: CD003803. DOI: 10.1002/14651858.CD003803.

Mennini, T. and Gobbi, M. (2004) The antidepressant mechanism of *Hypericum perforatum*. *Life Sciences* **75**: 1021–7.

Mental Health Foundation (1997) *Knowing our own Minds. A Survey of how People in Emotional Distress Take Control of Their Lives.* London: MHF.

MHRA (Medicines and Healthcare Regulatory Agency) (2006) *Kava Report: Report of the Committee on Safety of Medicines Expert Working Group on the Safety of Kava. July 2006.* Available at http://www.mhra.gov.uk (accessed July 2007).

Miyasaka, L.S., Atallah, A.N. and Soares, B.G.O. (2007) Passiflora for anxiety disorder. *Cochrane Database of Systematic Reviews* Issue 1. Art. No.: CD004518. DOI: 10.1002/14651858.CD004518.pub2.

Miyasaka, L.S., Atallah, A.N. and Soares, B.G.O. (2006) Valerian for anxiety disorders. *Cochrane Database of Systematic Reviews* Issue 4. Art. No.: CD004515. DOI: 10.1002/14651858.CD004515.pub2.

Moner, S.E. (1996) Acupuncture and addiction treatment. *Journal of Addictive Diseases* **15**(3): 79–100.

Moyer, C.A., Rounds, J. and Hannum, J.W. (2004) A meta-analysis of massage therapy research. *Psychological Bulletin* **130**(1): 3–18.

Mukaino, Y., Park, J., White, A. and Ernst, E. (2005) The effectiveness of acupunture for depression – a systematic review of randomised controlled trials. *Acupuncture in Medicine* **23**(2): 70–6.

Nathan, M.M. (2001) Overcoming barriers to spiritual care. *Sacred Space* **2**(4): 18–24.

National Institute for Health and Clinical Excellence (2004) *Depression: Management of Depression in Primary and Secondary Care. Clinical Guideline 23.* Developed by the National Collaborating Centre for Mental Health. London: NICE. Available at: http://nice.org.uk/CG023NICEguideline

Peng, W.N., Zhao, H., Liu, Z.S. and Wang, S. (2007) Acupuncture for vascular dementia. *Cochrane Database of Systematic Reviews* Issue 2. Art. No.: CD004987. DOI: 10.1002/14651858.CD004987.pub2.

Pilkington, K., Kirkwood, G., Rampes, H., Fisher, P. and Richardson, J. (2005a) Homeopathy for depression: a systematic review of the research evidence. *Homeopathy* **94**(3): 153–63.

Pilkington, K., Kirkwood, G., Rampes, H. and Richardson, J. (2005b) Yoga for depression: the research evidence. *Journal of Affective Disorders* **89**(1–3): 13–24.

Pilkington, K., Kirkwood, G., Rampes, H. and Richardson, J. (2006a) Aromatherapy and massage for depression: a systematic review. *Complementary and Alternative Medicine Evidence Online (CAMEOL) Database.* Available at: http://www.rccm.org.uk/cameol/Default.aspx (accessed July 2007).

Pilkington, K., Kirkwood, G., Rampes, H. and Richardson, J. (2006b) Aromatherapy and massage for anxiety: a systematic review. *Complementary and Alternative Medicine Evidence Online (CAMEOL) Database.* Available at: http://www.rccm.org.uk/cameol/Default.aspx (accessed July 2007).

Pilkington, K., Kirkwood, G., Rampes, H. and Richardson, J. (2006c) Reflexology for anxiety: a systematic review. *Complementary and Alternative Medicine Evidence Online (CAMEOL) Database.* Available at: http://www.rccm.org.uk/cameol/Default.aspx (accessed July 2007).

Pilkington, K., Kirkwood, G., Rampes, H. and Richardson, J. (2006d) Reflexology for depression: a systematic review. *Complementary and Alternative Medicine Evidence Online (CAMEOL) Database.* Available at: http://www.rccm.org.uk/cameol/Default.aspx (accessed July 2007).

Pilkington, K., Kirkwood, G., Rampes, H., Fisher, P. and Richardson, J. (2006e) Homeopathy for anxiety and anxiety disorders: a systematic review of the research evidence. *Homeopathy* **95**(3): 151–62.

Pilkington, K., Kirkwood, G., Rampes, H., Cummins, M. and Richardson, J. (2007) Acupuncture for anxiety and anxiety disorders – a systematic literature review. *Acupuncture in Medicine* **25**: 1–10.

Pittler, M.H. and Ernst, E. (2003) Kava extract versus placebo for treating anxiety. *Cochrane Database of Systematic Reviews* Issue 1. Art. No.: CD003383. DOI: 10.1002/14651858.CD003383.

Rampes, H. and James, R. (1995) Complications of acupuncture. *Acupuncture in Medicine* **13**(1): 26–33.

Rathbone, J. and Xia, J. (2005) Acupuncture for schizophrenia. *Cochrane Database of Systematic Reviews* Issue 4. Art. No.: CD005475. DOI: 10.1002/14651858.CD005475.

Rathbone, J., Zhang, L., Zhang, M. *et al.* (2005) Chinese herbal medicine for schizophrenia. *Cochrane Database of Systematic Reviews* Issue 4. Art. No.: CD003444. DOI: 10.1002/14651858.CD003444.pub2.

Resch, K.L., Hill, S. and Ernst, E. (1997) Use of complementary therapies by individuals with arthritis. *Journal of Clinical Rheumatology* **16**: 391–5.

Riley, D. (2004) Hatha yoga and the treatment of illness (commentary). *Alternative Therapies in Health and Medicine* **10**(2): 20–1.

Schachter, H.M., Kourad, K., Merali, Z. *et al.* (2005) Effects of Omega-3 fatty acids on mental health. *Evid Rep Technol Assess No. 116. AHRQ Publication No 05-E022–1.* Rockville, MD: Agency for Healthcare Research and Quality.

Smith, C.A. and Hay, P.P.J. (2005) Acupuncture for depression. *The Cochrane Database of Systematic Reviews,* Issue 3, Art No CD004046.pub2. DOI: 10.1002/14651858.CD004046.pub2, John Wiley and Sons.

Thomas, K. and Coleman, P. (2004). Use of complementary or alternative medicine in a general population in Great Britain. Results from the National Omnibus survey. *Journal of Public Health* **26**(2): 152–7.

Thomas, K.J., Fall, M. and Williams, B. (1993) Methodological study to investigate the feasibility of conducting a population-based survey of the use of complementary healthcare. Final Report to the Research Council for Complementary Medicine. Unpublished.

Thomas, K., Nicholl, J. and Coleman, P. (2001) Use and expenditure on complementary medicine in England – a population based survey. *Complementary Therapies in Medicine* **9**: 2–11.

Thorgrimsen, L., Spector, A., Wiles, A. and Orrell, M. (2003) Aroma therapy for dementia. *Cochrane Database of Systematic Reviews* Issue 3. Art. No.: CD003150. DOI: 10.1002/14651858.CD003150.

Tindle, H.A., Davis, R.B., Phillips, R.S. and Eisenberg, D.M. (2005) Trends in use of complementary and alternative medicine by US adults: 1997–2002. *Alternative Therapies in Health and Medicine* **11**(1): 42–9.

Tiran, D. (2002). Reviewing theories and origins, in P.A. Mackereth and D. Tiran (eds) *Clinical Reflexology: A Guide for Health Professionals.* London: Churchill Livingstone, pp. 5–15.

Unützer, J., Klap, R., Sturm, R. *et al.* (2000) Mental disorders and the use of alternative medicine: results from a national survey. *American Journal of Psychiatry* **157**(11): 1851–7.

Wang, P.S., Lane, M., Olfson, M. *et al.* (2005) Twelve-month use of mental health services in the United States: results from the National Comorbidity Survey Replication. *Archives of General Psychiatry* **62**(6): 629–40.

White, A., Hayoe, S., Hart, A. *et al.* (2001) Adverse events following acupuncture: prospective survey of 32,000 consultations with doctors and physiotherapists. *British Medical Journal* **323**: 485–6.

White, A. amd Moody, R. (2006) The effects of auricular acupuncture on smoking cessation may not depend on the point chosen – an exloratory meta-analysis. *Acupuncture in Medicine* **24**(4):149–56.

White, A.R., Rampes, H. and Campbell, J.L. (2006) Acupuncture and related interventions for smoking cessation. *Cochrane Database of Systematic Reviews* Issue 1. Art. No.: CD000009. DOI: 10.1002/14651858.CD000009.pub2.

Williams, A.L., Girard, C., Jui, D., Sabina, A. and Katz, D.L. (2005) S-adenosylmethionine (SAMe) as treatment for depression: a systematic review. *Clinical and Investigative Medicine* **28**(3): 132–9.

Wootton, J.C. (2005) Classifying and defining complementary and alternative medicine. *Journal of Alternative and Complementary Medicine* **11**(5): 777–8.

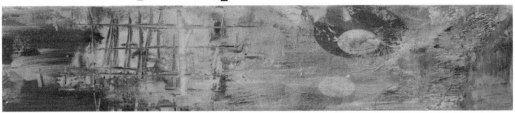

Chapter contents

CHAPTER 18

The person with a perceptual disorder

Geoff Brennan

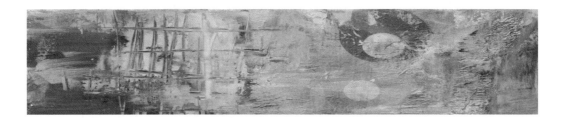

Chapter overview

66 At any one time one adult in six suffers from one or other forms of mental illness. In other words mental illnesses are as common as asthma. They vary from more common conditions such as deep depression to schizophrenia, which affects fewer than one person in a hundred. Mental illness is not well understood. It frightens people and all too often carries a stigma.

(DH 1999: 1) 99

So begins Frank Dobson's introduction to the *National Service Framework (NSF) for Mental Health*. This chapter aims to explore the 'not well understood' condition that is schizophrenia from the viewpoint that such a disorder involves an extension or subtraction of normal functioning. In order to do this we need to consider how a normal person perceives the world. But there is a problem here given that there is no such thing as a 'normal person'. All we actually have is our own experience of the world. Accordingly, this chapter will ask you to consider your own experience with reference to its content. As you read, please ask yourself:

■ How would this condition affect me?
■ Have I ever had experiences approximating those described in the chapter?

Stigma arises when we cannot understand a person or group and judge them to be deviant. Therefore, it is important for nurses or anyone interested in mental illness to attempt to 'get inside the mind' of the individual they are trying to assist and understand what it is like for them in a manner which brings empathetic understanding of their experiences. You may be surprised, as you read, how you can relate in some small or large way to the mental experiences of people deemed 'mad'.

This chapter covers:

■ What is a person?
■ Perception;
■ Schizophrenia;

- Symptom-focused treatments and interventions;
- Case studies.

What is a person?

It is often the simple questions that are the hardest. Psychiatry is awash with seemingly simple questions that are very complex. As a discipline which aims to promote health and well-being in society, it deals with *people*, either as an individual 'person' or grouped together into populations. But what makes a person a person? or What makes me '*me*'? Consider the following:

Imagine you are a judge in a legal system where only your opinion matters. You are hearing the trial of murder where the defendant freely admits to the crime, states they were of sound mind when they committed the crime and that the crime was premeditated with clear personal gain as a result of the victim's death. The defendant defiantly committed the murder. Their part in the crime was not discovered, however, until 20 years later. In that time, given the wonders of biology, every original cell in the defendant's body has been replicated in the natural process of cell regeneration. As a consequence their hotshot lawyer makes the defence that, although the person did, indeed, commit the murder, the present 'person' cannot be held responsible, as they are a completely different individual with different cells and therefore not responsible for the crime their earlier form committed. In his summing up the hotshot ends with the words 'How can we, in all seriousness, punish this person when it is true to say that not one cell was present when the murder was committed? How can we, when this hand was not there, when this brain was not there, when, by a process of clear logic, my client, in his present state, was not in that room, indeed, not even on the planet, when this crime was perpetrated?' The people await the verdict from you, the judge.

Obviously, you would find the defendant guilty, their hotshot lawyer would be chastened and you would be asked to join the House of Lords. But why?

In a nutshell, the hotshot lawyer's flaw is to argue that a person is a *body*. This does not take into account the mental, social, moral or spiritual aspects of an individual. While the body is *an aspect* of a person, it is only when this is combined with these other aspects, do we get the person, the 'me' that is a human being. The murderer committed the murder, and as the cells of the body changed, the person who committed the murder remained. If we accept the defence's argument, I did not pass (or fail) my exams, my wife is not married to the man she exchanged vows with, I am not the father of my children. Even my parents are impostors.

The aspects that are in addition to the body are often called the 'mental' aspects. The hotshot lawyer has omitted the fact that the mental aspects stay in place while the physical cells change. They are the threads that connect the cells together into the whole. If we are to really get technical, the cells of the body have a memory of the previous cells, so that, although the cells 'change', they do not become new, autonomous cells but replicas of the old cells, including carrying the memory of the previous. Hence scars are carried on the skin as a memory of previous trauma. Therefore, even the physical body has a 'memory'. While it is true that the physical state changes, the mental is carried along.

If we now agree that a person is a complex mixture of both the mental and the physical, we must acknowledge that there is some relation between them. The physical sense that we have, through our body's interaction with the world outside ourselves, feeds into the mental. This book exists in the real, physical world; the words exist as separate physical bits of ink on a physical bit of paper, which you are scanning with your eyes. The resulting images are carried through the optic nerve and are 'seen'. The meaning is then interpreted in the mental world of your thoughts as the words have mental meanings.

In turn our mental thoughts, ideas and drives influence our interaction with the world and can change this world as a result. For example, if your mental interpretation of what is written is that it is a load of rubbish, you can burn the book in the physical world.

As a consequence, our hotshot lawyer in disgrace has assisted us in getting nearer that very difficult question, 'What makes me "*me*"?' They have helped us to see that the mental and the physical are two aspects of a person and that the complete person is the totality of both the mental and the physical. Moreover, the person also exists within the world and can interact with it. The physical body exists in the world and allows the mental aspects access to the world. It is this interactive pathway between the mental and the physical that we know as perception.

Perception

Perception, as described above, is a complex process of interpretation, which is described in its simplest form in Figure 18.1.

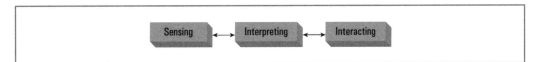

Figure 18.1 The process of perception

Sensing

We have five senses that operate on the edge of the mental physical interface. The mind without the senses would be like a computer without data. The potential to process would be there without anything to process. Provided you have no impairment to your senses, you can access all five of them easily. The sense you are using right now is sight. You are looking at the words on the page and literally seeing them. The other senses are there, but not so much in use. You are probably trying to not hear the world around you if you are concentrating on the words. If you wish to focus on hearing, you can do so effortlessly. Take a second to stop and listen. Likewise, your sense of smell and taste are there if you need them. What can you smell and taste?

Finally, close your eyes, pick up the book and feel the weight of it in your hand. Rub your fingers over the cover. All these senses are there and you can generally focus on them or ignore them as you wish.

Interpreting

You probably entered into interpretation in the last section. For example, it is virtually impossible just to *see* words. It is much more likely that you *read* them. You did not look at the sentence 'You are looking at the words on the page ...' and *see* the words as individual words, but rather read them as a complete sentence and therefore interpreted their meaning. Hence, if the sentence had said, 'You are looking at the elephants on the page ...' you would have reacted to the word 'elephant' because it was out of place. Thus you are interpreting the words that you are seeing. Also, when you were asked to listen, it is likely you would not have left it at just hearing, but thought: 'That was a police siren' or 'That was the television' or 'It's too quiet – the kids are up to no good/my partner has fallen asleep/I forgot to take my earplugs out.'

An important aspect of interpretation is that it is a purely mental activity. Once the eye has seen the words on this page and they pass the image into the brain, the process of sensing has finished, the interpretation of the image happens in the mind. Reading happens in the mind. Even if you read out loud, there is a point where the brain interprets the image and informs the mouth what to say. We know this because we can get a word wrong and read something that isn't there, but this isn't because we can't *read* but that we have *interpreted* wrongly.

There is an important aspect of interpretation that is summed up in the following:

> **❝** Instead of talking of seeing and knowing, we might do a little better to talk of seeing and noticing. We notice only when we look for something, and we look when our attention is aroused by some disequilibrium, a difference between our expectation and the incoming message. We cannot take in all we see in a room, but we notice if something has changed.
>
> (Gombrich 1960: 62) **❞**

A majority of what we sense is ignored as it is deemed unimportant. The process of interpretation has a filtration system that allows for the focusing noted earlier. If you had to stop reading for a minute to concentrate on hearing, this shows that the filtration system is working effectively. In other words, in order for you to focus on the words on the page, as you need to study and understand them, you need to lower your noticing of other senses. It would seem that the senses are wired into the brain like the control panel of a music studio, where certain inputs can be given higher or lower emphasis depending on the need. When you stopped and listened, you, in effect, turned up the hearing sense and lowered the seeing sense. While a conscious manipulation of the senses, the raising or lowering is an unconscious natural process necessary to function.

As we shall see, the process of filtration and focusing can be both a problem and a possible benefit if we wish to change things. We do have a complication in that the 'interpretation' we are discussing could be seen to be an aspect of brain functioning, which would make it a physical activity. In other words, we could say that the processes are based purely within the brain and are really just a chemical reaction within the neurones in response to the stimulus of the senses. The important thing within our discussion is that another person does not have access to this process. In other words, while you and I may 'see' the same thing, we could not agree that we 'interpret' it the same way. Imagine that we are both looking at a football match where we support opposite teams. Our interpretations of the event, while explicable by brain chemistry where our neurotransmitters will fluctuate depending on what is happening, will actually be at odds to each other. Similarly, we now know which chemicals are released in the brain if we see the person we love in a crowd of people, but why that person, and why doesn't everyone who sees them feel the same? Interpretation is in the eye of the beholder and brain function obeys it would seem.

Interacting

We live in and with the physical world. The purpose of sensing and interpreting is to keep us orientated within this world and to allow us to survive and thrive within it. An experience we all have in common is the reflex action of getting your hand off a hot object. There you are, the iron/cooker/bath water is too hot and will burn. Unaware, you place your hand on the hot object, sense it, interpret that this is dangerous (and if your mind was elsewhere, you certainly do now focus on your burning hand). What do you do next? You pull it away.

This simple reflex action sums up the purpose of interacting with the world. Our sensing and interpreting the world allows us to move and function to the best of our ability. Sometimes this interaction is as simple as moving our hand from a burning object (reaction), and sometimes it is as complex as changing our attitudes and beliefs (learning) or storing sensory data or interpretations to assist with future interactions (memory).

Where does it all go wrong?

> Are you just a complicated physical object? If not, are you a mind? If so, what are minds? What exactly is the relationship between the mind and the body? Are you a mind with a body, or a body with a mind? You are looking out of your body now. Does that mean you are your body or does it mean you are inside your body, or neither? Could we be immaterial souls, which survive our bodily death, or has that been ruled out by modern science? Are you your brain? How, if at all, is grey matter connected to our innermost thoughts and emotions? It is one of our peculiarities that we do not know what we are.
>
> (Priest 1991: xi)

This is how Stephen Priest begins an examination of the interaction between the physical and mental from a philosophical viewpoint. Psychiatry has also pondered this question and also has not come to any firm conclusion. The difference between the two examinations is that philosophy deals with the issue in a theoretical manner. Psychiatry, however, is a practical discipline, and one that has been set up (and set itself up) to deal with those aspects of the interaction between mental and physical which can go wrong and cause distress to individuals, family and social systems. Philosophy aims to make the world more understandable through detailed examination of basic assumptions while psychiatry aims to change the individual who has been identified as having difficulties existing within the world. Psychiatry, therefore, is necessary because things go wrong with people.

Psychiatry exists to correct the things that go wrong, or to reorientate the people for whom things go wrong to cope with the things that go wrong. Psychiatry also has the function of identifying what can cause things to go wrong and attempting to change them to stop things from going wrong. There is a problem here. How do we know when things go wrong? Given that the mental, as defined above, is a private realm only observable to another within the physical world of interaction and observation of the individual, how can psychiatry definitively say that things are wrong?

Psychiatry is a sibling of medicine. What I mean by this is that medicine, as a science, came into existence to address the ailments of the body, or the physical. As medicine developed, so did the awareness of the need to address the mental. Hence psychiatry. As we shall examine later, there are problems with this inception and affiliation and the link between medicine and psychiatry can be to the detriment of a clear understanding of mental issues. For now, however, let us take it that psychiatry decides what is wrong in roughly the same way as medicine does.

So how do you know you have a cold? Well, in honesty, you don't. You wake up in the morning and notice that certain things are different about you. In other words, you have an understanding of how you normally wake up and (remembering what we said earlier) ignore the fact that everything is as it usually is. Lost you for a second there? OK, how many times have you woken up and consciously thought, 'Oh good. I'm not ill today'? My guess is (unless you have had a recent experience of illness) you do not have this thought as your automatic introduction to each day. Rather you wake up and … nothing. You just go about your business. The only time you would notice your state of health is when there is something wrong. Then you notice the things that are wrong. In the case of a cold you may notice a 'runny nose', 'blocked sinus', 'sore throat', 'raised temperature', 'lack of energy' and, possibly, a general feeling of 'being a bit low in mood'. Given your previous knowledge of this combination of things you say, 'I have a cold.' Percentage-wise, your guess would probably be accurate, but in reality you cannot know for sure. You may have influenza, or any number of conditions which can start with this combination of things, or you may notice another thing wrong which you have not come across before in the 'I have a cold' combination, such as vomiting or some other nasty physical ailment.

The point is you notice something is wrong. Then you notice what is wrong. These are what we know as symptoms. Even if you visit the doctor or nurse, they will open with, 'Well, what is the matter with you then?' and you will not answer, 'My football team are rubbish, I hate my job and quite frankly, my partner better buck their ideas up!' Instead you know that they want a list of symptoms.

Psychiatry works in the same way with one massive difference. The similarity is that psychiatry also wants a list of the symptoms. The difference is that psychiatry will take a note of symptoms identified through the observation of a third party. This does not mean to say that medicine will not, but it is often the case that a disorder of perception can also extend to a person's perception of themselves, particularly in reference to how they are relating to the world and other people. In addition, if you look at the list of 'I have a cold' symptoms, my bet is that the one you are least likely to notice is the 'bit of a low mood', which often accompanies physical illness. It would seem we are not as good at noticing changes in our mental state as much as our physical state.

As a consequence, the world-view of the person with the disorder of perception is often at odds with the world-view of others. This is particularly true when it comes to relatives or close friends who notice changes in a person's demeanour, behaviour and attitude as a cause of concern. Hence, psychiatry places a value on what is known as 'taking a history' from those who are in close contact with the person. Usually the first part of this interview will begin with 'Have you noticed any change in X over the last few months?' Again, this is not without difficulty and we shall also come to this.

Another reason for calling on a secondary source of information to identify a mental health issue is that, where a physical illness can often call upon a secondary physical source to verify the presence or absence of symptoms, in psychiatry this is not possible. Disorders of perception are only elicited through the person relating their inner mental experiences. While there are various forms of behaviour that can be *associated* with mental disorders, *attributing* these to the presence of a mental disorder is guesswork until verified by the person exhibiting the disorder. What this means is that psychiatric examination should be an exceptionally cautious exercise. Every effort must be made to verify the validity of disorders suspected and check with the person being examined. In the absence of their individual testimony, everything else is second best, but sometimes all we have.

To get back to the symptoms and diagnosis of disorders of perception, we have one last dilemma before we can have a look at them. As with our example of waking up with symptoms that lead to a diagnosis of a cold, disorders of perception are categorized into diagnosis in the same way. In doing this, psychiatry attempts to emulate medicine's ability to clearly diagnose a problem in order to decide how best to manage it. The problem comes when we consider how much harder it is to categorize psychiatric symptoms because:

- They are harder to define given what we have already said about their reliance on a clear personal account of internal mental processes.
- There is huge crossover of symptoms between the diagnostic categories. This means that a specific symptom or even collection of symptoms can still meet several different diagnostic categories.
- There is an additional problem that many mental symptoms can be caused by physical problems. An example of this is confused thoughts caused by high or low blood sugar in diabetes or hallucinations caused by brain trauma or brain tumour.
- Some psychiatric diagnoses are not dependent on disorders of perception as much as identified issues with how the person relates to the world and other people. In this area it is less clear that the symptoms arise from disorders of perception so much as difficulties in interacting with others.

For the sake of clarity I am going to adopt the broad groupings of psychiatric diagnosis postulated by the psychiatrist philosopher Karl Jaspers (Table 18.1).

I am ignoring Group I conditions on the grounds that the symptoms that indicate these conditions are the result of physical illness and deterioration. Group III is also ignored, but for more complicated reasons. In these conditions, it is not how the world is sensed, interpreted and interacted with as a consequence, but rather how a person's personality is perceived by the world. It should be remembered, however, that people do not fit neatly into the above groups, and it is possible for people to have experiences applicable to more than one group.

The major psychoses, symptoms and perception

Psychosis is 'a severe mental disorder in which the person's ability to recognize reality and his or her emotional responses, thinking processes, judgement and ability to communicate are so affected that his or her functioning is seriously impaired' (Warner 1994: 4). If we look at this we can see that we are back in the realms of the process of perception: sensing, interpreting, interacting, and that things are going badly wrong. It's that first sentence that particularly gives the game away, where the ability to recognize reality comes in. To recap on the first section of this chapter, we recognize 'reality' through perception. So what sort of things can go wrong?

Group	Defining features	Notes
I	Cerebral illnesses, e.g. Trauma, Tumour, Infection of the brain and membranes, Hereditary illnesses which cause gradual damage to the brain, Mental deterioration due to age or age-related conditions	The root causes of these conditions are in the physical realm of the body. These are essentially psychiatric symptoms resulting from brain damage.
II	The major psychoses: Schizophrenia, Bipolar disorder/manic-depressive illness, Psychotic depression.	Jaspers originally included epilepsy in this category, which would now not be accepted. I have added psychotic depression, which would. Although the symptom presentation for these conditions is clear, there is huge sharing of symptom type between the three.
III	Personality disorders: Isolated abnormal reactions that do not arise from the recognized conditions in Groups I and II, Neuroses and neurotic syndromes, Abnormal personalities and their developments.	There are problems in representing some of these conditions as abnormal, since to do so would indicate that there are personality traits that are 'normal'.

Table 18.1 Psychiatric diagnoses
(Adapted from Jaspers 1963)

The major psychoses are a mixture of disorders of perception and disorders of mood. The main disorder of perception is schizophrenia, and the main disorder of mood is manic depression. To confuse matters, as indicated above, the actual symptoms, which are diagnostic of these conditions, have major crossovers. In other words, many of the symptoms listed below will be present in all three listed major psychoses. Having said this, schizophrenia is also the most commonly diagnosed of the major psychoses.

In the remainder of this chapter I will explore the major symptoms of schizophrenia to allow for a separate consideration of disorders of mood in Chapter 19.

Schizophrenia

Traditionally, symptoms of schizophrenia are categorized into two types: positive symptoms and negative symptoms.

If someone were to say to you that you had a symptom which was 'positive', what would you think? Would you think that there was perhaps, some benefit in having this particular symptom? Would you think that it meant that the symptom was the one that confirmed your diagnosis (like HIV positive), while a negative symptom meant the diagnosis was wrong? If you did, you would be incorrect in both instances. Many people who are given a diagnosis of schizophrenia with the phrase 'positive symptoms' respond with 'there is nothing positive about them!'. The 'positive' in this case means that the symptom is a mental experience, which would be considered as an *additional* experience to the norm, or an *exaggeration* of the norm. Given our exploration of perception above, this means the symptoms where mental events are generated independent of the physical world.

It follows that, if positive symptoms are an additional experience, negative symptoms are a *reduction* in normal experience. This can be seen from the list given in Box 18.1. As a general rule, however, the more a person is affected by negative symptoms, the more disabled they will be by schizophrenia.

Box 18.1   The two symptom groups of schizophrenia

- Hallucinations
- Delusions
- Thought disorder
- Catatonia

- Lack of volition
- Lack of excitement
- Poverty of thought
- Poverty of speech

Positive symptoms

Hallucinations

The archetypal symptom of mental illness has to be hallucinations. Hallucinations are traditionally defined as a person experiencing false sensory perception. With hallucinations a person experiences a sense which does not emanate from the world around them. As such, hallucinations are mental experiences that do not have the physical cause necessary from the experience to be a true sensory experience. Table 18.2 links the names of the hallucinatory types to the senses. Notice that hallucinations can come from physical trauma to the brain or other physical causes such as brain tumour, epilepsy, drugs and alcohol (the famous pink elephants!).

The fact that hallucinations are defined as 'false' in the real world does not mean to say that the mental experience is not 'true' in the person's mind, because it is. The person does, indeed, hear a voice, or see an object, but the voice or object is not real. Therefore, the experience is a true one, but there is no cause for it. The person would experience exactly the same as if the sense in question were activated by a true sensory experience. Therefore a noise or voice is 'heard' in the mind, despite there being no voice or noise in the physical world, an image is 'seen', despite there being no object to see in the physical world. To give some idea of how difficult this is to accept for the person experiencing a hallucination, imagine the following scenario happening to you. You are walking down the street and your mobile seems to vibrate in your pocket. You take it out and put it to your ear. After you say 'Hello', the person says, 'You won't get away with it you know.' The reception is a bit fuzzy, but the words are clear. When you ask who it is there is a silence on the other end. There is no more conversation. As you take the phone away from your ear, you notice that it is not switched on.

What would be your first reaction? Whatever the reason you came up with, you would not consider that the voice you had heard was anything but real.

Sense	Hallucination	Notes
Hearing	Auditory hallucination	Most commonly reported. Can be an individual voice, a combination of voices or simple noises.
Sight	Visual hallucination	Can be definite shapes, such as faces of people, or lights and flashes.
Smell	Olfactory hallucination	Often linked to other symptoms. Can be indicative of a physical problem such as brain tumour or epilepsy.
Taste	Gustatory hallucination	Often linked to other symptoms. Can be indicative of a physical problem such as brain tumour or epilepsy.
Touch	Tactile hallucination	Often linked to other symptoms. Can be indicative of a physical problem such as brain tumour or epilepsy.

Table 18.2 Types of hallucination noises

Although all senses can be falsely experienced, auditory hallucinations (often called 'voices') and visual hallucinations are the most reported.

Auditory hallucinations

If you had the experience with the mobile phone once, you would probably not even notice it as abnormal. If the experience does not happen again, you would gradually forget about it. If the experience happened again and again and again, you would begin, not only to notice it, but also become anxious and upset by it. If the voice started commenting on your actions in a derogatory way, or talked about you with another voice or threatened and abused you, then you might become extremely anxious. You may even confront the voice and start shouting at it to go away. The psychotic experience of having auditory hallucinations is not truly captured in the phrase 'hearing voices'. In psychotic experience the voice can often become a dominant factor in someone's life experience. In schizophrenia, auditory hallucinations are experienced over a long period of time, are intrusive, often abusive and disruptive and generally cause the person anxiety and distress.

In the case of auditory hallucinations a substantial amount of research has been conducted into both the experience of voice hearing and the means to assist voice hearers. This research has uncovered some very interesting facts, the most important of which is that auditory hallucinations are not confined to people who would be diagnosed as psychotic. The consequences of this are important, as it is evident that hearing voices alone will not indicate a 'full' psychosis. We need to explore this fact in more detail to get a clearer picture of the nature of auditory hallucinations.

Auditory hallucinations: a 'normal' mental experience?

Research indicates that the presence of auditory hallucinations is higher in people diagnosed with psychosis, but that they are present in the so-called normal population (see Table 18.3). As a consequence, auditory hallucinations have been explored as a separate mental experience as opposed to a symptom of schizophrenia.

Romme and Esher (1993) have undertaken what is probably the most illuminating work on auditory hallucinations alone. Their research investigated auditory hallucinations with a view to seeing if people experienced them in different ways. In a nutshell, they found that not all hallucinations were disabling in the manner that is assumed in a diagnosis of schizophrenia. What was clear in their discussions with people who experienced auditory hallucinations was that some people felt that they had control, or could cope with the experience of hearing voices, and some could not. Those who could cope experienced the voice in a pleasant way or had found methods to control the hallucinations and not allow it to disturb their lives. Those who were disabled reported being persecuted by the voice and/or feeling that they had little or no control. As we shall see, people who are grossly affected by the voice, or experience it along with other positive and negative symptoms are those who will be diagnosed with a psychosis. The experiences and techniques of those people who learn to cope with the auditory hallucination has also been utilized to assist voice hearers, becoming a standard approach in assisting people with psychosis (Downs 2001) (cf. Chapter 14).

Population	Percentage who experience auditory hallucination	Source
Diagnosed with schizophrenia	53	Landmark *et al.* 1990
Diagnosed with major affective disorder	28	Goodwin and Jamison 1990
The 'normal' population	2.3	Tien 1991

Table 18.3 Prevalence of auditory hallucinations

Other hallucinatory experience

Although auditory hallucinations are the most commonly experienced, other senses can also be falsely perceived. Visual hallucinations are the next most common after auditory hallucinations. The other sensory hallucinations are much less common and would lead to some concern that there may be a physical problem such as brain trauma, or that the hallucination is linked with other symptom types. An example is someone who believes a part of their body is dead when it is not and who gets an accompanying smell to confirm their thought, although no one else can smell anything (see somatic delusions below). Sometimes a brain scan or other physical tests can be carried out to rule out any physical cause for the hallucinatory experience.

A spanner in the works: pseudo hallucinations

There are a number of experiences which can be defined as false sensory perception, but which are not hallucinations. An example of this is an illusion (where the 'eyes play tricks on you'). Imagine it is a dark windy night and you are walking home. You suddenly see a black dog sitting under a lamp-post moving its head. As you draw nearer you realize you were mistaken and the 'dog' is a black binliner left out for the dustmen. This is an example of an illusion where the interpretation part of the perception system has got it wrong. This is not a hallucination, however, because, regardless of whether it was a binliner or a dog, there was something there.

In ordinary experience we also know that it is common to hear the voice of a loved one who has recently died, and that people are susceptible to hearing and seeing things in the process of falling asleep or waking up. It is fairly easy to see why these things should happen. A recently bereaved person is susceptible, as they are in a state of both shock and adjustment. It is common to hear bereaved people say, 'I keep expecting them to walk in the door.' It seems it is a short step from this feeling to a false perception that the person speaks to us, or gives us some form of message. Similarly, in the process of falling asleep and waking up, the mind is in a state of flux and again susceptible.

These experiences are called pseudo hallucinations. There is one very particular form of pseudo hallucination, which is worth knowing about. If a person says that they are hearing voices, but that the voice is inside their head as opposed to outside in the physical world, this is also thought to be a pseudo hallucination. This does not mean to say that there is not a problem, but rather that the problem is not an auditory hallucination. In this case an assessor would note the experience but look for some of the symptoms below to describe it, and would consider the voice inside the head to be part of the thought process, rather than the sensory experience process.

Delusions

A delusion is traditionally defined as a false belief based on an incorrect interpretation of an external reality, which is adhered to by a person despite evidence to the contrary. But what does this mean? Well, let us consider what a 'belief' is.

Beliefs

We come to believe something through a process. First, we perceive events as already discussed in perception. An example is that we see the sun in the sky every day and see it go down every night. We then draw an 'inference' from this. We infer that the sun goes up every morning and goes down every night. We then firm this inference into a belief. 'I believe that the sun will rise every morning and set every night.' This belief is further strengthened by new information:

- It always happens.
- We find factual information that confirms our belief. In school we are taught the science behind it.
- We are able to flesh out the belief into a wider belief system. We find out about the exception of eclipse. We find parts of the world where the sun is not in the sky for a long period and, again, understand the science behind this. Our belief becomes, 'The sun always rises and sets in the sky outside my home, although the occasional eclipse covers it up and I know that people living elsewhere do not experience the sun in the same way.'

Thus our beliefs become complex and are open to change. If we consider this process in a different way and consider the historical belief that the world is flat, we can see that people believed this because they perceived the horizon; that ships disappeared from sight, that the ships that went too far never came back and, besides, everyone else believed the world to be flat. In addition, some cultures had a model of the world which necessitated it being flat. The cultures that believed the world was carried on the back of a giant turtle had whole factual systems which told the people not only that the world was flat, but why, in the same way as our scientific system tells us it is not. That this belief would be considered wrong today is just an indication that beliefs can be wrong, but held as true by entire communities.

There are obviously far more complex beliefs which, given human beings ability to absorb information, have complex sources. If we are to consider the extent of religious belief in the world we can see that the powers of belief systems are amazing. These belief systems are passed from generation to generation as part of orientating children to the world, but then these children adopt the belief as their own and pass them on.

In some circumstances beliefs common to groups, such as a belief in witchcraft, can be misinterpreted as delusions. This is because in some cultures these beliefs are held with conviction among a significant number in the same way that a significant number of people in western culture believe in faith healing, crystallography, tarot cards, etc. Our definition of delusion needs to expand, then, to a false belief held with conviction that would be recognized as false within the cultural context of the individual.

Care should also be taken in considering delusional thinking as irrational. Often the delusion has a basis in a perceived reality, but the initial reality has been exacerbated to becomes bizarre. An example from the author's experience is a man who saw his friend stabbed to death who later believed that people were trying to kill him. While this might seem to be a perfectly reasonable, although horrible assumption, the incident had happened several years before, he was not directly threatened when it happened, and he had moved several hundred miles away and yet believed that the people had moved with him. In addition, he felt that the way the milk bottles were left outside various flats in his block were subtle signals among the group who were persecuting him. In a situation like this it is very important to acknowledge the previous real experience prior to discussing delusional thinking. In this situation the perception is based on a real and terrible incident, which would have left an indelible memory on any individual.

Types of delusion

The type of delusion a person experiences is important (Table 18.4). Traditionally delusions have also been considered fixed in a person's mind. It is now known that a person can come to have doubts about the validity of their delusional belief (Garety and Hemsley 1994). This can be useful if a skilled therapist can help the person to test and challenge their thinking. Bridget's story at the end of this chapter (p. 418) gives a clinical example of challenging and modifying beliefs.

Thought disorders

Delusional thinking is really a specific form of what is known as 'thought disorder'. In thought disorder a person experiences disruption or disturbance to normal thought patterns. These are usually named after the description given of the pattern observed. Hence, 'thought block' is a thought disorder described by the person as having thoughts that seem to get blocked in, as if they 'hit a wall in the mind' (client description). There are many other forms of thought disorder, and many individuals who experience thought disorder are aware of disruption to their thoughts.

Passivity phenomena

Passivity phenomena are a sub-type of thought disorder where a person feels their thoughts are being interfered with or accessed by the outside world. In our discussion of perception it would be a disorder of perception where the barrier between the mental and the world is felt to be breached.

Specific examples of passivity phenomena are listed in Table 18.5.

Delusional type	Note
Persecutory delusion	'They're out to get me' type of thought. These delusions are part of the lay person's stereotypical view of schizophrenia and many television or film portrayals use this stereotype. It is probable that we all have felt persecuted or harassed at some time in our lives, whether true or not. For the feeling to be delusional it must be a gross experience in that the conviction and feeling of danger and/or interference must be extreme. A personal example is a client who had moved house three times because neighbours were passing electric shocks through the walls and was asking for help with another housing transfer. My querying of this request and the simple fact that moving house three times had not stopped the experience was met with my being included as one of the persecutors. Therapeutic work could continue only when I agreed to write a letter to the housing department. It is sometimes very difficult to pin paranoia down as many people present with what I call 'plausible paranoia'. Examples are people who complain that they are being monitored by CCTV cameras, given that there has been a massive increased use of camera surveillance in England over the last ten years. Another example is people who fear terrorist attacks on their homes. Given the recent world events, this fear could seem plausible. The important distinction with a delusion is the irrationality when referred to the individual, so that they would feel the terrorists were targeting them specifically, or that the cameras could read their thoughts. Interestingly, in Western cultures, as the incidence of catatonia has gone down, the incidence of paranoid delusions has gone up, although no one knows why this is (Frangou and Murray 1996).
Ideas of reference	'They talk about me on the radio', 'David Bowie writes lyrics for me.' In this delusional type a person feels referred to, as in these examples. They can also feel that events or behaviours of others refer to themselves. A young client of mine who was a passionate supporter of a certain football club believed that certain goal celebrations related to whether he was accepted or rejected by the players.
Grandiose delusions	Where a client truly feels they have special powers, gifts or talents such as being able to heal the sick, change world events. The person can also believe that they influence powerful people or have powerful friends when they do not.
Religious delusions	Where the delusional type has a specific religious connotation. An example is a client who believed that God was communicating with him through various signs and asking him to do various things, which he would then do. A person can also believe that he or she is a religious figure, such as a profit or spiritual saviour.
Somatic delusions	Somatic means a physical manifestation or feeling. Hence a person can feel that they have cancer when they do not, or that a part of the body has died while they continue to live.

Table 18.4 Types of delusion

Thought disorder	Explanatory note
Thought broadcasting	The person feels as if the thoughts they have are broadcast and, become available to the outside world. In thought broadcast the person can often be suspicious of all social encounters and develop the belief that people react to them in such a way as to confirm the thought broadcast. An example is a client of mine who would interpret people smiling at them as people laughing at the thoughts being broadcast.
Thought insertion	As it sounds, this is where a person feels that thoughts are being inserted into the mind by someone or something else, although clients can often be unsure who or what is inserting the thought. In my experience, thoughts inserted in this way are often at odds with the individual's related beliefs. An example is a black female client who had anti-black racist thoughts inserted by her neighbours.
Thought withdrawal	Thoughts being taken out of the mind wilfully by a third party. Different from thought broadcast in that a specific agent will withdraw the thought but others will not be able to hear it.
Thought echo	Thoughts continue to sound in the mind as an echo, or repeat, either in full or part. The person feels that they have no control over this process.
Made feelings	An emotion is experienced which a third party has generated.
Made actions	Can be both simple and complex actions. 'Look, see my leg twitching? It's not me doing that – it's the freak getting me to look a fool.'

Table 18.5 Types of thought disorder

Catatonic behaviour

There is one symptom linked with schizophrenia that deserves separate consideration, and this is catatonic behaviour (also called catatonia). Catatonic behaviour is a recognizable symptom given that the person exhibits bizarre behaviour and seems lacking in physical or psychomotor movement, but the symptom is not considered to be a negative symptom. With catatonic behaviour, individuals can alternate between extreme agitation and stupor. In its most dramatic form, the stupor can result in statuesque behaviour with one posture maintained for a long time. The interesting aspect of catatonic behaviour is its gradual reduction in Western societies, but this is coupled with a concern that it has become under-diagnosed (Van der Heijden *et al.* 2005). Having said this, it is still a very rare condition. The theory given for this is that catatonia is a somatic form of a particular delusion called delusion of possession. In this delusional belief the person will believe someone or something has taken possession of the person's body and Western societies have developed the means to articulate these delusions verbally (Craig 2000). There is also doubt about the traditional diagnostic link to schizophrenia with many commentators rightly pointing out that it is more commonly found in people with disorders of mood, rather than disorders of perception (Rajagopal 2007).

Negative symptoms

Negative symptoms are harder to define and separate. They tend to be grouped together in the person's experience. The presence of negative symptoms usually results in changes in behaviour and functioning, as will be seen. For this reason, it is often negative symptoms that lay people such as family and friends tend to notice first. Great care should be taken as the loss of functioning associated with negative symptoms can often be viewed as within the individual's control, whereas the positive symptoms, with their bizarre, but noticeable difference from ordinary experience, are not. This misconception can lead to the person being criticized for 'being lazy'. Negative symptoms are not in the person's control but are a very real part of the disabling experience of schizophrenia.

The main types of negative symptom are summarized in Table 18.6. The strange words in the brackets are the complicated medical terms for the conditions. We need to be aware that the symptoms and behaviours in Table 18.6 could be attributed to other conditions or causes. The following would therefore need to be ruled out for a clearer understanding of the symptoms presented.

Negative symptom	Possible observed behaviour
Poverty of thought or speech (alogia)	Monosyllabic conversation. Inability to follow conversation. Repetitious topics of conversation.
Impaired volition (avolition)	Reductions in social care skills. Passive acceptance of situations.
Blunt affect (anhedonia)	Reduction in emotion and ability to enjoy.
Social withdrawal	Social isolation, avoidance of social interaction.

Table 18.6 Types of negative symptom

Behavioural consequences of positive symptoms

People who have positive symptoms can respond in many ways. Sometimes their behavioural response can look like negative symptoms. An example would be a person not leaving their room due to a voice telling them that they would be harmed if they were to do so or a person not talking because of a delusional belief that people were against them. A thorough assessment of the lived experience of the individual is obviously necessary in these circumstances to ensure we have a correct interpretation of the person's presentation.

Clinical depression

Sadly, having schizophrenia gives you no protection from other things. In fact, people with schizophrenia are prone to other health disabling conditions. You are more likely to be clinically depressed if you have schizophrenia than if you do not. There can be many causes for this, including living with all the positive and negative symptoms listed above, or simply stigma. Whatever the cause, if you are depressed, you will exhibit the above. A thorough assessment of functioning should attempt to assess mood as well as mental experience to explore the possibility of depression.

Side effects of medication

As discussed in Chapter 16, medication given to counteract the symptoms of schizophrenia can have side effects such as sedation and movement disorders. Again, a thorough assessment of medication is needed to rule out side effects. Having said this, recent advances in medication seem to cut down on those side effects, which can be mistaken for negative symptoms (Adams 1999).

The point was made earlier that a history could be taken from people who know the person well to elicit any changes in behaviour or functioning. It was also noted that there could be problems with this. It is clear from the above that care needs to be taken if assumptions are made on the basis of observed behaviour as there can be many causes for this behavioural change. If the behavioural change is due to negative symptoms the individual family and friends need to be informed that these symptoms are as much part of the condition as the more obvious positive symptoms. The negative symptoms can cause as much distress and disability as the positive symptoms if not acknowledged and taken into consideration when supporting the person.

It used to be thought that negative symptoms were also the result of people with a diagnosis of schizophrenia being treated in large institutions and loosing social skills as a consequence. The advent of community care has not eradicated the presence of negative symptoms, however, and their presence remains in people now living in group homes or independently (Hogg 1996).

So how do we diagnose schizophrenia?

Let us take stock. Schizophrenia is diagnosed through the presence of a number of symptoms. These symptoms are split into two groups, the positive and the negative. The positives are exceptional experiences which others would recognize as strange. The negative symptoms are the lack of skills, which lead people to seem flat and withdrawn, or who have limited social ability.

We have also seen that a large number of other factors have to be taken into consideration when considering any single symptom. Auditory hallucinations can be experienced by so-called 'normal' people. Brain damage can also account for some of the symptoms, along with other physical causes. Depression and even the medication given for schizophrenia can mirror some of the negative symptoms, and we are even unclear about whether or not catatonia is a positive or a negative symptom. So how do we put it all together and come up with a diagnosis?

Let us examine the World Health Organization classification criteria for a diagnosis of schizophrenia, often referred to as ICD-10, to see if we can find some answers (Box 18.2).

We can see from Box 18.2 that diagnosis following the experience is dependent on two things:

- *Time.* It is important that we are not talking about fleeting experiences but ones that are experienced for at least four weeks.
- *Gross disturbance.* In order for schizophrenia to be diagnosed there must be some gross disturbance to an aspect of functioning. The disturbance can be to the mental experience of perception as described above or social functioning and social performance.

Therefore, significant disorders of perception experienced over a long period of time is what schizophrenia actually means. In addition, the course of schizophrenia can take many forms depending on the prominent symptoms and if they remain after the first episode. As a consequence, it is better to view the overall care of people with schizophrenia with reference to their symptoms because:

1. There can never be one generic approach to 'schizophrenia' because the condition contains too many variables.
2. Research studies need to ensure that population samples have similar symptom presentation, and not just rely on diagnosis. In evaluating research into schizophrenia we need to ask if there has been an attempt to ensure comparability of sample selection in this regard.
3. Treatments and interventions should identify exactly which symptoms or group of symptoms they aim to influence.
4. The variation in prognosis between different ends of the spectrum of psychotic experience is vast. It is very likely that this is influenced by time of onset (i.e. at what age symptoms first become disabling, acceptance of treatment in early stages, time between first onset and treatment), symptom presentation, and ability to control symptoms.
5. We need to re-evaluate outcome measures in line with the above symptom variables. In this way services must move from pejorative terms such as 'revolving door clients' and 'treatment resistant clients' which seem to view the ineffectiveness of treatment as the clients fault, rather than the treatments.

(Brennan 2001)

Box 18.2   Diagnostic criteria for schizophrenia

At least one of the symptoms (a)–(d) or at least two of the symptoms (e)–(i) should have been present during a period of a month or more:

(a) thought echo, thought insertion or withdrawal, and thought broadcasting;
(b) delusions of control, influence or passivity, clearly referred to body or limb movements or specific thoughts, actions or sensations, delusional perception;
(c) hallucinatory voices giving running commentary on the patient's behaviour, or discussing the patient among themselves, or other types of hallucinatory voices coming from some part of the body;
(d) persistent delusions of other kinds that are culturally inappropriate and completely impossible, such as religious or political identity, or superhuman powers and abilities;
(e) persistent hallucinations in any modality, accompanied either by fleeting or half formed delusions without clear affective component, or persistent overvalued ideas, occurring every day for weeks or months on end;
(f) breaks in interpolations in the train of thought, resulting in incoherence or irrelevant speech or neologisms;
(g) catatonic behaviour, such as excitement, posturing, waxy flexibility, negativism, mutism and stupor;
(h) 'negative' symptoms such as marked apathy, paucity of speech and blunting or incongruity of emotional responses, usually resulting in social withdrawal and lowering of social performance; it must be clear that they are not due to depression or neuroleptic medication;
(i) a significant and consistent change in the overall quality of some aspects of the personal behaviour, manifest as loss of interest, aimlessness, idleness, a self-absorbed attitude and social withdrawal.

Symptom-focused treatments and interventions

It is important to have some understanding of the advances in treatment that have been made over recent decades, as the policy of community care behind the NSF for Mental Health can only be realized if we can assist people to live with their symptoms. The best way to approach the treatment of psychosis is as a *process* rather than as an *event*. This means that we take a long-term view of treatment. Recent research into effective interventions has accepted this reality and evaluated benefits on a long-term basis. Clinicians should also take this view. Any positive improvement on a person's ability to cope and manage the symptoms and consequences of schizophrenia can benefit the person long after the relationship with a particular clinician has ended.

Psychiatric medication

Treatments for schizophrenia need to focus on the symptom or symptom group they are intending to encounter. The most widely used treatment method remains the chemical treatments provided by medication (discussed in Chapters 16 and 32).

Medication is used to address changes in the activity of neurotransmitters in the brain. Schizophrenia has long been associated with neurotransmitter irregularities and it was once thought that it could be explained solely in terms of these abnormalities. We did not and do not, however, know enough about the action of neurotransmitters to justify this claim.

Mental health nurses can now prescribe medication as non-medical prescribers and under patient group directions, and this activity is set to increase in the future (National Prescribing Centre 2005). They also have a major role to play in monitoring medication and advocating medication review in multi-disciplinary teams. Monitoring medication is about ensuring the maximum benefit with the fewest possible side effects. To do this, we must ask ourselves:

1.   What symptoms are being targeted by the medication?
2.   What change in symptom has the medication achieved for the client?
3.   What side effects does the client experience?
4.   Does the benefit of the symptom change justify the side effect for the client?
5.   Can we further reduce the side effect?

We can only elicit this from constant discussion and negotiation with the client. To facilitate this, all clients should also be made aware of the specific side effects associated with any medication and encouraged to monitor these themselves.

Problem- and symptom-focused psychosocial interventions

One of the common complaints regarding psychiatric treatment of schizophrenia has been its over-reliance on psychiatric medication. Since the 1970s, however, various talking interventions have been used in conjunction with medication in an attempt to address symptoms. These interventions are discussed in detail in Chapter 14 and are evident within the case studies below.

Case one: Bridget's story

The following case studies illustrate the discussion above, and the human experience that is schizophrenia.

History and experience

Bridget was a middle-aged widow and mother who had lived with psychotic symptoms for nearly 30 years. Bridget was experiencing a relapse of her psychotic symptoms following the death of her husband, Cyril, the year before. Cyril died of cancer and was described by Bridget as a loving husband and father. Bridget's two adult children described their parents as loving and caring.

Bridget first experienced symptoms following the death of her mother and the birth of her second child. At the time her experiences took the form of a hallucinatory voice which called her a whore and a 'sex pig'. The voice accused her of being too sexual and yet suggested she perform various sex acts with various people. Bridget had a strong religious belief and found particularly distressing the voice's suggestion to seduce her priest. Gradually she gained control of her hallucinations through medication and what she termed 'the love of my family and my God'. Although Bridget gained control the voice stayed with her and her control fluctuated over the years. Accordingly, she needed admissions to hospital, which were always accompanied by a secondary guilt about not being a good mother. On analysis these admissions coincided with various stresses and life events. As a consequence Bridget, on assessment, felt that the voice had 'robbed her of years'.

In addition to the voice, Bridget also experienced various thought disorders, particularly passivity phenomena. At these times she experienced thought insertion and thought broadcast. The content of the insertion and broadcast would be predominantly anti-God. These experiences, in her account, were always the precursors to admission and had led to serious suicide attempts, one of which had left permanent organ damage.

Between highly florid episodes of positive symptoms, Bridget would also experience lowering of mood, energy and the ability to enjoy her children. It was unclear if these experiences were the result of depression or negative symptoms.

The death of her husband Cyril had, predictably, led to a crisis and an increase of all positive symptoms. What was particularly distressing her was the fact that she experienced the voice as Cyril abusing her 'from the grave' and saying he didn't love her, as she was a 'whore with a dirty mind'. At the time of referral there were serious concerns regarding Bridget's ability to keep herself safe. An increase in medication had not had the desired affect of reducing the positive symptoms.

Bridget, as can be seen from the above, was a remarkable woman who was very burdened by her symptoms, and was viewed as an amazing survivor in the face of extreme difficulties. Her schizophrenia was only one aspect of her life, an aspect which gained dominance over her abilities as a wife, mother and individual at times, but was not her defining feature.

Keeping Bridget safe

The first priority of work with Bridget was to keep her alive. This necessitated some clear and open discussions with Bridget as to whether she should receive care in her home or in an inpatient unit. She was adamant that she wanted to stay at home with her children. An open analysis of the risk that this posed had to be undertaken with the family. It was decided that Bridget could continue to receive care in her home, but under tight supervision and that admission (against her will) would not be ruled out should it become necessary.

Medication

A review was undertaken. Although the medication for positive symptoms was not changed, an anti-depressant was added. Bridget and her family were informed of the fact that the medication would take some weeks to start taking effect.

Dealing with the 'voice'

Two psychosocial techniques were used as indicated by the work of Romme and Esher. A system of distraction using a recording of the Pope saying the rosary (a sequence of prayers with relevance to the Catholic faith) was utilized where Bridget would listen to the recording when the voices became particularly bad. Distraction is a technique true to its name where the mind is 'distracted' from the voice experience by various alternative activities. If successful, distraction is really a short-term relief from the voice experience and teaches the individual that they can begin to control the voice experience themselves.

In addition to distraction, set sessions focused on the incongruity of Bridget's lived experience with her husband and the content of the hallucinatory voice. This technique is a direct challenge to the voice experience and is designed to show that the voice is not as powerful as it seems to the person.

Bridget was encouraged to reread old letters from her husband and to consider the possibility that the voice was not, in fact, his. Bridget was encouraged to ask the voice why she should believe it, as her real husband would not say these things. In these sessions it soon became evident that Bridget was frightened that if the voices stopped, even though it was negative and cruel, she would truly lose Cyril. This was felt to be a reasonable concern and in keeping with the process of grief.

Eventually Bridget regained control of her experiences and the voice became less frequent and, sometimes, reverted to its old form. The distraction was extremely effective in enabling her to gain control and she found herself getting so involved in prayer that she was able to block out the voice completely. Despite this, the thought insertion remained and Bridget came to the belief that 'God did not love me'. For Bridget this was a major concern, increasing the risk of suicide. As the belief was examined, Bridget stated that the only way she could prove to herself that God loved her was if a certain priest were to tell her. Bridget was encouraged to write to this priest explaining her situation. She did this and the priest duly responded with a letter and a set of rosary beads. The priest stated that the beads had been blessed and were to be used in 'times of hardship as an indication of God's love for you'. Bridget took great comfort in this letter and the beads and was able to use them to challenge her negative thoughts.

Although it took more than 12 months for Bridget to regain her normal level of mental experience, and even then she did have to continue in her grief, she was deemed as no longer presenting a suicide risk. More importantly, Bridget felt able to control her symptoms and experience pleasure in her family.

Bridget's story shows how a detailed knowledge of the lived experience can both help to understand and support a person with psychotic symptoms.

Bridget's greatest asset in the process of care was her ability to use positive mental experiences (her memory of Cyril and the reality of their marriage), beliefs (her religious faith) and relationships (her children) to combat negative false perceptions (her psychotic symptoms).

Case two: Brian's story

History and experience

Brian is a young man who was diagnosed with learning disabilities at age 4. Brian and his family have lived for many years on a council housing estate in a close-knit inner-city community. Given Brian's learning disability, he was marked as different from his older brother and sister at an early age. The family had been used to being involved with services as Brian had attended special school and a work programme for people with learning disability. It was in the work programme, when Brian was 21 years of age, that his mental health problems were first noted. Having said this, he was initially thought to be having difficulties adjusting to the work placement following leaving school.

At the time Brian's problems were coming to light he moved into a shared home for people with learning disabilities. It was in this home he experienced his first episode of florid psychotic symptoms, believing that other people in the house were attempting to poison him as they knew he was the son of a famous gangster, which he was not. Brian's family became so concerned that they took him back home, but his mental experiences did not change and he eventually needed admission, as he would stay up into the early hours to 'protect his family from harm'.

Eventually Brian was admitted to a special unit for people with mental health and learning disabilities. This unit was 60 miles away from his family and this further heightened his paranoia. Following assessment, Brian was transferred to a local inpatient unit where he improved on an atypical antipsychotic.

Brian was discharged following a CPA (care programme approach) meeting to a local mental health hostel. When his family went to visit him they again found him frightened and saying his room-mate was stealing his benefits and physically and verbally abusing him. Another resident verified Brian's story and his family again took him back home, very angry at services. They refused to take Brian back to see his psychiatrist and insisted that all medication and treatment be coordinated through the local general practitioner (GP). Brian's GP referred him and his family to a primary care mental health service run by a voluntary organization. The care plan for Brian and his family focused on assisting the family to care for him in their own home in order to build a rapport with them.

On assessment, Brian was suspicious and had reverted to sitting up at night watching the house. It was decided, given the effect his behaviour was having on the family, to meet him and his parents in joint sessions to address the wider family implications. Accordingly, the first sessions were spent in answering any questions the collective family members had regarding Brian's diagnosis of schizophrenia. It soon became clear that neither Brian nor his parents were aware of the long-term effects of schizophrenia, and that a person with learning disabilities could experience psychotic symptoms. In these sessions the family also expressed confusion as to the increased number of professionals they now had to deal with.

Collaborative work

Brian's suspicion transferred into his relationship with his care team. He would not talk in sessions, in spite of the best efforts of his family. After sessions, Brian would say that he was frightened that members of his care team wanted to 'experiment on him' or that the community nurse was motivated by homosexual feelings towards him. The family would then phone the care team to relate these feelings and talk about the strain caused by Brian's suspicion. It was clear to the care team that the only way to maintain Brian in any form of collaborative work was through the family, and, in particular, his mother who was a dominant force within the family.

Working with a family system

In order to work with Brian, a series of family meetings aimed at assisting his family in their caring roles were conducted. While he remained a quiet, suspicious presence in these meetings, his family were encouraged to discuss their experience and concerns in front of him. Eventually, he was able to articulate his thought processes and related a series of both positive symptoms and realistic fears due to his experiences. The positive symptoms were mainly in the form of delusions of reference (various television programmes referred to Brian and his family), passivity phenomena, which led to Brian feeling that his body had been taken over by a 'bad person with bad ideas'. The realistic fears were that he would be taken away from his family if he told people what he experienced. At this stage in the work, Brian's mother related that she had a brother born with a severe learning disability who had been admitted into a learning disabilities hospital shortly after his birth and 'abandoned'. The fear of separation, given the family's life experiences and previous treatment decisions was viewed as realistic.

Medication

It was clear in the early stages of family meetings that Brian had stopped all forms of medication due to a mixture of suspicion that the medication was aimed at drugging him so that he could be 'taken away' (related to family members and not the care team) and side effects. The medication was reviewed and changed to an atypical drug under the supervision of his GP, whom he still trusted. The family was encouraged to administer and supervise the medication. After a few weeks, clear gains in Brian's communication were being seen in meetings, and the family related that they were pleased with his response as there were no reported side effects.

Problem solving

The main area of concern, once the situation had been stabilized, was Brian's lack of socialization outside of the family. A plan was made that Brian would leave the house for planned activities with his father and brother, with whom he felt safe. As this proved effective, Brain was encouraged to carry out small tasks in the locality to build his confidence. This proved very effective and, with the gains attributed to his taking regular effective medication, Brian began to leave the house by himself.

There followed a period of unforeseen problems as Brian began to spend his days drinking alcohol in his room. His drinking became an issue as he would get intoxicated and get into arguments with family members.

Brain related that he was now bored and it was clear that he needed more focused activities during the day when other family members were at work.

Service problems

Both family and care team were frustrated by an inability to find appropriate activities for Brian. A mental health day unit proved to be unsuccessful as he was frightened of again being exploited and learning disability work and day units were uneasy at accepting him due to his mental health problems. In the process of working through these issues, Brian began to deteriorate. He was now at home for long periods by himself, continued to drink and began to omit medication doses. Eventually, following an argument with his sister during which the police were called, he was admitted to the local inpatient unit.

Conclusion

Following a short admission, Brian stabilized. He continued to remain well at home, but the struggle to find appropriate activities continued. At the time I left Brian's care team it was clear that if a solution could not be found, he would continue to go through a sequence of improvement and relapse with his family bearing most of the caring role.

Conclusion

These case studies attempt to put a human face on the collection of symptoms that is schizophrenia. Take another look at the stories and you will note that these are two very different people in terms of age, gender and position within the family, but they have in common a set of mental experiences which many do not have – psychotic symptoms.

It is right that people with schizophrenia live in the communities to which they belong and contribute. However, it is also right that these communities are assisted through quality mental health services run by professionals who are able to see the person through the disorders of perception that often mask their potential. Only then will we ever hope to overcome the fear and stigma still present in our society.

In summary, the main points of this chapter are:

- Mental processes can go wrong due to: physical processes affecting mental processes; problems with the formulation of personality; and problems with the process of perception.
- Schizophrenia is a mental disorder associated with serious problems with perception. The world-view of people suffering from schizophrenia may often be at odds with the world-view of others, in particular their relatives or close friends who notice changes in the person's demeanour, behaviour and attitude as a cause for concern.
- Traditionally, the symptoms of schizophrenia are classified as 'positive' symptoms – those that are an additional experience to the norm, or an exaggeration of normal experience – or 'negative' symptoms, which represent a reduction in normal experience. As a general rule, the more a person is affected by negative symptoms, the more disabled they will be by schizophrenia.
- Treatment of people suffering from schizophrenia is best regarded as a long-term process, rather than a one-off event. Medication and psychosocial interventions in combination can help clients to manage their symptoms while living in the community. Nurses have a major role to play with regard to both these types of interventions.
- Crucial to high quality care is the nurse's ability to relate to people suffering from psychosis as people, rather than as a collection of symptoms.

Questions for reflection and discussion

1   Reflect on your own mental experiences. Can you relate to any of the mental experiences outlined above?
2   Reflect on your own belief systems. Are there aspects of your beliefs, such as religious beliefs, that others would not share? Why are your beliefs not delusional?
3   Consider what your own beliefs and attitudes were to people with schizophrenia prior to your training. Where did these come from? Have they changed? What has changed them?
4   What do you feel is the prevalent attitude to schizophrenia among the general population? If you wished to change this, how would you go about it?
5   Review Standards 4 and 5 of the NSF for Mental Health (listed in Chapter 6) with regard to the above case studies. Are these standards relevant to Bridget and Brian and their carers?
6   Review Standard 6. How is this standard relevant to Bridget and Brian? Who is this standard most relevant to and why?
7   How has Standard 7 been met in Bridget's case?

Annotated bibliography

■   Chadwick, P. (2002) Understanding one man's schizophrenic experience. *Nursing Times* **98**(38): 32–3. In this short personal account, Peter Chadwick outlines his own experience of schizophrenia. The article gives a personal view of the issues presented here and is immensely worth the small effort that it takes to read. Peter Chadwick is an expert in many ways, being both a user of services and a teacher of professionals.
■   Deveson, A. (1991) *Tell Me I'm Here.* London: Penguin. This is a personal account from the carer's perspective. The book is uncomfortable reading at times, particularly some of the family's encounters with professionals. The book again allows us to consider the perspective of non-professionals who are experts in their own right.
■   Haddock, G. and Slade, P. (1996) *Cognitive Behavioural Interventions with Psychotic Disorders.* Routledge: London. A complex book, but a comprehensive exploration of talking interventions aimed at alleviating psychotic symptoms.

References

Adams, C. (1999) Drug treatments for schizophrenia. *Effective Health Care Bulletin: NHS Centre for Reviews and Dissemination* **5**: 6.
Brennan, G. (2001) Schizophrenia, diagnosis and introduction to interventions. *Mental Health Practice* **4**(7): 32–8.
Craig, T.K.J. (2000) Severe mental illness: symptoms signs and diagnosis, in C. Gamble and G. Brennan (eds) *Serious Mental Illness: A Manual for Clinical Practice.* London: Baillière Tindall.
Department of Health (1999) *The National Service Framework for Mental Health, Modern Standards and Service Models.* London: DH.
Downs, J. (ed.) (2001) *Starting and Supporting Hearing Voices Groups.* Manchester: Hearing Voices Network.
Frangou, S. and Murray, R. (1996) *Schizophrenia.* London: Martin Dunitz.

Garety, P. and Hemsley, D. (1994) *Delusions: Investigations into the Psychology of Delusional Reasoning.* Hove: Psychology Press.

Gombrich, E.H. (1960) *Art and Illusion: A Study of the Psychology of Pictorial Representation.* Princeton, NJ: Princeton University Press.

Goodwin, K. and Jamison, K.R. (1990) *Manic Depressive Illness.* New York: Oxford University Press.

Hogg, L. (1996) Treatment for negative symptoms, in G. Haddock and P. Slade (eds) *Cognitive Behavioural Interventions with Psychotic Disorders.* London: Routledge.

Jaspers, K. (1963) *General Psychopathology* (trans. J. Hoenig and M.W. Hamilton). Chicago, IL: University of Chicago Press.

Landmark, J., Merkskey, Z., Cernousky, Z. and Helmes, E. (1990) The positive trials of schizophrenic symptoms: its statistical properties and its relationship to thirteen traditional diagnostic systems. *British Journal of Psychiatry* **156**: 388–94.

National Prescribing Centre (2005) *Improving Mental Health Services by Extending the Role of Nurses in Prescribing and Supplying Medication.* Good practice guide. London: National Prescribing Centre/National Institute for Mental Health in England, http://www.npc.co.uk/pdf/mental_health_guide.pdf

Priest, S. (1991) *Theories of the Mind.* London: Penguin Books.

Rajagopal (2007) Catatonia. *Advances in Psychiatric Treatment* **13**: 51–9.

Romme, M. and Esher, S. (1993) *Accepting Voices.* London: MIND.

Tien, A.Y. (1991) Distribution of hallucinations in the population, *Social Psychiatry and Psychiatric Epidemiology* **26**: 287–92.

Van der Heijden, F.M., Tuinier, S., Arts, N.J. *et al.* (2005) Catatonia: disappeared or under-diagnosed? *Psychopathology.* **38**: 3–8.

Warner, R. (1994) *Recovery from Schizophrenia: Psychiatry and Political Economy.* London: Routledge.

CHAPTER 19

The person with an affective/mood disorder

Sue Gurney

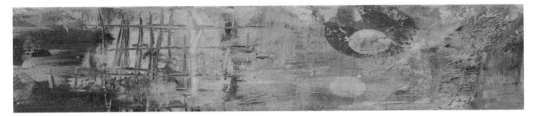

Chapter overview

The terms affective/mood disorder is a general expression used to describe a state of health where the predominant mood is viewed as distorted or inappropriate. Mood disorders are common and present a diverse picture, some are mild, others severe, some last a few weeks, others a lifetime, some are obvious while others are barely perceptible. This chapter gives an overview of the two main types of mood disorders, depression and bipolar disorder, and provides information for consideration in the application to mental health nursing practice. This chapter covers:

- Introduction and overview of mood disorders;
- What is depression?
- What is bipolar disorder?
- Types of depression and bipolar disorder;
- Reasons for depression;
- Screening and assessment;
- Approaches to care and treatment;
- Implications for mental health nursing practice.

Introduction

Within the UK the National Institute for Health and Clinical Excellence provides recommendations on promoting health and treating ill health. The specific recommendations related to mood disorders are located in a number of clinical guidelines and technology appraisals that are summarized in Table 19.1.

Clinical Guideline 16	Self-harm
Clinical Guideline 23	Depression
Clinical Guideline 28	Depression in children and young people.
Clinical Guideline 38	Bipolar disorder
Clinical Guideline 45	Antenatal and postnatal mental health
Technology Appraisal 59	Electroconvulsive therapy (ECT)
Technology Appraisal 97	Depression and anxiety computerized cognitive behavioural therapy (CCBT)

Table 19.1 Relevant NICE clinical guidance and technology appraisals
Source: NICE (2007).

The past ten years has seen an emphasis on the development of specialist mental health services, now there is to be a shift of this emphasis to the mental health of the community as a whole (DH 2007). Mental health problems are common and although most people experiencing mood disorders are seen in primary care, they may or may not be offered effective treatments (Boardman *et al.* 2004). Mental health nurses (MHNs) are the largest professional group providing both care to those with high severity-complex needs, or in supporting other workers in caring for those with less complex needs (DH 2006a). This places MHNs in a unique position to fully comprehend the needs and views of people who use our services; thus enabling MHNs to influence change in improving care and advancing practice.

People who use our services

Language is important. The mental health literature details an evolving language from the use of the term patient to: client, customer, user, user survivor and people who use services. These terms have associations to power structures within systems of care provision. The term patient relates to a paternalistic model; the client with a consumerist model; the user with an amended consumerist model (as people detained under the Mental Health Act have choice removed) and people who use services relating to a citizenship-community model (Hickey and Kipping 1998). The terms people, individual or people who use our services is used throughout this chapter to encompass the terms service user, client and patient.

What is depression?

Overview

Depression (low mood) is an umbrella term used to describe an experience that affects the whole person in terms of feelings, thoughts, judgements and behaviour (Lilja *et al.* 2006). Depression is often characterized by some, or many, of the following: sadness, anxiousness, hopelessness, pessimism, guilt, worthlessness, loss of confidence, low self-esteem, fatigue, decreased interest in activities, disturbance of sleep, changes in appetite with resulting loss or increase in weight, decrease and loss of libido, diminished concentration, irritability, restlessness, physical complaints and thoughts of death/suicide and self-harm/suicide attempts. Occasionally states of psychosis may be experienced and sometimes a tragic outcome of depression is suicide (NIMHE 2007).

If projections prove accurate, then by 2020, depression will become the second cause of the global disease burden (WHO 2001). Globally the estimated incidence of chronic depression is around 20 per cent (especially if inadequately treated). A reoccurrence rate on recovery from a first episode is estimated at around 35 per cent within two years and around 60 per cent at 12 years (WHO 2001). The incidence of depression is higher in those of middle age (Üstün *et al.* 2004) with prevalence estimations varying across populations (WHO 2001).

Medical classification of depression

Although the experience of depression is common for most people, particularly when experiencing adversity, a diagnosis is determined by medical classification. The ICD-10 (WHO 1992) describes ten symptoms of depression and grades the results in terms of severity; symptoms must be present for at least two weeks. If three symptoms are present, then there is no depression; four symptoms are classified as mild; five or six symptoms as moderate and seven or more as severe depression. Most experiences of depression are at the mild to moderate end of the depression spectrum and it is these that are mainly seen in primary care (Boardman *et al.* 2004). Terminology also refers to a spectrum of depression disorders such as postnatal depression (low mood following childbirth), seasonal affective disorder (low mood during winter) and dysthymia (persistent uncomfortable mood). The symptoms of depression may also present in combination with other mental health medically classified conditions such as anxiety and psychosis (WHO 1992).

What is bipolar disorder?

Overview

The term bipolar disorder is another umbrella term and refers to the experience of opposite states of mood, whereby depression alternates with the experience of mania (elevated/high mood). These cyclic mood changes may be gradual or rapid and dramatic; occasionally mania occurs on its own. Mania is marked with an elevation of mood, which is very different to the person's usual mood, and which is held over a significant period of time. This may be accompanied by some, or many, of the following: over-activity, increased energy, increased confidence, impaired concentration, pressure of speech, flights of ideas, grandiose ideas, racing thoughts and a decreased need for sleep, all of which may affect thinking, judgement and behaviour. Occasionally people experiencing bipolar disorder may also experience states of psychosis (Baker 2001; NICE 2006a).

The lifetime prevalence of bipolar disorder is estimated to be similar to schizophrenia, at around 1 per cent of the population (NICE 2006a). A genetic risk factor is also associated with condition (Craddock and Jones 2001) as are higher levels of physical morbidity and mortality than the general population (NICE 2006a; DH 2006b).

Medical classification of bipolar disorder

The ICD-10 (WHO 1992) classification system defines a spectrum of bipolar disorders in terms of mania, hypomania, mixed episodes and cyclothymic mood disorders. DSM-IV (APA 1994) classifies two sub-types of bipolar disorder: bipolar-1: generally the experience of a manic episode followed by a period of depression; and bipolar 11: generally the experience of severe depressive episodes alternating with hypomania.

Reasons for depression

Overview

There is a large volume of literature on the risk/causative factors associated with developing depression. Theories and evidence exist in supporting: psychosocial factors involving basic life experience, psychological attributes related to vulnerability and coping skills, changes in brain functioning, genetic predisposition, life events and stressors (particularly involving losses and major long-term difficulties), poor relationships, social, cultural and environmental factors (Piccinelli and Wilkinson 2000; Lilja *et al.* 2006). In most cases the roots of depression are generally accepted as multi-dimensional (Lilja *et al.* 2006).

Depression in children

An estimate of the prevalence of childhood and adolescent depression in the community ranges from 0.5 per cent to 10 per cent (NICE 2005). Mood disorders can be difficult to identify and may be masked by developmental stages (Meadus 2007). Research has identified risk factors to include: family discord, bullying, physical, sexual or emotional abuse, history of parental depression, ethnic and cultural factors, homelessness, refugee status and institutional living (NICE 2005).

Depression in women

Women experience depression almost twice as often as men (Üstün *et al.* 2004). In the past most research has tended to focus on the biological differences between the genders that possibly contribute to this increased rate. However, more recent research on biological, psychological and socio-political explanations is offering a more integrated approach to informing the development of appropriate prevention/treatment approaches (Corey and Goodman 2006).

Depression in men

Although men are less likely to suffer depression than women the rate of suicide in men is three to four times that of women, although more women attempt it (Gunnell and Lewis 2005). While a wide range of explanation and risk factors are proposed robust explanations for these gender differences have yet to be established (Piccinelli and Wilkinson 2000).

Depression in the elderly

The incidence of depression and suicidal intent, in combination with physical symptoms, is slightly higher in the elderly (NICE 2004a). Research has identified risk factors to include: poor social integration, loneliness, adverse life events, physical frailty/illness and lack of support from services (Mayall *et al.* 2004; Dennis *et al.* 2005).

Cultural issues

Although the experience of depression is recognized across different cultures, the challenge is in identifying genuine differences without being misguided by ethnic stereotyping (Kirmayer 2006). This research arena is complex and controversial 'a jungle of speculation but a desert of information' Bebbington (1993 cited in Bhugra and Mastrogianni 2004: 18). In this era of increasing globalization it is proposed that individual differences are as great as ethnic ones with the headline message of treating the individual (Bhugra and Mastrogianni 2004).

> 66   I wrote the Loony-bin Trip between 1982 and 1985. Now, when I reread it I find something in it rings false ... typing it over I want to say, wait a moment – why call this depression? – why not call it grief? You've permitted your grief even your outrage, to be converted into a disease (Kate Millett 1991).
>
> Ramsey *et al.* (2002: 4)   99

Screening and assessment

Overview

Screening

People experiencing mood disorders may turn for help to numerous informal and formal sources. The type of help seeking behaviour is generally influenced by the conceptual belief/model that the individual holds, e.g. a psychological model generally associated with self-help compared to a biological model with help seeking behaviours (Goldstein and Rosselli 2003). Occasionally, at risk situations require people to be detained for assessment/treatment under the Mental Health Act 1983 or 2007.

NICE (2004a) recommends routine screening in primary care of at-risk groups, such as people with a history of depression, the experience of recent major life events etc. An initial two-part screening question is recommended (CSIP 2006: 28):

- During the last month have you been feeling down, depressed or hopeless?
- During the last month have you often been bothered by having little interest or pleasure in doing things?

If depression is potentially identified then a more comprehensive assessment by an appropriately skilled professional is recommended (NICE 2004a, 2005).

Screening tools and assessment measures

In screening and reviewing progress the routine use of measures in informing clinical decisions is recommended (NICE 2004a, 2005, 2006a). Many measures are available and the art lies in choosing the measure that best fits the practice setting. Regardless of the measures employed it is the interpretation of results that require validation with the individual that is most important. Some examples of measures are given in Table 19.2.

Measure	Source
General measures	
The work and social adjustment scale	Mundt *et al.* (2002)
General Health Questionnaire	Goldberg and Williams (1988)
Brief Psychiatric Rating Scale (BPRS)	Lukoff *et al.* (1986)
The Client satisfaction Questionnaire	Attkisson and Zwick (1982)
Mini Mental State Examination (MMSE)	Folstein *et al.* (1975)
Disorder specific measures	
Patient Health Questionnaire (PHQ-9)	Spitzer *et al.* (1999)
Hospital Anxiety Depression Scale (HAD)	Zigmond and Snaith (1983)
Beck Depression Inventory (BDI-I)	Beck *et al.* (1961)
Beck Depression Inventory (BDI-II)	Steer *et al.* (2000)
Geriatric Depression Scale (GDS)	Sheikh and Yesavage (1986)
Edinburgh Postnatal Depression Scale (PDS)	Cox *et al.* (1987)
Mania Scale	Bech *et al.* (1979)
Beck Hopelessness Scale	Beck *et al.* (1993)
Case specific measures	
Case specific measures are highly personal and simple to use, e.g. scoring an experience/view on a scale of 0 to 10. However, they cannot be used for screening purposes or in comparison with treatment groups.	

Table 19.2 Examples of screening and assessment measures

Overview of assessment

Best practice follows a holistic, person-centred approach with clinical judgement informed by the *person's voice* and current best practice (Barker 2004; NICE 2004a, 2004b, 2005, 2006b; CSIP 2006). The reader is also referred to Chapters 10 on assessment, 11 on assessing and managing risk and 27 on engaging with clients in their care and treatment. The following outlines the core principles and key components of assessment:

■ effective communication skills in building, maintaining and closing person-centred relationships;

■ holistic assessment with the involvement of family and carers as appropriate;

■ taking full account of the voice and views of what is important to the person, families and carers and all those involved in the delivery of care;

■ acknowledging strengths and working with these.

The key components of assessment include:

■ physical assessment: presentation, health history, current treatments and lifestyle related to physical well-being;

■ mental health assessment: duration and severity of the current experience including: thoughts, self worth, self esteem, risk, coping abilities, mental health history and lifestyle related to mental well-being;

■ social circumstances: stressors in life, relationships, religious/spiritual needs, networks, employment, accommodation, finance, interests, potential support systems and identification of carers.

Risk

An element of the assessment process is routine exploration of risk. Although there are many forms of risk, suicidal thoughts are common. Table 19.3 outlines the broad themes in enquiring about risk.

It is also important to identify the risks of:

■ self-neglect, self-harm and sensitive enquiry of abuse from others (physical, sexual or emotional) and actual and potential risk to others, e.g. identifying a need for safeguarding children;
■ identifying past and current use of prescribed/non-prescribed drugs.

Risk can be generally categorized into:

Low risk: no current/infrequent thoughts;
Intermediate risk: frequent current thought but no intention/plan;
High risk: current thoughts/plans/preparations.

Intention – thoughts
Do things ever feel that bad that you think about harming or killing yourself?
Do you ever feel that life is not worth living?

Plans
Have you made plans to end your life?
Do you know how you would kill yourself?

Actions
Have you made any actual preparations to kill yourself?
Have you ever attempted suicide in the past?

Prevention
How likely is it that you will act on such thoughts and plans?
What is stopping you killing or harming yourself at the moment?

Table 19.3 Asking about risk
Source: CSIP (2006: 28)

Formulating a care plan

Overview

A comprehensive assessment will inform the formulation of an appropriate care plan which addresses the following broad themes:

■ All possible physical causes such as hormonal conditions, medication side effects, etc. have been excluded or been/being treated.
■ The 'diagnosis' and severity of the 'experience' is ascertained.
■ The level of risk is identified: low/medium/high.
■ Other relevant psychosocial factors are considered.

For most people in contact with specialist mental health services treatment and care is delivered through the Care Programme Approach process (DH 2008). This will be influenced by the needs of the individual, the care group, the care setting and the availability of appropriate treatments/interventions. The reader is also referred to Chapter 28 on problems, goals and care planning.

Approaches to care and treatment

Overview

Treatment is informed by the severity and complexity of the person's experience and clinical judgement based on current best evidence. Systematic monitoring and review are essential in deciding and delivering the most appropriate and effective care strategies.

Stepped care

Stepped care (summarized in Table 19.4) is a model of care originating from the USA (Scogin *et al.* 2003). It is recommended for the management of a number of conditions including depression (NICE 2004a, 2005, 2007) and other NICE pathways. The two principles of this approach are firstly in offering treatment likely to provide a significant health benefit, but is the least intensive of those available. Secondly that any decision to 'step up' care is informed by the findings of systematic monitoring, indicating that the current treatment is not achieving the desired gain.

Step	Who is responsible?	The focus	What they do
Step 5	Inpatient care, crisis teams	Risk to life, severe self neglect	Medication, combined treatments, ECT
Step 4	Mental health specialists including crisis teams	Treatment-resistant, recurrent, atypical and psychotic depression and those at significant risk	Medication, complex psychological interventions, combined treatment, case management
Step 3	Primary care team, primary care mental health worker	Moderate or severe depression	Medication, psychological interventions, social support
Step 2	Primary care team, primary care mental health worker	Mild to moderate depression	Watchful waiting, guided self help, computerized CBT, exercise, brief psychological interventions
Step 1	GP, practice nurse	Recognition	Assessment

Table 19.4 The stepped care model
Source: NICE (2004a: 28)

Treatment approaches

Overview

Diet, exercise and physical health

A somewhat obvious but neglected area with clear evidence existing on the positive impact of a balanced diet and exercise on overall well-being (NICE 2004a; Mental Health Foundation 2006). Structured exercise programmes have also proved beneficial as a distinct treatment approach for people with mild to moderate depression (NICE 2004a, 2005). The reader is also referred to Chapter 15 on physical health care.

Psychological approaches for depression

Psychological approaches/interventions for the treatment of depression are wide-ranging and include approaches such as cognitive behavioural therapy (CBT), psychotherapy, brief therapy, counselling, problem solving, education and self-help methods (NICE 2004a, 2005, 2006a, 2006b). CBT generally challenges negative styles of thinking and behaving associated with depression, whereas psychodynamic therapies are sometimes used to focus on resolving people's conflicting feelings. Although there are many forms of psychological intervention there is robust evidence on the efficacy of short-term CBT and interpersonal therapy in the treatment of depression (NICE 2004a, 2005, 2006b).

For the treatment of mild to moderate depression CBT/brief psychological approaches are recommended as a first-line treatment. This is generally around six sessions over six to nine weeks (NICE 2004a, 2005, 2006b). Currently an alternative computerized CBT approach for mild depression and anxiety is being introduced throughout the UK (NICE 2006b). Generally, as the severity of the depression increases the psychological intervention is extended over a longer period of time and may also involve other psychological approaches such as family therapy. The reader is referred to Chapters 30 and 31 on behavioural and cognitive techniques.

Psychosocial approaches for bipolar disorder

For people with bipolar disorder the treatment and management of depressive episodes is as described above. Over the last 20 years there have been developments in psychosocial interventions particularly in identifying prodromes that are unique to the individual. Once identified, coping strategies can be developed in decreasing the likelihood and severity of potential/future manic episodes (Baker 2001). The reader is referred to Chapter 14 on psychosocial interventions.

Medication

Chapters 16 and 32 are recommended reading for greater detail on pharmacological interventions and medication concordance.

Medication for depression

The two main neurotransmitters particularly thought to be associated with depression are serotonin, sometimes referred to as 5HT, and noradrenaline. Antidepressants generally work by increasing the concentrations of these. The three main groups of antidepressants used to treat depression are selective serotonin reuptake inhibitors (SSRIs), the tricylics and the monoamine oxidase inhibitors (MAOIs). The SSRIs are newer medications with fewer side effects compared to tricyclics. MAOIs are more rarely used and require dietary restriction as foods containing high levels of tyramine may precipitate a hypertensive crisis (Stahl 2000).

NICE (2004a, 2005, 2006a) outline prescribing recommendations; in routine care the antidepressant of choice is from the SSRI group. Antidepressants take time to establish therapeutic levels and so generally need to be prescribed for a minimum of six weeks, or more, before being considered ineffective.

Medication is recommended routinely in treating moderate and severe depression, in conjunction with a psychological therapy (NICE 2004a, 2005).

Augmentation of medication may be required in treating combinations of depression with anxiety, psychosis and other conditions. Specific arrangements need to be made for careful monitoring of progress, side effects, and adverse drug reactions with prescribed and un-prescribed drugs and when switching antidepressants. Generally, people who have had two or more depressive episodes in the recent past and who experience significant functional impairment are advised to continue medication for at least two years. Discontinuation should be gradual and depends on symptoms, support and current/potential stressors (NICE 2004a, 2005, 2006a).

Medication for bipolar disorder

Depressive episodes are treated as above and if a person is taking antidepressants at the acute onset of mania then they are generally stopped. People with a first episode of mania are usually, initially, offered an antipsychotic such as olanzapine, quetiapine or risperidone. If symptoms fail to improve then valporate, lithium or carbamazepine may be offered. These latter three preparations may also be the medications of choice for long-term treatment. Lithium needs careful monitoring as there is a small range between its efficacy and toxicity and in people with certain pre-existing physical conditions it may not be recommended (NICE 2006a).

Generally, treatment with anti-mania medication lasts around two years after the first episode and up to five years if the person has risk factors such as a history of frequent relapse, ongoing stressors (NICE 2006a). Once again specific arrangements need to be made for careful monitoring of progress as described in the previous section. However, particular awareness needs to be given to the toxicity of some of these preparations and when switching from one medication to another, titrating doses and discontinuing (NICE 2004a, 2005, 2006a).

Case study: Stephen

Stephen was in his late twenties, he had relationship difficulties, held a high pressured job, had some ongoing physical health problems and had recently moved house. At the request of his family he was referred to the crisis team by his GP. Stephen was seen and admitted to hospital for assessment under the Mental Health Act.

At school Stephen had mood swings but this was attributed to 'growing up'. Over recent years he had experienced several periods of depression for which he had seen a therapist and found it helpful. Over recent months he had become increasingly busy, then really busy and multi-tasking big time. He remortgaged the house and started recklessly spending and running up debt into tens of thousands of pounds, he had also started spending business funds. Stephen felt great, he had loads of energy and ideas, he hardly slept and ate and was becoming sexually promiscuous and disinhibited.

When Stephen arrived on the ward he was eccentrically and inappropriately dressed. He was restless, agitated, angry, frightened and talked so excessively fast that his speech was slurred. He had also lost a significant amount of weight. Following a thorough physical and mental health assessment a diagnosis of mania was made and medication suggested. Stephen was angry, and viewed the diagnosis as incorrect. Stephen's named nurse approached him to explore his 'world' and spent some time over the following week providing information and talking this through. Finally Stephen was willing to 'give it a try', he accepted the medication and 30 days later was discharged from hospital.

The community team and the nurse, his Care Programme Approach (CPA) care coordinator, supported Stephen's care and treatment which in the main was medication, a psycho-education package that included CBT and membership of a support group.

Stephen's life has changed, the experience resulted in the loss of a relationship, home and job. Eighteen months down the line and life is beginning to rebuild. Stephen has moved out of his parents' home into a small flat and is planning to move from voluntary work to commence a course in graphic design. Stephen self monitors his mood with a mood diary and holds ambivalent views about his family for the life-changing event that brought him into contact with mental health services.

Alternative and complementary therapies

A vast array of alternative or complementary therapies exist such as: light therapy, transcranial magnetic stimulation, vagus nerve stimulation (Shelton 2006), herbalism, aromatherapy, massage, traditional Chinese medicine, hypnosis (Mantle 2002), folate, St John's wort, meditation, acupuncture (Larzelere 2002), self-help and web and online sources (Stjernswärd and Ostmän 2006). The extent of usage of these interventions in primary and secondary care is currently constrained, as evidence to support their efficacy remains limited (Wu 2007). Because a number of people use such approaches as their main health care system, or in supplementing conventional treatments it is important for MHNs to have awareness and knowledge of these approaches. The reader is referred to Chapters 17 and 29 for further information on complementary and alternative therapies and self-help.

Electroconvulsive therapy

Overview

Electroconvulsive therapy (ECT) has been in use since the 1930s and how it works is still not fully understood. Guidelines for the use of ECT have been developed by the Royal College of Psychiatrists (RCP 2005) and NICE *Technology Appraisal No 59* (2003). The main themes from this guidance form the following overview and the reader is referred to the NICE website for current information.

ECT is undertaken under general anaesthetic and so general preparation and guidance for pre and post general anaesthetic care applies. While under anaesthesia electrodes are placed at precise locations on the head to deliver electrical impulses. The electrical stimulation causes a brief, about 30 seconds, seizure within the brain (NICE 2003).

Although the use of ECT in the UK is declining it is still administered within the UK to a substantial number of people (Ruthen 2006). NICE (2003) recommends ECT to be used as a treatment for people suffering from: a severe depressive illness, prolonged or severe mania, or catatonia, and must be used only for conditions which are life-threatening and unresponsive to existing treatment and after all other treatment options have failed. To achieve full therapeutic benefit it is recommended that several sessions of ECT be given each week over a three- to six-week period (NICE 2003). ECT is used for gaining fast or short-term improvement of very severe symptoms; it is not used as maintenance therapy (NICE 2003; RCP 2005).

In assessing the need for ECT a cost–benefit analysis needs to be undertaken of having/not having the treatment. This requires the consideration of valid consent in making a joint decision based on informed discussion of the situation taking into account such issues as advanced directives, advocacy, the risk of anaesthesia, current co-morbidities, adverse events such as potential cognitive impairment, pregnancy, age and risk of not receiving treatment (NICE 2003).

ECT remains one of the most controversial and contradictory medical treatments in theory and practice (Ruthen 2006).

> 66 On Mind's website a psychologist compares ECT to the 'assumption a broken television could be mended as readily with a sledgehammer as with a screwdriver: you might jog the right bit'. Well, if you don't have a screwdriver and you need the television, using the sledgehammer might be better than nothing. I feel I needed that sledgehammer, but I also needed to know all the risks involved in its use.
>
> Caroline Hearst (2007: 21) 99

Mental health nursing: caring for people with mood disorders

Overview

This section explores some emergent themes from the recent mental health nursing (MHN) literature in caring for people experiencing depression or bipolar disorder. Each theme concludes with a point for practice consideration.

Context of mental health nursing

Mental health nurses emphasize providing care and supporting people through their physical and emotional distress, while doctors are primarily concerned with diagnosis and cure (Feely and Long 2007). The context of MHN in England is set within the recommendations of the recent *Review of Mental Health Nursing* (DH 2006a). The review sets the direction of travel for MHN in moving from a traditional medical model to a psychosocial approach (DH 2006a). However, Gallop and Reynolds (2004) suggest that until recently the biological, psychological and sociological models have operated as distinct entities, and while we may refer to holistic care the reality is limited in practice and even more so in research.

Point for practice consideration

■ Achieving holistic integrated person-centred care is beset with challenges and opportunities.

Mental health nursing and stigma

A study of MHN students' attitudes towards people with depression found that they were similar to those held by the general public, that people with depression have some control of and responsibility for their experience. As the students progressed through their learning this attitude lessened and the students displayed increasing attitudes of help and pity. Although the desire to help is consistent with choosing a nursing career, feelings of pity although viewed positively can be viewed negatively as condescending and exclusionary (Halter 2004).

In caring for vulnerable people whose reality may be very different to the majority in the community, nurses may be at risk of developing 'despair and pity' (Finnema *et al.* 1996 cited in Lilja *et al.* 2006: 270). Some care settings are also challenging in attempting to meet all individuals' needs in remaining continuously empathic and understanding. Within this context MHNs may develop coping strategies that adopt a symptom/task approach to care with a resulting disassociation with the person (Hellzen *et al.* 2003 cited in Lilja *et al.* 2006). There is also evidence that MHNs hold positive views towards the 'good, unproblematic, trusting patient' and negative views to all others (Lilja *et al.* 2004: 552).

Point for practice consideration

■ People with mental health problems, particularly those in contact with mental health services, experience stigma and discrimination. Stigma and discrimination is also held by MHNs, with some care settings posing challenges to MHNs in remaining constantly empathic and understanding. These points have important relationships with structures such as supervision, reflective practice, professional development and opportunities for self-evaluation.

Fundamental nursing practice

MHN has championed an interpersonal context at its core (Peplau 1952; Altschul 1972) and so the concept of inspiring hope is also central to MHNs. However, inspiring hope generally appears to be achieved by the presence of certain aptitudes and traits in the MHN rather than 'technical skills' (Cutcliffe and Koehn 2007; Koehn and Cutcliffe 2007). Although the interpersonal context is central to MHN, there is also the issue that the nurse–person relationship may not always be a positive and enabling one (Lilja *et al.* 2004).

Point for practice consideration

■ The importance of self-awareness required by MHNs of their appearance, attitudes and behaviour on their relationship with people in 'interpreting and confirming the client's worthiness or worthlessness' (Hedelin and Jonsson 2003: 321).

What should mental health nurses do?

❝ Let's abandon the metaphor of metal distress being an illness and recognize what it actually is: our response to being hurt, betrayed, abandoned, shammed, humiliated and finding ourselves unable to make some kind of sense of our lives than we can live with happily.

Dorothy Rowe (2006: 15) ,,

Advanced nursing practice

Current research into the efficacy of treatments for depression supports, in the main, pharmacological and psychological approaches. MHNs may now prescribe and are routinely involved in the administration and monitoring of medication. However, there are reports that MHNs are often ill prepared for this aspect of practice (Gray *et al.* 2001). A similar situation is reflected in MHNs providing psychological support, of which it is also suggested that preparation is insufficient (Crowe and Luty 2005). Having time to spend caring and delivering psychotherapeutic care are two different things (McLaughlin 1999). Indeed, CBT and brief term psychological therapies have proven efficacy and MHNs are in a unique position in taking these forward (Beech 2000; DH 2006a).

Point for practice consideration

■   Advanced MHN practice is defined, in this domain, by the acquisition and employment of psychotherapeutic and pharmacological 'advanced/technical skills'. Some evidence suggests that some MHNs are ill prepared for these areas of practice.

The true expert

Acknowledging the negative impact of the experience of depression and contact with mental health services, it is proposed that for some people this experience reinforces a 'sick role' and hinders recovery (Millward *et al.* 2005). MHNs can gain invaluable learning from listening to the experiences of people who use mental health services. 'When we are able to hear all voices then nurses will be able to frame research and practice in ways that can profoundly impact on clients' lives' (Gallop and Reynolds 2004: 64).

Point for practice consideration

■   In delivering evidence-based care, it is important that the voice of true experts (patients) is heard (Feely *et al.* 2007: 400).

An understanding of the complexity of mood disorders

An understanding of cultural expectations and their relation to mental distress provides a reference for understanding the meaning of behaviours that may be regarded as mental disorders (Crowe 2002). Aware that 'depression' is experienced by nearly all of us we might conclude that this human commonality informs MHN practice; but this may not be so according to the following personal story:

  ❝   I do not believe that depression is instructive in many ways. It does not necessarily help you to understand others better, and it does not in my view, make you a better nurse. The danger with having a particular 'experience' is always that we can believe that other people's experiences may be the same: they may or may not be. It does occasionally, allow you to see things from two different perspectives: the health-care professionals' and the consumers'. And sometimes these are very different. I can still remember the sister in the psychiatric outpatient clinic who said: 'Oh you are a psychiatric nurse! Are they going to keep you on in your job?' At a time when I felt it difficult to carry on with very much at all, this was of little comfort. Recently, in asking me to recount my symptoms, a doctor asked me: 'Do you feel worthless?' I replied that, as a diagnostic question, I thought it was terrible.

(Burnard 2006: 245) **"**

Point for practice consideration
- The experience of living and overcoming depression is both complex and individual (Lilja *et al.* 2006).

Conclusion

This chapter has provided an overview of mood disorders. The chapter describes briefly what they are, possible causes, screening, assessment, diagnosis, common care and treatment approaches and some points for consideration for MHN practice. In the main these areas have been discussed in relation to the current NICE recommendations and the current context and strategic direction for MHN (2006). Within this context the nature, the art and science, and future of MNH will evolve.

In summary the main points from this chapter are:

- Depression and bipolar disorder are two umbrella terms describing a spectrum of mood experience.
- Mood disorders are multifaceted, complex phenomena. Medical diagnosis acts as a frame of reference and MHNs are adopting an integrated approach.
- The art and science of nursing: the core being of MHN lies in an enabling therapeutic alliance/relationship with people. However, care and treatments need to be delivered that are competency and evidence based.
- There are challenges for MHNs in particular care settings, in providing holistic, individualized person care.
- A more standardized and cohesive approach to effective care and treatments is being provided by NICE.
- There is a shift of focus from mental illness to mental wellness.
- The person's voice guides practice in offering person-centred care, preferences and choice.

Questions for reflection and discussion

1   Identify a recent loss. How did the experience affect you? How did you cope? How did you manage it?
2   Consider the treatment approaches that you observe in practice.

3   What do you think of the information provided to people about the service and treatment? Is choice offered?

4   Diet and exercise are important in maintaining physical and mental well-being. How do you observe this occurring in practice? What have you eaten over the last three days? How do you rate your general physical and mental health?

Annotated bibliography

- Koehn, C. and Cutcliffe, J. (2007) Hope and interpersonal psychiatric/mental health nursing: a systematic review of the literature – part one. *Journal of Psychiatric and Mental Health Nursing* **14**: 134–40 and Cutcliffe, J and Koehn, C. (2007) Hope and interpersonal psychiatric/mental health nursing: a systematic review of the literature – part two. *Journal of Psychiatric and Mental Health Nursing* **14**: 141–7. These two papers explore the concept of MHN hope inspiring in people with mental health problems.
- NICE www.nice.org.uk. Familiarize yourself with the website: mental health clinical guidelines, technology appraisals, and public health initiatives.
- Royal College of Psychiatry www.rcpsych.ac.uk. The mental health information pages of this website have a range of information leaflets, although aimed at the general public they are a useful resource.
- Moncrief, J. (2002) The antidepressant debate. *British Journal of Psychiatry* **180**: 193–4. An editorial feature that raises contrasting perspectives on the efficacy of antidepressants.

References

Altschul, A. (1972) *Patient-Nurse Interaction: a study of interactive patterns in acute psychiatric wards.* Edinburgh: Churchill Livingstone.

APA (1994) *Diagnostic and Statistical Manual for Mental Disorders*, 4th revision. Washington: American Psychiatric Association.

Attkisson, C. and Zwick, R. (1982) The client satisfaction questionnaire: Psychometric properties and correlations with service utilization and psychotherapy outcome. *Evaluation Program Planning* **5**: 233–7.

Baker, A. (2001) Bipolar disorders: an overview of current literature. *Journal of Psychiatric and Mental Health Nursing* **8**: 437–41.

Barker, P. (2004) *Assessment in Psychiatric and Mental Health Nursing: In Search of the Whole Person* (2nd edn). Cheltenham: Stanley Thornes Ltd.

Beech, B. (2000) The strengths and weaknesses of cognitive behavioural approaches to treating depression and their potential for wider utilisation by mental health nurses. *Journal of Psychiatric and Mental Health Nursing* **7**: 343–54.

Bech, P., Bowlig, T., Kramp, P. and Rafaelson, O. (1979) The Bech-Rafaelson Mania Scale and the Hamilton Depression Scale. *Acta Psychiatrica Scandinavica* **49**: 248–56.

Beck, A., Ward, C., Mendelson, M. *et al.* (1961) An inventory for measuring depression. *Archives of General Psychiatry* **4**: 561–71.

Beck, A., Steer, R., Beck, J. and Newman, C. (1993) Hopelessness, depression, suicidal ideation and clinical diagnosis of depression. *Suicide and Life-Threatening Behaviour*: **2**: 139–45.

Bhugra, D. and Mastrogianni, A. (2004) Globalisation and mental disorders. *British Journal of Psychiatry* **184**: 10–20.

Boardman, J., Henshaw, C. and Willmott, S. (2004) Needs for mental health treatment among general practice attenders. *British Journal of Psychiatry* **185**: 318–27.

Burnard, P. (2006) Sisyphus happy: the experience of depression. *Journal of Psychiatric and Mental Health Nursing* **13**: 242–6.

Corey, L. and Goodman, S. (eds) (2006) *Women and Depression.* USA: Cambridge University Press.

Cox, J., Holden, J. and Sagovsky, R. (1987) Detection of postnatal depression: development of the 10-item. Edinburgh Postnatal Depression Scale. *British Journal of Psychiatry* **150**: 782–876.

Craddock, N. and Jones. I. (2001) Molecular genetics of bipolar disorder. *British Journal of Psychiatry* **178** (suppl.41): s128–s133.

Crowe, M. (2002) Reflexivity and detachment: a discursive approach to women's depression. *Nursing Inquiry* **9**(2): 126–32.

Crowe, M. and Luty, S. (2005) Interpersonal psychotherapy: An effective psychotherapeutic intervention for mental health nursing practice. *International Journal of Mental Health Nursing* **14**: 126–33.

CSIP (2006) *Primary Care Services for Depression – A guide to best practice.* London: DH.

Cutcliffe, J. and Koehn, C. (2007) Hope and interpersonal psychiatric/mental health nursing: a systematic review of the literature – part two. *Journal of Psychiatric and Mental Health Nursing* **14**(2): 141–7.

Dennis, M., Wakefield, P., Molloy, C., Andrews, A. and Friedman, T. (2005) Self-harm in older people with depression. *British Journal of Psychiatry* **186**: 538–9.

Department of Health (2006a) *From Values to Action: The Chief Nursing Officer's Review of Mental Health Nursing.* London: DH.

Department of Health (2006b) *Reviewing the Care Programme Approach 2006: A consultation document.* London: DH.

Department of Health (2007) *Mental Health Ten Years on: progress on mental health care reform.* London: DH.

Department of Health (2008) Refocusing the Core Programme Approach. London: DH.

Feely, M. and Long, A. (2007) Naming of depression: nursing, social and personal descriptors. *Journal of Psychiatric and Mental Health Nursing* **14**: 21–31.

Feely, M., Sines, D. and Long, A. (2007) Early life experiences and their impact on our understanding of depression. *Journal of Psychiatric and Mental Health Nursing* **14**: 393–402.

Folstein, M., Folstein, S. and McHugh, P. (1975) Mini mental state examination: a practical method for grading the cognitive state of patients for the clinician. *Journal of Psychiatric Research* **12**: 189–98.

Gallop, R. and Reynolds, W. (2004) Putting it all together: dealing with complexity in the understanding of the human condition. *Journal of Psychiatric and Mental Health Nursing* **11**: 357–64.

Goldberg, D. and Williams, P. (1988) *A User's Guide to the General Health Questionnaire.* Windsor: NFER-Nelson.

Goldstein, B. and Rosselli, F. (2003) Etiological paradigms of depression: The relationship between perceived causes, empowerment, treatment, preferences and stigma. *Journal of Mental Health* **12**(6): 551–63.

Gray, R., Wykes, T., Parr, A-M. and Hails, E. (2001) The use of outcome measures to evaluate the efficacy and tolerability of antipsychotic medication: a comparison of Thorn graduate and CPN practice. *Journal of Psychiatric and Mental Health Nursing* **8**: 191–6.

Gunnell, D. and Lewis, G. (2005) Studying suicide from the life course perspective: implications for prevention. *British Journal of Psychiatry* **187**: 206–8.

Halter, M. (2004) Stigma and help seeking related to depression: a study of nursing students. *Journal of Psychosocial Nursing and Mental Health.* **42**(2): 42–53.

Hearst, C. (2007) Blasted into the present. *Openmind* **144**: 20–1.

Hedelin, B. and Jonsson, I. (2003) Mutuality as background music in women's lived experience of mental health and depression. *Journal of Psychiatric and Mental Health Nursing* **10**: 317–22.

Hickey, G. and Kipping, C. (1998) Exploring the concept of user involvement in mental health through a participation continuum. *Journal of Clinical Nursing* **7**: 83–8.

Kirmayer, L. (2006) Beyond the 'new cross-cultural psychiatry' cultural biology, discursive psychology and the ironies of globalization. *Transcultural Psychiatry* **43**(1): 126–44.

Koehn, C. and Cutcliffe, R. (2007) Hope and interpersonal psychiatric/mental health nursing: a systematic review of the literature – part one. *Journal of Psychiatric and Mental Health Nursing* **14**(2): 134–40.

Larzelere, M. (2002) Anxiety, depression and insomnia. *Primary Care* **2**: 339–60.

Lilja, L., Ordell, M., Dahl, A. and Hellzen, O. (2004) Judging the other: psychiatric nurses' attitudes towards inpatients as measured by the semantic differential technique. *Journal of Psychiatric and Mental Health Nursing* **11**: 546–53.

Lilja, L., Hellzen, M., Lind, I. and Hellzen, O. (2006) The meaning of depression: Swedish nurses' perceptions of depressed inpatients. *Journal of Psychiatric and Mental Health Nursing* **13**: 269–78.

Lukoff, D., Neuchterlein, K. and Ventura, J. (1986) Manual for the Expanded Brief Psychiatric Rating Scale (BPRS). *Schizophrenia Bulletin* **12**: 594–602.

Mantle, F. (2002) The role of alternative medicine in treating postnatal depression. *Complementary Therapies in Nursing and Midwifery* **8**(4): 197–203.

Mayall, E., Oathamshaw, S., Lovell, K. and Pusey, H. (2004) Development and piloting of a multidisciplinary training course for detecting and managing depression in the older person. *Journal of Psychiatric and Mental Health Nursing* **11**: 165–71.

McLaughlin, C. (1999) An exploration of psychiatric nurses' and patient care for suicidal patients. *Journal of Advanced Nursing* **29**(5): 1042–51.

Meadus, R. (2007) Adolescents coping with mood disorder: a grounded theory study. *Journal of Psychiatric and Mental Health Nursing* **14**: 209–17.

Mental Health Foundation (2006) *Feeding Minds.* London: Mental Health Foundation.

Millward, L., Lutte, A. and Purvis, R. (2005) Depression and the perpetuation of an incapacitated identity as an inhibitor of return to work. *Journal of Psychiatric and Mental Health Nursing* **12**: 565–73.

Mundt, J., Marks, I., Shear, M. and Greist, J. (2002) The work and social adjustment scale: a simple measure of impairment of functioning. *British Journal of Psychiatry* **180**: 461–4.

National Institute for Clinical Excellence (2003) *Technology Appraisal 59: Guidance on the use of electroconvulsive therapy.* Available from: www.nice.org.uk.

National Institute for Health and Clinical Excellence (2004a) *Clinical Guideline 23 Depression: management of depression in primary and secondary care.* Available from: www.nice.org.uk.

National Institute for Health and Clinical Excellence (2004b) *Clinical Guideline 16: Self harm: the short-term physical and psychological management and secondary prevention of self-harm in primary and secondary care.* Available from: www.nice.org.uk

National Institute for Health and Clinical Excellence (2005) *Clinical Guideline 28: Depression in children and young people.* Available from: www.nice.org.uk.

National Institute for Health and Clinical Excellence (2006a) *Clinical Guideline 38: Bipolar disorder: the management of bipolar disorder in adults, children and adolescents, in primary and secondary care.* Available from: www.nice.org.uk.

National Institute for Health and Clinical Excellence (2006b) *Technology Appraisal 97: Guidance on the use of computerised cognitive behavioural therapy for anxiety and depression. Review of technology appraisal 51.* Available from: www.nice.org.uk.

National Institute for Health and Clinical Excellence (2007) *Clinical guideline 45: Antenatal and postnatal mental health.* Available from: www.nice.org.uk.

NIMHE (2007) *National Suicide Prevention Strategy for England: Annual Report on Progress 2006.* Available from www.nimhe.csip.org.uk/our-work/suicide-prevention/annual-report-on-progress-2006.

Peplau, H. (1952) *Interpersonal Relations in Nursing.* London: Macmillan.

Piccinelli, M. and Wilkinson, G. (2000) Gender differences in depression. *British Journal of Psychiatry* **177**: 486–92.

Ramsey, R., Page, A., Goodman, T. and Hart, D. (2002) *Changing Minds: our lives our mental illness.* London: Gaskell.

Rowe, D. (2006) What should mental health nurses do? *Openmind* **141**: 15.

Royal College of Psychiatrists (2005) *The ECT Handbook* (2nd edn). London: Royal College of Psychiatrists.

Ruthen, P. (2006) Electroconvulsive therapy (ECT). The imposition of 'truth'? *SCRIPT-ed.* **3**(4): 12–36.

Scogin, F., Hanson, A. and Welsh, D. (2003) Self administered treatment in stepped-care models of depression treatment. *Journal of Clinical Psychology* **68**: 573–9.

Sheikh, J. and Yesavage, J. (1986) Geriatric Depression Scale (GDS). Recent evidence and development of a shorter version, in T.C. Brink (ed.) *Clinical Gerontology: A guide to Assessment and Intervention.* New York: Hayworth Press, pp. 165–73.

Shelton, R. (2006) Management of major depression following failure of first antidepressant treatment. *Primary Psychiatry* **13**(4): 73–82, 85–90.

Spitzer, R., Kroenke, K. and Williams, J. (1999) Validation and utility of a self-report version of PRIME-MD the PHQ Primary Care Study. *Journal of the American Medical Association* **282**: 1737–44.

Steer, R., Rissmiller, D. and Beck, A. (2000) Use of the Beck Depression Inventory-II with depressed geriatric patients. *Behaviour Research and Therapy* **38**(3): 311–18.

Stjernswärd, S. and Ostmän, M. (2006) Potential of e-health in relation to depression: short survey of previous research. *Journal of Psychiatric and Mental Health Nursing* **13**: 698–703.

Üstün, T., Ayuso-Mateos, J., Chatterji, S., Mathers, C. and Murray, C. (2004) Global burden of depressive disorders in the year 2000. *British Journal of Psychiatry* **184**: 386–92.

WHO (1992) *International Classification of Disease* (10th edn). Geneva: WHO.

WHO (2001) *The World Health Report. Mental Health: New Understanding, New Hope.* Geneva. WHO.

Wu, P. (2007) Use of complementary and alternative medicine among women with depression: results of a national survey. *Psychiatric Services* **58**(3): 349–56.

Zigmond, A. and Snaith, R. (1983) The Hospital Anxiety Depression Scale. *Acta Psychiatrica* **67**: 361–70.

CHAPTER 20

The person with an anxiety disorder

Phil Confue

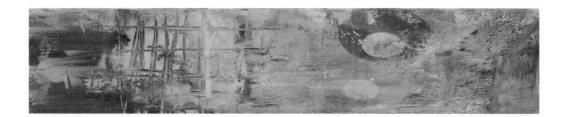

Chapter overview

Anxiety disorders are some of the most common mental disorders that occur. There is no longer any expectation that an individual with an anxiety disorder would be admitted to hospital purely as a result of anxiety, although many people who are admitted would have co-morbid anxiety symptoms. Within a four-tiered model of mental health services relating to the treatment of anxiety disorders, the majority of cases would be seen to fall within tiers one and two, around primary mental health care. 'Around 90 per cent of mental health care is dealt with in primary care. The most common mental health problems are depression, eating disorders and anxiety disorders' (DH 2001).

This chapter examines definitions of anxiety disorders and the service models for treatment response. There is a focus on the treatment interventions available for people with a common anxiety disorder such as phobias, panic disorder and generalized anxiety, along with background information on prevalence, definition and diagnosis, treatment effectiveness coupled with case studies. There is then a discussion of the main treatment models and self-help approaches.

The chapter has not been written as a guide to delivering cognitive behavioural therapy, some of which is provided elsewhere in this book, but rather to provide the reader with information to explore this disorder further and understand the context of treatment for people with an anxiety disorder. It draws on the anxiety disorder chapter from the first edition of this book, NICE guidance and evaluation work undertaken by Tribal Consulting to provide a baseline of information. This chapter will cover:

- Anxiety disorders;
- Phobias;
- Impact on lifestyle and social functioning;
- Assessment and treatment measures;
- Service models of intervention;
- Self-help and guided self-help.

Anxiety disorders

At a basic level fear is a universal human response to many difficult situations. The so-called 'fight or flight' response (Cannon 1929) is seen as a universal and fundamental response. The suggestion is that when placed in a situation perceived as an immediate danger the individual will either flee or remain to fight their corner. Later researchers have suggested that the response is more complex than this with a 'fight, flight, freeze or faint' response (Beck *et al.* 1988) and 'withdrawal, immobility, aggressive defence, or deflection of attack' (Marks 1987). These responses are seen as normal with the anxiety generated in a situation helping to drive a response, but where the response becomes inappropriate this may be the beginnings of an anxiety disorder. The main physiological systems involved in the anxiety response are the psychomotor system, autonomic nervous system and the neuroendocrine system (Marks 1987).

Historically most anxiety disorders have been seen as the responsibility of primary care with little to do with secondary care mental health services with their focus on severe and enduring mental illness. This ignores the fact that many people with a major psychotic illness also suffer from anxiety disorders which can be equally debilitating. The policy shift towards mental health and well-being means that these conditions that were often ignored by mental health services must now be considered and treated appropriately. The report by Lord Layard (Layard 2005) highlighted that anxiety disorders were a significant drain on the financial resources of England. This has led to an increased interest in the treatment of these disorders, culminating in the 'Improving Access to Psychological Therapies' programme (DH 2006).

Definition of anxiety and related concepts

It is important to separate out when fear or anxiety is useful and where it becomes a problem to the individual. It has been suggested that fear can be seen as a 'usually unpleasant response to realistic danger', where as anxiety is 'fear without an objective source of danger' (Marks 1987). There are a number of physiological, behavioural and cognitive symptoms associated with anxiety, these are outlined below:

Physiological symptoms

- *Cardiovascular*: palpitations, heart racing, increased blood pressure, faintness (and/or actual fainting);
- *Respiratory*: rapid breathing, shortness of breath, shallow breathing, lump in throat, choking sensation;
- *Neuromuscular*: Increased reflexes, muscle spasms, tremors, rigidity, fidgeting, wobbly legs;
- *Gastrointestinal*: abdominal discomfort, nausea, vomiting;
- *Urinary tract*: Pressure to urinate, frequency of urination;
- *Skin*: Face flushed or pale, localized and/or generalized sweating, itching, 'hot and cold spells'.

Behavioural symptoms

These include inhibition, tonic immobility, flight, avoidance, restlessness, impaired coordination, speech difficulties (for example, stammering) and hyperventilation.

Cognitive symptoms

- *Sensory-perceptual*: hazy, cloudy, foggy 'mind', feelings of unreality, hyper vigilance;
- *Thinking difficulties*: confusion, difficulty concentrating, distractibility, unable to control thinking;
- *Conceptual:* fear of losing control, fear of mental disorder, repetitive fearful ideation.

It should be noted that the symptoms of anxiety are not a product of modern society, they have existed and been identified throughout history (Berrios 1999).

Specific disorders

In December 2004 the then National Institute for Clinical Excellence (NICE) produced guidance on the treatment of people with an anxiety disorder (NICE 2004). They produced a clinical algorithm that split people into three different groups for treatment purposes. This algorithm is laid out in Figure 20.1 and it offers the best evidence-based approach to identifying the most appropriate diagnosis and thus treatment for an individual with an anxiety disorder.

Panic disorders

Panic disorders represent a significant disability for the person who experiences them. They differ from phobias and other anxiety-related conditions by merit of the fact that they can occur out of the blue, even when sleeping, making prediction of when an attack is likely to occur difficult. Ehlers (1993) suggests that panic disorders are brought about as a result of:

- greater physical reactivity;
- enhanced ability to perceive physiological sensations;
- increased attention.

Panic disorders are seen to be among the more common mental disorders, with a prevalence of approximately 1.5 per cent in a lifetime, this rate may be even higher in women. Panic disorder is seen as a marker of impaired quality of life (Markowitz *et al.* 1989), with it also being suggested that it can indicate an increased risk of suicidal ideation (Weissman *et al.* 1989) and thus an increased risk of self-harm and suicide. Much of the disorder is seen to relate to the cognitive perception of symptoms that an individual has and how these symptoms are interpreted, generally in a negative or catastrophizing way. Thus someone with an anxiety disorder who starts to experience palpitations will immediately assume that this is the indication of an imminent heart attack and seek treatment at a cardiac unit. Indeed in order to reduce pressure on cardiac services some have engaged mental health professionals to deal with those who repeatedly attend with panic disorders.

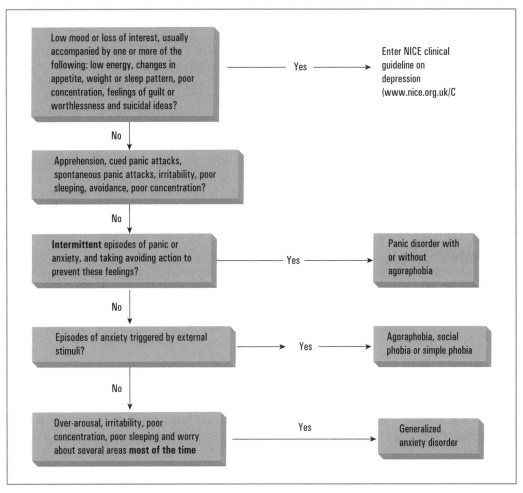

Figure 20.1 Anxiety classification

It has been identified that people with a panic disorder will look to use one of three different safety behaviours: avoidance, escape or subtle avoidance behaviour (Salkovskis *et al.* 1996).

Definition

The essential feature is recurrent attacks of severe anxiety (panic), which are not restricted to any particular situation or set of circumstances and are therefore unpredictable. As with other anxiety disorders, the dominant symptoms include sudden onset of palpitations, chest pain, choking sensations, dizziness and feelings of unreality (depersonalization or derealization). There is often also a secondary fear of dying, losing control or going mad. Panic disorder should not be given as the main diagnosis if the patient has a depressive disorder at the time the attacks start; in these circumstances the panic attacks are probably secondary to depression.

Case study: panic disorder

Bill was a man in his early thirties who was an accountant in a small building company. He had developed a history of panic attacks as a result of applying for a new job four years earlier. Prior to a presentation he was due to be making, as part of the interview process, he started to develop palpitations, dizziness, shortness of breath and sweating. He became convinced that he was suffering from a heart attack and did not participate in the interview but instead went to hospital. No physical causes were found to his symptoms and the hospital told him that he was having a panic attack. Since then he started to have more panic attacks when he engaged in new challenging situations, he began to avoid meeting new customers for the building company and being in situations where he had to talk to more than one person and made no further efforts to change his current job. He remains convinced that his symptoms represented the early warning signs of a heart attack, despite the evidence, and continuously monitors his pulse and blood pressure to spot the symptoms.

Treatment interventions

Benzodiazepine medication is associated with poor outcomes in the longer term and should not be prescribed for the treatment of individuals with panic disorder. Any of the following types of intervention should be offered and the preference of the person should be taken into account. The interventions that have evidence for the longest duration of effect, in descending order, are:

- psychological therapy (cognitive behavioural therapy (CBT));
- pharmacological therapy (a selective serotonin reuptake inhibitor (SSRI) licensed for panic disorder; or if an SSRI is unsuitable or there is no improvement, imipramine or clomipramine may be considered);
- self-help (bibliotherapy – the use of written material to help people understand their psychological problems and learn ways to overcome them by changing their behaviour – based on CBT principles).

Phobias

Fear of specific events or circumstances is a common feeling among the general population and can be a useful safety mechanism in the appropriate environment. Thus a fear of spiders in the UK can be seen as unreasonable in an environment where spiders are not poisonous; whereas the fear of spiders in a country with many poisonous spiders can be seen as a rational response. Even so it is when this fear becomes all-consuming and begins to interfere with aspects of a person's daily life that the issue becomes a phobia.

Definition (ICD-10)

A group of disorders in which anxiety is evoked only, or predominantly, in certain well-defined situations that are not currently dangerous. As a result these situations are characteristically avoided or endured with dread. The patient's concern may be focused on individual symptoms like palpitations or feeling faint and is often associated with secondary fears of dying, losing control or going mad. Contemplating entry to the phobic situation usually generates anticipatory anxiety. Phobic anxiety and depression often coexist. Whether two diagnoses, phobic anxiety and depressive episode, are needed, or only one, is determined by the time course of the two conditions and by therapeutic considerations at the time of consultation.

The main groupings in phobic anxieties are agoraphobia, social phobia, specific phobias (e.g. heights, dark). These are defined as:

- F40.0 (Agoraphobia) – A fairly well-defined cluster of phobias embracing fears of leaving home, entering shops, crowds and public places, or travelling alone in trains, buses or planes. Panic disorder is a frequent feature of both present and past episodes. Depressive and obsessional symptoms and social phobias are also commonly present as subsidiary features. Avoidance of the phobic situation is often prominent, and some agoraphobics experience little anxiety because they are able to avoid their phobic situations.
- F40.1 (Social phobia) – Fear of scrutiny by other people leading to avoidance of social situations. More pervasive social phobias are usually associated with low self-esteem and fear of criticism. They may present as a complaint of blushing, hand tremor, nausea or urgency of micturition, the patient sometimes being convinced that one of these secondary manifestations of their anxiety is the primary problem. Symptoms may progress to panic attacks.
- F40.2 (Specific (isolate) phobia) – Phobias restricted to highly specific situations such as proximity to particular animals, heights, thunder, darkness, flying, closed spaces, urinating or defecating in public toilets, eating certain foods, dentistry, or the sight of blood or injury. Though the triggering situation is discrete, contact with it can evoke panic as in agoraphobia or social phobia.

Case study: agoraphobia

Mary lived on a housing estate with her two children aged 5 and 8. She had recently been divorced by her husband who was in the Navy and had often been away for long periods of time. After her divorce she became increasingly reluctant to go outside so the children walked to the nearby school on their own and friends and family brought in shopping for her. If she left her house she would feel dizzy and suffer palpitations thinking she was going to have a heart attack. After a programme of graded exposure coupled with relaxation techniques Mary moved to a point where she was able to go to the local shops on her own and collect the children from school, finally achieving her goal of going to a local nightclub with friends one evening.

Case study: social phobia

Clair had always been a shy girl when at school, and had become pregnant at 18; she kept the child and remained living at home with her parents. While attending a playgroup meeting she knocked over a large jug of milk and she became aware that everyone was watching her. She then began to believe that the other mothers were laughing at her behind her back. As a consequence she stopped attending the playgroup and other mother and toddler events slowly isolating herself from other people. Clair continued to believe that if she met other people they would just laugh at her so she began to avoid all social situations. Clair did not engage in any social situation and her circumstances remained the same until her son reached the age of 5 when she was forced to confront her issues in order for her son to enrol in school.

Treatment interventions

A review of treatment interventions for specific phobias (Roth *et al.* 2005) identified that the main treatment approach that should be employed is that of exposure. While there are arguments that there is benefit from delivering this exposure with cognitive interventions, exposure remains the key element. The NHS Centre for Reviews and Dissemination (2002) published a critical assessment of treatments for social phobia which found that exposure and cognitive behavioural treatments resulted in 'significant and meaningful reductions in anxiety'. Furthermore, the review noted that the 'combination of psychological and pharmacological treatments was disappointing and did not exceed the effects of psychological treatments alone'.

Generalized anxiety disorders

Generalized anxiety disorder is a debilitating condition that leads to an individual feeling anxious and worried most of the time with little real ability to control their anxiety. While everyone may worry about their family, job and health, people with generalized anxiety disorder have unrealistic fears and worries. This can lead to people having a constant feeling of an impending disaster due to concerns that are out of proportion to the actual events. It occurs 'as a chain of thoughts, which have a negative affect component. It is concerned with future events where there is uncertainty over outcome' (Wells and Butler 1997).

Definition ICD-10

Anxiety that is generalized and persistent but not restricted to, or even strongly predominating in, any particular environmental circumstances (i.e. it is 'free-floating'). The dominant symptoms are variable but include complaints of persistent nervousness, trembling, muscular tensions, sweating, light headedness, palpitations, dizziness and epigastric discomfort. Fears that the patient or a relative will shortly become ill or have an accident are often expressed.

Case study: generalized anxiety disorder

Andrew was a 49-year-old tradesman who reported feeling worked up, tense and worried for most of his waking day. He had difficulty sleeping, particularly getting to sleep. His chief complaint was that he was unable to stop worrying about 'stupid little things' that, he considered, most people would take in their stride. Examples of current worries were his ability to do his job properly, where he should go on holiday, and whom he should invite to his 50th birthday party. He reported thinking things over and over in his head to try and plan and prepare but he always found that he could not stop the process once started. In addition he reported feeling low and sad at the impact his inability to stop worrying had had on his and his family's life. When he noticed these emotions he would try to think of ways of making things up to them, by attempting to plan special events or outings, but found that he was never able to settle on a suitable solution. Although his predominant emotion was anxiety he did experience episodes of irritability and annoyance with himself. His characteristic thinking process was reported as consisting of many 'What ifs', for example, 'What if I don't get this job done on time?', 'What if they (my family) don't like what I've done for them?' More detailed examination of his thinking suggested that he was particularly concerned that he would get things wrong, that he would not cope, or that he would never be able to switch his thoughts off.

Treatment interventions

Benzodiazepine medication should not usually be used beyond two to four weeks. For the longer-term care of individuals with generalized anxiety disorder, any of the following types of intervention should be offered and the preference of the person with generalized anxiety disorder should be taken into account. The interventions that have evidence for the longest duration of effect, in descending order, are

- psychological therapy (CBT);
- pharmacological therapy (an SSRI);
- self-help (bibliotherapy based on CBT principles).

Impact

The NSF for Mental Health states:

> Panic attacks, phobias, or persistent generalized anxiety can impede a person's ability to work, form relationships, raise children, and participate fully in life. GPs often see anxiety, mixed anxiety and depressive disorders, which may be associated with high levels of disability. People who have anxiety symptoms usually smoke more, and may drink more alcohol too, increasing their risk of physical ill health.
>
> (DH 2004: 30)

Assessment and treatment approaches

Treatment protocols have been laid out by the National Institute for Health and Clinical Excellence and the algorithm has been described earlier in this chapter. In essence, the evidence falls on the side of either a pharmaceutical-based solution or the use of cognitive behaviour therapy or a combination of both. With an increased growth in demand driven by a consumerist view of the NHS in England, there has been a steady increase in the demand of people for approaches such as cognitive behaviour therapy and other 'talking therapies'.

There are a number of different standardized assessment tools for anxiety disorder. One of the most commonly used and easiest to administer is Beck's Anxiety Inventory (Beck *et al.* 1988), which relies on a systematic rating scale of symptomology by the practitioners and the individual. This approach helps to assess the current level of anxiety but can also be used at a latter point in time to identify if the feelings of anxiety have increased or decreased as a result of interventions. Beck's Anxiety Inventory is effectively a self-reporting 21-point rating scale, reasonably easy to use and administer. There is also a Beck's Depression Scale (Beck 1961; Beck *et al.* 1988) using a similar approach to the Anxiety scale. Connecting for Health, the national programme for IT in the NHS, is developing a uniform IT system and computerized recording system in England. Within this system there are expected to be a number of standardized measuring tools to be used, but at this point in time it is not known which tools they will include.

Table 20.1 identifies a number of specific scales and some self-help resources.

Disorder	Specific measures	Self-help resources
All phobias	The fear questionnaire (Marks and Mathews 1979)	www.triumphoverphobia.com www.phobics-society.org.uk www.no-panic.co.uk
Agoraphobia	The mobility inventory for agoraphobia (Chambless *et al.* 1985) The agoraphobic cognitions questionnaire (Chambless *et al.* 1984)	www.triumphoverphobia.com www.phobics-society.org.uk www.no-panic.co.uk
Social phobia	Fear of negative evaluation scale (Watson and Friend 1969) Social phobia and anxiety inventory (Beidel *et al.* 1995) Social interaction anxiety scale and social phobia scale (Brown *et al.* 1997)	www.triumphoverphobia.com www.phobics-society.org.uk www.no.panic.co.uk
Specific phobias	Dental fear survey (McGlynn *et al.* 1987) Spider phobia beliefs questionnaire (Arntz *et al.* 1993)	www.needlephobia.co.uk (needle) www.beyondfear.org (dental)
Obsessive compulsive disorder	Yale-Brown obsessive compulsive scale (McKay *et al.* 1995) Maudsley obsessional-compulsive inventory (Hodgson and Rachman 1977) The Padua Inventory (Sanavio 1988)	www.obsessive-action.demon.co.uk www.ocfoundation.org www.no-panic.co.uk
Post-traumatic stress disorder	The clinician-administered PTSD scale (CAPS 2) (Blake *et al.* 1995) Impact of event scale (IES) (Horowitz *et al.* 1979) PTSD diagnostic scale (PDS) (Foa *et al.* 1997)	www.ncptsd.org/index.html
Panic disorder	The fear questionnaire (Marks and Mathews 1979)	http://mentalhelp.net www.cyberpsych.org/anxieties www.panicdisorder.about.com www.no-panic.co.uk

Disorder	Specific measures	Self-help resources
	The automatic thoughts questionnaire (Wells 1997)	
Health anxiety	Symptom interpretation questionnaire (Robbins and Kirmayer 1991)	http://healthanxiety.com
	The illness attitude scale (IAS) (Kellner 1987)	
Generalized anxiety disorder	Penn State worry questionnaire, the worry and anxiety questionnaire (Meyer *et al.* 1990)	http://mentalhelp.net www.cyberpsych.org/anxieties www.no-panic.co.uk
Body dysmorphic disorder	The Body Dysmorphic Disorder Examination (BDDE) (Rosen *et al.* 1995) Modified Yale-Brown obsessive compulsive scale (YBOCS) for BDD (Hollander *et al.* 1994)	www.worldcollegehealth.org/031199.htm http://mentalhelp.net

Table 20.1 Specific measures used for disorders and Internet self-help resources

Auditing interventions

In delivering treatment for any mental health problem it is important that there is a clear audit process undertaken to support the delivery of the most appropriate regime. NICE in their guidance on anxiety disorders has identified an audit protocol that ensures that interventions are being delivered effectively and in line with best practice. This audit protocol is laid out below. It identifies 15 key questions to ask about the provision of services to people with an anxiety disorder and in a time when evidence-based health care is a required standard this is an audit that services should be undertaking.

1. The patient shares decision-making with the health care professionals during the process of diagnosis and in all phases of care.
2. The patient and, when appropriate, his or her family and carer(s) are offered appropriate information on the nature, course and treatment of panic disorder or generalized anxiety disorder, including information on the use and likely side-effect profile of medication.
3. The patient and his or her family and carer(s) are informed of self-help groups and support groups and are encouraged to participate in programmes.
4. All patients prescribed antidepressants are informed that, although the drugs are not associated with tolerance and craving, discontinuation/withdrawal symptoms may occur on stopping or missing doses or, occasionally, on reducing the dose of the drug. These symptoms are usually mild and self-limiting but occasionally can be severe, particularly if the drug is stopped abruptly.
5. Necessary relevant information is elicited from the diagnostic process.

6. The treatment of choice is available promptly.
7. Individuals with panic disorder are not prescribed benzodiazepines.

A patient with panic disorder is offered any of the following types of intervention, and the person's preference is taken into account:

■ Psychological therapy;
■ Pharmacological therapy;
■ Self-help.

A patient with generalized anxiety disorder is not prescribed benzodiazepines for longer than two to four weeks.

A patient with longer-term generalized anxiety disorder is offered any of the following types of intervention, and the person's preference is taken into account:

■ Psychological therapy;
■ Pharmacological therapy;
■ Self-help.

■ A patient is reassessed if one type of intervention does not work, and consideration is given to trying one of the other types of intervention.
■ A patient who still has significant symptoms after two interventions is offered referral to specialist.
■ A thorough, holistic reassessment of the individual, his or her environment and social circumstances is conducted by specialist mental health services.
■ Outcomes are monitored using short, self-complete questionnaires.
■ A short self-complete questionnaire such as the panic subscale of the agoraphobic mobility inventory for individuals with panic disorder.

Practitioners should consider using this audit regularly in their work with people who experience anxiety disorders in order to help them reflect on their own clinical practice.

Service models

The recent developments of the 'Improving Access to Psychological Therapies' programme (Newham Primary Care Trust and East London and the City Mental Health NHS Trust 2006) means that CBT is likely to be the treatment of choice for people with anxiety disorders. There are, however, different models of service delivery for CBT that people will access. In understanding how treatment is delivered it is important to understand the impact of the different models. The delivery of CBT and other psychological therapies is seen to be through three specific models of service delivery:

■ a traditional outpatient model;
■ a stepped care model identified in improving access to psychological therapies (DH 2006);
■ psychological treatment centres as described by Layard (2006).

Traditional outpatient referral models

This approach is organized and delivered around a secondary care model. The majority of professionals providing cognitive behavioural therapy (CBT) are located within a specialist secondary care setting which forms the 'hub'. Under some forms of delivery however, such as shifted outpatients, CBT interventions may be delivered within primary care. The interface with primary care is facilitated through arrangements such as community mental health teams, primary care liaison teams or gateway workers.

Specialists in the secondary care setting (hub) receive referrals from primary care. Such referrals are often only made when a service user presents with a common mental health problem of moderate to severe intensity, mental illness and/or presenting with risk. Service users with less severe difficulties may be offered a range of interventions provided within primary care, placed on waiting lists or receive no treatment.

Since implementation of the Primary Care Graduate Mental Health Worker, a range of interventions such as self-help have become available within primary care. The extent to which these interventions have been interfaced with those available in secondary care is highly variable.

CBT is mainly provided within a 45–60 minute face-to-face weekly session format, with 8–20 sessions being initially scheduled for service users presenting with a range of common mental health problems, often of severe intensity. There is little evidence to ascertain whether this is the optimum session length and number to maximize efficiency.

CBT is provided by a range of qualified mental health (mental health nurses, clinical psychologists, psychiatrists) and allied health (occupational therapist, physiotherapist) professionals, although mental health nurses often prominently feature. The majority will have received training of at least one year in CBT which enables them to implement a range of CBT techniques within a more complex clinical approach.

Stepped care models

The stepped care model is a framework for using limited resources to their greatest effect. Interventions and professional care are 'stepped up' in intensity alongside the risks and complexities presented by the service user.

Low risk service users receive a range of low-intensity, high-volume interventions. If the service user is 'stepped up', i.e. fails to reach an acceptable outcome, the therapist input, level of clinical experience and intervention intensity increases.

Service users receive an individualized service according to their preferences and progress (service users are systematically monitored) and are assigned a health or mental health professional upon entry to the service.

These stepped care models are often combined with a collaborative approach to care, including elements of managed care. This is to ensure effective monitoring and facilitate effective and efficient links between mental health staff located within primary and specialist care.

Two large randomized trials evaluating stepped care models both showed improved outcomes in clinical response over six months (Katon *et al.* 1999; Hendrick *et al.* 2003).

Improving access to psychological therapies (IAPT)

The improving access to psychological therapies programme is a Department of Health initiative to examine the extent to which increasing access to psychological therapy (mostly CBT):

- improves well-being;
- reduces worklessness and the number of people claiming incapacity benefit;
- provides greater choices in treatment and care options for people with a range of mental health conditions.

The initial focus of the service is only on service users of working age with a special consideration upon those who claim incapacity benefits. There are two demonstration sites established in Doncaster and Newham, both of which adopt different stepped care approaches.

The Doncaster IAPT approach is organized according to a 'hub and spoke' model. Hub acts as a resource centre and administrative base for the service. The hub is located within the Doncaster Chamber of Commerce, making the service, in all but the higher more specialist steps, operate outside of a health setting. All referrals are channelled into the hub which is staffed by case managers who are available to speak to referrers and make quick contact, usually with one week, with service users. The hub operates on an extended hours basis.

Referrals are accepted from any member of primary care, specialist mental health, other associated service partners such as Job Centre Plus, occupational health departments, NHS Direct, and it also supports self-referral. An initial assessment then directs the service user towards the most appropriate step. A full specialist psychological assessment is undertaken only within higher steps.

The service provides a range of highly structured and progressive interventions, ranging from low-intensity, high-volume to high intensity, specialist face-to-face individual therapy (see Figure 20.2). There is significant focus upon the development of the community sector to support the low-intensity, high-volume interventions. Individuals from the community sector receive training from professionals within the IAPT initiative.

This model utilizes a diverse mix of appropriately trained personnel, varying in terms of skill level and competencies, from community-based individuals (including occupational health specialists), to 'case managers' (otherwise known as graduate mental health workers), to specialists in CBT.

Psychological treatment centre

The Newham model is informed by the Psychological Treatment Centre approach proposed under Layard (2004, 2005). Psychological treatment centres are based upon the proposition that savings made by providing psychological interventions will be paid for through increased economic output and reduced costs in terms of incapacity benefit. The Newham IAPT model operates along the lines of several proposals advanced by Layard.

It is also a hub and spoke model, like Doncaster, with specialist therapists based within one building, the Psychological Treatment Centre, which forms the hub. The majority of

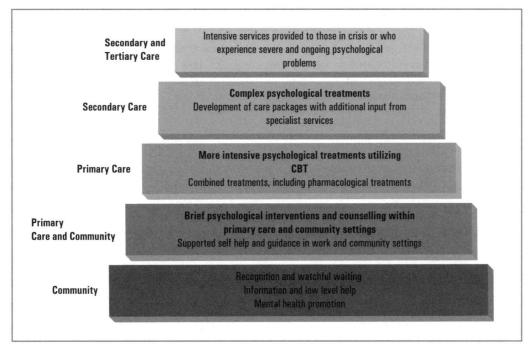

Figure 20.2 Range of interventions provided at different steps and within different settings within Doncaster IAPT model

therapy is delivered through low-intensity, high-volume interventions delivered in GPs' practices, job centres and other community locations (similar to Figure 10.2).

Referrals are made to the Psychological Treatment Centre by range of health professionals and include self referral. Full assessments made by senior specialist therapists form a central part of the service delivery and service users are directed towards the most appropriate step within the model on the basis of the assessment.

This model has shown that the workforce will need to have moderate to high levels of experience, with initial proposals suggesting a clinical psychologist-led service. The model has identified the need for an additional 10,000 professionals across the country, of which it is expected that 5000 will be clinical psychologists and another 5000 psychological therapists (nurses, occupational therapists, social workers and counsellors). This workforce would be given 'rigorous' training in (mostly) CBT, resulting in a one-year qualification in CBT for mild to moderate common mental health problems and a two-year qualification for a wider range of more complex difficulties. The hub within the psychological treatment centre will be responsible for ensuring that all staff receive effective training and supervision ensuring a continued growth in the workforce.

It is anticipated that these sites will help clarify the number of staff, the skills set and the training requirements needed to improve access to psychological therapies. The evidence from these demonstration sites is also supplemented by a national network of smaller, local IAPT projects and 20 national primary care mental health collaborative sites. These projects are being managed by the Care Services Improvement Partnership.

Comparison of approaches

The Doncaster IAPT and Newham Psychological Treatment Centre models along with the traditional outpatient referral model for delivering CBT have been rated using the information identified above and the criteria set out by Parry (1992) to evaluate mental health service delivery models (Table 20.2).

	Stepped Care (Doncaster IAPT)	Stepped Care (Newham – Psychological Treatment Centre)	Traditional Outpatient Referral
Acceptability (Service User)	Maybe	Maybe	Unlikely
Acceptability (Service Provider)	Maybe	Likely	Likely
Accessibility	Likely	Maybe	Unlikely
Equity	Likely	Maybe	Unlikely
Effectiveness	Maybe	Maybe	Likely
Efficiency	Maybe	Maybe	Unlikely

Table 20.2 Evaluation of three CBT service delivery models

The criteria employed by Parry (1992) are described below along with a rationale for the rating of each service model in Table 20.2.

Acceptability (service user): 'Extent to which the service delivery model is acceptable to service users and service providers alike. The predominant factor related to client acceptability towards a service is related to the extent to which the service is accessible.'

- Traditional: Service users generally positive towards specialist, intensive (face-to-face) forms of interventions. However, restricted access minimizes acceptability.
- Psychological Treatment Centre and Doncaster: Acceptability towards specialist, intensive forms of interventions, cannot imply that service users will find the range of low-intensity, high-volume interventions equally acceptable. Evidence specifically addressing acceptability towards such interventions is limited in number and quality. However, several studies highlight that some service users may find such interventions less acceptable, with higher drop out rates from services being reported.

Acceptability (service provider): 'The acceptability criteria can also be applied to assess the perspective of service providers.'

- Traditional: Generally seen as acceptable by many professionals with a background in secondary mental health services. Seen as providing effective, evidence-based interventions within a structure believed to manage risk. Obvious frustrations surrounding access.
- Psychological Treatment Centre: Proposals highlight a large expansion in specialist provision with organization maintaining a specialist (secondary care) focus. Satisfaction with the maintenance of risk management via full and specialist risk assessments.

Potentially some reservations surrounding effectiveness of low-intensity, high-volume interventions and effect that failure to improve following these interventions will have upon service users needing to step up.

- Doncaster: The lack of specialist, in favour of a brief assessment, undertaken by paraprofessionals may challenge many professionals with a specialist background. Reservations concerning low-intensity, high-volume interventions as above.

Accessibility: 'The ease and extent to which service users can gain timely access to appropriate and effective psychological interventions is the highest priority for service users.'

- Traditional: Focus upon specialist and intensive interventions would require an unrealistic expansion in professionals to provide services.
- Psychological Treatment Centre: Requirement for specialist and full assessment of service users prior to entering service may create bottlenecks and hence restrict access due to excessive demand upon number a limited number professionals undertaking assessments.
- Doncaster: Lack of initial specialist full assessment, combined with large expansion in low-intensity, high-volume interventions based both within the community and primary care settings likely to be able to meet demand.

Equity: 'Extent to which services are equally suited to users varying across a range of social, cultural or economic factors.'

- Traditional: Limited number and nature of specialist interventions unlikely to be equally suited to groups varying in social, cultural and economic factors. Requirement for referral into service prevents those not registered with GP (over-represented among Black, Minority Ethnic (BME) populations) from access. Predominant locating of services in health settings may be seen as stigmatizing.
- Psychological Treatment Centre: Referral from range of professionals, other organizations and self referral will likely enhance equity as long as access can be maintained. Issues concerning stigma remain if service maintains a secondary care focus and appearance.
- Doncaster: GP referral not required, with range of referral pathways, including self referral, supported. Large development of community-based interventions enables and empowers greater variability in service development and reduces stigma at lower levels of intervention.

Effectiveness: 'Extent to which interventions are effective in bringing about clinically reliable improvement in mental health state of service users or improve quality of life.'

- Traditional: Extensive and growing evidence base highlighting effectiveness of specialist CBT interventions.
- Psychological Treatment Centre and Doncaster: Extensive evidence base for specialist CBT interventions. Evidence base examining effectiveness of low-intensity, high-volume intervention currently limited in number and sometimes of lower methodological quality, although number and quality of studies increasing quickly. Available evidence highlights equivalence in effectiveness between simpler v. complex, brief v. intensive and face-to-face versus other (e.g. telephone) forms of delivery. Given the evidence, it is likely that the range of interventions provided in stepped care models will be effective.

Efficiency: 'Degree of input required by service to bring about clinically reliable improvement in service users. Measures such as service throughput, therapist input, use of additional services, and improvement in mental health derive an economic evaluation.'

- Traditional: Levels of effectiveness likely to make a positive contribution to efficiency, however limited clinic throughput and high therapist input likely to have adverse influence.
- Psychological Treatment Centre: Assuming good levels of effectiveness with low-intensity interventions, associated with less therapist input and high clinic throughput may result in good levels of efficiency. However this will be negatively affected by the requirement for specialist full assessment, and hence more experienced, and expensive workforce. Possibility that service users undertaking low-intensity interventions will engage an increasing number of additional services.
- Doncaster: Lack of specialist assessment will enhance efficiency, assuming interventions effective. Potential for higher rates of drop out and increased used of additional services may have a negative impact.

It is likely that the Doncaster approach to delivering services for people with anxiety will become the dominant model, although others may remain. This will be driven by delivering a model that can provide easy and rapid access combined with a relatively cost efficient model.

Treatment approaches

Principles and practice of exposure

Exposure involves the individual having to face the issue or situation that is causing them anxiety. There are a number of different approaches or methods of exposure, but these can be divided into two main groups, one where the exposure is carried out in the real life situation, and the other where it is carried out via simulation of some form. Simulation is most often used where access to the real situation is not easily obtainable, i.e. in the case of anxiety provoked by flying. The approaches involved can be:

- Flooding, the process where an individual is exposed to the most anxiety provoking stimulus. Much of this is built on a view that the fight/flight reaction cannot be held for long and that by flooding the anxiety will decrease.
- Implosion, where the principle of flooding is applied except that the individual is asked to imagine themselves in this most anxiety provoking situation.

Introceptive exposure is used where the anxiety relates to internal physical causes

- Systematic desensitization, this is a specific intervention that works to reduce the feelings of anxiety over a period of treatment or intervention. Developed by Wolpe (1958, 1990) it is based on the theory of 'reciprocal inhibition' in that you cannot be both anxious and relaxed.
- Modelling, this approach involves the therapist exposing themselves to the individual's anxiety stimulus to model the appropriate response.

The purpose of exposure techniques is to remove or reduce the level of anxiety that an individual suffers. It works to educate or train the individual to develop an alternative and more acceptable response to the anxiety provoking situation or stimulus. The term habituation is used by social scientists to describe the therapy goal, a decrease in stimulation under normal circumstances, excluding response decrements due to injury, drugs or other abnormal conditions. Alternatively, the term extinction is applied, meaning a reduction of previously learnt behaviours. Thus the goal of the exposure programme is to condition a more appropriate response. Much of this stems from the work of Pavlov in the 1920s (Pavlov 1927), but this classical conditioning approach has been refined and developed over the years. Most recently it has been reformulated through the theory of 'emotional processing' (Foa and Kozak 1986), where it is suggested that exposure-based treatments have an effect due to modification of internal fear structure, in which cognitive, affective and behavioural information about feared stimulus is contained.

In delivering an exposure programme there is a difference in the effectiveness and speed of response. To be exposed to the real/live situation is always more effective than having to use a guided fantasy approach. A longer period of exposure to the stimulus is always more effective than a short exposure. Self-directed exposure by the individual is as effective as the exposure guided by a therapist, although there are benefits to the presence of a therapist. It is suggested that exposure sessions should be in the region of 50 minutes although this may vary based on individual needs and responses. It should also be noted that flooding will yield better responses than a graded exposure, but the process should proceed at the rate acceptable to the individual not that of the therapist. The use of an anxiety diary helps both the individual and the therapist assess the success or not of the interventions, an anxiety diary should record the level of anxiety prior to the session, half way through and at the end of the session.

In conducting a session it is important that the individual fully understands the process and what the mental health practitioner is hoping to achieve. The explanation needs to be in a format that is easily understandable to the individual, thus explanations such as 'like driving a car, the more that you drive a car the easier it becomes' as an analogy to dealing with the anxiety provoking stimulus/situation. It is then important to identify what are the anxiety causing stimuli/situations and also what are the avoidance techniques deployed by the individual. These should be ranked in order to identify the intervention programme; this should really be a maximum of ten. Initially the aim should be to have a session working with one of the events that has been identified as moderate anxiety and then through a session be able to reduce this anxiety by 50 per cent based on the diary scores. It would be hoped that this early win would encourage the individual to persevere with the approach. Once the pattern of recording the anxiety and therapist lead sessions have been established it then becomes important to establish a programme of homework where the individual undertakes exposure activity between sessions and records the impact in their diary, thus moving to a more self-directed approach. It should be remembered throughout this process that the role of the mental health practitioner is to support and help the individual through the process, but it is for the individual with anxiety to work through all the stages.

Principles of cognitive behaviour therapy

Cognitive behaviour therapy (CBT) could be defined as a system of psychotherapy based on the premise that distorted or dysfunctional thinking, which influences a person's mood or behaviour, is common to all psychosocial problems. The focus of therapy is to identify the distorted thinking and to replace it with more rational, adaptive thoughts and beliefs.

For most mental health practitioners CBT can be seen as a short intervention over 10–12 sessions which involves:

- working with a structure to help the person understand the problems and challenges facing them, identifying the extreme and unhelpful thoughts and altered behaviour that keeps the problem of anxiety ongoing;
- working with problems on a step-by-step approach;
- working in a collaborative way supported by the practitioners;
- encouraging the individual to put into practice what they have learned (Williams 2004).

The approach seeks to encourage the individual to review their own cognitive processes by effecting how they appraise situations and how they then process that information. As an example an individual may have a selective, heightened attention to threat cues which will lead to an appraisal of greater risk than actually exists. In CBT the initial assessment would attempt to identify the automatic thoughts that lead to the incorrect appraisal and by the use of assessment diaries encourage the individual to assess and over time modify their own behaviour and responses.

Self-help

Given the shortage of qualified cognitive behavioural therapists there has been a move towards self-help and guided self-help approaches as interventions. The two main approaches are by structured self-help booklets and by computerized CBT (CCBT) interventions.

There has been a growth in the use of this approach with CCBT now being encouraged by NICE (2006). These approaches are seen as working well for people with mild to moderate conditions. The approach also fits with the main principles behind CBT in that it is for the individual themselves to do the work with the therapist only supporting that process.

The advent of both graduate primary care mental health workers and the development of the IAPT programmes, with their inclusion of low intensity interventions, have lead to greater interest in this area. These developments have significantly increased the number of people who can access these interventions.

Conclusion

This chapter has highlighted a policy shift toward mental health and well-being that requires anxiety disorders, which were often ignored by mental health services, to be considered and treated appropriately. An overview of those disorders has been provided with a specific focus on panic, phobias and generalized anxiety. The evidence base for specific interventions has been reviewed and contemporary service models have been presented and appraised. The increased development of stepped care in delivering services for the treatment of anxiety disorders will lead to a greater input by all professional groups and an increase in the use of cognitive behaviour therapy.

In summary the main points are:

- Anxiety is a normal human response to stressful stimuli. If the response is inappropriate to the risk posed by a stimulus then this may be indicative of an anxiety disorder.
- Although often seen as 'non-severe' anxiety disorders can be extremely disabling and have significant effects on a person's life and relationships.

■ Anxiety symptoms affect physiology, behaviour and cognitions and people can be grouped into different types of anxiety disorder according to their symptoms, each with their own treatment implications.

■ There has been an increasing recognition of the value of talking therapies as an intervention for anxiety disorders and a corresponding reluctance to rely on anxiolytic medications.

■ Stepped care programmes provide an important framework for service delivery and match interventions to service user levels of need.

Acknowledgements

Thanks in developing this chapter go to Paul Rogers, Joe Curran and Kevin Gourney who authored the original chapter in the first edition, Paul Farrand senior lecturer at the University of Plymouth and Emma Gibbard at Tribal Consulting.

Questions for reflection and discussion

Following the treatment efficacy evidence for CBT that has been offered in this chapter, consider the last five patients that you have seen with an anxiety disorder and ask yourself:

1   Did they have access to CBT?
2   What local services are on offer and do they provide good access?
3   What could be done to improve CBT access in your clinical area for this often neglected population?
4   Consider the anxiety measures that have been highlighted. Do you routinely use these measures in your practice? If not, then could you improve your measurement and assessment of anxiety disorders in your practice and in the practice of others?
5   Consider the skills required within the core components of exposure and CBT. Do you have these skills as core components of your nursing knowledge and experience? If so, what relevance do they have for your current working practices and what areas of learning can you identify for further professional development?
6   Considering the audit of services for people with anxiety disorder. Is this audit being undertaken in your area or can you consider undertaking this audit?

Annotated bibliography

■ Marks, I.M. (1987) *Fears, Phobias and Rituals: Panic, Anxiety and their Disorders.* Oxford: Oxford University Press. A classic text, which although in need of update in regards to the analyses of the clinical trials that are reviewed, still contains arguably the best psychopathological review of the field. Professor Marks was one of the main researchers/clinicians who was responsible for exposure therapy as it is practised today and a great supporter of nurse-led therapy.

■ Wells, A. (1997) *Cognitive Therapy of Anxiety Disorders: A Procedural Manual and Conceptual Guide*. Chichester, West Sussex: Wiley. An excellent, pragmatic text which provides an invaluable theoretical and clinical review. Wells provides a number of questionnaires and measures which readers are free to use. Predominantly CBT in focus, and includes exceptional chapters on interventions for panic and worry which are hard to find.

■ Rachman, S. (2004) *Anxiety* (2nd edn). Hove: Psychology Press. Written by a leading researcher and clinician in the field of anxiety disorders this book provides a detailed, yet concise, account of the nature of anxiety, the main theoretical approaches and the clinical presentations seen in practice. The book is thoroughly referenced throughout, summarizing the research to date. Specific attention is given to panic and anxiety, agoraphobia, obsessions and compulsion, social anxiety and generalized anxiety disorder. The book is relatively easy to read and is likely to be useful to student mental health practitioners.

■ Leahy, R.L. and Holland, S.J. (2000) *Treatment Plans and Interventions for Depression and Anxiety Disorders*. New York: Guilford Press. As the title suggests this book's main emphasis is on treatment, although each chapter contains descriptive and diagnostic information for all of the disorders covered. The book is rich in practical detail and advice, including flow-charts to aid diagnosis, session-by-session treatment options to the 'Information for Patients' handouts. All forms and supplementary information, which are contained on an accompanying CD-ROM, can be printed by purchasers for their, and their clients', use. The treatment approaches are specifically cognitive behavioural and written for practising clinicians. Being American, occasional reference is made to the 'managed care' system, although this does not affect the relevance of the text to the practising (or soon to be practising) UK mental health practitioner.

References

Arntz, A., Lavy, E., van den Berg, G. and van Rijsoort, S. (1993) Negative beliefs of spider phobics: A psychometric evaluation of the Spider Phobic Beliefs Questionnaire. *Advances in Behaviour Research and Theory* **15**: 257–77.

Beck, A.T. (1961). An inventory of measuring depression. *Archives of General Psychiatry* **4**: 561–71.

Beck, A.T., Epstein, N., Brown, G. and Steer, R.A. (1988) An inventory for measuring clinical anxiety: psychometric properties. *Journal of Consulting and Clinical Psychology* **56**: 893–7.

Beidel, D., Turner, S. and Morris, T. (1995) A new inventory to assess social anxiety and phobia: The Social Phobia and Anxiety Inventory for Children. *Psychology Assessment* **7**: 73–9.

Berrios, G. (1999) Anxiety disorders: a conceptual history. *Journal of Affective Disorders* **56**: 83–94.

Blake, D.D., Weathers, F.W., Nagy, L.M. *et al.* (1995) The development of a clinician-administered PTSD scale. *Journal of Traumatic Stress* **8**: 75–90.

Brown, E., Turovsky, J., Heimberg, R., Juster, H., Brown, T. and Barlow, D. (1997) Validation of the social interaction anxiety scale across the anxiety disorders. *Psychological Assessment* **9**: 21–7.

Cannon, W.B. (1929) *Bodily Changes in Pain, Hunger, Fear, and Rage* (2nd edn). New York: Appleton-Century-Crofts.

Chambless, D.L., Caputo, G.C., Bright, P. and Gallager, R. (1984) Assessment of 'fear of fear' in agoraphobics: The Body Sensations Questionnaire and the Agoraphobic Cognitions Questionnaire. *Journal of Consulting and Clinical Psychology* **52**: 1090–7.

Chambless, D.L., Caputo, G.C., Jasin, S.E., Gracely, E.J. and Williams, C. (1985) The Mobility Inventory for Agoraphobia. *Behaviour Research and Therapy* **23**(1): 35–44.

Department of Health (2001) *Treatment Choice in Psychological Therapies and Counselling.* London: Department of Health.

Department of Health (2004) *Organizing and Delivering Psychological Therapies.* London: Department of Health.

Department of Health (2006) *Improving Access to Psychological Therapies (IAPT) Programme National Learning Event – 28 February 2006.* London: Department of Health.

Ehlers, A. (1993) Interoception and panic disorder. *Behaviour Research and Therapy* **15**: 3–21.

Foa, E.B. and Kozak, M.J. (1986) Emotional processing of fear: exposure to corrective information. *Psychological Bulletin* **99**(1): 20–35.

Foa, E.B., Cashman, L.A., Jaycox, L. and Perry, K. (1997) The validation of a selfreport measure of posttraumatic stress disorder: The Posttraumatic Diagnostic Scale, *Psychological Assessment* **4**: 445–51.

Hendrick S.C., Chaney, E.F., Felker, B. *et al.* (2003) Effectiveness of collaborative care depression treatment in Veterans' Affairs primary care. *Journal of General Internal Medicine* **18**: 9–16.

Hodgson, R.J. and Rachman, S. (1977) Obsessive-compulsive complaints. *Behaviour Research and Therapy* **15**: 389–95.

Hollander, E. Cohen, L., Simeon, D., Rosen, J., DeCaraia, C. and Stein, D. (1994) Fluvoxamine treatment of body dysmorphic disorder. *Journal of Clinical Psychopharmacology* **14**: 75–7.

Horowitz, M., Wilner, N. and Alvarez, W. (1979) Impact of Event Scale: A measure of subjective stress. *Psychosomatic Medicine* **41**: 209–18.

Katon, W. *et al.* (1999). Stepped collaborative care for primary care patients with persistent symptoms of depression: a randomized trial. *Archives of General Psychiatry* **56**: 1109–15.

Kellner, R. (1987) *Abridged Manual of the Illness Attitude Scale.* Albuquerque: University of New Mexico.

Layard, R. (2004) *Mental Health: Britain's Biggest Social Problem?* The Strategy Unit, http://www.strategy.gov.uk/downloads/files/mh_agenda.pdf

Layard, R. (2005), *Therapy For All On The NHS,* Sainsbury Centre Lecture, http://www.scmh.org.uk/80256FBD004F3555/vWeb/flKHAL6H3D4F/$file/layard+lecture+scmh+120905.doc

Layard, R. (2006) *The Depression Report – A New Deal for Depression and Anxiety Disorders.* The Centre for Economic Performance's Mental Health Policy Group, London School of Economics.

Markowitz, J.S., Weissman, M.M., Ouelette, R., Lish, J.D. and Klerman, G.L. (1989) Quality of life in panic disorder. *Archives of General Psychiatry* **46**: 984–92.

Marks, I.M. (1987) *Fears, Phobias and Rituals: Panic, Anxiety and their Disorders.* Oxford: Oxford University Press.

Marks, I.M. and Mathews, A.M. (1979) Brief standard self-rating for phobic patients. *Behaviour Research and Therapy* **17**: 59–68.

McGlynn, F., McNeil, D., Gallagher, S. and Vrana, S. (1987) Factor structure, stability and internal consistency of the dental fear survey. *Behvioural Assessment* **9**: 5728–66.

McKay, D., Danyko, S., Neziroglu, F. and Yaryura-Tobias, J. (1995) Factor structure of the Yale-Brown Obsessive-Compulsive Scale: a two dimensional measure. *Behavioural Research and Therapy* **33**: 865–9.

Meyer, T.J., Miller, M.L., Metzger, R.L. and Borkovec, T.D. (1990) Development and validation of the Penn State worry questionnaire. *Behaviour Research and Therapy* **28**: 487–95.

NHS Centre for Reviews and Dissemination Reviewers (2002) The treatment of social phobia: a critical assessment. *Database of Abstracts of Reviews of Effectiveness, University of York,* Vol. 2, June 2002.

National Institute for Clinical Excellence (2004) Management of anxiety in primary and secondary care. London: NICE.

National Institute for Health and Clinical Excellence (2006) *Computerised cognitive behavioural therapy for depression and anxiety: TA97.* London: NICE.

Newham Primary Care Trust and East London and The City Mental Health NHS Trust (2006) *Improving Access To Psychological Therapies, National Demonstration Pilot – Newham Site, Project Outline,* London.

Parry, G. (1992) Improving psychotherapy services: applications of research, audit and evaluation. *British Journal of Clinical Psychology* **31**: 3–19.

Pavlov, I.P. (1927) *Conditioned Reflexes* (trans. G.V. Anrep). London: Oxford University Press.

Robbins, J. and Kirmayer, L. (1991) Attributions of common somatic symptoms. *Psychological Medicine* **21**: 1029–45.

Rosen, J.C., Reiter, J. and Orosan, P. (1995) Assessment of body image in eating disorders with the body drymorphic disorder examination. *Behaviour Research and Therapy* **33**(1): 77–84.

Roth, A., Fonagy, P. and Perry, G. (2005) *What Works for Whom?: A Critical Review of Psychotherapy Research*. New York: Guilford Publications.

Salkovskis, P.M., Clark, D.M. and Gelder, M.G. (1996) Cognition-behaviour links in the persistence of panic. *Behaviour Research and Therapy* **32**: 1–8.

Sanavio, E. (1988) Obsessions and compulsions: The Padua Inventory. *Behavioural Research and Therapy* **26**: 169–77.

Watson, B. and Friend, R. (1969) Measurement of social-evaluate anxiety, *Journal of Consulting and Clinical Psychology* **33**: 448–57.

Weissman, M.M., Klerman, G.L., Markowitz, J.S. and Ouellette, R. (1989) Suicidal ideation and suicide attempts in panic disorder and attacks. *New England Journal of Medicine* **321**: 1209–14.

Wells, A. (1997) *Cognitive Therapy of Anxiety Disorders: A Procedural Manual and Conceptual Guide*. Chichester: Wiley.

Wells, A. and Butler, G. (1997) Generalized anxiety disorder, in D. Clark and C. Fairburn (eds) *Science and Practice of Cognitive Behaviour Therapy*. Oxford: Oxford Medical Publications, ch. 7, pp. 155–78.

Williams C (2004) *Alternative Methods of Treatment Delivery for Anxiety Disorders*. Abingdon: The Medicine Publishing Company Ltd.

Wolpe, J. (1958) *Psychotherapy by Reciprocal Inhibition*. Stanford: Stanford University Press.

Wolpe, J. (1990) *The Practice of Behaviour Therapy*. Tarrytown, NY: Pergamon Press.

CHAPTER 21

The person with an eating disorder

Chris Prestwood

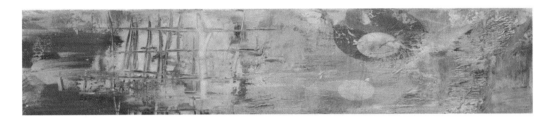

Chapter overview

This chapter provides an introduction for nurses to the eating disorders anorexia nervosa and bulimia nervosa as defined in the International Classification of Diseases (ICD-10) (WHO 1992). The chapter also covers 'eating disorder not otherwise specified' (EDNOS) (APA 1994) and includes the diagnostic category 'binge eating disorder'. The chapter does not address the management of obesity, loss of appetite or psychogenic disturbance of appetite due to known physical illness.

This chapter covers:

- An introduction to the eating disorders;
- The main physical, psychological and behavioural features of the eating disorders;
- The aetiology of eating disorders;
- Approaches to the assessment, treatment and management of care of a person with an eating disorder, including an overview of recent guidelines produced by the National Institute for Clinical Excellence;
- The skills needed by the nurse to develop a therapeutic relationship with a person with an eating disorder;
- A case study which highlights the importance of maintaining a client-centred approach.

Introduction

As a pattern of self-regulation, properly controlled eating contributes to psychological, biological and sociocultural health and well-being (Cochrane 2000). Adaptive eating responses are characterized by balanced eating patterns, appropriate calorific intake, and a body weight that is appropriate for height. However, food can also be used in an attempt to satisfy unmet emotional needs, moderate stress, and provide rewards and punishment. Illnesses associated with maladaptive eating regulation responses are known as eating disorders.

Eating disorders are complex, life-threatening conditions which can affect anyone. They are best understood as a way of coping with unmanageable feelings, thoughts and emotions.

Until relatively recently awareness of the eating disorders was limited. Bulimia nervosa was first described in 1979 (Russell 1979) and although anorexia nervosa has been known for well over a century (Gull 1874), until the 1960s it was thought of as a rarity. The increased prominence of the eating disorders has been a phenomenon of the late twentieth century (Palmer 2000).

The term 'eating disorder' refers to a group of conditions characterized by:

- severe disturbances in eating;
- emotional and psychological distress;
- physical consequences.

The behaviour of a person with an eating disorder revolves around food and eating, consequently eating disorders are often mistakenly believed to be solely about food. It is important to recognize that the behaviour around eating is an outward sign of emotional distress. Eating disorders are not primarily about food and weight issues or about 'slimming'. For long-term recovery to be possible the psychological issues and emotional distress as well as the physical symptoms must be addressed. The distress of a person experiencing an eating disorder, whether or not it is acknowledged, will have a considerable impact on family and friends (www.bodywhys.ie).

Although the term 'eating disorder' is applied to a wide range of disturbed eating behaviours; only three conditions are listed in official classifications of eating disorders: anorexia nervosa, bulimia nervosa and binge eating disorder (APA 1994).

What is anorexia nervosa?

Anorexia nervosa is an eating disorder characterized by the deliberate refusal to eat enough to maintain a normal body weight. As a result, both the body and the mind are starved of the nutrients needed for healthy, balanced functioning.

Although the word 'anorexia nervosa' literally means loss of appetite, this does not accurately describe what a person experiences. Appetite is suppressed rather than lost and an intense interest in food is retained. Self-starvation and weight loss/control represent an attempt to feel more in control of one's life and gives the person a much needed sense of effectiveness and achievement. Other means of maintaining low body weight might include fasting, excessive exercise, self-induced vomiting, the use of laxatives, diuretics or appetite suppressants.

Anorexia nervosa can affect both males and females of all ages. It is most common among girls and young women. Around 10 per cent of people with anorexia nervosa are male (Pawluck and Gorey 1998).

The main features of anorexia nervosa are:

- Weight is maintained at least 15 per cent below that expected.
- Restriction of food intake.
- Intense fear of putting on weight.
- Preoccupation with body weight, size and shape.
- Perception of body shape and size are disturbed (body image distortion).

■ Disruption of hormonal balance. In women and adolescent girls the menstrual cycle is upset: periods become irregular and eventually cease (amenorrhoea). In men there can be a loss of libido (American Psychiatric Association (APA) 1994)

Other signs and symptoms of anorexia nervosa are listed in Table 21.1.

Physical
■ Over-activity and excessive exercising.
■ Bloating of stomach, fluid retention.
■ Constipation and abdominal pain.
■ Restlessness, inability to settle.
■ Difficulty sleeping, tiredness.
■ Dry, thinning hair.
■ Dry, discoloured skin.
■ Growth of fine, downy hair (lanugo) on the face and body resulting from the body's efforts to keep warm.
■ Loss of periods.
■ Decreased interest in sex.
Psychological and social
■ Low self-esteem.
■ Irritability and mood swings.
■ Difficulty resolving conflict.
■ Social isolation.
■ Inflexible 'black or white'/'right or wrong' thinking.
■ Depression.
■ Obsessive and/or compulsive behaviour.
Food related
■ Rigid, limited diet.
■ Frequent weighing.
■ Excessive thinking and talking about food and related issues.
■ Lying about food intake, claiming to have already eaten or to have plans to eat elsewhere.
■ Moving food around the plate, taking a long time over meals.
■ Cooking for others.
■ Reading and collecting recipes.
■ Rituals around food and eating.
■ Increased use of spices, condiments, chewing gum.
■ Increased consumption of fluids.
■ Secret disposal of food.

Table 21.1 Other signs and symptoms of anorexia nervosa

Most symptoms of the disorder will resolve with weight gain and normalization of diet and eating habits.

Health consequences of anorexia nervosa

To deal with the effects of starvation, the body is forced to slow down all its processes and find ways of conserving energy.

The physical effects of starvation include:

- Dehydration → risk of kidney failure.
- Muscle weakness → risk of muscle loss.
- Tiredness and overall weakness → risk of fainting.
- Abnormally slow heart rate and low blood pressure produces changes in the heart muscle → risk of heart failure.
- Loss of bone density resulting in dry, brittle bones (osteoporosis) → risk of postural problems and risk of fracture.

Starvation also affects a person's thinking and behaviour. Poor nutrition and dehydration produce changes in brain chemistry. It is thought that these changes in brain chemistry contribute to sustain the distorted thinking, disturbed perception and obsession with food associated with anorexia nervosa. Intellectual ability can also be affected resulting in reduced concentration, poor memory, difficulties with abstract thinking, problem solving, decision-making and planning. In some cases, these changes can also increase vulnerability to depression, anxiety and other psychiatric disorders such as obsessive compulsive disorder. If the depression is severe, there is a risk of suicide. Other means of weight control such as self-induced vomiting, use of laxatives or diuretics and excessive exercise can also have serious health consequences and a significant impact on a person's capacity to function effectively.

What is bulimia nervosa?

Bulimia nervosa is characterized by repeated episodes of binge-eating followed by behaviour aimed at compensating for the out of control eating. These compensatory behaviours can include fasting, self-induced vomiting, the use of laxatives and diuretics or appetite suppressants and excessive exercising. In many cases, bulimia nervosa begins with dieting but the preoccupation with food and weight becomes obsessive and can take over the person's life. A compulsive cycle of bingeing and purging (getting rid of the food) develops and attempts to break the cycle often fail. The person begins to feel more and more out of control. On the outside, a person with bulimia nervosa may seem very capable, positive, successful and on top of things. However, on the inside, they may be struggling desperately with feelings of guilt, shame, self-loathing and ineffectiveness. For some people, bulimia nervosa develops after a period of anorexia nervosa. In such cases, diagnosis is not always clear-cut and treatment can be more complex.

Many people with bulimia nervosa maintain a normal body weight. As a result, the disorder can sometimes go unnoticed and untreated for a long time. The longer the binge-purge cycle remains in place, the harder it becomes to overcome it.

The main features of bulimia nervosa are:

- Repeated episodes of binge eating, i.e. eating larger than normal quantities of food in a short space of time.
- Compensating for binges – this can take the form of purging.

- Exercising or using laxatives and/or diuretics.
- Preoccupation with body weight, shape and size.
- Self-evaluation is influenced significantly by body weight, size and shape.
- Hormonal disturbance including irregular menstruation (APA 1994).

Other signs and symptoms of bulimia nervosa are listed in Table 21.2.

Physical

- Frequent changes in weight.
- Lethargy, tiredness and insomnia.
- Dehydration.
- General digestive problems (cramps, wind, constipation, diarrhoea)
- Poor skin condition.
- Headaches, tension.
- Sore throat and mouth ulcers, husky voice.
- Calluses on fingers.
- Irregular periods.
- Enlarged salivary glands.
- Erosion of tooth enamel, tooth decay.

Psychological

- Feeling emotional, irritability, mood swings.
- Dissatisfaction with body image.
- Feeling out of control.
- Feelings of inadequacy and worthlessness.
- Feelings of guilt and shame.
- Depression and related symptoms.
- Anxiety.

Other behavioural signs

- Preoccupation with dieting.
- Regular binges (uncontrollable overeating).
- Being sick after meals.
- Disappearing to the lavatory after meals in order to get rid of food.
- Secret hoarding of food.
- Secret disposal of vomit (e.g. bags of vomit hidden in bedroom).
- Abuse of laxatives.
- Excessive exercising.
- Lying.
- Risk-taking behaviours such as alcohol or drug misuse, shoplifting, promiscuity or self-harm.
- Problems dealing with social situations and interaction with others.

Table 21.2 Other signs and symptoms of bulimia nervosa

Health consequences of bulimia nervosa

Frequent vomiting and the use of laxatives, in particular, can lead to dehydration and to the depletion of electrolytes (body salts). When this occurs, it can seriously affect the body's ability to function properly. All organs can be affected. The heart is particularly at risk. A simple blood test will indicate the level of dehydration and electrolyte depletion. Dietary advice can then be sought to help correct these problems. If a person is severely dehydrated or depleted of essential nutrients, hospitalization may be required. Frequent vomiting can also cause erosion to tooth enamel and dental decay.

Depression and high levels of anxiety and periods of emotional overwhelm often accompany bulimia nervosa. Addressing these and other psychological aspects of the disorder is crucial to recovery.

What is binge eating disorder?

Binge eating disorder or compulsive overeating is characterized by periods of compulsive binge eating or overeating. There is no purging (getting rid of the food) but there may be sporadic fasts or repeated diets. Weight may vary from normal to significantly overweight.

In binge eating disorder, food is not used to nourish the body, but to manage emotional need. Overeating becomes a way of coping. A person with binge eating disorder becomes caught up in a vicious cycle of bingeing and dieting or restricting their food intake.

People with binge eating problems often experience some of the following:

- Eating is out of control.
- Eating much more quickly than usual during binges.
- Eating until uncomfortably full.
- Eating large amounts of food, even when not hungry.
- Eating alone due to embarrassment about the amount eaten.
- Feelings of disgust, guilt, self loathing and shame after overeating.
- Depression and anxiety (APA 1994).

Complications of binge eating disorder

Binge eating puts a lot of stress on the digestive processes and on the metabolism which can become chaotic. Digestive problems such as bloating, stomach cramps, constipation or diarrhoea can be experienced. Disordered eating patterns can also affect the body's capacity to absorb the nutrients it needs for healthy functioning and can have a marked effect on energy levels.

The medical complications associated with binge eating disorder tend to be the same as those associated with obesity:

- high blood pressure;
- high cholesterol levels;
- heart disease;
- diabetes;
- gallbladder disease.

Depression and anxiety can become severe and may require specialist intervention.

How many people suffer from the eating disorders?

Estimates of the community prevalence of the eating disorders are complicated by their relative rarity and the reluctance of many sufferers to declare their disorder in surveys. There are often problems of sampling or of studying particular populations and then generalizing the results too widely (Palmer 2000). However typical results for anorexia nervosa suggest a prevalence of between 10 and 30 per 100,000 (van Hoeken *et al.* 1998). Bulimia nervosa has a prevalence of 100 per 100,000. Similar figures are suggested for binge eating disorder but these are tentative as it is a relatively new disorder, estimates vary widely and it is not clear how stable the untreated syndrome is over time (Cachelin *et al.* 1999).

The aetiology of eating disorders

The aetiology of eating disorders is generally considered to be multi-factorial; no single aetiological factor in isolation can account for the development of these disorders in an individual, nor can it be seen to account for the variation among individuals (Cooper and Steere 1995). We really do not know what causes an eating disorder (Palmer 2000). NICE guidance recognizes that much of the research in this area suffers from methodological limitations (NCCMH 2004). Where the onset of the disorder is insidious, it is not always clear whether recognized factors are causes or consequences of the disorder. One recent study (Tozzi *et al.* 2003) suggested that those with anorexia nervosa perceived dysfunctional families, dieting behaviour and stressful life events as the main causes of their condition.

Whether or not a person develops an eating disorder will depend on their individual vulnerability, consequent on the presence of biological or other predisposing factors, their exposure to particular provoking risk factors and on the operation of protective factors. Following the establishment of the disorder a further combination of risk and protective factors may act to maintain the condition or determine whether an individual recovers (NCCMH 2004).

What follows is a brief appraisal of many of the issues that have been invoked as playing some part in the causation of the eating disorders. This is largely based on a meta-analysis of prospective and experimental studies reviewing the evidence for aetiological and maintaining factors in the eating disorders (Stice 2002).

Genetic factors

The majority of family studies have shown that eating disorders run in families. Female relatives of those with anorexia nervosa are 11.4 times as likely to suffer the disorder than relatives of control subjects, while female relatives of those with bulimia nervosa are 3.7 times as likely to suffer with bulimia (Strober 1995). A twin study of anorexia nervosa has estimated the heritability to be 58 per cent (Wade *et al.* 2000) but the relative contribution of genetic to other factors is unclear (Bulik *et al.* 2000).

It appears that specific genetic factors are important in the aetiology of anorexia nervosa but we are far from knowing what these could be. The clinical presentation and the familial context of bulimia nervosa are both much more heterogeneous than for anorexia nervosa and it is unlikely that a unique biological abnormality will be present in bulimia nervosa (Treasure and Holland 1995).

Physical risk factors

A history of premorbid obesity is evident with both anorexia nervosa (7–20%) and bulimia nervosa (18–40%) (Cooper and Steere 1995). There is prospective evidence that this experience leads to a propensity to an increase in body dissatisfaction and likelihood of dieting behaviour (Stice 2002). Although a range of neuro-endocrine and metabolic disturbances occurs in those with eating disorders, the evidence suggests that these disturbances are secondary rather than primary to the disorder. Early menarche has long been considered a risk factor for eating disorders through the relationship with adiposity and body dissatisfaction (NCCMH 2004).

The dietary restraint model suggests that calorie restriction increases the risk for binge eating and bulimia nervosa. The concept of restrained eating refers to a state in which the individual deliberately eats less than his or her hunger or drive to eat would otherwise lead him or her to do (Palmer 2000). Although dieting appears to increase negative affect and may contribute to eating difficulties, dieting has a small effect in the contribution to the development of eating pathology (Stice 2002). However, some of the physiological features of the eating disorders, for example delayed gastric emptying, act to sustain the behaviour of fasting even though these features are the consequences of dietary restraint not precipitating causes (Robinson and McHugh 1995). The obvious therapeutic implication of these consequences is that renourishment is emphasized as a first step in treatment.

Adverse life events and difficulties

Severe life stresses have been implicated in the aetiology of both anorexia nervosa and bulimia nervosa, with approximately 70 per cent of cases been triggered by severe life events or difficulties (Schmidt et al. 1997). These stresses most commonly occur in the area of close relationships with family or friends (Welch et al. 1997). There is little persuasive evidence that sexual abuse is a specific predisposing factor for eating disorders rather than psychiatric disorder per se (Vogelantz-Holm et al. 2000).

Family factors

In spite of a growing number of empirical studies, most beliefs about families of eating disordered clients have their origin in clinical observations (Gull 1874; Minuchin et al. 1978). These provide a rich source of insight into the functioning of these families but can also give a misleading picture (Eisler 1995). The notion that there is a particular type of family arrangement or style of family functioning that is invariably associated with the eating disorders is unlikely to be found. There is also difficulty in recognizing whether any observed differences in family functioning are consequences rather than causes of the illness (Dare and Eisler 1992).

Evidence from family studies suggests increased rates of affective disorder among first and second degree relatives of people with both anorexia nervosa and bulimia nervosa (Cooper and Steere 1995). A family history of substance abuse may be a specific risk factor for bulimia nervosa (Cooper and Steere 1995).

Although a number of studies have looked at family environment and functioning there is no evidence to support the causative role of dysfunctional family systems (Stice 2002). However this does not mean that we should stop investigating how families function.

Understanding how families cope with adversity will tell us more about how to help them rather than about the role of families in the aetiology of eating disorders (Eisler 1995).

Many people with eating disorders are aware that they are causing deep distress to parents or others close to them. However, they feel helpless to bridge the gulf between themselves and others; too much has to be concealed, too little can be understood and furthermore, the starved state breeds a self-interest which is all-consuming. The client's area of private distress, her capacity to keep secret her inner fears and preoccupations, stems partly from her sense of the precariousness of her defensive stance and her inability to risk exposure (Crisp 1980).

Socio-cultural factors

A number of socio-cultural theories have been put forward to explain the aetiology of eating disorders. Rarely has a notion of social processes as causes of psychiatric disorder received more attention than in anorexia nervosa. Such theories include the meaning of weight and shape for women in different cultures and the impact of advertising and other media. It is argued that societal pressure to be thin fosters an internalization of a thin ideal and body dissatisfaction, which in turn leads to dieting behaviour and places the person at risk for eating pathology (Striegel-Moore *et al.* 1986). This perceived pressure does appear to predict dieting and eating pathology (Stice 2002).

Although not conclusive, evidence suggests that there has been an increase in anorexia nervosa and bulimia nervosa over recent decades consistent with the operation of social forces (Szmukler *et al.* 1995).

Perfectionism

Perfectionism has long been considered a risk factor for eating pathology as it may promote the relentless pursuit of the 'thin ideal'. A variety of studies support the notion of perfectionism as a risk factor for bulimic pathology and a maintenance factor for more general eating pathology (Stice 2002). Cognitively, people with eating disorders often display an 'all or nothing' thinking style. Eating can be 'all or nothing' but this style extends beyond food and weight and involves other behaviours such as studying, exercise, relationships, attitudes to the self, and attitudes to others (others may be idealized or vilified) (Crisp 1980).

Self-esteem

Most people with eating disorders seem to have low self-esteem (Palmer 2000). However, whether low self-esteem is a risk factor or part of the disorder is hard to ascertain. There is some evidence to suggest that low self-esteem is a risk factor both for slimming and for the development of an eating disorder (Fairburn *et al.* 1999). People with eating disorders are very dependent on external phenomenon for the maintenance of their self-esteem. Performance and achievement are tied to pleasing others rather than pleasing oneself.

Other models

Many other models, usually incorporating a number of the risk factors outlined above, have been proposed to help understand the aetiology of the eating disorders. Observations and speculations abound but, as yet, no one model has a sufficient evidence base.

One model that has received much support from those working in the eating disorders field is that proposed by Arthur Crisp (Crisp 1980). Crisp developed a model based on biological issues that informed assessment and treatment protocols that produced good health outcomes. Crisp saw anorexia nervosa as a problem relating to the difficulties of progressing through adolescence. His model emphasizes that adolescence is driven by puberty and that puberty triggers developmental events, such as changes in body shape. These developmental events can be welcomed or feared by an individual. For a young person struggling with the process of growing up, losing weight and reversing the process of puberty can be a welcome response to these developmental changes. Crisp suggested that anorexia nervosa sufferers fear maturity because of the increased personal responsibility that maturity requires. Clients fail to develop a sense of mastery or control over their own world and dieting then becomes an isolated area of personal control (Crisp 1980). Furthermore eating disorder clients have a relative lack of awareness of bodily processes, including inner feelings and changes in one's body shape. They often perceive their body as something foreign and something that must be artificially controlled (Bruch 1973).

In summary, although theories which explain the development of eating disorders have a limited evidence base, we can identify many risk factors which can guide care and treatment.

Assessment

Clients with maladaptive eating regulation responses should receive a comprehensive assessment, including complete biological, psychological and sociocultural evaluations (Cochrane 2000). In completing a comprehensive nursing assessment the following information should be obtained:

- actual and desired weight;
- onset and pattern of menstruation;
- food restrictions and fasting patterns;
- frequency and extent of binging and vomiting;
- use of laxatives, diuretics, diet pills etc.;
- body image disturbance;
- food preferences and peculiarities;
- exercise patterns.

It is also helpful to explore the client's understanding of how the illness developed and its impact on school, work and social relationships so that an holistic view of the client's world can be obtained (Cochrane 2000).

NICE guidance on treatment and care management

The National Collaborating Centre for Mental Health was commissioned by the National Institute for Clinical Excellence to produce guidelines on the treatment and management of anorexia nervosa, bulimia nervosa and related eating disorders which were first published in 2004 (NCCMH 2004). This guidance was based on the available evidence and identified a number of key priorities for implementation. Nearly all of these were based on expert opinion rather than on clinical studies, and many of the priorities related to appropriate use of the care programme approach and risk management tools. This section focuses on those guidelines that are particularly relevant to the nursing care of eating disorder sufferers.

Key priorities of care across all eating diorders are as follows:

- Assessment of people with eating disorders should be comprehensive and include physical, psychological and social needs, and a comprehensive assessment of risk to self.
- Clients and, where appropriate, carers should be provided with education on the nature, course and treatment of eating disorders.
- Health care professionals should acknowledge that many people with eating disorders are ambivalent about treatment.
- People with eating disorders seeking help should be assessed and receive treatment at the earliest opportunity.
- Clients who are vomiting should have regular dental reviews and avoid brushing teeth after vomiting (to stop brushing stomach acid into the teeth).
- Health care professionals should advise people with eating disorders and oesteoporosis or related bone disorders to refrain from physical activities that significantly increase the likelihood of falls.
- Family members should be included in the treatment of children and adolescents with eating disorders.
- In children and adolescents growth and development should be closely monitored.
- Health care professionals assessing children and adolescents should be alert to indicators of abuse.

Anorexia nervosa

The treatment plan for a client with anorexia nervosa needs to consider the appropriate service setting, and the client's psychological and physical management. The appropriate setting depends on the assessment of risk and the client's wishes, but, in general, the client will be treated initially in a secondary care outpatient service, moving into a day or inpatient setting if required. Psychological therapy is crucial in addressing the underlying behaviours and cognitions. In children and adolescents some family-based psychological intervention is essential. Physical treatments comprise nutritional interventions and psychopharmacological agents. The latter are used to support psychological treatments or for the management of comorbid conditions, rather than being first-line treatments.

The treatment options should be discussed fully with the client to ensure informed choice. Given the ambivalence inherent in the disorder, engagement and efforts at motivational enhancement may be helpful in maximizing adherence to treatment. A small number of clients do not have the capacity to make decisions about their own health and safety and in these cases provision for their admission to hospital and treatment is under the remit of the Mental Health Act 1983 and the Children Act 1989 (NCCMH 2004).

NICE guidance identifies the following key priorities in the treatment of anorexia nervosa:

- Weight and body mass index (BMI, calculated as weight in kilograms divided by height in metres squared) should not be considered the sole indicators of physical risk.
- Psychological therapies to be considered include cognitive analytical therapy (CAT), cognitive behaviour therapy (CBT), interpersonal psychotherapy (IPT), focal psychodynamic therapy and family interventions focused explicitly on eating disorders.
- The aims of psychological treatment should be to reduce risk, to encourage weight gain and healthy eating, to reduce other symptoms related to an eating disorder, and to facilitate psychological and physical recovery.
- Outpatient psychological treatment should normally be of at least six months duration.
- Dietary counselling should not be provided as the sole treatment.

Bulimia nervosa

Psychological interventions

As a possible first step clients should be encouraged to follow an evidence-based self-help programme, e.g. Getting Better Bit(e) by Bit(e) (Schmidt and Treasure 1998). Cognitive behavioural therapy for bulimia nervosa (CBT-BN), a specifically adapted form of CBT, should be offered to adults with bulimia nervosa. The course of treatment should be for 16 to 20 sessions over four to five months. Adolescents may be treated with CBT-BN adapted as needed to suit their age, circumstances and level of development, and include the family as appropriate. Self-help programmes and CBT-BN have been well researched, focus on the psychological and sociocultural aspects of the bulimia nervosa to reduce symptomology, and have good clinical outcomes.

Pharmacological interventions

As an alternative or additional first step to using an evidence-based self-help programme, adults with bulimia nervosa may be offered a trial of an antidepressant drug. Selective serotonin reuptake inhibitors (SSRIs) (specifically fluoxetine) are the drugs of first choice in terms of acceptability, tolerability and reduction of symptoms.

Management of physical aspects

Clients who are vomiting regularly or taking large quantities of laxatives (especially if underweight) should have their fluid and electrolyte balance assessed. When electrolyte balance is detected it is usually sufficient to focus on eliminating the behaviour responsible.

The great majority of clients can be treated as outpatients. There is a very limited role for the inpatient treatment of bulimia nervosa. This is primarily concerned with the management of suicide risk or severe self-harm.

Role and function of the mental health nurse

Eating disorders are multi-factorial in origin and therefore assessment and management needs to include medical, psychiatric, nutritional, behavioural and psychosocial components. Any treatment approach to the eating disorders has to be multi-professional given the multi-factorial nature of the illness, within which the mental health nurse has an important role to play.

The successful treatment of the eating disorders depends upon the creation and maintenance of an adequate treatment alliance between the sufferer and the clinician who seeks to help her recover (Palmer 1989). The primary role of the nurse is likely to be less clearly defined than some other members of the multi-disciplinary team, but needs to focus on developing a therapeutic nurse–client relationship within which the nurse uses personal attributes and clinical techniques in working with the client to bring about insight and behavioural change. This is more likely to take place in a community rather than an inpatient setting. To develop this role the nurse must: have good knowledge of the eating disorders to understand what is motivating the client's actions; convey empathy and understanding to the client; and be self-aware and able to form an intimate, interdependent, interpersonal relationship which involves a capacity to give and receive respect.

In developing the relationship, various aspects of the client's life experiences are explored, the nurse allowing the client to express thoughts, feelings and emotions and relating these to observed and reported actions. Together, the client and nurse correct communication problems and modify maladaptive behaviour patterns by testing new patterns of behaviour and more adaptive coping mechanisms. This section identifies important aspects of this relationship in the context of the care of people suffering from eating disorders.

Developing skills to engage in a therapeutic relationship

Self-awareness

Crisp, writing nearly 30 years ago, specifically about inpatient eating disorder units, suggested that within the nursing team there needs to be those who are still in touch with their own adolescent struggles so that they can be of greater help, supporting the client through a friendship within which they appropriately share their own experiences. He says that such contact will require expert supervision, not least because it is the nurse's lot, while on duty, to be permanently responsible for and involved with the client (Crisp 1980). If the nurse is to facilitate the expression of thoughts and feelings and achieve authentic, open and personal communication, then the nurse must have an understanding of his or her own self. Many nurses working with eating disorder clients may find themselves identifying with the needs of the client to relapse into the anorectic position. The nurse may himself or herself eat little carbohydrate or wish that he or she ate less. The effect of this is that the nurse may align himself of herself with the anorexia nervosa and hinder recovery for the client by not recognizing the importance of renourishment in the treatment of the disorder.

Many clients with an eating disorder are struggling with issues of sexuality or sexual identity. The nurse often develops intimate relationships with clients where these issues are discussed. The feelings generated for the nurse should be identified and verbalized through supervision. Only then can nurses resolve them in a constructive manner. Failure to do so can lead to inappropriate relationships between staff and clients which may result in the client being drawn into an abusive relationship.

Nurses will function as role models for their clients with an eating disorder. Therefore, a nurse has an obligation to model adaptive and growth producing behaviour. This can be challenging because the client will often view the nurse closely and subtly try to understand the nurse's view on food, weight and body shape. The nurse has a responsibility to respond in a way that encourages the client to modify maladaptive behaviour. For example, a client may ask a nurse why he or she does not eat anything at lunchtime. The nurse's response could help the client understand that for somebody without an eating disorder, eating is driven by hunger and satiation rather than avoided as a way to lose weight.

Nurses often have a strong desire to help others. This is understandable, to be respected and can be a worthy attribute of a professional nurse. However, care must be taken that the wish to help is not confused with a wish to be liked or exist to an extent that denial or self-sacrifice is practised. A nurse who ignores a client's weight loss because he or she does not want to confront a client is not helping the client recover from his or her eating disorder. Alternatively a client may ask a community nurse to visit on a daily basis. This may not be practical or needed but the nurse may agree rather than manage the client's potential rejection of him or her. A nurse who is unable to care for himself of herself by recognizing and addressing his or her own needs is unlikely to develop the therapeutic relationship that is necessary to help somebody with an eating disorder. The nurse is not modelling the social skills that need to be developed by the client to function without his or her eating disorder. A balance between the needs of the client and the needs of the nurse has to be discussed with the client. This will be helpful to the client in developing relationships with others as the client recovers from his or her illness.

Working with eating disorder clients usually involves setting firm but fair boundaries particularly over weight gain. Once these are agreed upon, the client needs to feel that he or she can trust these boundaries. It is not helpful to the client if the nurse ignores any breach of these agreements due to a wish to be liked by the client. The client is likely to feel unsafe and will lessen his or her trust in the nurse and the overall treatment plan, especially if the client is able to recognize that breaking the agreement is driven by the eating disorder rather than his or her own wish to recover. Many clients with an eating disorder have little trust in health care professionals, who may be thought to be interested in controlling them rather than alleviating their suffering. Often they also mistrust themselves, particularly with regard to their ability to control bodily functions naturally. A useful therapeutic stance to take is that you can trust an individual but you cannot trust an eating disorder. From personal experience most clients tell me that they do not trust their eating disorder and when recovered have expressed how important it was to have people around them who helped them confront their eating disorder.

Therapeutic communication

Communication involving verbal and non-verbal communication and listening is the essence of a therapeutic relationship; it is the means by which people influence the behaviour of each other.

For a client suffering from an eating disorder and almost constantly focusing on issues relating to food and weight it is easy to misunderstand the meaning of what a nurse might say. For example, to say to a person who is recovering from anorexia nervosa that 'she looks well' may be perceived as being told that she looks fat.

It is not uncommon for clients with eating disorders to be functioning emotionally at a younger age than their chronological age. Anorexia nervosa, in particular, hinders emotional development as the illness provides a protection from developing meaningful relationships. This places a demand on the nurse to ensure he or she is communicating effectively. This can be further complicated by the changes in emotional age that can occur within the recovery process and confused by the client's intellectual capacities which will be intact or enhanced.

Interpreting non-verbal communication can present difficulty to the nurse. The nurse should respond by referring to the specific behaviour observed and attempt to confirm its meaning and significance with the client. Discussing the meaning of a client's shape or weight can help the client identify his or her conscious or unconscious motivations.

Attentive listening is a sign of respect for the client and is a powerful reinforcer. Most clients with an eating disorder are unused to verbalizing their thoughts, feelings and emotions because their illness has helped them avoid their feelings. Many clients will see this as part of their personality rather than a consequence of their illness. Many forms of creative therapies can help the client to express their feelings and it can be particularly useful if the client with anorexia nervosa is encouraged to regularly write of his or her experiences as a way to encourage further exploration of his or her feelings.

For the more impulsive bulimic type of client, a 'food diary' can be utilized. Clients are encouraged to write down all behaviours relating to the control of food and weight, helping the client to recognize the behaviours he or she is using, such as bingeing, vomiting etc. If this process includes the opportunity to write down the feelings, thoughts and emotions that accompany these behaviours, then the client has a valuable opportunity to make connections, which can be explored with the nurse. For example, the client may recognize that his or her bingeing behaviour is associated with feeling angry. Often these associations may be obvious to the nurse but less obvious to the client.

Therapeutic problems

It is not unusual for people with eating disorders to refuse help. They may believe that they have found a solution to their problems through the eating disorder. The nurse will attempt to help the client give up the eating disorder and find a more fruitful way of living. This involves suggesting to the client that they change their way of life. Not surprisingly, this can be a very frightening prospect for the client.

The client's fear of giving up their eating disorder should not be underestimated. It means facing up to known and unknown fears: Who am I? How will I fill my life if I give up my eating disorder? This is a daunting prospect, and even the most motivated client will have ambivalent feelings and may want to resort to eating disorder pathology when facing his or her fears. Often clients feel trapped and will be looking for any way to avoid getting into a relationship with the nurse, who may be seen as a threat to his or her current way of coping.

This resistance by the client can block the progress of the nurse – client relationship and provoke intense feelings in both the nurse and the client. Resistance can be a reaction by the client to the nurse who has moved too quickly or too deeply into exploration of the client's feelings or who has intentionally or unintentionally communicated a lack of respect. Resistance can result from the client's need to avoid the social pressures inherent in giving up the disorder. The need to avoid unpleasant situations, to gain increased sympathy, to escape from responsibility and to attempt to control people can always result in resistance.

Working with resistance

Resistance can pose difficult problems for the mental health nurse who must be prepared to be exposed to powerful negative and positive emotional feelings coming from the client, often on what would appear an irrational basis.

Sometimes resistance occurs because the nurse and client have not arrived at mutually acceptable goals or plans of action. The appropriate action here is to jointly review the goals, purpose and roles of the nurse and client in treatment. Therapeutic work might then be directed towards increasing the client's awareness of their motivations and learning to be responsible for their actions and behaviour. It is not sufficient to merely recognize that resistance is occurring. The behaviour must be explored and possible reasons for its occurrence analysed.

It is vital for the nurse to continually convey to the client an understanding that the illness makes the client do things that are out of character when they are fearful of gaining weight and to reassure them that they will be not be allowed to behave in these self-defeating ways.

Motivational interviewing, developed by Miller and Rollnick (1991), is one of several techniques of enhancing motivation that the nurse can develop in helping him or her to work with the ambivalent client. The spirit of motivational interviewing includes:

- Motivation to change is elicited from the client and not imposed from without.
- It is the client's task, not the nurse's, to articulate and resolve his or her ambivalence.
- Direct persuasion is not an effective method for resolving ambivalence.
- Readiness to change is not a client trait but a fluctuating product of interpersonal interaction.

The aims of motivational interviewing are to:

- improve internal motivation; not external pressure;
- make the individual aware of the discrepancy between current behaviours and long-term personal values/goals;
- express empathy and support;
- support self-efficacy and optimism;
- improve self-esteem (Miller and Rollnick 1991).

Garner and Garfinkel (1997) point out that throughout treatment, staff must be understanding and supportive but firm. A punitive and angry approach will merely increase the client's resistance and destroy any therapeutic alliance. A client who has been deceptive about weight, hiding food, vomiting or excessive exercising must be confronted in a non-judgemental manner. Staff members must act sympathetically, and convey support and understanding, yet always with recognition of the reality of the situation and maintaining consistency in their approach. Treatment success may be jeopardized if one staff member 'bends the rules' to win the client's favour. Because of the difficulty people with anorexia nervosa have in seeing in-betweens, they tend to view staff members as being all good or all bad. Some may be consistently idealized; others may be severely criticized. Staff members often recognize these as reflections of the client's disordered thinking, but may become caught in their desire to win the client's favour. The client's attempt to split their perceptions and project them onto the staff must be recognized by all staff members.

Problems within the nursing staff team and the wider multi-disciplinary team can be minimized if all staff share a clear understanding of the treatment philosophy and the rationale upon which it is based. Regular staff seminars and clinical supervision are important in this regard, as is a sense of open communication within the treatment team.

Concerned family members or carers are usually the ones who identify a problem and attempt to obtain help. People with anorexia nervosa are usually angry or impatient with the concern shown by others. Family members, including siblings, should normally be included in the treatment of children and adolescents with eating disorders. Interventions may include sharing of information, advice on behavioural management and facilitating communication (NCCMH 2004).

Prognosis

The eating disorders are ego-syntonic disorders. Sufferers welcome many of the symptoms of their disorder which results in about 15 per cent of clients failing to engage in treatment and about 33–50 per cent dropping out of treatment (Mahon 2000).

The prognosis for individuals with anorexia nervosa is variable and depends on a variety of prognostic factors such as: age of onset – younger do better; severity of weight loss – less weight loss do better; duration of symptoms – shorter duration do better; duration of inpatient care – shorter duration do better; and state of family relationships – good relationships do better. Onset of anorexia nervosa before adulthood carries a more favourable outcome. However, when onset occurs at an age younger than 11 years the prognosis is poor (Liburd 2001). The mortality rate in anorexia nervosa is 10–20 per cent. In general, 50 per cent of individuals with anorexia nervosa recover completely, while 20 per cent remain emaciated, 25 per cent are thin (BMI<18.5) and 5–10 per cent die of starvation (Crisp *et al.* 1992).

The prognosis for individuals with bulimia nervosa is also variable. A ten-year follow-up study found that 52 per cent of people with bulimia nervosa had recovered fully and 9 per cent continued to experience symptoms of bulimia nervosa (Collings and King 1994). A study of 222 individuals treated with antidepressants and intensive group therapy found that after 11.5 years, 70 per cent were in full or partial remission, but 11 per cent still met the criteria for bulimia nervosa (Keel *et al.* 1999). Although cognitive behavioural therapy and medication have shown to benefit those with bulimia nervosa, they fail in approximately one-third to one-half of cases. Relapse rates are around 30 per cent (Walsh and Devlin 1998). A good prognosis has been associated with shorter duration of illness, younger age of onset, and higher social class (Sayetta 1996). Poor prognosis has been associated with a history of substance abuse, premorbid and paternal obesity, and personality disorder (Keel *et al.* 1999).

Box 21.1 presents a brief case study of Sally who suffers from anorexia nervosa, together with guidance on assessment and initial management.

Box 21.1   Case study: Anorexia nervosa

Sally is 19 years of age and has recently returned home to live with her mother and father, leaving university after one term. She has reluctantly come to see you and says it's only to keep mum happy. You have been asked to see her because her GP is worried about her weight and has made a provisional diagnosis of anorexia nervosa. Sally's mother has accompanied her to the meeting. Sally tells you that she feels great and can't understand why people are worried about her. She is adamant that her weight is fine. She is vague about why she left university but says something about being worried about mum. She tells you that she has loads of friends and an active social life. Mum shakes her head at this point, but doesn't say anything. The letter from the GP says that Sally has lost nearly 10 kg in recent months and is continuing to lose weight. The letter also states that Sally has recently finished a relationship with a longstanding boyfriend, and that the parental relationship is going through a difficult time. From observation it is evident to you that Sally is underweight, she doesn't have eye-contact with you when she speaks and she is restless and impatient throughout the interview.

How to respond

It is difficult to assess and treat somebody who doesn't want your help. The first task is to try to begin to establish a therapeutic relationship with Sally. Although Sally says that she has only attended for her mother's benefit she is present and this may be part of a wish for help. It may be beneficial to ask to see Sally on her own to discuss her motivation to change. It is important to stress that you will not make her gain weight; that is her choice. However it can be helpful to share with Sally the physical and psychological consequences of being at a low weight and what could happen if she continues to lose weight. Many of the questions that need to be asked in an assessment can be done in a conversational style and need to reflect a genuine curiosity on the part of the nurse to understand the client. Sally could be asked to identify the advantages and disadvantages of her present behaviour to evaluate her insight, coping resources and issues for further discussion. It is probable that there will be a small part of Sally that recognizes that her way of coping, i.e. the anorexia nervosa, is destructive and is stopping her moving forward in life. It is the task of the nurse to engage with this part of Sally. This can be done by using many of the techniques outlined above. It is also important to complete a physical assessment which will usually be more acceptable to Sally after you have engaged with her.

In addition to focusing on what to do to engage and motivate Sally it can also be useful to look at what not to do.

How not to do it!

- Argue with Sally;
- Be an authoritarian expert;
- Direct initial attention to 'the right way';
- Threaten or order;
- Talk too much;
- Focus on intellectual debate;
- Use moral judgements;
- Use closed or multiple questions;
- Prescribe solutions.

Conclusion

This chapter has:

- provided an overview of what the eating disorders are, how many people suffer from them and explored the factors of their causation;
- highlighted approaches to assessment, treatment and care and reviewed aspects of recently published NICE guidance on eating disorders;
- explored the role and function of the nurse and focused on developing practical skills to help the nurse engage and work with the client with an eating disorder;
- recognized the inherent difficulties in helping someone with an eating disorder and explored evidence-based practical responses to address these challenges;
- acknowledged the need to place the client at the centre of any treatment plan and to develop a therapeutic relationship that is based on an understanding of the client and the theoretical knowledge of eating disorders that is presently available to us;
- highlighted the importance that the eating disorders are about the individual's thoughts, feelings and emotions and not simply about the client's food intake and their preoccupation with weight.

Questions for reflection and discussion

1   Consider your own views on why people develop an eating disorder and reflect on how these views may affect the therapeutic relationship you have with a client.
2   Given that many people with an eating disorder are reluctant to give up their illness, discuss different techniques you may use to help somebody give up something that is important to them. (Think outside eating disorders, e.g. smoking, alcohol etc.)
3   Consider your own attitude to food and weight and how this may affect your work with this client group.

Annotated bibliography

- Bruch, H. (1973) *Eating Disorders: Obesity, Anorexia Nervosa and the Person Within.* London: Routledge and Kegan Paul. A very readable client-centred approach which helps to understand the illness from the client's perspective.
- Crisp, A.H. (1980) *Anorexia Nervosa: Let Me Be.* London: Academic Press. A seminal book which was the first to explore the idea that anorexia nervosa results as a response to adolescent adjustment. The first few chapters are strongly recommended.
- Palmer, R. (2000) *Helping People with Eating Disorders: A Clinical Guide to Assessment and Treatment.* Chichester: Wiley. A concise, comprehensive and practical guide to understanding eating disorders. Includes many case studies and an invaluable tome for all practitioners working with the eating disorders.

■ Garner, D.M. and Garfinkel, P.E. (eds) (1997) *Handbook of Treatment for Eating Disorders* (2nd edn). New York: Guilford Press. An extensive, comprehensive approach to treatment. Often follows a manual type format including numerous case illustrations and examples of therapist–client dialogue.

Useful websites

■ www.edauk.org. Information and help on all aspects of eating disorders, including anorexia nervosa, bulimia nervosa, binge eating disorder and related eating disorders. The eating disorders association of UK website.

■ www.bodywhys.ie. The eating disorders association of Ireland website.

■ www.something-fishy.org. A comprehensive American website on all aspects of eating disorders. Even includes music and poetry relating to the eating disorders.

References

APA (1994) *Diagnostic and Statistical Manual of Mental Disorders* (4th edn). Washington DC: American Psychiatric Association.

Bruch, H. (1973) *Eating Disorders: Obesity, Anorexia Nervosa and the Person Within.* London: Routledge and Kegan Paul.

Bulik, C.M., Sullivan, P.F., Fear, J.L. and Pickering, A. (2000) Twin studies of eating disorders: A review. *International Journal of Eating Disorders* **28**(2): 139–47.

Cachelin, F.M, Striegal-Moore, R.H, Elder, K.A, Pike, K.M, Wilfley, D.E and Fairburn, C.G. (1999) Natural course of a community sample of binge eating disorder. *International Journal of Eating Disorders* **25**: 45–54.

Cochrane, C.E. (2000) Eating regulation responses and eating disorders, in G.W. Stuart and S.J. Sundeen (eds) *Principles and Practice of Psychiatric Nursing.* St Louis: Mosby.

Collings, S. and King, M. (1994) Ten year follow-up of 50 clients with bulimia nervosa. *British Journal of Psychiatry* **164**: 80–7.

Cooper, P.J. and Steere, J.A. (1995) Comparison of two psychological treatments for bulimia nervosa: Implications for models of maintenance. *Behaviour Research and Therapy* **33**: 875–85.

Crisp, A.H. (1980) *Anorexia Nervosa: Let Me Be.* London: Academic Press.

Crisp, A.H., Callender, J.S., Halek, C. and Hsu, L.K.G. (1992) Long-term mortality in anorexia nervosa: a 20-year follow-up of the St George's and Aberdeen cohorts. *British Journal of Psychiatry* **161**: 104–7.

Dare, C. and Eisler, I. (1992) Family therapy for anorexia nervosa, in P.J. Cooper and A. Stein (eds) *Feeding Problems and Eating Disorders in Children and Adolescents.* Reading: Harwood.

Eisler, I. (1995) Family models of eating disorders, in G. Smukler, C. Dare and J. Treasure (eds) *Handbook of Eating Disorders.* Chichester: John Wiley.

Fairburn, C.G, Cooper, Z., Doll, H.A and Welch, S.L. (1999) Risk factors for anorexia nervosa: three integrated case comparisons. *Archives of General Psychiatry* **56**: 468–76.

Garner, D.M. and Garfinkel, P.E. (eds) (1997) *Handbook of Treatment for Eating Disorders* (2nd edn). New York and London: Guilford Press.

Gull, W.W. (1874) Anorexia nervosa (apepsia hysterica, anorexia nervosa hysterica). *Transactions of the Clinical Society of London* **7**: 22–8.

Keel, P.K., Mitchell, J.E., Miller, K.B., Davis, T.L. and Crow, S.J. (1999) Long term outcome of bulimia nervosa. *Archives of General Psychiatry* **56**: 63–9.

Liburd, J.D.A. (2001) Eating disorder: anorexia. *eMedicine Journal* **2**(9): 1–13.

Mahon, J. (2000) Dropping out from psychological treatment from eating disorders: What are the issues? *European Eating Disorders Review* **8**(3): 198–216.

Miller, W.R. and Rollnick, S. (1991) *Motivational Interviewing: Preparing People for Change to Addictive Behaviours.* New York and London: Guilford Press.

Minuchin, S., Rosman, B.L. and Baker, L. (1978) *Psychosomatic Families: Anorexia Nervosa in context.* Cambridge, Mass: Harvard University Press.

National Collaborating Centre for Mental Health (2004) *Eating Disorders: Core interventions in the treatment and management of anorexia nervosa, bulimia nervosa and related eating disorders.* Leicester: British Psychological Society.

Palmer, R. (1989) *Anorexia Nervosa: A Guide for Sufferers and their Families.* London: Penguin.

Palmer, R. (2000) *Helping People with Eating Disorders: A Clinical Guide to Assessment and Treatment.* Chichester: Wiley.

Pawluck, D.E. and Gorey, K.M. (1998). Secular trends in the incidence of anorexia nervosa: integrative review of population-based studies. *Psychiatry Research* **119**(2): 145–54.

Robinson, P.H. and McHugh, P.R. (1995) A physiology of starvation that sustains eating disorders, in G. Smukler, C. Dare and J. Treasure (eds) *Handbook of Eating Disorders.* Chichester: John Wiley.

Russell, G.F.M. (1979) Bulimia nervosa: an ominent variant of anorexia nervosa nervosa? *Psychological Medicine* **9**: 429–48.

Sayetta, R.B. (1996) Pica: an overview. *American Family Physician* **7**: 174–5.

Schmidt, U. and Treasure, J. (1998) *Getting Better Bit(e) by Bit(e).* London: Lawrence Erlbaum Associates.

Schmidt, U., Humfress, H. and Treasure, J. (1997) The role of general family environment and sexual and physical abuse in the origins of eating disorders. *European Eating Disorders Review* **5**: 184–207.

Stice, E. (2002) Risk and maintenance factors for eating pathology: A meta-analytic review. *Psychological Bulletin* **128**: 825–48.

Striegel-Moore, R.H., Silberstein, L.R. and Rodin, J. (1986). Towards an understanding of risk factors for bulimia. *American Psychology* **41**(3): 246–63.

Strober, M. (1995) Family genetic perspectives on anorexia nervosa and bulimia nervosa, in K.D. Brownell and C.G. Fairburn (eds) *Eating disorders and obesity: A comprehensive handbook.* London: Guilford Press.

Szmukler, G.I., Young, G.P., Miller, G., Lichtenstein, M. and Binns, D.S. (1995) A controlled trial of cisapride in anorexia nervosa. *International Journal of Eating Disorders* **17**: 345–57.

Tozzi, F., Sullivan, P., Fear, J., McKenzie, J. and Bulik, C.M. (2003) Causes and recovery in anorexia nervosa: The client's perspective. *International Journal of Eating Disorders* **33**: 143–54.

Treasure, J. and Holland, A. (1995) Genetic factors in eating disorders (2000). Longitudinal predictors of binge eating, intense dieting and weight concerns in a national sample of women. *Behavior Therapy* **31**: 221–35.

Van Hoeken, D., Lucas, A. and Hoek, H. (1998). Epidemiology, in H.W. Hoek, J.L. Treasure and M.A. Katzman (eds) *Neurobiology in the Treatment of Eating Disorders.* New York: Wiley, pp. 97–126.

Vogelantz-Holm, N., Wonderlich S.A, Lewis, B. *et al.* (2000) Longitudinal predictors of binge eating, intense dieting, and weight concerns in a national sample of women. *Behaviour Therapy* **31**: 221–35.

Wade, T.D., Bulik, C.M., Neale, M. and Kendler, M.D. (2000) Anorexia nervosa and major depression: shared genetic and environmental risk factors. *American Journal of Psychiatry* **157**: 469–71.

Walsh, B.T. and Devlin, M.J. (1998) Eating disorders: progress and problems. *Science* **280**(5368): 1387–90.

Welch, S.L., Doll, H.A. and Fairburn, C.G. (1997) Life events and the onset of bulimia nervosa; a controlled study. *Psychological Medicine* **27**: 515–22.

World Health Organization (1992) *International Statistical Classification of Diseases and Related Health Problems*, 10th Revision (ICD-10). Geneva: WHO.

CHAPTER 22

The person with co-existing mental health and substance misuse problems ('dual diagnosis')

Cheryl Kipping

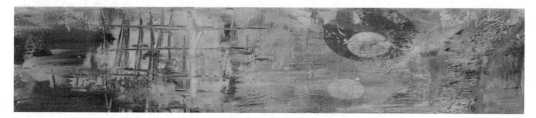

Chapter overview

Dual diagnosis has been identified as one of the most challenging clinical problems faced by mental health services (DH 2004). This chapter begins with an examination of terms and concepts associated with dual diagnosis and substance misuse. The possible relationships between substance misuse and mental illness are examined, as are the clinical difficulties encountered by people with a dual diagnosis and the challenges faced by service providers. Detailed descriptions of commonly misused substances and an overview of the foundations for working with people with a dual diagnosis are described before specific assessment and treatment issues are considered.

This chapter covers:

- Introduction and overview of dual diagnosis and substance misuse;
- Commonly misused substances, modes of use, effects and complications;
- Assessment and treatment.

Introduction

Although substance misuse has traditionally been thought of as a specialist area of mental health practice it is now accepted that *all* mental health professionals need knowledge and skills in this area. This is because drug and/or alcohol use is common among people with mental health problems and, regardless of clinical area, practitioners will inevitably work with people who are misusing substances. The National Director of Mental Health has stated that provision for dual diagnosis should be central to modern mental health care (University of Manchester 2006). Nurses have a key role in achieving this goal. The Chief Nursing Officer's Review of Mental Health Nursing (DH 2006a) recommended that mental health nurses in all settings be able to respond to the needs of people with a dual diagnosis. This chapter focuses on working with people who misuse substances as a core component of mental health care provision.

Concepts and terminology

'Dual diagnosis' has been adopted as a convenient term for the coexistence of mental health and substance misuse problems. Some people think this is unhelpful because of its link to the medical model and focus on two problem areas – mental health and substance misuse – when in reality people with a 'dual diagnosis' usually have multiple needs, for example housing, financial, physical. The term 'complex needs' is sometimes used as an alternative. This points to the range of needs which people with a dual diagnosis often have and the challenges faced by service users, carers and service providers. Despite its limitations, given its widespread usage, 'dual diagnosis' will be used in this chapter.

Focusing more specifically on substance mis/use, substance use is a broad concept. Use in itself may not be problematic. Many people experiment with substances or use them on a recreational basis. However, adverse physical, psychological, psychiatric, interpersonal, social or legal consequences are often experienced, particularly with regular use. The 'problem', however, may not be perceived as such by users but may be by those close to them or the wider society. Substance misuse can be thought of as use that is not socially or medically approved, or which is illegal. What is socially acceptable, medically approved or illegal in one culture, or at one point in time, may not be in another or at another time. Although a distinction is often made between drugs and alcohol, alcohol is a drug which happens to be legal. Other legal drugs include tobacco and caffeine – while caffeine is socially acceptable, tobacco is becoming less so.

Dependence has a more precise meaning, suggesting a compulsion to continue taking a substance on a regular, repetitive basis. Physical dependence indicates that the person's body has adapted to repeated doses of the drug and withholding it will result in withdrawal symptoms. Some substances do not create physical dependence but do create psychological dependence. Specific criteria for a diagnosis of substance dependence are identified in the DSM-IV (Diagnostic and Statistical Manual of Mental Disorders) (American Psychiatric Association 1994) and ICD-10 (International Classification of Diseases) (World Health Organization 1992). Criteria for a diagnosis of 'substance abuse' (DSM-IV) and 'harmful substance use' (ICD-10) have also been identified.

Reflecting on one's views about substance misuse can be important. Negative attitudes towards people who use substances have been identified as a potential barrier to working effectively with this group. Regardless of personal opinion, people who use substances should receive high quality care and are entitled to the same care and respect as others (DH 2006a; NICE 2007a).

Overview of dual diagnosis

Defining dual diagnosis as the coexistence of mental health and substance misuse disorders may seem straightforward but the range of people who might be categorized in this way is diverse. The Department of Health (DH 2002) has suggested that the scope of dual diagnosis can be conceptualized as two intersecting continua, where one represents severity of mental illness and the other severity of substance misuse (Figure 22.1). Personality disorder is conceptualized as a separate dimension, which can coexist with a mental illness, a substance misuse problem, or both.

Severity of substance misuse

High	
e.g. dependent drinker who experiences anxiety	e.g. a person with schizophrenia who smokes cannabis on a daily basis

Severity of mental illness

Low	**High**
e.g. recreational user of ecstasy who has begun to experience low mood after weekend use	e.g. a person with bipolar disorder whose occasional binge drinking destabilized their mental state
	Low

Figure 22.1 Scope of coexistent psychiatric and substance misuse disorder (Department of Health 2002)

Further complexity is added when the relationship(s) between mental illness and substance misuse is considered. Crome (1999) has suggested that:

- substance use or withdrawal can produce psychiatric symptoms or illness;
- dependence, intoxication or withdrawal can produce psychological symptoms;
- psychiatric disorder can lead to a substance misuse disorder;
- substance misuse may exacerbate a pre-existing psychiatric disorder.

In clinical practice it can be difficult to identify which of these mechanisms is operating.

Research studies conducted to establish the prevalence of dual diagnosis vary in their definitions of mental illness and substance misuse, their sample selection, measurement tools and timeframes. It is generally accepted that 30–50 per cent of people with a severe mental illness also have substance misuse problems. Summaries of prevalence studies conducted with mental health populations are available in Banerjee *et al.* (2002) and Maslin (2003). Substance misuse services also work with large numbers of people with a dual diagnosis. Rates of coexisting mental health problems of 75 per cent or more have been found (Weaver *et al.* 2002). Psychiatric diagnoses among this population tend to be anxiety and mood disorders.

People with a dual diagnosis are a vulnerable group. In comparison to people with a mental illness alone, people who also use substances have:

- higher rates of homelessness;
- increased rates of suicidal behaviour;
- increased rates of violence;
- worsening of their psychiatric symptoms;
- poorer adherence with medication;
- increased rates of HIV and hepatitis infection;
- greater contact with the criminal justice system;
- make greater use of institutional services (e.g. Banerjee *et al.* 2002; DH 2002).

Three service models have been identified for working with this group: serial, parallel and integrated. In the serial model mental health and substance misuse disorders are treated consecutively by different services. Each expects the person to deal with the other 'problem' first. In the parallel model, mental health and substance misuse interventions are provided by the two services concurrently. In the integrated model mental health and substance misuse interventions are provided concurrently, in the same setting, by one team. This is the model advocated by the Department of Health (DH 2002) and in the dual diagnosis literature (e.g. Drake *et al.* 2001; Mueser *et al.* 2003; Graham 2004). Although there is some evidence to supports this model the Cochrane review, which considered 25 randomized controlled trials that evaluated interventions designed to meet the needs of people with a severe mental illness and substance misuse problem, was inconclusive. It noted that there was no compelling evidence to support any one psychosocial treatment over another in reducing substance use or improving mental state (Cleary *et al.* 2008).

Reasons for substance use and aetiological theories

People have many reasons for using substances regardless of whether or not they have mental health problems. These include: dealing with negative feelings or situations (e.g. anger, anxiety, boredom, lack of sleep, blocking out past painful experiences, avoiding withdrawal symptoms); promoting positive feelings (e.g. enjoying the 'buzz', to give energy, aid relaxation, boost confidence) and responding to social pressures (e.g. it is the norm within the peer group).

In people with mental health problems the notion of 'self-medication' has received particular attention. A literature review conducted by Phillips and Johnson (2001) found evidence of people using drugs to self-medicate negative symptoms, mood problems, anxiety and insomnia but the findings related to managing positive symptoms and medication side effects were inconsistent.

Several theoretical models have been proposed to explain the high levels of comorbid substance misuse and mental health problems. These include:

■ common factor – a common vulnerability factor increases the risk of mental illness and substance misuse (e.g. genetic, childhood sexual abuse);
■ secondary substance misuse – mental illness is a vulnerability factor for substance misuse;
■ secondary psychiatric illness – mental illness develops as a consequence of substance misuse;
■ bidirectional, both disorders are present and likely to interact.

While these models provide a conceptual framework for understanding co-morbidity evidence to support them is equivocal (Mueser *et al.* 1998; Phillips and Johnson 2001).

Commonly misused substances

This section identifies commonly misused substances, describes how they are used, their effects, complications and categorization under the Misuse of Drugs Act 1971. This knowledge underpins assessment, care planning and treatment interventions. Having an understanding of the language associated with substance misuse can also be useful. Some drug users' jargon is included, indicated by the word being in italics and inverted commas (for example, *'gear'*). Substances most commonly used by people with mental health problems are alcohol, cannabis and stimulant drugs (e.g. cocaine, crack cocaine, amphetamine) (Maslin 2003; Graham 2004).

Alcohol

Alcohol is widely available and over 90 per cent of adults drink. Alcoholic drinks come in different strengths, indicated by the 'alcohol by volume' (ABV), the percentage of the total liquid that is alcohol. Consumption can be measured in units. One unit is the equivalent of half a pint of standard strength beer (3–4% ABV), a pub measure of spirits (40% ABV) or a small (125 ml) glass of wine (8–10% ABV). However over recent years the strength of many drinks and the size of glasses has increased. So, for example, half a pint of 5% ABV beer is 1.4 units and a 175 ml glass of wine of 12% ABV is two units. Units can be calculated by multiplying the volume of the drink in millilitres by the percentage ABV and dividing by 1000.

$$\text{Units} = \frac{\text{volume of drink in millilitres} \times \text{ABV}}{1000}$$

Unit calculators can be obtained free of charge from www.drinkawaretrust.org.uk or the Department of Health Publications orderline: www.orderline.dh.gov.uk/ecom_dh/public/home.jsf Type alcohol into the keyword prompt. Government advice on 'sensible' drinking levels (i.e. levels unlikely to cause significant harm to self or others) is that men should not regularly drink more that three to four units daily and women more than two to three. Pregnant women are encouraged to avoid alcohol (DH *et al.* 2007).

The effects of alcohol will depend on how much the person is used to drinking. Tolerance develops (i.e. more is needed to gain the same effect). With small amounts the person is likely to feel less inhibited, more sociable and relaxed. Their heart rate will increase and they may appear flushed (due to vasodilation). As consumption increases slurred speech and a lack of coordination may be evident. The drinker's emotions may become labile. With heavy use the person may experience double vision, stagger, lose balance and lose consciousness. Severe intoxication may result in vomiting which can prevent fatal overdose but impaired consciousness can lead to death if vomit is inhaled.

With regular, heavy use some people become physically dependent and, in the absence of alcohol, experience withdrawal symptoms, typically in the morning, when the alcohol level in their body has fallen. Restlessness, sweatiness, shaking, nausea and vomiting are common symptoms. Delirium tremens, a state characterized by rapid pulse, raised blood pressure, feverishness, sweating, shaking, confusion, disorientation, agitation, hallucinations, and sometimes also paranoid delusions may be experienced. Typically this occurs about 24 hours after the last drink. Seizures are another complication of alcohol withdrawal. These occur in 5–15 per cent of dependent drinkers, 7 to 48 hours after stopping drinking. Delirium tremens and withdrawal seizures can be fatal (Edwards *et al.* 2003).

While some people drink heavily every day, others drink in binges. A binge is defined as more that six units a day for a women and more than eight for a man. Many people drink at much higher levels. Patterns of binges vary, for example, some people will drink heavily for several weeks and remain abstinent for several months, others drink heavily for two- or three-day periods and remain abstinent throughout the remainder of the week. Even this latter pattern can pose health risks. A range of mental and physical health problems are associated with heavy alcohol use. Depression is common, but it can be difficult to assess whether this is independent of, or secondary to, alcohol use. If abstinence is achieved and the depression is secondary to drinking, symptoms should improve after two to three weeks. A similar picture exists with anxiety. Many drinkers experience problems with both.

The risk of suicide is high in people with alcohol problems. The depressive symptoms associated with drinking can be a trigger, and, when intoxicated, inhibitions are likely to be reduced, making people more likely to act on suicidal thoughts. To add to these risks, various factors which can be typical of the lifestyles of problem drinkers are associated with suicidal thoughts: having major financial problems (spending money on alcohol can become the priority); difficulties with the police or courts (through alcohol-related convictions); problems with close friends/relatives (the person's drinking may create tensions and arguments); and a lack of social support (relationships break down) (Meltzer *et al.* 2002). Alcohol, in combination with other drugs which are central nervous system (CNS) depressants, significantly increases the risk of intentional and accidental overdose.

Other health problems associated with heavy drinking include: brain damage (which may be irreversible), gastritis, pancreatitis, ulcers, oesophageal varices, peripheral neuropathy, liver damage (for example, alcoholic hepatitis, cirrhosis), Wernicke's encephalopathy and Korsakoff's syndrome. 'Black outs', transient memory loss induced by intoxication, can be experienced by both dependent and non-dependent drinkers. Some people have total memory loss for a period of time, which may last from a few hours to several days.

Because alcohol affects judgement and coordination, drinkers may be particularly prone to accidents, potentially putting themselves and others at risk of harm. Some of the social consequences of drinking have been highlighted. Others include: school exclusion, lost employment, violence (within and outside the home), neglect of children, engaging in unsafe sex, drinking and driving, homelessness (e.g. Alcohol Concern 2000). Women who drink when pregnant risk complications and damage to their unborn child.

Opiates

Opiates are derived from the opium poppy. Synthetically produced opiates are known as opioids. Therapeutically these drugs can be used as painkillers (for example, pethidine, dihydrocodeine), cough suppressants (for example, codeine linctus) and anti-diarrhoea agents (for example, kaolin and morphine mixture). Methadone and buprenorphine are opioids used to treat opiate dependency.

Although all opiates have misuse potential, heroin is the most widely misused and will be the focus here. It is a class A drug under the Misuse of Drugs Act. People caught in possession, or dealing may face imprisonment. Heroin ('*gear*', '*smack*', '*brown*', '*scag*') is a brownish white powder that can be snorted, smoked or injected. Smoking ('*chasing*', '*booting*') involves placing heroin on aluminium foil and heating it. The vapours given off are inhaled through a tube. Occasionally heroin is mixed with tobacco and smoked in a cigarette. To prepare heroin for injection it is mixed in a spoon with water and citric acid (to help dissolve the powder) and heated. The liquid preparation is drawn up into a syringe through a filter, often a cigarette filter, which removes undissolved material. Heroin can then be injected into the tissue under the skin ('*skinpopping*'), into muscle, or into a vein (intravenous use). Many heroin users never inject. Of those that do, it is common to start by smoking and move to injecting as tolerance develops.

Heroin is usually bought in '*bags*'. It induces feelings of well-being, warmth and relaxation. The initial euphoria ('*buzz*'), particularly following intravenous use, is intense. When intoxicated, the person is likely to have small '*pinned*' pupils, heavy eyelids, and appear drowsy. With repeated use physical and psychological dependence develop. Heroin is then needed to stave off withdrawal symptoms: dilated pupils, watery eyes, sneezing, runny nose, yawning, goose flesh, feeling cold and shivery, muscle aches and cramps, diarrhoea and vomiting, raised pulse, blood pressure and respiratory rate. Symptoms begin 6–8 hours after last use and peak 32–72 hours after. While they can be very distressing, they are not life-threatening but the discomfort experienced can be a strong motivator to use again. Not all heroin users become physically dependent, but for many, heroin becomes the focus of their life. Everything else (for example, relationships, possessions, paying bills, self-care, eating) becomes less important. Borrowing, stealing from family and friends, selling possessions, involvement in prostitution, drug dealing, and a range of other criminal activities from shoplifting to armed robbery are all ways in which money may be raised to fund use.

Although heroin itself does not have an adverse effect on mental state, psychological and psychiatric symptoms are common in opiate misusers. The National Treatment Outcome Research Study (Gossop *et al.* 2001), which followed the progress of 1075 primarily opiate users, reported that, at the start of the study, anxiety and depressive mood were 'common'. Furthermore, 29 per cent of the sample had thought about suicide in the previous three months, 10 per cent had received psychiatric inpatient treatment (for a problem other than drug dependence) in the past two years and 14 per cent had received community psychiatric treatment. Lifestyle factors such as those outlined above may contribute, as may underlying problems, for example, childhood sexual abuse.

Death from accidental overdose is another possible consequence of heroin use. This risk increases if the person is injecting, using other CNS depressant drugs or has a reduced level of tolerance (for example, after a period of abstinence in a treatment programme). Variability in the purity of illicit heroin means that overdose is always a risk. As with alcohol, other accidents may be precipitated due to slowed reactions.

Intravenous use brings further complications. Sharing injecting equipment (this includes spoons, filters and water, as well as needles and syringes) may result in blood-borne virus transmission (e.g. HIV and hepatitis B and C). Puncturing the skin to inject can introduce bacteria into the body causing local or systemic infections (for example abscesses or septicaemia). Vein damage and thromboses are further complications. In the early stages of use people generally inject into veins in their arms but as these collapse they move to other sites. It is not uncommon for people to inject into their groin. This can be particularly dangerous as there is a risk of hitting an artery or nerve rather than the vein.

Smoking heroin can precipitate or exacerbate respiratory problems. Other health concerns associated with opiate use are constipation, reduced libido and amenorrhoea. Women who continue to use during pregnancy risk their baby being opiate dependent.

Methadone (physeptone) and buprenorphine are used in the treatment of opiate dependency (NICE 2007a, c). Both have misuse potential. Methadone is available in liquid, tablet and injectable form but is most commonly prescribed in its liquid formulation. Risk of overdose is particularly high during the first two weeks of initiation onto methadone due to methadone toxicity (DH (England) and the devolved administrations 2007). Complications can also arise from injecting liquid and tablet formulations. Buprenorphine comes as a sublingual tablet. Overdose is possible with both drugs, particularly when used in combination with other CNS depressants.

Benzodiazepines

Benzodiazepines are prescribed for their therapeutic effects in relieving anxiety and promoting sleep, as a muscle relaxant and an anticonvulsant. Diazepam, temazepam and nitrazepam are examples. Benzodiazepines are most commonly available in tablet form but when misused may be injected (after crushing). Tolerance develops to both therapeutic and non-therapeutic effects. Physical and psychological dependence can occur. Benzodiazepines are class C drugs.

Benzodiazepines may be misused by the person to whom they were prescribed, or by others who have obtained illicit supplies. Reasons for use include: the effects they have if used alone (relieving anxiety, inducing feelings of calmness and relaxation, inducing sleep); enhancing the effect of other substances (for example opiates and alcohol); countering the effects of stimulant drugs; and as a substitute for, or to help cope with withdrawal symptoms of, other substances.

In excess, benzodiazepines cause drowsiness, slurred speech, poor coordination and a glassy-eyed appearance (with dilated pupils). When taken in high doses some people experience a paradoxical effect, characterized by aggression and hostility. Withdrawal symptoms include: anxiety, sweating, tremor, irritability, headache, nausea, insomnia and perceptual distortions. Sudden cessation of benzodiazepines in someone who has used high doses for a lengthy time period can induce withdrawal seizures.

Anxiety disorders are common in people who misuse benzodiazepines. Detoxification can be extremely difficult as anxiety is also a withdrawal symptom and people are likely to be highly anxious about detoxification.

As with other CNS depressants a risk of accidents is associated with use. Overdose is possible but unlikely to be fatal unless other CNS depressants are taken. Injecting potentially brings the problems associated with intravenous use outlined above. There is a risk to the foetus if pregnant women continue to use heavily.

Stimulants

Stimulant drugs include amphetamine, cocaine and crack cocaine. Some amphetamine and amphetamine-like drugs are used therapeutically. For example, dexamphetamine (dexedrine) and methylphenidate (ritalin) are prescribed for children with attention deficit hyperactivity disorder.

Amphetamine sulphate ('*speed*', '*whizz*', '*sulphate*') is illicitly produced amphetamine. It is a whitish (pink/grey) powder that can be snorted, swallowed or injected. Other forms of amphetamine are amphetamine base and methylamphetamine (or methamphetamine), ('*ice*', '*crystal meth*'). Amphetamine is a class B drug unless prepared for injection when it becomes a class A. Crystal meth has been classified as a class A.

Amphetamines cause arousal (increasing heart and respiratory rate), and dilate the pupils. Users seek the feelings of alertness, energy, confidence, exhilaration and reduced fatigue which the drug brings. To the observer they are likely to appear excitable, speak rapidly and have poor concentration. Appetite will be diminished. The effects last three to four hours. Following repeated use, tolerance and psychological dependence may develop.

Cocaine ('*coke*', '*charlie*') is a white powder that is usually snorted but can be injected, swallowed or smoked. When cocaine powder is dissolved in water and heated with baking soda small crystals of crack cocaine ('*rocks*' or '*stones*') are produced. Crack is usually smoked using a crack pipe (often made from a plastic water bottle or cola can) where the rock is heated and the vapours inhaled. It can also be injected. Cocaine and crack are class A drugs.

Like amphetamine, crack and cocaine produce physiological arousal and feelings of well-being, alertness and exhilaration. The effects are much shorter than those of amphetamine, reaching a peak after about 20–30 minutes for cocaine, and almost immediately for crack. This means that it must be used frequently to sustain the effect.

A range of psychological and psychiatric complications are associated with stimulant use. In contrast to the desired effects, users may experience anxiety, agitation, irritability and restlessness. After regular, repeated use a '*come down*' or '*crash*', typified by feelings of lethargy, sleepiness and depression, is common as the body adjusts to the absence of the drug. The depression can be severe and suicide is a risk.

A drug-induced psychosis may be precipitated. This would usually follow high levels of use over several days and be characterized by hallucinations, feelings of paranoia and delusions. Symptoms resolve as the drug is eliminated from the body. In people with pre-existing mental disorders stimulant use may precipitate relapse.

Crack users who are smoking are prone to respiratory problems due to the build-up of fluids in the lungs. Wheezing, shortness of breath, coughing and chest pains are common, a condition known as 'crack lung'. Cardiovascular problems such as high blood pressure, irregular heartbeat and strokes can occur with both cocaine and crack. Seizures may also occur with high levels of use.

Prolonged use of any stimulants can have detrimental effects on the user's general physical health due to lack of food and sleep. When injected the problems associated with intravenous drug use can occur. Use during pregnancy may bring complications for mother and child.

Significant amounts of money may be required to sustain use, particularly of cocaine or crack, and people may engage in a variety of illegal activities to raise money. Gun crime has particularly been associated with crack use.

Cannabis

Although not widely available for therapeutic use research into the medicinal benefits of tetrahydrocannabinols (THC), the psychoactive ingredient in cannabis, is in progress. 'Savitex', a treatment for neuropathic pain in people with multiple sclerosis, is now available.

Cannabis can come as a green/brown block of compressed resin ('*hash*', '*blow*', '*draw*') or as herbal cannabis, the leaves, stalks and seeds of the plant ('*marijuana*', '*grass*', '*weed*'). '*Skunk*' is a particularly strong variety. Cannabis is usually smoked with tobacco in a '*joint*' or '*spliff*', but can be smoked in a pipe. It can also be made into a tea or eaten. Cannabis is the most commonly used illicit drug in the UK. Debate continues about the appropriate classification of cannabis. At the time of writing it is class C but is due for reclassification to class B in 2009.

The effects of cannabis depend to a large extent on the expectations and mood of the user and the amount taken. Effects start within a few minutes and may last several hours. Feelings of relaxation, euphoria and a greater appreciation of sensory experiences are commonly described. When intoxicated cognitive and motor skills will be impaired.

Psychological dependence on cannabis can develop and withdrawal symptoms, including restlessness, anxiety, irritability and insomnia, have been documented. Cannabis induces feelings of anxiety and paranoia in some users. Use can precipitate psychotic episodes and exacerbate pre-existing psychiatric symptoms. There is now strong evidence to indicate that cannabis use increases the risk of developing a psychotic illness such as schizophrenia and the greater the level of use the greater the risk. There is also evidence to suggest that cannabis use increases the risk of affective disorders. See Castle and Murray (2004) for a comprehensive overview of the psychiatry and neuroscience of cannabis and Moore *et al.* (2007) for a systematic review of the research literature on cannabis use and mental illness.

The physical health problems associated with cannabis are mainly those linked to smoking tobacco. Use during pregnancy is associated with low birth weight. For further information about the effect of substance misuse during pregnancy see Johnson *et al.* (2003).

Other substances which may be used by people with mental health problems include: ecstasy, khat (quat), LSD, solvents/gases and ketamine. Information about these and other substances can be found at www.drugscope.org.uk and www.talktofrank.com.

Assessment and treatment

Foundations for working with people with a dual diagnosis

Before considering specific assessment and treatment issues attention will be given to the foundations upon which work with people with a dual diagnosis is based. An integration of principles from the mental health and substance misuse fields is required (Osher and Kofoed 1989; Drake *et al.* 2001; DH 2002; Graham 2004). This is because people's substance misuse and mental health will almost certainly impact on each other so working on one area in isolation from the other is unlikely to be effective. 'Closing the Gap' the dual diagnosis capability framework (Hughes 2006) identifies capabilities required for working with this group across three domains: values, knowledge and skills, and practice development, and at three levels: core, generalist and specialist. Level two, 'generalist', capabilities are required by post-qualification staff in regular contact with people with a dual diagnosis.

The values associated with motivational interviewing (MI) (Miller and Rollnick 2002) build on those identified in the capability framework (accepting that working with people with dual diagnosis is part of one's role, maintaining therapeutic optimism, accepting the uniqueness of the individual, being non-judgemental and empathic) and can be seen as essential for working effectively with this group. In addition to these core values, to provide a framework to inform assessment and treatment, an understanding of Prochaska and DiClemente's transtheoretical model of change (1986) and Osher and Kofoed's (1989) staged treatment model is required.

Core values: the spirit of motivational interviewing

MI is a counselling and communication style, which, at its heart, is 'a way of being with people' (Miller and Rollnick 2002: 34). MI is collaborative, the nurse works in partnership with, and respects the autonomy of, the service user. Service users make choices about whether or not to make changes and if they do, what those changes will be. The decision to change is contingent on the person's motivation to attain desired values and goals. The nurse's role is to help elicit motivation. Although specific techniques are associated with MI, Miller and Rollnick argue that the 'spirit' is more important that the techniques.

The spirit of MI contrasts with the way in which mental health professionals often work with people with a dual diagnosis. MI does not confront people, suggest that they are 'in denial' or 'unmotivated', or advocate that the professional takes an expert stance advising what should be done and persuading service users to follow the solutions proposed. Rather the service user is seen as the expert about their own situation. Evidence suggests that the nature of the relationship between the nurse and service user is important to treatment effectiveness, a confrontational approach is associated with poorer outcomes (e.g. Miller and Rollnick 2002; Raistrick *et al.* 2006).

As well as being an essential component for working with people with a dual diagnosis (e.g. Barrowclough *et al.* 2001; Drake *et al.* 2001) MI is a skill which mental health nurses should possess (DH 2006b).

Transtheoretical model of change

Prochaska and DiClemente's (1986) model of change is widely used in the substance misuse field but is applicable to any type of behaviour change (Figure 22.2). Change is seen as a process where the person moves from precontemplation, where their behaviour is not seen as problematic and change is therefore not considered, through contemplation, where there is some acknowledgement of difficulties and the possibility of change is considered, on to preparation/determination where plans to make change are made, and then action when change is made. Finally maintenance concerns sustaining long-term change. Of course, people are often unable to maintain change and relapse. Because both mental illness and substance misuse are chronic relapsing conditions people may move backwards and forwards round the cycle several times (Prochaska *et al.* 1992) and a long-term perspective, often several years, is therefore needed (Drake *et al.* 2001).

Understanding where the person is in the change process is important as this will inform the approach taken and interventions used.

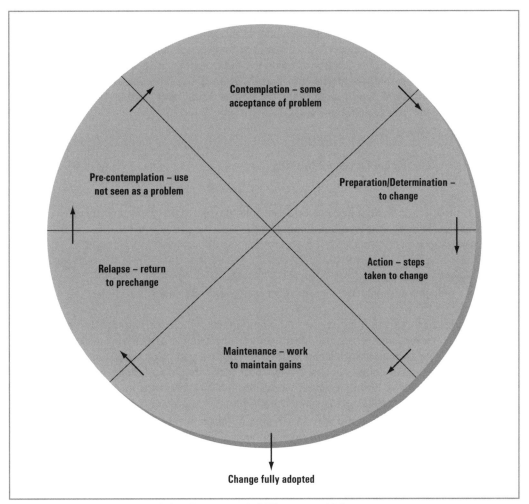

Figure 22.2 Cycle of change (After Prochaska & DiClemente 1986)

Staged treatment model

Osher and Kofoed's (1989) model for working with people with a dual diagnosis comprises four stages: engagement, persuasion, active treatment and relapse prevention. These reflect

Prochaska and DiClemente's stages of change and provide a framework for identifying specific interventions appropriate to the change stage. See Figure 22.3. More detail is provided later.

Knowledge about the substances which people are using, an approach underpinned by the core values identified, and an understanding of the cycle of change and staged treatment model provide the foundations for working with people with a dual diagnosis. The next section looks more specifically at assessment.

Assessment

Assessment should not be thought of as separate from treatment as it can be important for engaging the person, building a therapeutic relationship, providing information and advice, and enhancing motivation. Assessment of substance use should be integral to any mental health assessment (DH 2002) but evidence indicates that it is often inadequately assessed and therefore under-detected (e.g. Barnby *et al.* 2003; Noordsy *et al.* 2003). This may result in misdiagnosis and inappropriate treatment (Carey and Correia 1998).

Key components of a comprehensive assessment are:

■ current and recent use;
■ past use;
■ physical health (including sexual health);
■ mental health;
■ prescribed medication;
■ social situation (including accommodation, relationships, family circumstances – especially children, employment, finances);
■ legal situation;
■ personal and family history;
■ risk assessment;
■ client's perception of situation, reasons for using and motivation for change.

The remainder of this section focuses on the components which are particularly pertinent to substance use: current and recent use; past use; and the client's perception, reasons for using and motivation for change. As indicated, substance misuse can have significant physical, mental, social and legal complications; evidence of these should be sought and this information incorporated into that which would routinely be obtained for other assessment domains. Risk assessment and management are extremely important when working with this group. As well as considering the way in which substance misuse may increase risks such as suicide and violence, it is important to take account of risks specifically associated with substance misuse such as withdrawal seizures and blood-borne viruses. The impact which parental substance misuse can have on children should also be considered. Risk management plans should incorporate the full range of risks.

Assessment is an ongoing process. It will take time to build a full picture of the person's use, the way it has developed over time and its impact on various aspects of the person's life. Furthermore, patterns of use change so assessment of substance use needs to be regularly reviewed.

Current and recent use

Information about which substances are being used, the quantity and frequency of use, route of administration and length of time the person has been using at the current level is needed. People should be asked about alcohol and drugs – illicit and prescribed. Prompting for specific substances and further questioning to gain clarification (for example, what type/strength of lager is consumed, whether prescribed medication is taken as directed) may be necessary. If a person is injecting, information about the injection site(s), whether they share equipment, and whether they know where to obtain clean equipment should be obtained. Injection sites should be inspected.

Taking a history of the past five to seven days use, starting with 'today' and working back can indicate whether the person's use is reasonably stable from day to day, or fluctuating. A more detailed picture of use over the course of the day may also be desirable (for example, establishing what time drinking usually begins, whether it continues steadily throughout the day, or whether there are breaks). Other factors which may influence patterns of use should also be explored, for example, use may be heavy after receipt of benefit payments, the person may use one drug to counteract the effects of another.

Details of withdrawal symptoms are needed to establish whether or not the person is physically dependent on any substances. Previous experiences of withdrawal seizures and delirium tremens should be noted, as should any overdoses (accidental and intentional). Information about how use is funded should also be obtained.

Observation of the person's physical appearance and non-verbal communication is integral to assessment. Factors to observe include: whether there are signs of intoxication or withdrawal, evidence of injuries, signs of jaundice, whether the person appears underweight, they are dishevelled or unkempt, agitated or anxious. Objective tests provide another important source of information, for example, urinalysis, breathalyser readings and blood tests (e.g. liver function).

Throughout the assessment process opportunities for providing health education/harm minimization information (for example, advising alcohol-dependent people not to stop drinking immediately because of the risk of withdrawal seizures and delirium tremens, advising on safer injecting practices) should be taken.

Past use

A substance misuse history will be required. This should establish when the person began taking each of the substances they have used (or are currently using), what prompted use, how it developed over time, its impact on different aspects of the person's life (for example, education and employment, relationships, finances, physical and mental health, contact with the criminal justice system), whether there have been periods of abstinence, how these were achieved and maintained, and details of any previous substance misuse treatment (what was provided, what was helpful and the outcome). Bringing together a chronological account of a person's substance misuse and mental health history in a 'time line' may provide insights into the interrelationship of the two.

Client's perception of situation, reasons for use and motivation to change

Information about the person's perception of their situation and motivation to change is likely to emerge during the assessment and, on the basis of this, their position on Prochaska and

DiClementi's cycle of change can be identified. For example, a person may report that he is fed up with his wife and GP nagging him about his drinking when all he does is go down to the pub with his mates a few nights each week, and his only reason for attending this appointment is to get them off his back. This man is probably at the precontemplation, or perhaps, contemplation stage (he has, at least, attended the service). Someone else might tell you that as a consequence of his drinking he has lost his job, his marriage has broken down, he is feeling depressed and his GP has told him he has liver damage. He has now had enough, wants to address his alcohol use and yesterday went to Alcoholics Anonymous. This man has probably reached the active change stage. Future work is likely to proceed very differently with these two people.

Standardized instruments

Although the most common way of obtaining assessment information is asking the person, standardized instruments may complement this process. Many have been developed for the drug and alcohol treatment population but few specifically for people with a dual diagnosis. Each instrument has a different purpose, some are screening tools, others assess problem severity and some are intended as outcome measures.

AUDIT, the Alcohol Use Disorders Identification Test (Babor et al. 1989), a widely used screening tool, assesses use in the past 12 months. It has been shown to be effective for use with people with mental health problems (Hulse et al. 2000). Other examples of screening tools are CAGE (King 1986) (alcohol), CAGE-AID (Brown and Rounds 1995) (alcohol and drugs) and MAST, Michigan Alcoholism Screening Test (Selzer 1971), all of which assess lifetime use. A particular risk when using screening tools with people with a dual diagnosis is that they may not be sufficiently sensitive to detect problematic use. As use is often low in this population scores may not meet the threshold criteria, but even low level use can have serious consequences for people with severe mental illness. The DALI, Dartmouth Assessment of Lifestyle Instrument (Rosenberg et al. 1998) is a drug and alcohol screening tool designed for people with a dual diagnosis. Although validated in the USA its use in a medium secure setting in the UK was found to be limited (Ford 2003).

Examples of tools which assess the severity of substance misuse problem are SADQ, Severity of Alcohol Dependence Questionnaire (Stockwell et al. 1983) and the LDQ, Leeds Dependence Questionnaire (Raistrick et al. 1994). The LDQ has been shown to be valid for use with people with a severe mental illness (Ford 2003). The Drug Use Scale – Revised, and Alcohol Use Scale – Revised (Mueser et al. 2003) assess drug and alcohol use in people with severe mental illness. Clinical case managers/care coordinators collate information from various sources and across different domains. This is scored and the person allocated to one of five categories (abstinence, use with impairment, abuse, dependence or dependence with institutionalization).

Services are increasingly being expected to report treatment outcomes. Tools which assess severity can be used to assess change over time potentially providing an indicator of treatment effectiveness. Instruments designed specifically for monitoring the outcomes of substance misuse treatment, include the Christo Inventory for Substance Misuse Services (Christo et al. 2000) and the TOP, Treatment Outcomes Profile (Marsden et al. 2007). The Time Line Follow Back uses a calendar to compile information on substance use over a period of time (Sobell and Sobell 1996) and can therefore also monitor changes over time.

Approaches to treatment using the four staged treatment model

The stages of Osher and Kofoed's (1989) treatment model provide the framework for this section. In practice, flexibility is required, movement between the stages can be fluid and aspects of the various interventions are likely to be utilized at each stage, as illustrated in Figure 22.3. The emphasis in this section is on substance misuse interventions but these cannot be seen in isolation from mental health interventions which are also crucial. Many components of treatment are essential regardless of whether the person has mental health, substance misuse or co-morbid problems, for example, provision of safe accommodation, development of meaningful daytime activity, building support networks.

Engagement

This stage focuses on development of a therapeutic alliance with the person. While some people approach services seeking help, others, often those with a severe mental illness, may not want treatment. Such people have often been difficult to engage in services. To promote engagement clinicians need to work flexibly, seeing people at times of day and locations convenient to them, such as at home or in a café. Helping sort out practical issues (for example, benefit payments, housing difficulties) can promote contact and relationship development. Although MI has been most closely associated with the persuasion stage of Osher and Kofoed's model it can be useful in engaging and retaining people in treatment (e.g. Swanson *et al.* 1999; Zuckoff and Daley 2001; Handmaker *et al.* 2002).

Focusing on substance use, and in particular reducing use, is not the main aim at this stage, rather there is an emphasis on reducing harm. Harm reduction has been defined as policies, programmes, services and actions to reduce health, social and economic harms to individuals, communities and societies (United Kingdom Harm Reduction Alliance 2007). This approach derives from the substance misuse field, where the focus has been on reducing the harms associated with injecting drug use, but the principles are applicable to other forms of substance use and to broader issues associated with mental health, e.g. homelessness, physical health, exposure to violence.

While long-term engagement and treatment will be required for many people, especially those with more severe mental health problems, in some circumstances contact between service user and service provider may be brief, for example in primary care, at a needle exchange scheme, in a community mental health team assessment clinic. Brief interventions, which focus on offering information and advice (written and verbal), and may include motivational enhancement strategies are recommended as they have a sound evidence base (e.g. Raistrick *et al.* 2006; NICE 2007b). Information provided may include: safe drinking limits, the effects various substances can have on physical and mental health, transmission routes of blood-borne infections. The acronym FRAMES has been used to summarize the elements of brief interventions (Bien *et al.* 1993).

> F – *feedback* of current status and risk.
> R – emphasis on the client having *responsibility* for change.
> A – *advice* to change.
> M – a *menu* of change options.
> E – an *empathic* manner.
> S – reinforcing the client's *self-efficacy*.

Stage of change (Prochasks and DiClemente 1986)	Treatment stage (Osher and Kofoed 1989)	Possible treatment approaches/interventions

Precontemplation	Engagement	Building relationships
		Assertive outreach
		Flexible working practices
		Identifying needs
		Address practical issues, e.g. housing, benefits
		Motivational interviewing
		Harm minimization
		Brief interventions
		Provision of information and advice
		Pharmacotherapy–for stabilization
		  of psychiatric symptoms
		Assessment of carers' needs
		Obtain initial information to begin
		  building comprehensive assessment

Contemplation	Persuasion	Continue building relationship Motivational interviewing Comprehensive assessment Building motivation Decision matrices Readiness rulers Diaries Pharmacotherapy–for psychiatric symptoms

Action	Active treatment	Motivational interviewing
		Strengthening commitment to change
		Goal setting and planning
		Solution focused approach
		Diaries
		Development of new skills and lifestyle
		  changes, e.g. budgeting, building social
		  networks, enhancing social skills, developing
		  leisure interests, developing vocational skills
		Activity scheduling
		Pharmacotherapy–for psychiatric symptoms–
		  for detox from substances: inpatient or
		  community reduction
		Adjunctive therapy to address specific
		  problems, e.g. bereavement issues, childhood
		  sexual abuse
		Self-help groups, e.g. AA, NA

Maintenance	Relapse prevention	Motivational interviewing
		Pharmacotherapy–for psychiatric symptoms–
		  for substance misuse relapse prevention
		Relapse prevention mental health and
		  substance misuse
		Day programmes, residential programmes
		Consolidation of skills and lifestyle
		  changes Self-help groups, e.g. AA, NA

Figure 22.3 Stages of change, treatment stage and possible treatment approaches/interventions

Persuasion

Once a positive relationship has been developed and regular contact established attention can be given to building motivation for change. 'Persuasion' suggests that the nurse persuades the service user to change. This is *not* the case, the person themselves needs to identify reasons for change. It is the nurse's role to elicit these. This stage matches the contemplation stage of the cycle of change, so ambivalence, being in two minds, is characteristic. There will be some reasons for making changes and others for not doing so.

All of us experience ambivalence when contemplating behaviour change. For example: 'I may want to go to the gym to improve my health and help me lose weight. However, I work long hours and by the time I get home I'm tired and it is difficult to summon up the energy to go. I need to unwind and a glass of wine in front of the television is a reward for the work of the day.'

The experience of people with a dual diagnosis is similar, they too have reasons for and against making changes. An example from John, a service user who smokes cannabis and has a diagnosis of schizophrenia is: 'I accept that cannabis might be having a negative impact on my mental health and when I've been smoking a lot I've ended up in hospital but I like the buzz and all my mates puff.'

In both examples there are reasons for and against change. Ambivalence is a normal part of the change process. 'Persuasion' is about resolving ambivalence in favour of change so that the perceived benefits of change outweigh the perceived benefits of not doing so. MI is key to this process.

Miller and Rollnick (2002) identify four principles of MI:

- *Express empathy*. Being client centred and empathic is central. The nurse focuses on the person's concerns, tries to understand his/her way of seeing things and conveys this understanding to the person. Asking open question (e.g. what? how?) and use of reflection are key skills.
- *Develop discrepancy*. Change is motivated by a mismatch between the person's goals and values and their present behaviour. The importance of change increases as the person becomes more aware of the discrepancies between where they are and where they want to be. The nurse amplifies the discrepancy by eliciting 'change talk', the service user's reasons for changing.

Picking up the example of John …

John	I accept that cannabis might be having a negative impact on my mental health and when I've been smoking a lot I've ended up in hospital but I like the buzz and all my mates puff.
Nurse	Being in hospital isn't somewhere you want to be.
John	No way. Last time I ended up on the intensive care unit, being held down and injected. I was locked up there for weeks. I didn't have any contact with my son. My flat got broken into when I was away too.
Nurse	It sounds like it was a difficult time.
John	It was. I definitely don't want to go back there.

By exploring John's experiences of hospital the nurse is eliciting 'change talk'. Developing the discrepancy between what he wants (not to be in hospital), and where he is (smoking cannabis, the consequence of which may be another admission) may help to tip the balance in favour of a decision to change.

During the contemplation stage, where there are both reasons for and against change, use of decision matrices can be useful. They provide a structured way of exploring the advantages and disadvantages (pros and cons) of continued use and of change. Figure 22.4 is John's decision matrix.

Discussion of the material from a decision matrix will provide opportunities for eliciting change talk. This is selectively reflected back reinforcing the person's own reasons for change and enhancing motivation.

Continuing to use cannabis	
Advantages/Pros	*Disadvantages/Cons*
Like the buzz. Helps me to relax. Enjoy puffing with mates. Messes my head up less than when I was using crack. It's part of my routine.	May be having bad effect on mental health. May end up in hospital again. Spending more money than I can afford. Might have electricity, phone, gas cut off. Arguments with mum. Less contact with son. It's illegal. Bad effect on physical health.

Stopping cannabis use	
Advantages/Cons	*Disadvantages/Cons*
Less likely to end up back in hospital. Could buy new clothes, music. Could buy presents for son. Less rows with mum. Might get to college. Stop getting into debt. Might get into going to gym.	Wouldn't be part of the group with mates – would feel left out and could be lonely. Might have to cut down contact with my mates. Boredom. Would be tense and irritable.

Figure 22.4 Example of a Completed Decision matrix

■ *Roll with resistance.* Resistance is likely to occur if the person feels that change is being imposed or if a suggestion or recommendation that has not been asked for, or is not helpful to the person at their stage of change, is provided. If the nurse is presenting one side of an argument then it is likely the service user will take the other and change is less likely.

For example:

Nurse	You've said that smoking cannabis probably has a negative impact on your mental health and that you don't want to end up in hospital again so it would make sense for you to stop using.
John	Yes but I can't imagine not getting together and puffing with my mates.
Nurse	Well you'll probably need to stop seeing your mates.
John	There's no way I could do that, I've known some of them since I was a kid.

John is now putting forward reasons for not changing. The more the nurse argues for change, the more John is likely to argue against it. The nurse has jumped ahead of John. He has indicated some acceptance that cannabis may be detrimental to his mental health but has not indicated that he is planning for change. More work needs to be done on exploring and understanding his reasons for using and the difficulties use is causing him. Unless the nurse shifts direction scope for further exploration of these issues may be lost.

Rather than dealing with resistance head on by arguing or challenging a different approach is needed. The nurse could have reflected 'Your friends are really important to you'. This might open up discussion about John's friends and his relationships with them, which could be important to explore.

- *Support self-efficacy.* Belief in the possibility of change, on the part of the person themselves and the nurse, is an important motivator for change. Given that people with a dual diagnosis often have low self-esteem affirming their accomplishments can be important in boosting confidence in their ability to change.

To gauge the person's motivation to change the readiness ruler can be helpful. Readiness to change is conceptualized as comprising two components: importance and confidence. The person is asked to rate themselves on each using a scale of 0–10.

0	1	2	3	4	5	6	7	8	9	10
Not at all important								Very important		

0	1	2	3	4	5	6	7	8	9	10
Not at all confident								Very confident		

If someone is ready to change they need to be willing (it is important for them to change) and able (confident that they can change). If importance is low the nurse needs to focus on building importance. If importance is high but confidence low the focus will be on building confidence. Using the ruler as a tool provides further scope for enhancing motivation. The following excerpt shows how it might be used with John.

Some time later:

Nurse	You said you've been thinking about cutting down your cannabis. Is it okay to talk a bit more about that?
John	Yeah
Nurse	If I asked you how important it is for you to make some changes to your use, on a scale of 0–10, where 0 is not at all important and 10 is very important, where would you put yourself?
John	I'd say about a 5.
Nurse	Five, okay. Why a 5 and not, say, a 1 or 2?
John	Well I'm worried about the impact on my mental health and I really don't want to go back into hospital, it was such an awful experience.
Nurse	Anything else?
John	Well I'm probably spending more on it than I can afford, sometimes I haven't got enough money to pay my bills.

Having explored further and elicited other reasons John might have for thinking it important to change the nurse might ask:

Nurse	What would need to happen for the 5 to become a 6 or 7?
John	Well if I started feeling that I was becoming unwell again and I thought I was going to end up back in hospital that would make it more important. I guess if I ended up having my electricity cut off again, like I did before when I didn't pay my bill, especially if my mum wouldn't pay it for me – she's said she's not going to bail me out again if I spend all my money on cannabis.

More reasons for change are being elicited. Note that in this excerpt, rather than making suggestions about the changes John should make, the nurse asks permission to talk more about his thoughts about cutting down. This demonstrates respect for his autonomy and enables him to have some control over the direction of the discussion. John then identifies more reasons for changing. Perhaps he would end up saying:

John	Having thought about it a bit, perhaps I am at more of a 7, there are a lot of reasons for me to change.
Nurse	So change is important to you.
John	Yes, yes it is.
Nurse	If you do decide to have a go at cutting down how confident do you feel about being able to succeed – again thinking about 0 being not at all confident and 10 being very confident.
John	Well I think about 5. It would be difficult to have less contact with my mates and I do like a spliff at least at the end of the day to chill before I go to bed.

Exploring why John has rated himself as a 5 and not lower on the scale would again produce change talk.

Nurse	What would need to happen to make you feel more confident, say a 6?
John	Well maybe if I spent some time with my cousin who doesn't puff it would be easier and if I could prove to myself that I could get through one day without, then maybe I could do it again.

These latter statements are further examples of change talk. John is expressing some optimism about the possibility of change.

When importance and confidence are high the person is probably ready to plan for change. This could be confirmed by asking for an overall rating of how ready they feel.

Although MI is identified as a core component for working with people with a dual diagnosis, some adaptations may be required to accommodation the cognitive impairment, and positive and negative symptoms commonly experienced by people with mental health problems. These include: keeping open questions simple; refining reflective listening skills by using simple language, reflecting and paraphrasing often; increased emphasis on affirming people's qualities and efforts to change, simplifying the structure of decisional matrices, presenting information in visual format (Martino *et al.* 2002; Martino and Moyers 2008).

Active treatment

In this stage goals are identified and plans put in place to pursue them. While abstinence from substances is likely to be the ideal goal for people with a severe mental illness, many people are unwilling or unable to achieve this. Gains can be made by reducing the harm associated with use, so reducing, or changing the pattern of use can be beneficial. In keeping with MI, the goals and decisions about strategies for achieving them must be those of the service user. It is important that realistic goals are set. Ambitious goals (e.g. wanting a job) need to be broken down into a series of smaller steps. Achieving small goals can encourage the person, build confidence and provide a platform upon which future change can be built. Not achieving can create a sense of failure and trigger a return to precontemplation or contemplation stages. The nurse should help elicit the service user's suggestions about how goals might be achieved. The pros and cons of various options can be explored (the decision matrix framework may be used for this) and the person can make an informed decision about which will be pursued. Information about services that may be helpful, or suggestions about strategies can be offered but only after the service user's solutions have been sought and after permission to pass on information, or make suggestions, has been obtained.

Returning to John, a realistic target might be for him to abstain from cannabis one day each week, or perhaps to reduce use during the day (he noted that it would be difficult for him not to have a spliff before going to bed). Planning how he will achieve his goal may include reflection on a typical day, consideration of what may need to change if he is to avoid use, consideration of whether a particular day(s) of the week would be a good (or bad) day to try to make this change, deciding how he might plan his time, identifying people or situations he might avoid and people who would be supportive of him, and anticipating difficulties he may encounter and how these might be managed.

If ongoing change is to be achieved it is likely that all the material in the decision matrix will need to be explored as it can provide pointers to areas for further interventions. For example, John indicated that cannabis helped him to relax; work may need to be done on identifying other ways of relaxing. He also suggested that he might feel bored if he wasn't smoking cannabis. Work on structuring his time may be required. He has suggested some ways in which this could be achieved, indicating that he might be interested in going to college and to the gym. If he subsequently decides to pursue these options then he may need support in doing this.

It may be helpful for John to keep a diary of his cannabis use. Figure 22.5 is a standard drink diary. This format can be adapted to meet individual needs. Information gained in diaries can provide baseline data about level of use and insights into motivations for using. Additional columns can be added to monitor psychiatric symptoms. A person with depression might rate their mood alongside their alcohol intake. John may want to record any psychotic symptoms he experiences. Diaries are also a means of monitoring progress and, if gains have been made, looking back can provide encouragement and boost the person's confidence in their ability to make further changes.

It can take many months, and sometimes years, before people are ready to address their use. Pharmacological interventions may be needed to enable people to stop using safely if they are dependent on alcohol, opiates or benzodiazepines. Some people will detoxify in the community, others will require inpatient admission. Factors influencing this decision include: the number and quantity of substances being used, previous withdrawal experiences, physical and mental health, availability of support in the community, family responsibilities (for

Day	How much and what type of alcohol	Times drinking started and ended	Who with	Where drinking took place	Number of units	Thoughts, feelings and consequences	Cost (£s)
Monday							
Tuesday							
Wednesday							
Thursday							
Friday							
Saturday							
Sunday							

Fig 22.5 Drink diary

example, childcare) and personal preference. Maintaining the person's safety is essential. People who are using dangerous combinations of substances, have experienced withdrawal seizures, delirium tremens or whose physical health is very poor must be admitted to hospital. For people whose mental health tends to be unstable this is also likely to be the best option, and once detoxified, time in an inpatient setting can allow a more thorough mental health assessment to be made.

Alcohol detoxification is achieved by prescribing a reducing regimen of a long-acting benzodiazepine (chlordiazepoxide or diazepam) over a period of about a week. Close monitoring is required because of the risks if the person drinks alcohol while taking benzodiazepines, and because of the severe complications that can be associated with withdrawal (for example, seizures).

Detoxification from opiates is usually undertaken by prescribing methadone or buprenorphine (both opioids). Lofexidine may be considered in some cases. Contingency management, the offering of incentives to promote positive behaviours, is recommended as an adjunct. NICE have published guidelines on pharmacological interventions and contingency management (NICE 2007a, b). More detailed practical guidance on the clinical management of drug misuse and dependence is available in DH (England and the devolved administrations) 2007).

People using stimulants, cannabis or ecstasy do not need pharmacological interventions to stop using. However, antidepressants are sometimes useful for people who have been using crack and cocaine, as low mood can persist for many weeks.

Benzodiazepine detoxification is achieved by prescribing diazepam, a long-acting benzodiazepine, at an equivalent dose to the drug which was being taken and then reducing the dose. The reduction rate can be more rapid at the beginning, but people are often extremely anxious about detoxification. A slow gradual reduction, that the person feels is achievable, is preferable to a more rapid one which makes the person overly anxious and may result in them obtaining illicit supplies.

Relapse prevention

As mental illness and substance misuse are chronic relapsing conditions once use has been reduced or abstinence achieved interventions should address prevention of future relapses so that gains are maintained. Clearly relapse of substance misuse and mental illness may be interrelated.

A specific approach for preventing and managing substance misuse relapse has been developed by Marlatt and his colleagues (Marlatt and Gordon 1985; Marlatt and Donovan 2005). A cognitive behavioural framework is used to identify high-risk situations and triggers for use and the development of strategies for coping with them. Effective coping enhances the person's sense of self-control. If substance use does occur this is seen as a lapse or 'slip-up' that can be overcome, and from which learning can take place. In terms of Prochaska and DiClemente's (1986) model, the person returns to active treatment rather than precontemplation, or contemplation. Such a perspective contrasts with the sense of failure and hopelessness which can be engendered if drinking or using drugs is seen as a relapse which has put the person 'back to square one'.

Situations/triggers for relapse will be many and varied. These include: negative emotional states (for example, anger, anxiety, depression, boredom), positive emotional states (for example, celebrations), interpersonal conflicts (for example, with partner, family members, employer), social pressures (for example, at a party) and associations with particular places, people, times/dates or situations. Diaries and decision matrices can be used to help identify triggers. Exploring the chain of events which has led to past (re)lapses can also highlight triggers as well as points at which the person could have acted differently. Strategies for managing risk situations will require the development of new coping skills as well as lifestyle changes. Like all new skills they will require practice. Family and friends can be a source of support. For example, they may accompany the person to cash their benefit cheque and do their shopping to break the routine of buying drugs when money has been received, they may invite them to a social outing to help structure their time and kindle a new interest (e.g. theatre, football match), they may be willing to be available on the phone to provide a listening ear at times of low mood, or craving for drink/drugs, they may give the person a lift to an Alcoholics Anonymous meeting.

Planning to prevent psychiatric relapse is also essential. A process for identifying a 'relapse signature', the unique pattern of early warning signs likely to indicate impending relapse, and development of a 'relapse drill', the coping strategies to manage emergence of these relapse indicators, has been described by Birchwood et al. (2000). Use of substances may be a part of a person's relapse signature. Bringing together the approaches of Marlatt and Birchwood provides scope for taking a comprehensive approach to relapse prevention in people with a dual diagnosis.

Ongoing pharmacological management of psychiatric symptoms can be important in preventing substance misuse relapse as substances may be used to deal with troubling symptoms. Pharmacological interventions can also play a direct part in preventing substance misuse relapse. People with opiate problems may find naltrexone helpful as it blocks the effects of opiates (NICE 2007d). For people with alcohol problems acamprosate may be beneficial as it can reduce craving when used in conjunction with psychosocial interventions (Raistrick et al. 2006). Disulfiram (antabuse) acts as a deterrent to drinking as adverse consequences are experienced if alcohol is consumed (flushing, headache, palpitations, nausea and vomiting – in large amounts cardiac arrhythmias, hypotension and collapse may occur). Although there is a risk that it can trigger depression and psychotic symptoms Raistrick *et al.* (2006) concluded that it could be used by people with a psychotic illness, although caution should be exercised.

At present, there are few projects specifically for people with a dual diagnosis. While some substance misuse projects will accept people with a dual diagnosis their programmes may not be sufficiently flexible to meet the specific needs of this group. Many services, particularly residential projects, exclude people with severe mental health problems. Similarly, residential projects specifically for people with mental health problems may exclude people with substance misuse problems. Those that do accept them generally do not address substance misuse as an integral part of a mental health recovery programme. Given these service deficits it is important that nurses working in community mental health services are able to address needs associated with both problems.

Older people

There is a tendency to think of substance misuse as an issue mainly concerned with younger people. Many people do stop using substances as they get older but some do not and others develop problems with substances in later life. Substance misuse in this group can have serious consequences as it is associated with falls, depression, suicide and possible interaction effects with prescribed medications (UK Inquiry into Mental Health and Wellbeing in Later Life 2007).

Meeting the needs of families and carers

Carers and family members of people with a dual diagnosis will also have needs which nurses have a role in addressing. They often bear the brunt of the distress and difficult behaviour of the person with a dual diagnosis, for example, being the victim of aggression, being coerced into handing over money for substances. Carers may also feel frustrated with service providers. They may feel their relative is not getting the care needed, for example, because they are being 'bounced' between mental health and substance misuse services and neither is adequately addressing their problems. They may also feel excluded from decisions about care or that they are being fobbed off by providers who say they cannot pass on information because of confidentiality.

Although often keen to support their relative, carer and family behaviour can have a negative impact. Arguing and confrontation can increase resistance and service users' distress and may contribute to relapse. Enabling behaviours such as buying drink or drugs for the person, and helping them pay bills can prevent change.

All carers and family members will need information. Even if service users do not want their family involved in their treatment, information can be provided, for example, about substances, their effects and complications, mental illnesses and their signs and symptoms, the impact of substance use on mental illness, the nature of care and treatment, and information about what to do and who to contact in a crisis.

To enable family members to be more effective in helping their relative Barrowclough *et al.* (2001) found that it was important for them to develop an approach consistent with the stages of change model and motivational interviewing style. For example, leaving responsibility for change to the individual, recognizing that confrontation about use may create resistance to change. Setting boundaries to limit the impact use may have on family life was also important, for example, no use in the home, not bailing the person out financially when all their money has been spent on substances.

Information about family and carer support groups should be made available. National organizations providing support for the families of people with substance misuse problems include:

■ Al-Anon and Al-Ateen (both on 020 7403 0888) – these work with family members of problem drinkers, the latter is targeted at teenagers.

■ Families Anonymous (020 7498 4680) – this focuses on the families of drug users.

Groups which support the carers of people with mental health problems are available in most areas. As yet, there are few, if any, groups which specifically focus on the carers of people with a dual diagnosis. A DVD and accompanying booklet have been produced to highlight the needs of this group (Care Services Improvement Partnership 2007). People providing 'regular and substantial' amounts of care and support should be offered a carer's assessment (DH 1999) and steps taken to address the needs identified.

Conclusion

This chapter has provided an overview of substance misuse within the context of mental health care. Concepts and terminology relating to dual diagnosis and substance misuse were explored. Information was provided about commonly misused substances, their mode of use, effects and complications. The foundations for working with people with a dual diagnosis were described and assessment and treatment issues considered.

In summary, the main points of this chapter are:

■ Substance misuse is common in people with mental health problems and all mental health professionals need knowledge and skills in this area.

■ Dual diagnosis is a broad concept, which encompasses a wide range of people with varying levels of mental illness and substance use.

■ The relationship between psychiatric illness and substance misuse is complex.

■ A range of physical, psychiatric, interpersonal, social and legal complications can be associated with substance misuse.

■ A variety of risks are associated with dual diagnosis.

■ Assessment of substance misuse should be integral to mental health assessments.

■ An integration of mental health and substance misuse interventions is needed for working with people with a dual diagnosis.

■ A client's readiness to change should guide treatment interventions.

■ Working with people with a dual diagnosis requires flexibility and a long-term perspective.

■ Attention should be given to the needs of families and carers.

■ The various services in contact with people with a dual diagnosis need to develop partnership working so that, as far as possible, the person's experience is of seamless care provision.

Acknowledgements

Thanks to colleagues at South London and Maudsley NHS Foundation Trust who commented on earlier drafts of the chapter.

Questions for reflection and discussion

1 List the substances you have used over recent days and identify your reasons for using them.
2 Identify any ethical issues which might be encountered when working with people with a dual diagnosis.
3 Think of someone you are working with who has a dual diagnosis. What stage of change are they at? How do you know? From which stage of Osher and Kofoed's (1989) treatment model would appropriate treatment interventions be selected? Does this reflect the way you are working with the person? If not, what needs to change?
4 Think about a behaviour change you would like to make and complete a decision matrix, identifying the advantages and disadvantages of changing and not doing so.

Annotated bibliography

- Turning Point/Rethink (2004) *Dual Diagnosis Toolkit.* London: Rethink and Turning Point. This is a practical guide to working with people with a dual diagnosis. It is a useful introductory text which is presented in an accessible format. It can be downloaded from www.rethink.org/dualdiagnosis/toolkit.html
- Graham, H.L., Copello, A., Birchwood, M.J. and Mueser, K.T. (2003) *Substance Misuse in Psychosis: Approaches to treatment and service delivery.* Chichester: Wiley. This excellent volume comprises 20 chapters written by recognized experts in the dual diagnosis field. It will be useful for those who want a more in-depth understanding of dual diagnosis.
- Graham, H.L. (2004) *Cognitive-Behavioural Integrated Treatment (C-BIT): A treatment manual for substance misuse in people with severe mental health problems.* Chichester: Wiley. This manual sets out a framework for the delivery of integrated treatment for people with severe mental illness and substance misuse problems. Step-by-step guidance on how to deliver interventions appropriate to the person's stage of change are described and case material is included for illustration.
- Miller, W. and Rollnick. S. (2nd edition) (2002) *Motivational Interviewing: Preparing people for change.* London: Guilford Press. This is the bible for MI. The first half of the book provides a detailed account of what MI is and how to work in a motivational way, the second brings together chapters written by leading MI practitioners describing its application to a variety of groups and settings.
- Rollnick, S., Miller, W. and Butler, C. (2008) *Motivational Interviewing in Health Care: Helping patients change behaviour.* New York: Guilford Press. This is a shorter, simpler introduction to MI.

Useful websites

■ 'Frank' www.talktofrank.com
■ Drugscope www.drugscope.org.uk
■ Alcohol Concern www.alcoholconcern.org.uk

All provide up-to-date information for professionals and the public. As well as information which can be downloaded, some publications can be ordered free of charge.

References

Alcohol Concern (2000) *Britain's Ruin?* London: Alcohol Concern.

American Psychiatric Association (1994) *Diagnostic and Statistical Manual of Mental Disorders.* Washington, DC: American Psychiatric Association.

Babor, T., de la Fuente, J., Saunders, J. and Grant, M. (1989) *AUDIT, The Alcohol Use Disorders Identification Test: Guidelines for Use in Primary Care.* Geneva: World Health Organization.

Banerjee, S., Clancy, C. and Crome, I. (eds) (2002) *Co-existing Problems of Mental Disorder and Substance Misuse (dual diagnosis): An information manual.* London: Royal College of Psychiatrists Research Unit.

Barnby, B., Drummond, C., McLeod, A. *et al.* (2003) Substance misuse in psychiatric inpatients: comparison of a screening questionnaire survey with case notes. *British Medical Journal* **327**: 783–4.

Barrowclough, C., Haddock, G., Tarrier, N. *et al.* (2001) Randomised control trial of motivational interviewing, cognitive behaviour therapy, and family interventions for patients with co-morbid schizophrenia and substance use disorders. *American Journal of Psychiatry* **158**(10): 1706–13.

Bien, T.H., Miller, W.R. and Tonigan, J.S. (1993) Brief interventions for alcohol problems: a review. *Addiction* **88**(3): 315–35.

Birchwood, M., Spencer, E. and McGovern, D. (2000) Schizophrenia: early warning signs. *Advances in Psychiatric Treatment* **6**: 93–101.

Brown, R.L. and Rounds, L.A. (1995) Conjoint screening questionnaires for alcohol and drug abuse. *Wisconsin Medical Journal* **94**: 135–40.

Care Services Improvement Partnership (2007) *What It Means to Make a Difference: Caring for people with mental illness who use alcohol and drugs.* London: Care Services Improvement Partnership.

Carey, K.B. and Correia, C.J. (1998) Severe mental illness and addictions: assessment considerations. *Addictive Behaviours* **23**(6): 735–48.

Castle, D. and Murray, R. (eds) (2004) *Marijuana and Madness.* Cambridge: Cambridge University Press.

Christo, G., Spurrell, S. and Alcorn, R. (2000) Validation of the Christo Inventory for Substance Misuse Services (CISS): A simple outcome evaluation tool. *Drug and Alcohol Dependence* **59**: 189–97.

Cleary, M., Hunt, G.E., Matheson, S.L. *et al.* (2008) Psychosocial interventions for people with both severe mental illness and substance misuse. *Cochrane Database of Systematic Reviews 2008*, Issue 4.

Crome, I. (1999) Substance misuse and psychiatric co-morbidity: towards improved service provision. *Drugs: Education, Prevention and Policy* **6**: 151–74.

Department of Health (1999) *National Service Framework for Mental Health.* London: DH.

Department of Health (2002) *Mental Health Policy Implementation Guide: Dual Diagnosis Good Practice Guide.* London: DH.

Department of Health (2004) *The National Service Framework – Five years on.* London. DH.

Department of Health (2006a) *From Values to Action: The Chief Nursing Officer's review of mental health nursing.* London: DH.

Department of Health (2006b) *Best Practice Competencies and Capabilities for Pre-registration Mental Health Nurses in England: The Chief Nursing Officer's Review of Mental Health Nursing.* London: DH.

Department of Health, Home Office, Department for Education and Skills, Department of Culture, Media and Sport (2007) *Safe, Sensible, Social: The next steps in the National Alcohol Strategy.* London: DH.

Department of Health (England) and the devolved administrations (2007) *Drug Misuse and Dependence: UK Guidelines on Clinical Management*. London: Department of Health (England), the Scottish Government, Welsh Assembly Government and Northern Ireland Executive.

Drake, R., Essock, S., Shaner, A. *et al.* (2001) Implementing dual diagnosis services for clients with severe mental illness. *Psychiatric Services* **52**: 469–76.

Edwards, G., Marshall, E.J. and Cook, C.C. (2003) *The Treatment of Drinking Problems* (4th edn). Cambridge: Cambridge University Press.

Ford, P. (2003) An evaluation of the Dartmouth Assessment of Lifestyle Inventory and the Leeds Dependence Questionnaire for use among detained psychiatric inpatients. *Addiction* **98**: 111–18.

Gossop, M., Marsden, J. and Stewart, D. (2001) NTORS *After Five Years: The National Treatment Outcome Research Study*. London: National Addiction Centre.

Graham, H. (2004) *Cognitive-Behavioural Integrated Treatment (C-BIT): A treatment manual for substance misuse in people with severe mental health problems*. Chichester: Wiley.

Handmaker, N., Packard, M. and Conforti, K. (2002) Motivational interviewing in treatment of dual disorders, in W. Miller, and S. Rollnick (2002) *Motivational Interviewing: Preparing People to Change Addictive Behaviour* (2nd edn). New York: Guilford Press.

Hughes, L. (2006) *Closing The Gap: A capability framework for working effectively with combined mental health and substance use problems (dual diagnosis)*. Mansfield Centre for Clinical and Workforce Innovation, University of Lincoln.

Hulse, G., Saunders, J., Roydhouse, R. *et al.* (2000) Screening for hazardous alcohol use and dependence in psychiatric in-patients using the AUDIT questionnaire. *Drug and Alcohol Review* **19**: 291–8.

Johnson, K., Gerada, C. and Greenough, A. (2003) Substance misuse during pregnancy. *British Journal of Psychiatry* **183**: 187–9.

King, M. (1986) At risk drinking among general practice attenders: validation of the CAGE questionnaire. *Psychological Medicine* **16**: 213–17.

Marlatt, G.A. and Gordon, J.R. (1985) *Relapse Prevention: Maintenance Strategies in the Treatment of Addictive Behaviours*. New York: Guilford Press.

Marlatt, G.A. and Donovan, D.M. (2005) *Relapse Prevention: Maintenance Strategies in the Treatment of Addictive Behaviours* (2nd edn). New York: Guilford Press.

Marsden, J., Farrell, M., Bradbury, C. *et al.* (2007) *The Treatment Outcome Profile*. London: NTA.

Martino, S. and Moyers, T. (2008) Motivational interviewing with dually diagnosed patients, in H. Arkowitz, H.A. Weston, W.R. Miller and S. Rollnick (eds) *Motivational Interviewing in the Treatment of Psychological Problems*. New York: Guilford Press.

Martino, S., Carroll, K., Kostas, D. *et al.* (2002) Dual diagnosis motivational interviewing: a modification of motivational interviewing for substance abusing patients with psychotic disorders. *Journal of Substance Abuse Treatment* **23**: 297–308.

Maslin, J. (2003) Substance misuse in psychosis: contextual issues, in H.L. Graham, A. Copello, M.J. Birchwood and K.T. Mueser (eds) *Substance Misuse in Psychosis: Approaches to Treatment and Service Delivery*. Chichester: Wiley.

Meltzer, H., Lader, D., Corbin, T. *et al.* (2002) *Non-Fatal Suicidal Behaviour Among Adults Aged 16–74 in Great Britain*. London: The Stationery Office.

Miller, W. and Rollnick, S. (2002) *Motivational Interviewing: Preparing People to Change Addictive Behaviour* (2nd edn). New York: Guilford Press.

Moore, T.H., Zammit, S., Lingford-Hughes, A. *et al.* (2007) Cannabis use and risk of psychotic or affective mental health outcomes: a systematic review. *Lancet* **370**: 319–28.

Mueser, K.T., Drake, R.E. and Wallach, M.A. (1998) Dual diagnosis: a review of aetiological theories. *Addictive Behaviour* **23**(6): 717–34.

Mueser, K.T., Noordsy, D.L., Drake, R.E. and Fox, L. (2003) *Integrated Treatment for Dual Disorders: a guide to effective practice*. New York: Guilford Press.

National Institute for Health and Clinical Excellence (2007a) *Drug Misuse: opiate detoxification*. NICE clinical guideline 52. London: NICE.

National Institute for Health and Clinical Excellence (2007b) *Drug Misuse: psychosocial interventions*. NICE clinical guideline 51. London: NICE.

National Institute for Health and Clinical Excellence (2007c) *Methadone and Buprenorphine for the Management of Opioid Dependence*. NICE technology appraisal 114. London: NICE.

National Institute for Health and Clinical Excellence (2007d) *Naltrexone for the Management of Opioid Dependence.* NICE technology appraisal 115. London: NICE.

Noordsy, D.L., McQuade, D.V. and Mueser, K. (2003) Assessment considerations, in H.L. Graham, A. Copello, M.J. Birchwood and K.T. Mueser (eds) *Substance Misuse in Psychosis: Approaches to Treatment and Service Delivery.* Chichester: Wiley.

Osher, F. and Kofoed, L. (1989) Treatment of patients with psychiatric and psychoactive substance abuse disorders. *Hospital and Community Psychiatry* **40**: 1025–30.

Phillips, P. and Johnson, S. (2001) How does drug and alcohol misuse develop among people with psychotic illness? A literature review. *Social Psychiatry and Psychiatric Epidemiology* **36**: 269–76.

Prochaska, J. and DiClemente, C. (1986) Towards a comprehensive model of change, in W. Miller and N. Heather (eds) *Treating Addictive Behaviours: Processes of Change.* New York: Plenum.

Prochaska, J., DiClemente, C. and Norcross, J. (1992) In search of how people change: applications to addictive behaviours. *American Psychologist* **47**: 1102–12.

Raistrick, D., Bradshaw, J., Tober, G. *et al.* (1994) Development of the Leeds Dependency Questionnaire (LDQ): a questionnaire to measure alcohol and opiate dependence in the context of a treatment evaluation package. *Addiction* **89**: 563–72.

Raistrick, D., Heather, N. and Godfrey, C. (2006) *Review of the Effectiveness of Treatment for Alcohol Problems.* London: National Treatment Agency.

Rosenberg, S., Drake, R., Wolford, G. *et al.* (1998) Dartmouth Assessment of Lifestyle Instrument (DALI): A substance use disorder screen for people with severe mental illness. *American Journal of Psychiatry* **155**: 232–8.

Selzer, M. (1971) The Michigan alcoholism screening test. *American Journal of Psychiatry* **127**: 1653–8.

Sobell, L.C. Sobell, M.B. (1996) *Timeline Follow Back User's Guide: A calendar method for assessing drug and alcohol use.* Toronto: Addiction Research Foundation.

Stockwell, T., Murphy, D. and Hodgson, R. (1983) The severity of alcohol dependence questionnaire: its use, reliability and validity. *British Journal of Addiction* **78**: 145–55.

Swanson, A.J., Pantalon, M.V. and Cohen, K.R. (1999) Motivational interviewing and treatment adherence among patients with psychiatric and dually diagnosed patients. *Journal of Nervous and Mental Disease* **187**: 630–5.

UK Inquiry into Mental Health and Wellbeing in Later Life (2007) *Improving Services and Support for Older People with Mental Health Problems.* London: Age Concern.

United Kingdom Harm Reduction Alliance (2007) www.ukhra.org.harm_reduction_definition.html

University of Manchester (2006) *Avoidable Deaths: Five year report of the national confidential inquiry into suicide and homicide by people with mental illness.* Manchester: National Confidential Inquiry into Suicide and Homicide by People with Mental Illness.

Weaver, T., Charles, V., Madden, P. and Renton, A. (2002) *Co-morbidity of Substance Misuse and Mental Illness Collaborative Study (COSMIC): A study of the prevalence and management of co-morbidity amongst adult substance misuse and mental health treatment populations.* London: DH/NTA.

World Health Organization (1992) *ICD-10 Classification of Mental and Behavioural Disorders.* Geneva: World Health Organization.

Zuckoff, A. and Daley, D. (2001) Engagement and adherence issues in treating persons with non-psychosis dual disorders. *Psychiatric Rehabilitation Skills* **5**(1): 131–62.

CHAPTER 23

Mental health problems in childhood and adolescence

Robin Basu and Jane Padmore

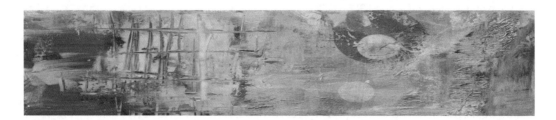

Chapter overview

Child and adolescent mental health services are concerned with the assessment and treatment of behavioural and emotional problems in people below the age of 18 years. During childhood, for the majority of the disorders, the symptoms shown by a child only become significant if these are of unusual intensity or duration, but are otherwise seen in most children at some point of their development. Prevalence studies differ in their estimates of mental health problems in young people. Having at least one psychiatric disorder by the age of 16 is thought to be much higher than point estimates would suggest (Costello *et al.* 2004). In their longitudinal community study Costello *et al.* (2004) found that although during a three-month period any disorder averaged 13.3 per cent, during the whole study period 36.7 per cent of participants had at least one psychiatric disorder. Adolescent mental health problems have increased for both boys and girls since the mid 1980s and this trend does not appear to be stopping (Hagell 2004).

People who have had mental health problems in adolescence are known to have an increase in mental health problems as adults. Long-term follow-up studies of depression in adolescents have emphasized the increase risk of adult depression (e.g. Fombonne *et al.* 2001). These studies have also shown that young people who have had an early onset psychosis (under 18) are more likely to go on to have mental health problems as adults.

The bulk of this chapter is devoted to describing the manifestations of mental distress and disorder in childhood and adolescence that nurses may encounter in the course of their work in a variety of practice settings. The chapter begins, however, with a discussion of those aspects of assessment that are particularly relevant when working with children and adolescents, since a full and comprehensive assessment is a prerequisite to successful treatment.

In summary this chapter covers:

- Assessment;
- Manifestations of mental health problems in childhood, specifically:
  - pre-school problems
  - hyperactivity
  - autistic disorders
  - conduct disorders
  - emotional disorders of childhood
  - disorders of social functioning
  - elimination disorders
  - child maltreatment
  - Tourette's syndrome;

- Psychiatric disorders in adolescence, specifically:
  - obsessive compulsive disorder
  - suicide and deliberate self-harm;

- Psychiatric disorders in childhood:
  - major affective disorders
  - adolescent schizophrenia
  - substance misuse in adolescence
  - eating disorders;

- Somatizing in children and adolescence;
- Treatment of child and adolescent psychiatry;
- Prevention of child psychiatric disorders;
- Child and adolescent mental health problems in primary care;
- The nurses' role in child and adolescent services.

Classification of child and adolescent psychiatric disorders

The present system of classification for child and adolescent psychiatric disorders has focused primarily on symptomatology rather than aetiology. In child psychiatry, organic disorders in which psychiatric disorders arise secondary to physical causes are rare. Multi-axial classification takes into account different aspects of a patient's disorder and classifies the disorder along different axes giving a composite picture of the condition. The commonly used axes from the International Classification of Diseases (ICD) of the World Health Organization are:

- Axis 1   Clinical psychiatric syndromes;
- Axis 2   Specific disorders of psychological development;
- Axis 3   Intellectual level;
- Axis 4   Medical conditions;
- Axis 5   Associated abnormal psychosocial situations;
- Axis 6   Global assessment of psychosocial disability.

Classification should not be an end in itself and to be effective should be clinically relevant and aid communication on possible aetiology, treatment and prognosis classification.

The two main systems in use are the International Classification of Diseases (ICD) of the World Health Organization (1996) and the Statistical Manual (DSM) of the American

Psychiatric Association (1994). The DSM-IV and the ICD-10 provide clear descriptive criteria that must be met before a diagnosis can be made. The ICD-10 classification of Behavioural and Emotional Disorders with onset usually occurring in childhood and adolescents is coded separately (F90–F98) (see Table 23.1).

F90 Hyperkinetic disorders
Examples of these are:
F90.0 – Disturbance of activity and attention
F90.1 – Hyperkinetic conduct disorder

F91 Conduct disorders
Examples of these are:
F91.0 – Conduct disorder confined to the family context
F91.1 – Unsocialized conduct disorder
F91.2 – Socialized conduct disorder
F91.3 – Oppositional defiant disorder

F92 Mixed disorders of conduct and emotions
An example of this is:
F92.0 – Depressive conduct disorder

F93 Emotional disorders with onset specific to childhood
Examples of these are:
F93.0 – Separation anxiety disorder of childhood
F93.1 – Phobic anxiety disorder of childhood
F93.2 – Social anxiety disorder of childhood
F93.3 – Sibling rivalry disorder

F94 Disorders of social functioning with onset specific to childhood and adolescence
F94.0 – Elective mutism
F94.1 – Reactive attachment disorder of childhood
F94.2 – Disinhibited attachment disorder of childhood

F95 Tic disorders
F95.0 – Transient tic disorder
F95.1 – Chronic motor or vocal tic disorder
F95.2 – Combined vocal and multiple motor tic disorder (Gilles de la Tourette's syndrome)

F98 Other behavioural and emotional disorders with onset usually occurring in childhood and adolescence
Examples of these are:
F98.0 – Nonorganic enuresis
F98.1 – Nonorganic encopresis

Table 23.1 F90–F98 Behavioural and emotional disorders with onset usually occurring in childhood and adolescence (After ICD-10, WHO 1996)

Issues to be addressed in a comprehensive CAMHS assessment are listed in Figure 23.1.

Presenting circumstances
Nature of problem, onset, frequency and duration
What lead them to coming to the assessment
What remedies have been tried
Who is affected by the problem
Sleep pattern
Appetite

Family history
Personal history of parents
Relationship to parents, carers, siblings and others
in the household
The families approach to parenting and children
Extended family
Mental health problems
Physical health problems
Patterns of communication
Forensic history in the family
Cultural background of the family
Domestic Violence

Personal history
Pregnancy, labour and delivery
Developmental milestones (physical, social and emotional)
Any disruptions to and reaction to attachment/separation
Preschool
Education including Academic ability and performance
History of involvement with mental health services
History of invovement with social care
Forensic History
Sexual History
Substance Misuse
Personality including interests and relationships
Emotions and Behaviour

Physical health
Height and Weight
History of physical health problems
Immunization history
Dental care

Social circumstances
Diversity issues-Ethnicity, sexuality, religion, gender,
disability and age
Financial situation
Accommodation
Activities of daily living
Relationship with others–in and out of school

Mental State

*How the child or young person is observed whilst in
the assessment appointment.This is more relevant to
older children and adolescents but it can be helpful to
think about some of the domains with the younger
children too.*

Appearance and Behaviour
Facial appearance
Dress and self care
Manner
Posture and Movement
Appropriateness
Speech
Mood and Affect including suicidal ideation.
Thoughts
Form
Content
Perception
Cognition
Orientation
Attention and Concentration
Memory
Insight

Risk assessment

Care plan

Fig 23.1 Issues to be addressed in a comprehensive CAMHS assessment

Mental health problems in childhood

When considered within a developmental context different patterns of mental health problems can be observed. Angold and Egger (2007) describe five patterns:

1. Disorders that manifest early and continue in the same form with more or less improvement or deterioration.

2. Disorders that manifest early in life, but tend to disappear by adulthood.
3. Disorders that may begin in childhood that wax and wane without significant changes in prevalence over time.
4. Disorders that are more common early in life, but decline in prevalence with age.
5. Disorders that are rare or even non-existent in early life, but become more common in later childhood, adolescence or adulthood.

Pre-school problems

There is much controversy and discussion about whether it is possible or appropriate to give pre-school children a mental health diagnosis. The most common problems are emotional and behavioural disturbances and eating, sleeping and adjustment disorders and regulatory disorder (Skovgaard *et al.* 2007) but studies have also suggested prevalence rates for depression are 0.3–1.4 per cent (e.g. Egger and Angold 2006).

'Lack of appropriate stimulation in the early years may result in language delay and together with inappropriate child-rearing practices, especially if characterized by neglect or inconsistency, may lead to emotional or behavioural disorders' (DH/DES 2004). Pre-school problems such as sleep problems, tantrums and feeding problems are relatively common. Boys of pre-school age in Western society have been found to have behavioural problems and irritability more often than girls (Coplan *et al.* 2003). Disorders starting in pre-school years can persist into later life. Children with difficult temperaments are more likely to react to adverse family factors and present psychological difficulties beyond their pre-school years.

Hyperactivity

The essential features of this disorder are developmentally inappropriate degrees of inattention, impulsiveness and hyperactivity. For a diagnosis to be made these need to cause impairment and be exhibited in different settings. The British have used more stringent criteria in the diagnosis of 'hyperkinesis' whereas North Americans use a wider criteria for 'attention deficit hyperactivity disorder' (ADHD). UK epidemiological studies have suggested prevalence rates were 1.4 per cent for ADHD and 1 per cent for ICD-10 hyperkinetic disorder although some studies have found rates of up to 5–6 per cent (National Statistical Office 2005; Thapar and Munoz-Solomando 2008).

There are many factors associated with ADHD but the causes remain unclear. The environmental risk factors occur early in a child's development supporting the idea that ADHD is a neurodevelopmental condition (Banerjee *et al.* 2007). Risk factors include genetics, prenatal influences, exposure to lead, maternal alcohol use and stress in pregnancy, maternal smoking, negative parent–child relationships, parental negative discipline, poor social support, and speech and language difficulties (e.g. Thapar *et al.* 2007). Research has found food additives and watching television are not associated with ADHD (e.g. Stevens and Mulsow 2006).

Marked restlessness, inattention and impulsiveness are characteristic features of hyperactivity. The children wriggle and squirm in their seats, find it hard to sit still in one place or experience difficulty persisting with any activity. In situations requiring attention and concentration, the child is easily distracted and seems not to listen when spoken to directly. Socially, such children find it hard awaiting their turn in activities or conversation, often blurting out answers before questions have been completed. For a diagnosis of hyperkinesis, the hyperactivity must be pervasive across different settings, for example, at home and at school. Diagnosis requires a chronicity of at least six months of symptoms and onset before the age of 7.

Assessment

A full child and adolescent mental health assessment needs to be taken with particular emphasis on attention, activity levels and impulsiveness. The history should include details on parenting style, developmental history, attachment patterns and social relationships. School reports and a school observation, by a CAMHS professional, are a valuable source of information and to ensure symptoms are present across all areas. Details of classroom behaviour, organizational skills and peer relationships can often confirm concerns about hyperactivity. The assessment is usually supported by using the Conners' Teacher's and Parent's Questionnaires (Conners 1973) and Strength and Difficulties Questionnaire (Goodman 1997). The scores on the questionnaires are not diagnostic and cannot be used as a substitute for clinical assessment.

Treatment

Current guidelines support multimodal treatment packages including medication, behaviour management, parent training programmes, psychoeducation, classroom interventions and support. Support for the family is crucial regarding management of the child. Parents need to adopt a consistent attitude to parenting with clear guidelines for acceptable behaviour. Simple time-out procedures can be used for unacceptable behaviour. Encouraging the child's sustained attention on jigsaws and Lego can increase the child's attention span. Psychoeducation for education staff may be required regarding the nature of the problem and the management of children with ADHD. Most children with hyperactive disorder require high levels of supervision and encouragement to remain on task.

Medication is the most effective treatment for hyperactivity. Psychostimulants, such as methylphenidate, have a beneficial effect on restlessness, inattentiveness and impulsiveness. Improvement in concentration and attention can increase academic performance leading to improved self-esteem and confidence. Common side effects of psychostimulant drugs include reduced appetite, weight loss and difficulty in falling asleep. Most children will need to continue medication at least until their early teens. Those on medication need to have their growth checked regularly as there is clear evidence that psychostimulates can effect a child's growth (Poulton 2005) and blood pressure should be monitored using gender specific blood pressure charts.

The MTA Co-operative Group (1999) demonstrated that where patients had a combined intervention of medication and behavioural therapy symptoms improved, their families benefited and there were less challenging behaviours, resulting in a reduction in medication. Behaviour therapy alone did not have such positive results leading to this approach alone not typically being recommended. Outcome can be determined by the presence of other concurrent disorders such as Asperger's syndrome, autism and conduct disorders.

Pervasive developmental disorders

Pervasive developmental disorders (PDD) represent a group whose difficulties are generally in social interaction, communication and behaviour particularly where the difficulties have manifested themselves before 3 years of age. PDD includes autism, Rett's disorder, childhood disintegrative disorder, overactive disorder associated with mental retardation and stereotyped movements, Asperger's disorder, and other PDD (WHO 1996). Prevalence rates vary but the general view is of 1 in 500 (Fombonne 1999). Boys are affected three times as much as girls. Asperger's syndrome is regarded by some as a milder version of autism. These children are often aloof, distant and lacking in empathy. There is usually no delay in the development of vocabulary and grammar, though other aspects of language are abnormal as in autism.

Autism has a high genetic loading and there is an extended phenotype in families with subtle social and language defects, and circumscribed interests. It is associated with a number of medical conditions and there is strong evidence of prenatal abnormality (Taylor 2006). The MMR vaccination has been incriminated as a cause of autism but this has been ruled out by extensive research (Smeeth *et al.* 2004; Honda *et al.* 2005).

Assessment

A comprehensive assessment is needed by a multi-disciplinary team. This involves a thorough neurological assessment and in-depth cognitive and language testing as well as observation of the child's behaviour and social communication skills.

The impairment of social development often reveals itself in infancy as the child appears aloof, fails to seek comfort from adults and generally shows a lack of interest in people. In half of the children with autism, some social interest and competence develops, although problems with empathy and social reciprocity remain. Roughly 50 per cent of children fail to acquire useful speech. Acquisition of language is delayed and, when present, language abnormalities are common, including poor comprehension, intonation and pronominal reversal (for example using 'you' for 'I').

Common abnormalities include resistance to change, stereotyped, narrow and repetitive patterns of play (for example, lining up toys). Some children show intensive attachment to unusual objects or preoccupation and interests (train timetables, cricket scores). Early signs of a lack of social interest may be missed but, by the second or third year of life, their social deficits become more noticeable. Some children go through a stage when they lose previously acquired skills.

Treatment

Treatments for children with PDD involve intensive, coordinated programmes involving education, language, development and behaviour intervention (Hurth *et al.* 1999). Intensive early intervention in optimal educational settings results in improved outcomes in most young children with autism (Rogers 1998) although complete resolution of symptoms is generally not achieved. Medication is sometimes also used, particularly to manage anxiety, depression, hyperactivity and obsessive compulsive disorder. Children with autism do well in a structured educational setting with behavioural programmes to reduce ritualistic behaviour, tantrums and aggressive behaviour while encouraging the child in task-orientated work. The prognosis is better in children with higher intelligence and for children who acquire useful speech by the age of 5 years.

Conduct disorders

Conduct disorders consist of repetitive and persistent patterns of behaviour which are age-inappropriate and violate accepted social norms. Children with conduct disorder often bully, intimidate or threaten others. Physical fight, cruelty to animals and people, serious violation of rules, such as truanting, staying away from home and damage to property and involvement in the Youth Justice System are not uncommon for this group. A category of family-based conduct disorders may be present where there is no significant disturbance or abnormality of social relationships outside the family. Disruptive behaviour in the classroom is common leading to repeated exclusion from schools, poor interpersonal relationships and poor academic achievement. Oppositional defiant disorder is a sub-type of conduct disorder in younger children. Usually there is an absence of behaviour that violates the law or seriously interferes with the rights of others.

Assessment

When assessing a child alternatives to conduct disorder need to be considered such as hearing problems, hyperkinetic disorder, chronic dental pain and specific learning difficulties. Co-morbid mental health problems are often present (Thomas 2006) and it is important to be mindful of focusing solely on the 'bad' behaviour.

Treatment

NICE (2006) recommend parent training, group sessions based on social learning theory where parents identify their own goals including role play and homework. This is only recommended for children aged 12 or under.

School refusal

Children who present with problems of school attendance are sometimes referred to CAMHS. The school refusal may be linked to a conduct disorder, where the child may be engaging in other activities without the knowledge of their parents. Alternatively the school refusal may be linked to a school phobia or separation anxiety. With the latter the problem can present in a variety of ways including abdominal pain and headaches in the mornings before setting out for school. Onset may be abrupt in which case a precipitating factor is likely to be found, or gradual with the child increasingly reluctant to attend school. The child is often fearful of separating from the parent and leaving home. There is often a lack of authority on the part of the parents to enforce attendance. Emotional over-involvement by the parents can also play a part. Treatment and management involves dealing with the underlying condition and working with the parents to enable them to enforce school. Effective liaison with the school is essential to deal with issues such as bullying and to harness teachers' support. Change of schools rarely helps unless there are particular problems, for example, distance from school, academic ability, necessitating change.

Emotional disorders

Emotional disturbances, such as anxiety and depression, are associated with poor outcomes for children. Up to 18 per cent of children meet the diagnostic criteria for an anxiety disorder (e.g. Costello *et al.* 2004). Anxiety and depression are associated with immaturity, inattention and concentration problems, academic difficulties, poor peer relations, low self-esteem and low social competence as well as mental health problems in later life (e.g. Bittner *et al.* 2007).

Separation anxiety arises in response to separation from parents and other attachment figures. It is most prominent during the pre-school years. When the intensity of anxiety is developmentally inappropriate and handicapping, separation anxiety disorder is diagnosed. Children with this condition are reluctant to let their parents out of their sight and complain of physical symptoms, for example, headaches, stomach ache and nausea when separation is enforced (in the mornings before setting out for school).

Generalized anxiety disorders are present in roughly 3 per cent of children who experience persistent anxieties and worries which are not related to a particular event or situation. Somatic complaints are common.

Specific phobias are common in early childhood. Animal phobias are common before the age of 2–4. Anxiety leads to avoidance and distress. It is more common in girls.

Treatment

Cognitive behavioural therapy has been shown to be helpful in the treatment of anxiety disorders, and is the first line of treatment (cf. Chapter 20), but there remain 20–60 per cent of children in research trials who do not show an improvement (Liber *et al.* 2008). In addition, family-based treatments, such as parent training programmes (Eisen *et al.* 2008), group programmes (Flannery-Schroeder *et al.* 2005) and antidepressants (Madden 2005) are effective.

Depression

There is now general acceptance that children can suffer from depression. Studies have demonstrated depressive symptomology starting before puberty, continuing into adolescence and adulthood. There are, however, some important developmental differences with children being relatively more reactive to their environment than adults. Depressed children are more likely to have parents with depression. Parents with depression are also more likely to have children who are depressed. Studies suggest a strong genetic loading while environmental factors clearly play an important role. About 1–2 per cent of prepubertal children and about 3–8 per cent of adolescents have experienced a depressive episode by the time they reach adulthood (e.g. Zalsman *et al.* 2006).

Young people will present with changes in mood, thinking and activity but may not have the emotional literacy to portray what they are experiencing. Instead they may describe somatic symptoms such as musculoskeletal pains and headaches. Poor concentration, low self-esteem and guilt are also common features. As with adult depressive disorder, depressed mood, hopelessness, misery and tearfulness are common. Changes in the young person's experience of school and social life may often herald the onset of depression. The presence of behavioural problems is common in depressed children and may mask an underlying depression. Changes in appetite and weight loss are less common than in adults. Suicidal thoughts and behaviour may lead to referral by worried parents or teachers.

The onset of depression in adolescence may be acute or insidious. While brief periods of low moods are not uncommon in children, evidence of sustained low mood needs to be elicited for a diagnosis of depressive disorder. It is not uncommon for parents to be unaware of depression in their children: there is often a precipitant for the episode of depression and some children may have been victims of physical or sexual abuse.

Treatment

NICE (2005a) have produced guidelines for depression in children and young people. The major aims of treatment are to reduce depression, to promote social and emotional functioning and help the family in understanding and dealing with their child's illness. Within three months 10 per cent will recover spontaneously and a further 40 per cent will within a year. Therefore a period of watchful waiting is recommended for mild depressions. Watching for any signs of deterioration and offering support.

In severe cases of depression where there is a high risk of self-harm the child may need admission to an inpatient unit. In the community, cognitive behavioural therapy (CBT) has been shown to be effective. CBT helps develop cognitive strategies for dealing with negative thoughts and helps in developing problem-solving techniques. Programmes have been researched and validated that are computer based as well as in manual form.

Antidepressant medication has been found to increase the risk of suicidal behaviour in adolescents and so should not be the first line of treatment. When it is offered it should be fluoxetine in the first instant, as this is the only one where the benefits have outweighed the risk of side effects. Also medication should be given in combination with a psychological therapy such as CBT unless the therapy has been declined. When taking the antidepressant the young person needs to be monitored for suicidal behaviour, deliberate self-harm and aggression.

Disorders of social functioning

This category includes selective mutism, reactive attachment disorders of childhood and disinhibited attachment disorders of infancy.

Selective mutism

The main problem in this condition is the child's refusal to talk in certain situations while conversing normally in others. Generally, normal speech is present while in a minority there are problems of articulation and speech production. Milder forms present themselves at the start of school life and are usually transitory. High levels of social phobia have been found in children who are selectively mute (Manassis *et al.* 2003). A speech and language assessment forms an important part of the assessment (Manassis *et al.* 2007).

Treatment

Treatment similar to that for anxiety has provided some success. There is also some evidence for anxiolytic medications in selective mutism (Dummit *et al.* 1996).

Attachment disorders

The motion of attachment in infants was strongly influenced by the writings of John Bowlby (1980). According to these theories, a child needs to be attached to a protective figure as biologically adaptive. Children develop attachments to a relatively small number of figures. This relationship offers a secure base from which the child explores the world around them. Although all children develop attachments, the quality of the attachments vary greatly and can be measured by how distressed the child becomes when separated and by the child's response to reunions. Children with attachment disorders have significantly more behavioural and psychosocial problems (Buckner *et al.* 2008).

Treatment

A number of treatments have been put forward, principles of interventions have been outlined and research is under way but, to date, no clear evidence-based practice has been identified (Newman and Mares 2007).

Elimination disorders

Enuresis

Primary enuresis is when bladder control has never been achieved and secondary is when bladder control is lost after a child has acquired it for at least six months. Boys are more prone to nocturnal enuresis (bed wetting at night) while girls are to diurnal enuresis. Once continence is achieved relapse occurs most commonly around the age of 5 or 6. About 70 per cent of enuretic children have a first degree relative with a history of wetting. Girls with enuresis are more likely to suffer from urinary tract infections.

It is arguable whether enuresis is a mental health problem. Enuresis is associated with stressful life events at the age of 3–4 years including early separations, birth of siblings, accidents and admissions to hospital as well as with with social disadvantage and institutional care (Douglas 1973). It is also thought culture has a role in the prevalence of enuresis (Safarinejad 2007) but In Europe, the reported rate of prevalence of nocturnal enuresis is 9–19 per cent at 5 years, 7–22 per cent at 7 years, 5–13 per cent at 9 years, and 1–2 per cent at 16 years (Butler 1998).

Treatment

Physical causes need to be excluded prior to mental health service involvement. Treatment is unlikely to be successful unless the child and family are motivated. A multifaceted treatment package is recommended (Robson 2008) including behaviour therapy and good bladder health education. Also treatment of nocturnal polyuria and reduced functional bladder control is recommended. A disorder of sleep arousal may also be present and alarm therapy can be considered.

Encopresis

Encopresis or faecal soiling is the voiding of faeces in inappropriate places and usually involves the soiling of the child's clothes. At the age of 7, the prevalence in boys is 2.3 per cent and 0.7 per cent in girls. By the age of 11, less than 1 per cent of children soil themselves once a month (Hersov 1994).

Faecal soiling can occur for a variety of reasons. Some children fail to achieve continence as they have never learned bowel control and this is termed primary faecal soiling. This is usually found in the context of inconsistent or coercive toilet training practice. Treatment involves educating parents in proper toilet training methods on realistic targets and reinforcement of achievement by the child. Star charts can be used to record success. Fear of using the toilet can lead to some children soiling their clothes. General reassurance and rewards for appropriate use of the toilet can help resolve the problem.

In some children encopresis may occur as a result of long-standing faecal retention. The original cause may be emotional or physical but, in time, leads to constipation. Chronic constipation can lead to hard faeces acting as a plug. Liquid and semi-solid stools eventually leak past the plug causing soiling. This form of soiling arises as a result of constipation with overflow leading to soiling. Soiling can occur in children who have achieved continence when they experience stressful situations such as physical or sexual abuse. The main aim of treatment is to reduce stress.

The provocative or aggressive soiler deliberately defecates onto furniture or smears walls with faeces. There is an association with dysfunctional family systems based on social disorganization and coercive and abusive child-rearing practices. Management and treatment usually needs the coordinated input of several agencies including social services and education.

Treatment

A combination of family education, disimpaction and maintenance medications, a well-balanced diet, and behavior management is essential (Philichi 2008).

Child maltreatment

There are wide variations in the reported incidence of child abuse and neglect based on variation in definition and methods used to estimate prevalence. Types of abuse include:

- physical abuse – non-accidental injury, burns, fractures, bruises;
- emotional abuse – threats, hostility, failure to protect;
- sexual abuse – penetrative, non-penetrative;
- neglect – lack of appropriate care and nurture, stimulation and supervision.

The causative factors are complex and multi-factorial. Parents who abuse children have often been victims of abuse themselves. Perpetrators often have problems in a number of areas including vocational and social skills, substance abuse, poor education and low income. Abuse is often seen as a part of dysfunction formerly with poor parent–child bonding and attachment. Abuse may also take place in institutional care, schools and children's homes.

Management

The primary aim is to prevent further abuse by safeguarding the child. A referral to the social care services is of utmost importance where an assessment and investigation can take place to ensure the safety and protection of the child. The second aim is to work in partnership with the other agencies to help meet the child's social, emotional and psychological needs while providing support to the family.

Mental health in adolescence

Although adolescence is often associated with a period of stress and turmoil, most adolescents manage the transition between childhood and adulthood without major problems. It is a period, however, during which there are major changes in body image, self-esteem, relationships with parents and mood. Awareness about sexual orientation and identity are also heightened. The rate at which children mature differs with early maturing boys showing some social advantage over boys who mature later. Early maturing girls, on the other hand tend to experience some depression and anxiety compared with late maturers.

Discomfort and embarrassment about body shape and size are comparatively greater in this group. Conflicts with parents and emotional and behavioural problems are also more commonly experienced.

The term 'identity crisis' was used originally by Erikson (1968), to describe the process of development during adolescence, leading to a well-developed notion of self. Experimentation with different roles and beliefs is not uncommon. There are large differences in the rate and pace of change in the development of personal identity. Adolescence is a period of transition between childhood and adulthood and, in most cultures, is heralded by the onset of puberty while termination is often socially and culturally determined. The interplay of social and biological influences play an important part in the disorders of adolescence.

Emotional conduct disorders are the most commonly diagnosed and, in a proportion of adolescents, are the continuation of unresolved disorders in earlier childhood. Conduct problems become more pronounced with the onset of adolescence and may result in forensic involvement. Substance misuse is also more evident. Anxiety disorders related to school attendance, phobias and agoraphobia may have its onset in adolescence. Obsessive compulsive disorders presenting with obsessional ideas, ruminations and ritual and can be associated with anxiety, depression or Tourette's syndrome. Depressive disorders, mania and bipolar disorders are more common during adolescent than in childhood. Self-harm and suicide rates also show an increase. A proportion of children with pervasive developmental disorders develop epilepsy during adolescence. Behavioural disturbance can increase and children may show difficulties in understanding and expressing sexual behaviour.

Although schizophrenia can occur in younger children, its onset before puberty is rare. Males are more vulnerable and it is usually preceded by a stage of behavioural and social difficulties and this may make early diagnosis difficult. Eating disorders, such as anorexia nervosa and bulimia nervosa have their onset during adolescence. In anorexia nervosa onset before puberty is uncommon. The prevalence rises from 0.1 per cent in 11- to 15-year-olds to 1 per cent in 16- to 18-year-olds; the male/female ratio being 1:10. Bulimia peaks a few years later (Steinhausen 1994).

Obsessive compulsive disorder

While there are striking similarities between the phenomenology of obsessive compulsive disorder (OCD) in children and adults, significant differences exist in terms of gender distribution, co-morbidity, familial contribution and developmental issues. Roughly a third of adults have their first symptoms before the age of 15. Prevalence studies suggest rates of 1.9–4 per cent in children (Zohar 1999) with onset averaging at 7–12 years but the age of onset is not predictive of outcome (Piacentini *et al.* 2002).

Obsessions are recurrent, intrusive thoughts, ideas or images or impulses that the person experiences as ego-dystonic and intensely distressing. One of the core characteristics of obsession in adults is that they are resisted. Resistance to obsessions and compulsions in children is, however, not always present. Common obsessions in childhood focus on contamination, harm or death, and symmetry. Compulsions are repetitive physical or mental acts that the person feels driven to perform in response to that obsession. The purpose of the compulsion is usually to reduce anxiety or magically prevent a dreaded event. Compulsive behaviour can become so extreme that it interferes with normal social functioning. Common examples are checking, touching, washing and repeating acts.

Normal childhood ritual such as bedtime routine and collecting are not uncommon in early childhood. Symptoms of OCD can present secondary to primary depressive disorders. Children with the autistic spectrum group of disorders may present with repetitive behaviour and sometimes develop full-blown symptoms of OCD. Symptoms of OCD can be associated with schizophrenia and anorexia. Obsessive compulsive symptoms occur in up to two thirds of patients with Tourette's syndrome.

Treatment

OCD is a chronic condition and needs long-term commitment to its management. Cognitive behavioural therapy including exposure and response prevention, involving the family (NICE 2005b; Freeman *et al.* 2008) is the first line of treatment. Medication, such as SSRIs, have all shown to be effective and is used when CBT has not had the desired effect. Good insight is related to better outcomes from treatment (Storch *et al.* 2008).

Suicide and deliberate self-harm

Suicide is the third leading cause of death in adolescence (Belfer 2008). Completed suicide is rare before puberty but its incidence increases during older adolescence. Suicidal behaviour and the meaning given to it are thought to be culturally specific (e.g. Borges *et al.* 2007; Apter *et al.* 2008) and religion tends not to act as a protective factor, as it does in adults (Murthy 2000). The most consistent correlates of suicidal ideas are psychiatric disorders, child sexual abuse, and maladaptive personality traits (Brezo *et al.* 2007). Studies have rejected the idea that music genres cause suicide although it may be suggestive of a vulnerability (e.g. Rustad *et al.* 2003).

Deliberate self-harm

Deliberate self-harm (DSH) peaks at adolescence and is generally low in childhood. Suicidal ideation is relatively common in adolescence with 10–20 per cent experiencing such thoughts over the past year. During early adolescence, DSH rates are far higher in females than males tending to start at around 12 years (Hawton and Harriss 2008). Common risk factors include previous DSH, alcohol misuse, sexual activity (Patton *et al.* 2007). A history of sexual abuse or physical abuse and parental psychiatric disorder may be present.

Assessment

All children who self-harm should have a full CAMHS assessment including a careful assessment of risk, taking into account family history of mood disturbance and past attempts at self-harm. Children who commit DSH may be seen in accident and emergency departments and admitted to an inpatient ward where they can be seen the following day for a full assessment once the toxic effects of an overdose have been dealt with. They should be seen by appropriately trained professionals. Some hospitals now have a Paediatric Liaison Service. Clear protocols need to be in place to meet the needs of these children so that they do not fall into the gaps between the medical and mental health services for children and those for adults. Factors indicating the suicide risk of children following an incident of DSH are shown in Table 23.2. Most children who self-harm should be offered follow-up after assessment.

Treatment

NICE (2004a) have published guidelines for the management of deliberate self-harm. Where repeated self-harm occurs up to six sessions of group psychotherapy can be offered. Involvement of the family is beneficial. They should be encouraged to see DSH as serious and play a role in minimizing further risk of DSH. Individual therapy aimed at helping the children to refrain from the problem and adopt a problem-solving approach has shown to be beneficial.

	Low risk	High risk
Location of overdose	In public, for example, on school bus	Isolated in the woods, locked room
Timing	Intervention likely	Intervention unlikely
Precipitants	Impulsive – following argument with girl/boyfriend	Extensive premeditation
Preparations in anticipation of death	No suicide note	Suicide notes stating arrangements for funeral, etc.
Attitude following overdose	Relieved about safe outcome	Still expressing suicidal intent
Revaluation of problems precipitating DSH	Positive, for example, school taking problems more seriously	Negative – outlook pessimistic

Table 23.2 Suicide risk assessment in children following deliberate self-harm (DSH)

Tourette's syndrome

This condition has been recognized for over 150 years. Tourette's syndrome affects 3–5 per 10,000 children. Prevalence is ten times greater in children than it is in adults and occurs four times more commonly in males than in females (Robertson 1989).

The mean age of onset of symptoms is 7 years and the essential features of the illness are the existence of multiple motor tics and at least one vocal tic. The most common symptoms involve eye-blinking, and tics affecting the face, neck or head. The onset of vocalization usually occurs later than the motor tics. Coprolalia, the inappropriate and involuntary uttering of obscenities, is seen in about a third of patients seen at the clinic. The manifestation of the tics varies in response to different conditions. Anxiety, stress and fatigue can aggravate tics. Concentration on controlling the symptoms can lead to temporary disappearance of symptoms. Children with Tourette's syndrome are disproportionately likely to be obsessional. Attention deficit hyperactivity disorder occurs in roughly 25–50 per cent.

Treatment

For the milder versions, explanation and reassurance to teacher, parents and the child has been shown to be helpful as well as self-help groups. Treatment is either medication (Robertson 1989) or habit reversal (HR) based on social learning theory (Verdellen et al. 2004). Progressive Tourette's syndrome runs a lifelong course with symptoms waxing and waning over time. In up to a third, the tics symptoms remit by late adolescents while an additional third show significant improvement in symptoms.

Mania and bipolar affective disorder

Manic disorders are rare before puberty. In pre-pubertal children, symptoms of mania may be confused with attention deficit hyperactive disorder. Manic patients present with irritability, euphoria or elated mood and insomnia. They tend to be hyperactive and may engage in reckless and impulsive behaviour. Mania may be part of a bipolar affective disorder with episodes of depression and mania. Onset is usually during adolescence or early adulthood. Neuroleptic drugs or lithium are commonly used to control acute episodes.

Psychosis

As discussed in Chapter 18 schizophrenia first presents typically in early adult life and is relatively rare in childhood. The majority of cases tend to have an onset in adolescence. Making a firm diagnosis is often difficult because of the limited verbal skills of the child and the confusion between vivid normal fantasy life and psychotic thinking. It can also be difficult to distinguish the prodromal stages of the illness from other disorders. Cannabis use has also been associated with the incidence of prodromal symptoms of psychosis (Miettunen *et al.* 2008).

About 40 per cent of males and 23 per cent of females have an onset of schizophrenia before age 19 (Schulz *et al.* 1998). Children with schizophrenia often present with earlier developmental delays and poor premorbid functioning. Developmental delays are particularly common in the areas of language development, reading and bladder control. A third of children also show difficulties in forming socio-emotional relationships. The onset of schizophrenia is usually insidious. There is usually a strong family history of psychosis/schizophrenia.

The main features of the clinical picture are described in Chapter 18.

Treatment
Before starting treatment it is important to seek consent from the patient and adults holding parental responsibility. Assessment of competence to give consent needs to be tailored to the young person's age and understanding of the purpose, nature and likely effects and risks. Inpatient admission should be considered where there is serious risk to the safety of the young person or others. Lack of insight and poor compliance with treatment are other factors which need to be considered. Alternatively, the patient may be treated as a day patient or an outpatient.

The NICE (2006) guideline for schizophrenia does not include children. Medication is the first line treatment of choice. Olanzapine and risperidone have been used with good effect. During the acute phase, benzodiazepine may be used to relieve distress or reduce behavioural disturbances. Psychoeducation of parents and the patient about the illness, treatment and prognosis is an essential part of treatment, aiding their understanding of an illness which can be frightening and stigmatizing. Cognitive behavioural strategies and supportive counselling may be beneficial.

Substance misuse in adolescence

There is increasing evidence of a rise in substance abuse among British adolescents. A survey of British 15- to 16-year-olds found that almost half had tried illicit drugs at some time (Fergusson and Horwood 2000). While most children who experiment with illicit drugs do not go on to habitual abuse of drugs, the earlier the onset, the more persistent the habit becomes and some will become substance dependent as adults. When compared to adults, young people experience more rapid progression from first use to abuse and dependence, shorter time from first to second dependence diagnosis, and an increase in other mental health problems (Winters 1999). Drug use is also a major risk in completed suicide. Among adolescent females involved in drug misuse, affective symptoms are likely to be more common while, in males, conduct disorders predominate.

While a proportion of illicit drug-abusing children go on to adult dependence, there are significant differences in the pattern of abuse among adolescents and adults. Children with conduct disorders are more likely to misuse drugs. The risk is increased in children with conduct disorder and hyperactivity. Adult role models and peer group drug use have a strong influence on adolescent drug abuse. Inhaling organic solvents is particularly associated with adolescent abuse and social adversity. There is some evidence to suggest that multiple drug use is more common among adolescents than adults with an irregular pattern of abuse rather than chronic use, as a result, dependence among adolescents in relatively uncommon.

Treatment

While substance misuse is more likely to respond to early treatment in adolescence, motivation in accepting treatment is generally poor. It is often the concern of others which leads to referral and young people do not readily present themselves for treatment. Only 10 per cent of young people who would meet the criteria for treatment are actually referred to services (Substance Abuse and Mental Health Services Administration (SAMHSA) 2007). An assertive approach therefore needs to be adopted, usually involving other agencies such as youth offending services, social services and education.

Although alcohol dependence is uncommon, in cases where dependence has developed, detoxification is required. Evidence-based protocols are available and research has emphasized the importance of maintaining a strong fidelity to the programmes (Hogue *et al.* 2008). Family influences play a significant role in the onset and progression of drug misuse; and family therapy approaches using techniques such as the multi-dimensional family therapy have been shown to be beneficial. Adolescents need considerable support to abstain from drug use. Interagency support and help with education, accommodation and training is important. Drug and alcohol use is discussed in detail in Chapter 22.

Eating disorders in children and adolescents

Eating disorders are conditions in which there is excessive preoccupation and concern with control of body weight and shape, with grossly restricted food intake or binging and vomiting. There are medical concerns particular to children with eating disorders due to the impact on their physical development. The term 'eating disorder' in children and adolescents covers a range of early onset conditions where one or all of the psychological, social and physical areas of functioning is involved. The spectrum of eating disorders in childhood and early adolescence covers the following: early onset anorexia nervosa, bulimia nervosa, food avoidance emotional disorder (FAED), selective eating, and pervasive refusal syndrome. It is important to note that eating disorders can arise secondary to other disorders such as depression, and obsessive compulsive disorders. Eating disorders are covered also in Chapter 21 of this volume and this should be considered alongside NICE (2004b) guidelines for the management and treatment of children with eating disorders.

Assessment

Individual psychopathology is best assessed through a structured interview such as the Eating Disorders Examination (EDE) (Fairburn and Cooper 1993) or child EDE for those under 13 years of age (Bryant-Waugh *et al.* 1996). The family should be assessed but the child should also be offered individual sessions during the assessment and throughout treatment. It is important that age appropriate height and weight charts are used.

Childhood onset anorexia nervosa

Anorexia nervosa can develop from about 8 years of age, reaching a peak around 15–18 (Bryant-Waugh and Lask 2007). In adolescent populations the prevalence of anorexia is estimated to be 0.1–0.2 per cent, and is lower in younger children. Among adolescents, 5–10 per cent of cases occur in males while in younger male children the numbers may be up to a third.

The features of childhood onset anorexia nervosa are:

- failure to maintain weight or gain weight with age and development or actual weight loss in relation to age;
- determined food avoidance;
- abnormal concerns/preoccupation with weight and shape;
- amenorrhoea in post-menarcheal adolescents or delayed or arrested puberty.

Although a number of psychological and familial factors have been implicated as playing a role in the pathogenesis of anorexia nervosa, there is insufficient empirical evaluation for these hypotheses. Cultural and social factors are also important. Generally, eating disorders are reported more frequently in societies where food is plentiful and thinness is valued. The risk of anorexia is high in occupations such as modelling and ballet dancing where there is an emphasis on slimness.

The onset is usually insidious and the most significant feature is food avoidance leading to severe weight loss. Patients are often secretive and adolescents are likely to avoid unsupervised meals such as school lunches. Distortions of body image are common, with denial of weight loss even when grossly underweight. Other associated symptoms include excessive physical activity in an attempt to lose weight and burn calories. Preoccupation with preparing food and feeding others is not uncommon. With decreasing weight the physical effects of starvation become evident. Patients complain of tiredness, lethargy, constipation and cold extremities. It is important to bear in mind that in severe cases death may occur and use of the Mental Health Act or the Children Act may be needed particularly when both the carer and the young person are refusing treatment and the situation is critical.

Treatment

NICE (2004b) recommend that family interventions directly addressing the eating disorder should be offered. The benefits of inpatient care, into age appropriate facilities, should be balanced against the effect on the young person's education and social needs. Dietary education and monitoring should aim at ensuring nutrients necessary to support the child's development are being consumed.

Bulimia nervosa

Bulimia nervosa is rare below the age of 13 but becomes more common than anorexia by young adulthood (Bryant-Waugh and Lask 2007). This is an eating disorder characterized by episodes of binge eating. During these episodes large amounts of food are consumed over short periods. The condition should not be diagnosed in patients with a diagnosis of anorexia nervosa up to 50 per cent of whom also binge eat. Periods of binge eating are usually preceded by intense craving or preoccupation with food and intractable urges to overeat. Although fear of becoming fat and concerns about body weight are common, usually body weight is close to normal.

The majority of patients are female. Patients usually describe loss of control over eating as the most significant problem. Up to 50 per cent vomit and binge eat or both on a daily basis. As this behaviour is associated with shame and guilt, self-induced vomiting is usually secretive. Disorders of mood with depression guilt and suicidal thought may be present. Impulsiveness in the form of promiscuousness and shoplifting of food is present in some cases.

Treatment

Most adolescents can be treated on an outpatient basis. Cognitive behaviour therapy that has been adapted to suit the young person's age, circumstances and level of development has been shown to be effective.

Somatizing in children and adolescents

Most professionals accept the need to take a holistic approach bringing together the physical and psychological dimensions in the assessment and treatment of children and adolescents. Complaints of somatic symptoms are common in children presenting with psychological problems. This chapter deals more specifically with conditions in which the main complaints are of somatic symptoms and where there is inadequate explanation in terms of a physical cause.

Developmental factors play an important role in the presentation of these disorders. Parental and cultural attitudes to 'illness behaviour' in children influence if and how children somatize. Very young children are less able to convey psychological distress based on their verbal competence and cognitive development. 'In the general population, 2–10 per cent of children have aches and pains, which are mostly unexplained, and 5–10 per cent of children and adolescents report distressing somatic symptoms or are regarded by their parents as 'sickly' (Garralda 2008).

The categories of somatic disorder differ based on the nature, chronicity and impact of unexplained somatic symptoms. There are certain factors associated with an increased reporting of physical symptoms; girls consistently report more symptoms, the gender difference becoming more marked during adolescence. This may, in part, be related to the increase in symptom reporting associated with the onset of menarche. Other factors, including temperament and conditions such as anxiety and depression, family discord, major life events, poor parental care and experience of abuse are also significant factors.

Dissociative disorders

The most common symptom in young people is loss of motor function but loss of function in any modality may be reported. Complaints of sensory loss involving sight, hearing or consciousness are not uncommon. The symptoms present as an 'epidemic' particularly involving girls where large numbers of children in a class report the same symptoms. True prevalence is difficult to estimate as transient disorders are not brought to medical attention. Unlike the individual form, the disorder may arise in a number of individuals within a closed community, such as a school or children's home. This variety of disorder is often described as 'epidemic hysteria'.

Diagnosis of the condition is fraught with difficulties as a proportion of children diagnosed on follow-up have been shown to be suffering from an organic condition. Children who are referred usually have had extensive physical investigations. It is important to engage the family in exploring the psychological stressor without stigmatizing the patient as malingering. Individual and family work has been shown to be helpful.

Chronic fatigue syndrome

This is a condition in which severe disabling fatigue persists for over six months (three months in children) and is associated with a variety of other associated symptoms unexplained by primary physical or psychiatric causes. The most significant complaint on presentation is one of fatigue often preceded by a flu-like illness from which complete recovery has not been made. Associated low mood, mental fatigue and inability to concentrate are not uncommon. Girls are more affected than boys.

The aetiological model is complex and physical and psychological factors have been suggested. The presence of persistent viral infection, muscular dysfunction, immune dysfunction and electrolyte imbalance have all been implicated. Low mood, anxiety and depression are not uncommon and, in up to a third of cases, depression may be present. While most cases remain ambulant, in very severe forms, children may be confined to a wheelchair and remain disabled from taking part in normal activity over a period of years. These children often present in paediatric clinics and may be resistant to transfer to child and adolescent mental health services as they see the principle cause of the problems as organic. It is best to adopt a supportive role while remaining open to discussion about the relative contribution of physical and psychological factors involved. Individual work with the child in using behavioural and cognitive strategies in goal-setting and encouraging graded rehabilitation has been found to be beneficial. It is important to involve the family in examining attitudes to illness and in encouraging compliance with treatment plans.

Factitious disorders

These present from middle childhood and are seen more commonly in girls. Existing minor physical problems are often exaggerated through interference to make the condition look more dramatic. There is often a need for medical attention with repeated presentation at accident and emergency departments. There is an overlap with other somatizing disorders.

In the severe and chronic forms, difficulties in attachment and bonding, temperamental traits and abusive experience have been found. Low self-esteem and poor social skills and peer relationships may be present. Individual work addressing these difficulties has shown to be of help.

Principles of treatment in child and adolescent mental health

Once a comprehensive assessment has been completed, the child and parents need to be involved in drawing up a treatment plan. The successful rate of treatment will depend on the extent to which they feel their wishes, fears and anxieties have been addressed during the initial meetings. It is useful for the therapists and the family/child to set out some goals for what will be seen as a successful outcome of treatment. A model, such as the Family Partnership Approach (Davis *et al*. 2002), can be used to facilitate this throughout the families contact with the service.

Diagnostic labels are helpful if parents and the child have an understanding of the criteria used for making a diagnosis and its potential for treatment. Caution needs to be exercised, however, as diagnostic labels can be seen as stigmatizing and parents often withdraw from treatment for fear of being 'labelled'. Diagnosis has potential benefits as it is a concise way in which information, regarding the nature, origin and prognosis for a particular child, can be conveyed. It also allows for special provisions to be made to meet the child's needs (special school, statementing).

Comprehensive CAMHS

National Service Framework for Children Young People and Maternity Services: The Mental Health and Psychological Well-being of Children and Young People: Standard 9 (2007) sets out what CAMHS should look like. The underlying principles are that it is accessible, effectively commissioned, driven by a multi-agency assessment of needs and commissioned to meet the needs of the population safely, timely and effectively.

The NSF details what the services should look like. For example, there should be appropriately trained staff through tiers 1–4 delivering child and adolescent mental health services for all 0–18-year-olds including those with a learning disability with 24 hour specialist CAMHS care should be available. The workforce should have the appropriate skills, competencies and capabilities.

Multi-agency working

Mental health problems are not just the remit of child and adolescent mental health services; commitment, input and investment are required from everyone involved in delivery of services to adolescents (Hagell 2004). Collaborative practices are now seen as the most efficient way of delivering high quality services and ensuring their effectiveness in being responsive to service user needs (Miller and Ahmed 2000). There is a need for non-health workers to understand the importance of the need for treatment as part of working towards reducing the risk of reoffending, to protect the public and to increase life chances for the young person.

Following the inquiry into the death of Victoria Climbié (Laming 2003) *Every Child Matters* (DES 2003) was published and a number of measures to reform and improve children's care were proposed. The most crucial of these is the requirement for all local authorities to set up Children's Trusts that will integrate social services, education and health and the introduction of the Common Assessment Framework (CAF) and the Team Around the Child (TAC). The CAF is a standardized approach to conducting an assessment of a child's additional, rather than universal, needs and deciding how those needs should be met.

The TAC are the professionals that work with a child. TAC meetings are held following the completion of a CAF and at regular intervals thereafter. This meeting is generally attended by all the relevant professionals, the child and the parents or carers. At this meeting a plan is drawn up with the family and the CAF tends to be distributed, with consent from the family. A lead professional is allocated to the child, this may be the CAMHS professional.

Youth Justice

The Youth Justice System, in its current form, was established by the Crime and Disorder Act 1998; its aim is to prevent offending by children and young people. There are Youth Offending Teams (YOTs) in every geographical area of England and Wales. Various agencies are represented, some with statutory responsibility, including police, probation, social services, education, health, housing department, voluntary sector and youth services. The Crime and Disorder Act 1998 stipulates YOTs should include 'a person nominated by a health authority any part of whose area lies within the local authority's area'; frequently this is a mental health nurse. This person is expected to ensure young people are provided with 100 per cent access to health assessments.

As many as 23.7 per cent of young people who are offenders have reported a prior suicide attempt (Howard *et al.* 2003). Prevalence studies of young offenders suggest conduct disorders, suicide, depression, substance misuse, post-traumatic stress disorder and attention deficit and hyperactivity disorder are more common (e.g. Dixon *et al.* 2004). Depression is associated with long-term maladjustment and interpersonal difficulties in adolescence but there are poorer social outcomes and higher risk of suicide for those that are also offenders (Fombonne *et al.* 2001). 'Young people at the interface of the criminal justice system and mental health services risk double jeopardy for social exclusion, alienation and stigmatisation' (Bailey 1997) both from being involved in the criminal justice system and from having mental health problems.

Factors that are strongly associated with mental health problems, such as childhood trauma, in the form of abuse or loss, were found in high rates in young offenders who were convicted of offences of a serious nature (Bailey 1996). Affective disorders also play some role in youth violence (Pliszka *et al.* 2000) and 'depression in adolescence can manifest itself as anger, which in turn is correlated with aggression' (Bailey 2002). Therefore it could be suggested that a substantial number of young people are not referred for treatment they require as the depression is misinterpreted as a conduct disorder.

Primary care

Although childhood psychiatric disorders are relatively common, only one in ten of cases is seen in specialist mental health services for children. Around 2 to 5 per cent of children attending primary care during any one year present with emotional or behavioural disorders. Pre-school children present predominantly with oppositional deficient disorder, while school-age children present with emotional and conduct disorders. Primary care recognition of disturbance is an important factor in referral to specialist mental health services. Children are less likely to be referred unless they present with overt psychological problems.

GPs are often the first point of contact in the referral system. They are in a unique position to implement preventative intervention and deal with less severe psychological problems. They have knowledge of the family's circumstances and can offer a service which is less stigmatizing. There is an increasing emphasis on collaborative support from specialist mental health services and paediatric services focusing on primary care intervention targeting high risk populations.

Many primary care practices employ counsellors, community psychiatric nurses and psychologists offering consultation and assessment in primary care settings. The appointment of primary care mental health workers offering consultation-liaison has helped reduce referrals to increasingly long waiting lists for specialist child mental health services. They also have an input in enhancing GP skills in managing milder cases and making more appropriate referrals to specialist services.

Prevention of childhood mental health problems

The Department of Health publication *Saving Lives* (1999), emphasized disease prevention and health promotion as one of its objectives. Specific mention was made of the reduction of suicide as a mental health target. The paper also acknowledged the importance of the mental health of children and adolescents and their vulnerability to physical, intellectual and emotional behaviour disorders which, if untreated, could have serious implications for adult life. This, along with the introduction of the Common Assessment Framework, has lead to an increase in CAMHS Early Intervention Services. The remit of these teams tend to be tier 2 assessment and treatment, mental health promotion and mental health education.

Three types of prevention are recognized. The aim of primary prevention is to reduce the possible incidence of a disorder in a population before its onset. Secondary prevention is aimed at early diagnosis and intervention to minimize the impact on the patient and carers. Tertiary prevention has the goal of limiting the physical social effects of the disorder (Caplan 1964). In undertaking primary preventative intervention, several factors need to be considered and these include risk factor, protective factors and the vulnerability of the individual to a particular disorder. Risk factors may arise from the genetic background, problems during pregnancy and maternal infection or malnutrition. Good antenatal care can help to minimize these risks. Primary preventative work can also protect the child from the adverse effects of birth trauma, accidents, exposure to infection, deprivation and abuse through timely intervention.

Protective factors include adaptable temperament, a good relationship with a significant adult caretaker and experience of areas in which the child has a good experience such as sports or school. Several studies (Rutter 1990) have shown that a proportion of children exposed to gross deprivation and severe stress are resilient to developing psychiatric disorder, although the precise reasons why some children are resilient is not understood. The formation of secure attachments and the ability to be self-reflective are seen as protective factors. Health promotion and illness prevention is the focus of Chapter 2.

The role of nurses in child and adolescent services

New Ways of Working (NWW) (DH 2007) aims to develop teams and services based on capabilities required to meet service user and carer needs, rather than based on a profession. Within NWW there is a need for nursing to reconsider its very essence and whether it is grounded enough to survive. The workforce could consist of generic CAMHS professionals, regardless of professional background. Nursing is a remarkably diverse discipline in CAMHS, with many identities, led by an increasingly well-qualified group of individuals who fulfil a wide range of responsibilities.

The Audit Commission document *Children in Mind* (1999) described a four-tier model for the delivery of child and adolescent services. Although still relevant, local services have interpreted the operational meaning of the tiers in different ways. Tier 1 services are provided by primary care and other front-line services, such as schools, offering advice for mild to moderate problems and promoting mental health. Tier 2 services are generally provided by specialist professionals working on their own with links to primary care (Tier 1 services), the Team Around the Child and the specialist multi-disciplinary CAMHS services (Tier 3). Tier 4 services deal with complex severe cases with links to inpatient child and adolescent beds.

As with all nursing posts, commitment to ongoing continuing professional development and lifelong learning is essential. There are a range of courses and developmental opportunities for registered nurses working within child and adolescent mental health services. Nurses with specialist training in child and adolescent psychiatry are uniquely placed to work in all four tiers of the service. At Tier 1, nurses are able to take on the role of primary care mental health workers (PMHWs). Besides providing first line intervention they have a role to support other professionals working in primary care and provide links between Tier 1 and specialist services. PMHWs also play an important role as gatekeepers to specialist services.

The core nursing skills and competencies such as assessment, health promotion and education, risk assessment and management, physical health care and medication management are of value throughout CAMHS. Nurses can also develop specialist training in a range of therapies, including cognitive behavioural therapy and family therapy, as well as working as nurse prescribers. Nurses will continue to play a central role in the services for adolescents with first onset psychosis and ADHD. While there is an emphasis on multi-disciplinary working in inpatient adolescent units, nurses provide care and therapeutic input as the core group of specialists who outnumber other professionals. Children admitted to such units often need medication for serious psychotic problems, and careful assessment of risk and monitoring of the effects of medication is an important role for nurses. Nurses are also taking on leadership roles in CAMHS with the development of the Modern Matron and Nurse Consultant posts.

Health visitors and school nurses with training in child development and assessment of children are uniquely placed to provide a service at Tier 2 level with support from specialist CAMHS services and are seen as less stigmatizing services for mild to moderate cases.

Users' views

Users of child and adolescent mental health services represent a large group of stakeholders including children, their families, schools, social services and others. Primary care trusts and social care are important stakeholders as the commissions of the CAMHS Grant. User organizations, focus groups and meetings of stakeholders are increasingly involved in decisions about service planning and delivery. Views from such meetings indicate a need for greater clarity about the range of services offered by child and adolescent mental health services and the roles of professionals working within the service. Problems with access to the service and waiting times for first appointments are also concerns. Parents have indicated a need for greater support in their role of parenting.

The appointment of primary care mental health workers based in primary care has made it possible for the mild and moderate cases to be seen within the primary care setting. Trained health visitors and school nurses are able to provide a less stigmatizing service with the support of specialist services offering consultation and liaison. Schools are increasingly offering Tier 2 services. There is still a need however to involve stakeholders and users more widely in the planning, delivery and evaluation of services provided by children's services.

Conclusion

In summary, the main points of this chapter are:

- Nurses may encounter mental distress and mental illness in children and adolescents in a wide variety of clinical practice settings. This chapter describes the manifestations of the more common mental health problems that children may experience and treatment approaches.
- Compared with the high profile of adult mental health, the significance of the mental health needs of children has only recently been recognized. A National Service Framework for Children has been published setting out national standards for a comprehensive CAMHS.
- There are substantial areas of overlap between childhood mental health and physical health particularly during the pre-school and early school years. A tiered service offers nurses a variety of roles in primary care and in specialist teams.
- Service users' views are important in guiding the future development of child and adolescent mental health services (CAMHS). They have highlighted concerns with access to the service and waiting times, and the need for greater support to people in their parenting role.

■ Increasingly there is an emphasis on preventive work and pressure to allocate an increasing proportion of resources to primary prevention, that is to measures taken to reduce the incidence of specific disorders in a population not currently suffering from those disorders (Caplan 1964).

Questions for reflection and discussion

1   Consider what more might be done to improve services for children and adolescents presenting with mental health problems in a primary care setting with which you are familiar.
2   Should children's services be provided under one umbrella? What are the potential benefits? What are your feelings about children's services being provided by a Children's Trust?
3   Should CAMHS align itself with community paediatrics, education and social care or adult mental health?
4   What specialist roles could nurses play in bridging the gap between services for adolescents and adult mental health?
5   What services could be nurse led? Is there scope for generic workers to be trained to undertake most of the functions within child and adolescent mental health services (CAMHS)?

Annotated bibliography

■ http://www.everychildmatters.gov.uk. A useful website which details *Every Child Matters*, the CAF and the TAC.
■ Rutter, M. and Taylor, E. (eds) (2008) *Child and Adolescent Psychiatry* (5th edn). Oxford: Blackwell Publishing. The fifth edition is one of the most comprehensive textbooks in child and adolescent psychiatry and is highly recommended for readers wishing to research topics in depth. It outlines recent research findings and current thinking in the field.

References

Angold, A. and Egger, H.L. (2007) Preschool psychopathology: lessons for the lifespan. *Journal of Child Psychology and Psychiatry and Allied Disciplines* **48**(10): 961–6.
American Psychiatric Association (1994) *Diagnostic and Statistical Manual of Mental Disorders, DSM-IV* (4th edn). Washington, DC: American Psychiatric Association.
Apter, A., King, R.A., Bleich, A., Fluck, A., Kotler, M. and Kron, S. (2008) Fatal and non-fatal suicidal behavior in Israeli adolescent males. *Archives of Suicide Research* **12**(1): 20–9.
Audit Commission (1999) *Children in Mind: Child and Adolescent Mental Health Services*. Portsmouth: Holbrooks Printers.
Bailey, S. (1996) Adolescents who murder. *Journal of Adolescence* **1**: 19–39.
Bailey, S. (1997) Adolescent offenders. *Current Opinion in Psychiatry* **10**: 445–53.
Bailey, S. (2002) Violent children: a framework for assessment. *Advances in Psychiatric Treatment* **8**: 97–106.

Banerjee, T.D., Middleton, F. and Faraone, S.V. (2007) Environmental risk factors for attention-deficit hyperactivity disorder. *Acta Paediatrica, International Journal of Paediatrics* **96**(9): 1269–74.

Bittner, A., Egger, H.L., Erkanli, A., Jane Costello, E., Foley, D.L. and Angold, A. (2007) What do childhood anxiety disorders predict? *Journal of Child Psychology and Psychiatry and Allied Disciplines* **48**(12): 1174–83.

Borges, G., Nock, M.K., Medina-Mora, M.E. *et al.* (2007) The epidemiology of suicide-related outcomes in Mexico. *Suicide and Life-Threatening Behavior* **37**(6): 627–40.

Bowlby, J. (1980) *Attachment and Loss: III. Loss, Sadness and Depression.* London: Basic Books.

Brezo, B., Paris, J., Tremblay, R., Vitaro, F., Hébert, M. and Tureck, G. (2007) Identifying correlates of suicide attempts in suicidal ideators: a population-based study. *Psychological Medicine* **37**: 1551–62.

Buckner, J.D., Lopez, C., Dunkel, S. and Joiner Jr., T.E. (2008) Behavior management training for the treatment of reactive attachment disorder. *Child Maltreatment* **13**(3): 289–97.

Bryant-Waugh, R. and Lask, B. (2007) Overview of the eating disorders, in B. Lask and R. Bryant-Waugh (eds) *Eating Disorders in Childhood and Adolescence* (3rd edn). Hove: Psychology Press, pp. 35–50.

Bryant-Waugh, R., Cooper, P., Taylor, C. and Lask, B. (1996) The use of the eating disorder examination with children: a pilot study. *International Journal of Eating Disorders* **19**: 391–7.

Caplan, G. (1964) *Principles of Preventative Psychiatry.* New York: Basic Books.

Conners, C.K. (1973) Rating scales for use in drug studies with children. *Psychopharmacology Bulletin: Special issue on Pharmacotherapy with children* **9**: 24–84.

Coplan, R.J., Bowker, A. and Cooper, S.M. (2003) Parenting daily hassles, child temperament, and social adjustment in preschool. *Early Childhood Research Quarterly* **18**: 376–95.

Costello, E.J., Egger, H.L. and Angold, A. (2004). Developmental epidemiology of anxiety disorders, in T.H. Ollendick and J.S. March (eds) *Phobic and Anxiety Disorders in Children and Adolescents.* Oxford: Oxford University Press, pp. 61–92.

Davis, H., Day, C. and Bidmead, C. (2002) *Working in Partnership with Parents: The Parent Adviser Model.* London: The Psychological Corporation.

Department for Education and Skills (2003) *Every Child Matters.* Nottingham: DfES.

Department of Health (1999) *Saving Lives: Our Healthier Nation.* White Paper, July. London: DH.

Department of Health (2007) *Creating capable teams approach – best practice guidance to support the implementation of new ways of working.* Executive Summary. London: The Stationery Office.

Department of Health, Department for Education and Skills (2004) *National Service Framework for Children Young People and Maternity Services: The Mental Health and Psychological Well-being of Children and Young People.* London: DH/DfES.

Dixon, A., Howie, P. and Starling, J. (2004) Psychopathology in female juvenile offenders. *Journal of Child Psychology and Psychiatry* **45**(6): 1150–8.

Douglas, J.W.B. (1973) Early disturbing events and later enuresis, in I. Kolvin, R. Mackeith and S.R. Meadow (eds) *Bladder Control and Enuresis, Clinics in Developmental Medicine*, Nos 48/49, 109–17. London: Heinemann/Spasibics International Medical Publications.

Dummit, E.S. III, Klein, R., Tancer, N.K., Ashe, B. and Martin, J. (1996) Fluoxetine treatment of children with selective mutism: an open trial. *Journal of the American Academy of Child and Adolescent Psychiatry* **35**: 615–21.

Egger, H.L. and Angold, A. (2006) Common emotional and behavioral disorders in preschool children: Presentation, nosology, and epidemiology. *Journal of Child Psychology and Psychiatry and Allied Disciplines* **47**(3–4): 313–37.

Eisen, A.R., Raleigh, H. and Neuhoff, C.C. (2008) The unique impact of parent training for separation anxiety disorder in children. *Behavior Therapy* **39**(2): 195–206.

Erikson, E.H. (1968) *Identity: Youth and Crisis.* New York: Norton.

Fairburn, C.G. and Cooper, Z. (1993) The eating disorders examination, in C.G. Fairburn and G.T. Wilson (eds) *Binge Eating: Nature, Assessment and Treatment* (12th edn). New York: Guilford Press.

Fergusson, D.M. and Horwood, L.J. (2000) Does cannabis use encourage other forms of illicit drug use? *Addiction* **95**: 505–20.

Flannery-Schroeder, E., Choudhury, M.S. and Kendall, P.C. (2005) Group and individual cognitive-behavioral treatments for youth with anxiety disorders: 1-year follow-up. *Cognitive Therapy and Research* **29**: 253–9.

Fombonne, E. (1999) The epidemiology of autism: a review. *Psychosocial Medicine* **29**: 769–89.

Fombonne, E., Wostear, G., Cooper, V., Harrington, R. and Rutter, M. (2001) The Maudsley long term follow up of child and adolescent depression. 2. Suicidality, criminality and social dysfunction in adulthood. *British Journal of Psychiatry* **179**: 218–23.

Freeman, J.B., Garcia, A.M., Coyne, L. *et al.* (2008) Early childhood OCD: Preliminary findings from a family-based cognitive-behavioral approach. *Journal of the American Academy of Child and Adolescent Psychiatry* **47**(5): 593–602.

Garralda, E. (2008) Somatization and somatoform disorders. *Psychiatry* **7**(8): 353–6.

Goodman, R. (1997) The Strengths and Difficulties Questionnaire: A research note. *Journal of Child Psychology and Psychiatry* **38**: 581–6.

Hagell, A. (2004) Time trends in adolescent well being. Seminars on children and families: evidence and implications. 6. London: The Nuffield Foundation.

Hawton, K. and Harriss, L. (2008) The changing gender ratio in occurrence of deliberate self-harm across the lifecycle. *Crisis* **29**(1): 4–10.

Hersov, L. (1994) Faecal soiling, in M. Rutter, E. Taylor and L. Hersov (eds) *Child and Adolescent Psychiatry: Modern Approaches* (3rd edn). Oxford: Blackwell Science, pp. 520–8.

Hogue, A., Dauber, S., Chinchilla, P. *et al.* (2008) Assessing fidelity in individual and family therapy for adolescent substance abuse. *Journal of Substance Abuse Treatment* **35**(2): 137–47.

Honda, H., Shimizu, Y. and Rutter, M. (2005) No effect of MMR withdrawal on the incidence of autism: a total population study. *Journal of Child Psychology and Psychiatry* **46**: 572–9.

Howard, J., Lennings, C.J. and Copeland, J. (2003) Suicidal behaviour in a young offender population. *Crisis* **24**(3): 98–104.

Hurth, J., Shaw, E. and Izeman, S. (1999) Areas of agreement about effective practices among programs serving young children with autism spectrum disorders. *Infants and Young Children* **12**: 17.

Laming, H. (2003) *The Victoria Climbié Inquiry. Report of an inquiry by Lord Laming.* London: The Stationery Office.

Liber, J.M., Van Widenfelt, B.M., Utens, E.M.W.J. *et al.* (2008) No differences between group versus individual treatment of childhood anxiety disorders in a randomised clinical trial. *Journal of Child Psychology and Psychiatry and Allied Disciplines* **49**(8): 886–93.

MTA Co-operative Group (1999) A 14-month randomized clinical trial of treatment strategies for attention-deficit/hyperactivity disorder: the multimodal treatment study of children with ADHD. *Archives of General Psychiatry* **56**(12): 1073–86.

Madden, S. (2005) Managing anxiety disorders in children and adolescents. *Medicine Today* **6**(5): 14–19.

Manassis, K., Fung, D., Tannock, R., Sloman, L., Fiksenbaum, L. and McInnes, A. (2003) Characterizing selective mutism: is it more than social anxiety? *Depression and Anxiety* **18**: 153–61.

Manassis, K., Tannock, R., Garland, E.J., Minde, K., Mcinnes, A. and Clark, S. (2007) The sounds of silence: language, cognition, and anxiety in selective mutism. *Journal of the American Academy of Child and Adolescent Psychiatry* **46**(9): 1187–95.

Miettunen, J., Törmänen, S., Murray, G.K. *et al.* (2008) Association of cannabis use with prodromal symptoms of psychosis in adolescence. *British Journal of Psychiatry* **192**(6): 470–1.

Miller, C. and Ahmed, Y. (2000) Collaboration and partnership: An effective response to complexity and fragmentation or solution built on sand? *International Journal of Sociology and Social Policy* **20**: 1–39.

Murthy, R.S. (2000) Approaches to suicide prevention in Asia and the Far East, in K. Hawton and K. Van Heeringen (eds) *International Handbook of Suicide and Attempted Suicide*. London: Wiley, pp. 625–37.

National Statistical Office (2005) *UK 2005 – The Official Yearbook of the United Kingdom of Great Britain and Northern Ireland*. London: National Statistical Office.

Newman, L. and Mares, S. (2007) Recent advances in the theories of and interventions with attachment disorders. *Current Opinion in Psychiatry* **20**(4): 343–8.

National Institute for Health and Clinical Excellence (2004a) *Self Harm*. London: NICE.

National Institute for Health and Clinical Excellence (2004b) *Eating Disorders in Children and Adolescence*. London: NICE.

National Institute for Health and Clinical Excellence (2005a) *Depression in Children and Young People*. London: NICE.

National Institute for Health and Clinical Excellence (2005b) *Obsessive-Compulsive Disorder.* London: NICE.

National Institute for Health and Clinical Excellence (2006) *Schizophrenia.* London: NICE.

Patton, G.C., Hemphill, S.A., Beyers, J.M., Bond, L., Toumbourou, J.W., and McMorris, B.J. (2007) Pubertal stage and deliberate self-harm in adolescents. *Journal of the American Academy of Child and Adolescent Psychiatry* **46**: 508–14.

Philichi, L. (2008) When the going gets tough: pediatric constipation and encopresis. *Gastroenterology Nursing* **31**(2): 121–30.

Piacentini, J. Bergman, R.L. Jacobs, C. McCracken J.T. and Kretchman, J. (2002) Open trial of cognitive behavior therapy for childhood obsessive-compulsive disorder. *Journal of Anxiety Disorders* **16**: 207–19.

Pliszka, S.R., Sherman, J.O., Barrow, M.V. and Irick, S. (2000) Affective disorder in juvenile offenders: a preliminary study. *American Journal of Psychiatry* **157**: 130–2.

Poulton, A. (2005) Growth on stimulant medication; clarifying the confusion: a review. *Archives of Disease in Childhood* **90**: 801–6.

Robertson, M.M. (1989) The Gilles de la Tourette syndrome: the current status. *British Journal of Psychiatry* **154**: 147–69.

Robson, W.L.M. (2008) Current management of nocturnal enuresis. *Current Opinion in Urology* **18**(4): 425–30.

Rogers, S.J. (1998) Empirically supported comprehensive treatments for young children with autism. *Journal of Clinical Child Psychology* **27**: 168–79.

Rustad, R., Small, J.E., Jobes, D.A., Safer, M.A. and Peterson, R.J. (2003) The impact of rock videos and music with suicidal content on thoughts and attitudes about suicide. *Suicide and Life Threatening Behavior* **33**: 120–31.

Rutter, M. (1990) Psychosocial resilience and protective mechanisms, in J. Rolf, A.A. Masten, D. Cicchetti, K.H. Neuchterlein and S. Weintraub (eds) *Risk and Protective Factors in the Development of Psychopathology.* New York: Cambridge University Press, pp. 79–101.

Safarinejad, M.R. (2007) Prevalence of nocturnal enuresis, risk factors, associated familial factors and urinary pathology among school children in Iran. *Journal of Pediatric Urology* **3**(6): 443–52.

Schulz, S.C., Findling, R.L., Wise, A., Friedman, L. and Kenny, J. (1998) Child and adolescent schizophrenia. *Psychiatric Clinics of North America* **21**: 43–56.

Skovgaard, A.M., Houmann, T., Christiansen, E. *et al.* (2007) The prevalence of mental health problems in children 1½ of age – The Copenhagen Child Cohort 2000. *Journal of Child Psychology and Psychiatry and Allied Disciplines* **48**(1): 62–70.

Smeeth, L., Cook, C., Fombonne, E. *et al.* (2004) MMR vaccination and pervasive developmental disorders: a case–control study. *Lancet* **364**: 963–9.

Steinhausen, H.-C. (1994) Anorexia and bulimia nervosa, in M. Rutter, E. Taylor and L. Hersov (eds) *Child and Adolescent Psychiatry: Modern Approaches* (3rd edn). Oxford: Blackwell Science, pp. 425–40.

Stevens, T. and Mulsow, M. (2006) There is no meaningful relationship between television exposure and symptoms of attention-deficit/hyperactivity disorder. *Pediatrics* **117**: 665–72.

Storch, E.A., Milsom, V.A., Merlo, L.J. *et al.* (2008) Insight in pediatric obsessive-compulsive disorder: Associations with clinical presentation. *Psychiatry Research* **160**(2): 212–20.

Substance Abuse and Mental Health Services Administration (2007) *Results from the 2006 National Survey on Drug Use and Health: National Findings* (NSDUH Series H-28, DHHS Publication No. SMA 05–4062). Rockville, MD: Office of Applied Studies.

Taylor, B. (2006) Vaccines and the changing epidemiology of autism. Review. *Child: Care, Health and Development* **32**(5): 511–19.

Thapar, A. and Munoz-Solomando, A. (2008) Attention deficit hyperactivity disorder. *Psychiatry* **7**(8): 340–4.

Thapar, A., Langley, K., Owen, M.J. and O'Donovan, M.C. (2007) Advances in genetic findings on attention deficit hyperactivity disorder. *Psychological Medicine* **37**(12): 1681–92.

Thomas, C.R. (2006) Evidence-based practice for conduct disorder symptoms. *Journal of the American Academy of Child and Adolescent Psychiatry* **45**(1): 109–14.

Verdellen, C.W.J., Keijsers, G.P.J., Cath, D.C. and Hoogduin, C.A.L. (2004) Exposure with response prevention versus habit reversal in Tourettes's syndrome: A controlled study. *Behaviour Research and Therapy* **42**(5): 501–11.

Winters, K.C. (1999) Treating adolescents with substance use disorders: An overview of practice issues and treatment outcome. *Substance Abuse* **20**: 203–24.

World Health Organization (1996) *Mulitaxial classification of child and adolescent psychiatric disorders: The ICD-10 Classification of Mental and Behavioral Disorders.* Geneva: World Health Organization.

Zalsman, G., Brent, D.A. and Weersing, V.R. (2006) Depressive disorders in childhood and adolescence: an overview epidemiology, clinical manifestation and risk factors. *Child and Adolescent Psychiatric Clinics of North America* **15**: 827–41.

Zohar, A. (1999) The epidemiology of obsessive-compulsive disorder in children and adolescents. *Child and Adolescent Psychiatric Clinics of North America* **8**: 445–60.

The person with dementia

John Keady, Sean Page and Kevin Hope

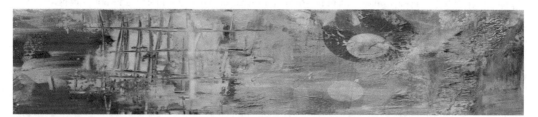

Chapter overview

The care of people with dementia has formed an integral part of the discourse and practice of mental health nursing from the times of asylum and attendant-based duties (Nolan 2003) right through to present-day descriptions of evidence-based practice and therapeutic effort in a range of primary, secondary and tertiary care environments (e.g. Keady *et al.* 2007). Moreover, community dementia care nursing formed part of the 'new wave' of innovative service designs and (re)configurations in the late 1950s that challenged the hegemony and primacy of institutional, task-based care as the 'only way' to deliver nursing and mental health services (Greene 1968). Indeed, this innovation was to prove so popular that by the mid-1980s Simmons and Brooker (1986) reported that when community psychiatric nurses specialized with a client group it tended to be with 'elderly mentally ill people' (1986: 46), thus emphasizing the rewards, opportunities and investment in working with some of the most vulnerable members of society.

Fast forward to mid-2007 and while policy imperatives, care priorities and service demographics have radically altered since the mid-1980s, the mental health profession's commitment to dementia care nursing has recently been confirmed in two separate, national reviews (DH 2006; Scottish Executive 2006), a standpoint we fully endorse and welcome. This chapter draws together some of the main issues that face mental health nurses in their work with people with dementia and their families and takes as its anchor point the publication of the National Institute for Health and Clinical Excellence (NICE) and the Social Care Institute for Excellence (SCIE) guideline *Dementia: Supporting people with dementia and their carers in health and social care* (NICE clinical practice guideline 42: NICE/SCIE 2006) and their promotion of a biopsychosocial model of dementia. We therefore divide the chapter into three sections: a *biological* perspective, including reference to demography, prevalence and clinical features; a *psychological* perspective, including a review of person-centred and relationship-centred care; and a *social* perspective that will articulate the social model of disability together with an appreciation of the place of language and ageism as barriers to the full integration of people with dementia into mainstream services and societal values. We develop the biopsychosocial model by separately highlighting the importance of family work and therapeutic effort, the latter of which includes an overview of palliative care practice. First, though, we set out the shifting policy context of dementia care in the United Kingdom (UK) which provides a foundation and framework for contextualizing dementia care nursing.

Dementia: UK policy perspective

At the turn of the 1980s, UK government policy and initiatives in dementia care were fragmented and poorly developed and consisted mainly of recommendations of good practice and service design by, for example, the Royal College of Physicians (1981), the Health Advisory Service (1982) and the King's Fund Centre (1984). As the decade wore on, government concern over the costs of funding the National Health Service (NHS) stimulated a major debate over its purpose and priorities. A fundamental review led by Sir Roy Griffiths (1988), the publication of two White Papers: *Caring for People* (DH 1989a) and *Working for Patients* (DH 1989b) – which were to form the blueprint of the NHS and Community Care Act 1990 – were to change the landscape of dementia care practice and assessment. In particular, the separation of 'health' and 'social' care within the NHS and Community Care Act 1990 spelt out new challenges and responsibilities for case management, and transferred primary assessment responsibilities for the social care needs of older people to local authorities (DH 1991a, b). In addition, for the first time, the NHS and Community Care Act 1990 legitimized and located carers' needs as a policy imperative, a recognition that eventually led to a sequence of dedicated legislation and practice guidance (DH 1995a, 1999, 2000, 2004). The NHS and Community Care Act 1990 also put into place a 'business' and 'accountability' culture within the health service and championed the voice of the consumer in management and quality control processes so that 'user perspectives' took centre stage in all aspects of service design, delivery and evaluation.

While the NHS and Community Care Act 1990 undoubtedly challenged contemporary thinking and attitudes, it did not specifically address the needs of people with dementia. Indeed, it was not until the mid-1990s that the Health of the Nation report *Building Bridges* provided a definition of severe mental illness and attached it to individuals who were 'diagnosed as suffering from some sort of mental illness (typically people suffering from schizophrenia or a severe affective disorder, but including dementia)' (DH 1995b: 11).

While this alignment undoubtedly helped to define service and practice parameters, and tied dementia into a 'severe mental illness' category, the need to set, and measure, standards of good practice was absent from the report's recommendations.

From the start of this century to the time of writing this chapter (mid-2007), UK government policy has relentlessly addressed this knowledge deficit and brought forward a language of performance indicators, measurement and targets into the culture of mental health practice, including that of dementia care. An early example of this focus was apparent in the Audit Commission's (2000) report *Forget Me Not: Mental health services for older people*. Conducted in 12 areas of England and Wales this influential study used a range of instruments to measure current practice in primary, secondary and tertiary care settings, including surveys of general practitioners (GPs), carers' individual case information and case file analysis. Three key aims of a mental health service for older people were stated as being able to:

1. Maintain the mental health of older people and to help preserve their independence;
2. Support family carers as well as older people themselves;
3. Provide intermittent or permanent residential care for those who are so disabled that it is the most practical and humane way of looking after them (Audit Commission 2000: 15).

In their follow-up report in February 2002, the Audit Commission (2002) synthesized the results of a series of local audits conducted on mental health services for older people. These audits were all conducted in England and the report (Audit Commission 2002) continued to highlight the problems experienced by GPs in identifying mental health problems early in their course, particularly dementia. Similarly, encouragement was given to health and social care agencies to develop joint plans for commissioning and delivering integrated services based on good information and involving key partners. We return to other aspects of this report later in this chapter.

The need to start benchmarking national service standards for the mental health care of older people was also reflected, in England, in the publication and dissemination of the *National Service Framework (NSF) for Older People* (DH 2001) and in Wales by the *NSF for Older People in Wales* (Welsh Assembly Government 2006). The *NSF for Older People* (DH 2001) set out a ten-year programme for action and reform to deliver higher quality services for older people and contained eight standards, as follows:

1. Rooting out age discrimination;
2. Person-centred care;
3. Intermediate care;
4. General hospital care;
5. Stroke;
6. Falls;
7. Mental health in older people;
8. The promotion of health and active life in older age.

While each of these standards has an impact upon the life of an older person, Standard 7 specifically addressed 'mental health in older people' with the overarching aim: 'to promote good mental health in older people and to treat and support those older people with dementia and depression' (DH 2001: 90).

Later on in its pages, Standard 7 aligned its recommendations to the cause of younger people with dementia and provided a salient reminder that under-detection of mental illness in older people is 'widespread' and complicated by the fact that many older people live alone without a close support network. Standard 7 also emphasizes the need to 'treat and support' older people with mental health needs around a community-orientated model that is underpinned by three key interventions, namely:

1. promoting good mental health;
2. early recognition and management of mental health problems;
3. access to specialist care (DH 2001: 91).

As also highlighted in the Audit Commission reports from 2000 and 2002, early recognition and management was identified as particularly important when a person with an (undiagnosed) condition first comes into contact with a member of the primary care team, usually their GP. Within Standard 7 advice is given also on the treatment of dementia (DH

2001: 98); this is repeated in Table 24.1 as it provides a baseline for establishing good mental health nursing practice in community and residential settings.

Treatment of dementia always involves:

- Explaining the diagnosis to the older person and any carers and where possible giving relevant information about sources of help and support.
- Giving information about the likely prognosis and options for packages of care.
- Making appropriate referrals to help with fears and worries, distress, practical and financial issues that affect the person and their carer.
- At all stages emphasizing the unique qualities of the individual with dementia and recognizing their personal and social needs.
- Using non-pharmacological management strategies such a mental exercise, physical therapy, dietary treatment alongside drug therapy.
- Prescribing antipsychotic drugs for more serious problems, such as delusions, and hallucinations, serious distress or danger from behaviour disturbance.

Table 24.1 Treatment of dementia
Source: DH (2001: 98)

To support these objectives, Standard 7 also suggested that there should be a specialist mental health service for people with dementia if, for instance, their diagnosis is uncertain, there are safety concerns or a risk assessment is necessary.

In 2005 the Department of Health published *A New Ambition for Old Age* (DH 2005a) which outlined progress in the *NSF for Older People* (DH 2001). Of particular interest in this document was a discussion on complex needs (programme 6 of the report) and an acknowledgement that many older people have 'one or more long-term condition' and have difficulty in maintaining their independence, well-being and quality of life. For mental health nurses this is a salient reminder that their profession is just one of many which have a vested interested in supporting people with dementia and their families; accordingly, the need to define and evaluate role performance, and tailor care interventions to individual/family circumstances, is paramount.

Contemporaneous with the publication of *A New Ambition for Old Age* (DH 2005a), the Care Services Improvement Partnership (CSIP) published a service development guide called *Everybody's Business: Integrated mental health services for older adults* (CSIP 2005). This guide argued against the artificial 'health' or 'social' divide created under the NHS and Community Care Act 1990. It emphasized that the needs of people with dementia did not fall neatly into either category and that mental health and mainstream services had to work in partnership with the aim of:

- improving older people's quality of life;
- meeting complex needs in a coordinated way;
- providing a person-centred approach;
- promoting age equality.

Each of these statements were later incorporated into the NICE/SCIE guideline *Dementia: Supporting people with dementia and their carers in health and social care* (NICE clinical practice guideline 42: NICE/SCIE 2006), a document that was published in November 2006.

This comprehensive and authoritative clinical practice guideline critically synthesizes evidence from controlled and qualitative studies as they pertain to key priorities for implementation. As the NICE clinical practice guideline 42 weighs in at 417 pages, it is simply not possible to do justice to the document in the space available and we would recommend that interested readers access the NICE website (www.nice.org.uk) to download the full and 'quick reference' guideline documents. In brief, however, the NICE clinical practice guideline 42 outlines nine 'key priorities' for implementation, these being:

1   *Non-discrimination*, i.e. the need not to exclude people with dementia from any service because of their diagnosis, age or coexisting learning disabilities.
2   *Valid consent*, i.e. for health and social care professionals to always seek valid consent from people with dementia, and if capacity is compromised, the provisions of the *Mental Capacity Act* (Ministry of Justice 2007) are to be followed.
3   *Carers*, i.e. the need to ensure that the rights of carers to receive an assessment are conducted, and that psychological therapy is offered to carers who are experiencing psychological upset and distress.
4   *Coordination and integration of health and social care*, i.e. the necessity for joint planning, policy, procedures and reviews. Joint planning should include the involvement of local service users and carers.
5   *Memory services*, i.e. the recommendation that memory assessment services (either through a dedicated clinic or through a community mental health team) should be the single point of referral for all people with a possible diagnosis of dementia.
6   *Structural imaging for diagnosis*, i.e. the use of magnetic resonance imaging (MRI) as the preferred modality to assist in establishing an early diagnosis.
7   *Behaviour that challenges*, i.e. early assessment should be offered to pinpoint the likely factors that may generate, aggravate or improve such behaviour.
8   *Training*, i.e. the requirement that all staff (including voluntary staff) working with people with dementia have access to dementia care training consistent with their roles and responsibilities.
9   *Mental health needs in acute hospitals*, i.e. the need for acute and general hospital trusts to plan and provide services that address the needs of people with dementia who use acute hospital services.

The NICE clinical practice guideline 42 also underpins the 'key priorities' with a set of 'principles of care' that range from person-centred care, to the preferred support option of community-based care and on to respecting diversity, equality, ethical treatment and the impact of dementia on relationships.

However, it is worth restating that a clinical practice guideline, no matter how comprehensive or authoritative, is *not* a substitute for professional knowledge and clinical judgement/decision-making. It is, in our opinion, vital that a mental health nurse acts with an informed knowledge about the content of the clinical guideline (NICE/SCIE 2006), but retains space in their care planning for creative and intuitive decision-making based upon a detailed understanding of the person's biography, presenting needs and social environment.

We now outline the biopsychosocial model of dementia, split into its three component parts.

Biomedical perspective

Cells, proteins and neurotransmitters

Arguably, the most powerful and persistently influential perspective of dementia is the biomedical one that highlights the physiological and cognitive nature of the condition. This is evident in all-encompassing definitions, such as that provided by the World Health Organization (WHO 2007):

> " Dementia is a syndrome due to disease of the brain, usually of a chronic or progressive nature, in which there is disturbance of multiple higher cortical functions, including memory, thinking, orientation, comprehension, calculation, learning capacity, language, and judgement. Consciousness is not clouded. The impairments of cognitive function are commonly accompanied, and occasionally preceded, by deterioration in emotional control, social behaviour, or motivation. This syndrome occurs in Alzheimer's disease, in cerebrovascular disease, and in other conditions primarily or secondarily affecting the brain. "
>
> (www.who.int/classifications/apps/icd/icd10online/: accessed 4 June 2007)

In this definition, the word 'dementia' relates to a syndrome, one that is used to describe a variety of conditions with similar, or common, features. Consequently, 'dementia' alone cannot tell the whole story and more precise diagnostic sub-categories are required to be identified in order to inform practice. The most common forms of dementia are shown in Box 24.1.

Box 24.1 Most common forms of dementia

Type of Dementia	Percentage of cases
Alzheimer's disease	62
Vascular dementia	17
Mixed dementia (Alzheimer's disease and vascular dementia)	10
Dementia with Lewy bodies	4
Frontal temporal dementia, including Pick's disease	2
Parkinson's dementia	2
Other types of dementia, e.g alcohol-related, AIDS-related	3

(Adapted from Alzheimers Society 2007 p29).

Note:
Alzheimer's disease reported as being more common in women than men.

As can also be seen from the WHO (2007) definition, memory impairment is only one of a range of important consequences of the illness and the nature, and interrelationship, of neurological impairment with subsequent symptoms is a central concern. At post-mortem this process is evident to the naked eye through an atrophied and shrunken brain. At a cellular level, the presence of senile (latterly named amyloid) plaques (AP) and neurofibrillary tangles (NFT) were first described by Alois Alzheimer at the turn of the last century (Alzheimer 1907) who reported on the presence of a 'peculiar substance' (AP) and 'dense bundles' (NFT). To develop this point further, APs are toxic to cells and the 'amyloid hypothesis' promotes the view that the disease process results from an imbalance between the production and clearance of amyloid precursor protein (APP). APP is cleaved by an enzyme (secretase) resulting in different forms of amyloid. The beta form is prone to self-aggregation resulting in plaques and subsequent cell death.

Treatment options focus on modifying the production, destruction and impact of beta amyloid, and mental health nurses will become increasingly aware of these as laboratory and clinical work progresses in relation to vaccination and new drug therapies (for a more complete discussion see Walker and Rosen 2006). In contrast, NFTs comprise of paired helical filaments made up of tau, an insoluble protein which makes up the cytoskeleton that supports the shape of the cell being necessary for intracellular transport. The aggregation of tau impairs transport mechanisms leading to cell death.

While therapeutic outcomes relating to the basic pathological processes continue to be explored, nurses may be more familiar with the treatment options based on the 'cholinergic hypothesis' which maintains that as a result of the underlying pathological processes, neurons that use acetylcholine, critical to memory and learning, are more prominently affected. The biological presentation of dementia is as a consequence of their selective degeneration. Recent advances have seen the development of acetylcholinesterase inhibitors, drugs that increase the amount of the neurotransmitter available by inhibiting the action of the enzyme responsible for its degradation: clinical practice guideline 42 (NICE/SCIE 2006) provides additional information related to this type of medication.

Demography

The prevalence of dementia in the UK is estimated to be around 700,000 representing one person in every 88 of the UK population. Age and female gender are associated with increased incidence, the former showing a notable impact with one person in 1000 aged 40–65 years; one person in 20 aged over 65 years; and one person in five over 80 years of age having a dementia (Alzheimer's Society 2007). The total number of people with dementia in the UK is forecast to increase to 940,110 by 2021 and 1,735,087 by 2051, an increase of 38 per cent over the next 15 years and 154 per cent over the next 45 years (Alzheimer's Society 2007).

It is estimated that 24.3 million people have dementia worldwide with 4.6 million new cases of dementia every year. Projections indicate that the number of people affected will double every 20 years to 81.1 million by 2040 (Ferri *et al.* 2005).

Presentation

As highlighted in Box 24.1, the most commonly occurring form of dementia is Alzheimer's disease. Its clinical presentation can be understood by considering the '5 A's of Alzheimer's', these being as follows:

Amnesia

Most people understand that memory loss (amnesia) is an element of Alzheimer's disease, but this may prove a superficial understanding as there are several types of memory that have a direct bearing on the person's presentation:

■ *Immediate or short-term memory* is the brain's 'notepad' and helps us to repeat things that are perceived, such as restating a telephone number for instance. It is required for communication and its impairment can lead to the person losing track of what is said or of what they are saying. This is demonstrated by unfinished utterances, repetitive and tangential conversation or unexpected changes of topic. Lengthy or complex speech is difficult to understand for the person with dementia as is repetitive use of references such as 'he', 'she' and 'it'.

■ *Episodic memory* is part of long-term memory. It involves our conscious recollection of past events including time, place and associated emotions and is frequently impaired in Alzheimer's disease. Problems in new learning, difficulty in temporal sequencing (e.g. elements of yesterday's memories inter-linked with one week ago) and repeating statements are reported as are examples, such as mislaying personal possessions or forgetting appointments.

■ *Semantic memory* is language-based and describes memory for facts and words. Its impairment leads to difficulty generating (word finding) or recognizing familiar words. The person might 'talk around' the word, e.g. telling you what a spoon is for but without being able to name the implement itself.

Aphasia

Alzheimer's disease is more than a 'problem of memory'. Aphasia is a loss or impairment of the ability to produce and/or comprehend language and includes an inability to read, write, speak, form words and name objects. The presentation of aphasia can readily be seen to be confused with memory impairment and neuropsychological assessment is necessary precursor to aid specificity.

Apraxia

Apraxia is impairment in the ability to perform purposeful acts or to manipulate objects not attributable to muscle deficit or lack of comprehension. There are several types and a detailed consideration of which is beyond the scope of this chapter. However, in addition to recall, constructional apraxia, the inability to draw or construct simple shapes, is assessed as part of the Mini-mental State Examination (Folstein *et al.* 1975), the most frequently used test to probe for cognitive loss and functioning. Additionally, spatial impairment in Alzheimer's disease is commonplace and demonstrated in the person having difficulty in visually locating objects in space and judging spatial relationships.

Agnosia

Agnosia refers to an inability to understand the significance of sensory stimuli, in spite of sensory pathways being intact. Prosopagnosia is a specific example in which the person does not recognize familiar faces, including their own.

Associated (*non-cognitive*) *features*

The four areas above are described as cognitive symptoms of Alzheimer's disease. Non-cognitive symptoms – or associated features – include a range of 'behavioural and psychiatric symptoms of dementia' (BPSD). Behavioural disturbances include agitation, aggression, wandering, sleep disturbances, inappropriate eating behaviour and inappropriate sexual behaviour. Psychiatric symptoms include delusions, hallucinations, paranoid ideas, depression, anxiety and misidentifications (for a more detailed exploration of BPSD, see IPA 2007).

The final consideration regarding presentation is related to the impact that such problems have. Diagnostic criteria for Alzheimer's disease make reference to impaired activities of daily living and altered patterns of behaviour. As a consequence, any comprehensive assessment process of the person presenting with dementia needs to take account of the range of cognitive factors, the broad spectrum of non-cognitive features as well as the impact of both of these on daily activities as a necessary precursor to care planning.

Other forms of dementia

While Alzheimer's disease is recognized as the most frequently occurring form of dementia, the mental health nurse needs to be aware of other forms and their implications for care. It is not practical to do justice to the full range and types of dementias within the space available, but we have summarized below specific examples that are most likely to be encountered in clinical practice.

1. The primary difference in the presentation of *frontal temporal dementia* relates to language and behavioural difficulties such as stereotypic and eating behaviour, mood changes and loss of social awareness. Barber *et al.* (1995) have provided a helpful summary comparing behaviour associated with Alzheimer's disease and frontal temporal dementia.
2. *Dementia with Lewy bodies* is a form of dementia which, in addition to the cognitive features, is associated with three core features: fluctuating cognition; recurrent visual hallucinations; and Parkinsonism (McKeith *et al.* 2005). Of particular importance is the potential for severe neuroleptic sensitivity in people with dementia with Lewy bodies, and antipsychotic medication is contra-indicated for mild to moderate non-cognitive symptoms.
3. In *vascular dementia*, the progression of the condition reflects cerebrovascular episodes so acute deterioration may be evident following a stroke, or a more stepwise pattern might be apparent. Diagnosis requires the presence of neurological symptoms indicative of such episodes, such as hemiparesis or lower facial weakness for instance. Significantly, if cardiovascular risk factors are managed, there is an increased potential for preventing the onset and/or limiting deterioration in this form of dementia.

While this section has considered the different types of dementia as single entities, in reality clinical presentation often assume a 'mixed form'. As such, an understanding of the various threads is necessary to begin to untie the (often) complicated 'knot' of presenting symptoms prior to care planning.

Critique of biomedical model

So far, consideration has been placed upon the disease processes and the range of signs and symptoms associated with the diagnostic category of 'dementia'. Conspicuous by its absence has been a consideration of what it might be like for the person who experiences such changes, or those close to him/her. Within the biomedical perspective, neither the person with the dementia nor those around him/her are seen as active agents in the disease process. Indeed, natural progression and deterioration are emphasized and the person is potentially framed as not having a sense of self or agency. We now balance this viewpoint by outlining the psychological and social perspectives.

Psychological perspective

For many of the reasons identified above, the dominant position of the biomedical model to dementia has begun to be questioned and alternative approaches put forward. These alternatives represent either a social or psychological model and each has a direct focus upon promoting the importance of 'the person' who has a dementia while exploring their 'lived experience'. Usage of the term 'lived experience' immediately begins to counter the 'illness-centred' narrative of the biomedical model and puts into motion the belief that any dementia can be approached through a positive lens; all that is needed is the 'right' social environment, cues and language to illuminate the value of this contribution.

The psycho-social perspective reminds us that a person with dementia is no less a person than anyone else, and that dementia care should be oriented around efforts to improve quality of life while recognizing and preserving a sense of that individual's personhood. Thus, in essence, dementia care should be focused upon an understanding of what dementia means to those who have it, rather than to those of us who are not affected. This argument was succinctly captured by Tom Kitwood, a leading figure in the psycho-social movement in dementia care, who argued that it was necessary to rebalance the 'technical framing' of dementia and complement it with a philosophy that was constructed from personhood and person-centred values (Kitwood 1988). As Kitwood and his colleagues cogently argued, 'the dementia' is not the problem, it is 'our' (individual, carer, professional, society) inability to accommodate 'their' view of the world. This, Kitwood and Bredin (1992) suggested, creates a 'them' and 'us' dialectic tension, a tension reinforced over the years by the devalued status of someone who is 'demented'.

We now elaborate the underpinning theoretical concepts of personhood, person-centredness and person-centred care.

Personhood

In his award-winning and seminal text before his untimely death, Kitwood (1997) defined personhood as:

> A standing or status bestowed upon one human being, by others, in the
> context of a relationship and social being. It implies recognition, respect and

> trust. Both the according of personhood, and the failure to do so, have consequences that are empirically testable.
>
> (page 8) ,,

Personhood, therefore, is the recognition of the absolute value of all human beings (regardless of age, disability, race, sex, cognitive ability and so on) and is a status that one individual bestows upon another. As such, it is a fragile process as 'the other' may not regard the individual in a positive, holistic or humanistic way. Regrettably, the nursing profession is not immune from holding such negative attitudes as repeated inquiry reports outlining institutional abuse towards people with dementia can testify (see for example: Commission for Health Improvement 2003). Furthermore, if 'the other' does not act to promote personhood, then the individual may be compelled to assert his/her own sense of self and self-identity (Sabat 2001, 2002) by demonstrating to others, in whatever communication or behavioural style has relevance and/or meaning, what it is that is unique and important about that themself. Within the care home sector, Kitwood (1997) used the term 'malignant social psychology' (see Table 24.2) to describe the ways in which the 'well intentioned other' often misinterprets communication approaches by people with dementia, often assigning labels such as 'challenging' or 'attention-seeking' to describe the meaning of such encounters and devalue the status of the person with dementia.

The necessity to modify (or remove) the professionally orchestrated mind-set, and view the world from the perspective and communication style of the person with dementia, upholds a sense of agency and personhood and should be a goal of all communication.

Person-centredness

As Morton (1999) argues, person-centredness is a concept that articulates the principles and practices associated with the promotion of personhood; as such, it has a direct influence upon the delivery of care. Thus person-centredness is a way of thinking about and behaving towards others that is derived from work on person-centred counselling first outlined by Carl Rogers (1961) and initially introduced into the dementia care field by Kitwood (1988). Person-centredness reflects a way of being that shows respect for each person's unique individuality and acknowledges that each person has the same human value, shares the same human rights and has the same varied human needs as any other person. Developing such thinking offers the potential to impact upon the care that is delivered and culminates in what is termed 'person-centred care'.

Treachery:	the use of dishonest representation or deception in order to obtain compliance;
Disempowerment:	doing for a dementia sufferer what he or she can still do, albeit clumsily or slowly;
Infantilization:	implying that a dementia sufferer has the mentality or capability of a baby or young child;
Condemnation:	blaming; the attribution of malicious or seditious motives, especially when the dementia sufferer is distressed;
Intimidation:	the use of threats, commands or physical assault; the abuse of power;
Stigmatization:	turning a dementia sufferer into an alien, a diseased object, an outcast, especially through verbal labels;
Outpacing:	the delivery of information or instruction at a rate far beyond what can be processed;
Invalidation:	the ignoring or discounting of a dementia sufferer's subjective states; especially feelings of distress or bewilderment;
Banishment:	the removal of a dementia sufferer from the human milieu, either physically or psychologically;
Objectification:	treating a person like a lump of dead matter; to be measured, pushed around, drained, filled and so on;
Ignoring:	carrying on (in conversation or action) in the presence of a person as if they were not there;
Imposition:	forcing a person to do something, overriding desire or denying the possibility of choice on their part;
Withholding:	refusing to give asked-for attention, or to meet an evident need;
Accusation:	blaming a person for actions or failures that arise from their lack of ability, or their misunderstanding of the situation;
Disruption:	intruding suddenly or disturbingly upon a person's action or reflection; crudely breaking their frame of reference;
Mockery:	making fun of a person's 'strange' actions or remarks; teasing, humiliating, making jokes at their expense; and
Disparagement:	telling a person that they are incompetent, useless, worthless and so on, giving them messages that are damaging to their self-esteem.

Table 24.2 Main features of a 'malignant social psychology'
Source: Kitwood (1997: 46–7)

Person-centred care

Person-centred care balances the negative effects of 'malignant social psychology' (see Table 24.2) by eradicating the excess disability that comes from poor quality of care and facilitates an appreciation of abilities that remain. It is, therefore, a philosophy of care that places emphasis upon empowerment, enablement and independence. Whether this may be achieved in reality is open to debate. For example, Brooker (2004) suggests that in recent years the notion of person-centred care has become 'all pervasive' as it is incorporated into national policy guidance – as outlined earlier in the list of the eight standards that comprise the *NSF for Older People* (DH 2001) – and is found in the everyday language of heath care, often becoming a vacuous watchword for quality service provision. Despite this, Brooker argues that person-centred care means 'different things to different people in different contexts' (2004: 216) and offers the following equation as a means of explanation:

$$PCC = V + I + P + S$$

PCC = person-centred care

V = the 'valuing' of people with dementia and those who care for them

I = the 'individuality' of treatment

P = the belief that we must attempt to view the world from the 'perspective' of that person

S = the value and importance of a positive 'social' environment which permits well-being

While this may be a helpful framework to consider the meaning and application of person-centred care, we should be mindful that the concepts underpinning person-centred care may not be universally understood and may consequently be misapplied or simply exist as evangelical rhetoric (Packer 2000). Arguably, the greatest obstacle to person-centred care may well be in the retention of 'traditional' (old culture) values rooted in a universal dislike and fear of change, and an uncertainty over how to progress the person with dementia's autonomy (Edwards 2004).

Relationship-centred care

Exploring concerns about the validity of person-centred care has led to a consideration of alternative approaches that remain rooted in core values, but which also consider the interpersonal reality of dementia care and human behaviour. Nolan *et al.* (2004, 2006) argue that while person-centred care places its emphasis upon autonomy and individualism, these may not be the best foundations for enhancing the quality of care. Instead, attention is drawn towards a 'relationship-centred' model of care in which emphasis is placed upon three specific prerequisites: respecting personhood; valuing interdependence; and investing in care giving as a choice.

Relationship-centred care is proposed as a new model of care delivery rooted in the belief that it is the interaction and dialogue between individuals that should be the cornerstone of all therapeutic activities. Essentially, the delivery of nursing care is determined by two people (patient and nurse) interacting and negotiating with each other, reaching agreement upon how care is to be provided. Surrounding this dynamic is a recognition that both the nurse and patient are engaged in relationships with others who may have a stake in how that care is delivered and that ultimately all must come to a shared understanding and decision over how to proceed.

Nolan *et al.* (2004) suggest that if such relationships are to realize their potential then there is a need to 'identify the fundamental similarities that characterize such inter-relationships' (2004: 49) and offer a framework to assist in this. The 'Senses Framework' (Nolan *et al.* 2006) is offered as a means of capturing the important dimensions of caring relationships and reflects the dynamic processes of giving and receiving care. The 'Senses Framework' is constructed around a belief that all parties (person with dementia, in this instance, family and statutory care provider) should experience the kind of relationship that offers a sense of:

- security;

- belonging;
- continuity;
- purpose;
- achievement;
- significance.

Negotiating and working within relationships through a 'senses' approach helps to address equality within a biopsychosocial model and also measures the impact of dementia on relationships, as required through the underpinning 'principles of care' of clinical practice guideline 42 (NICE/SCIE 2006).

Social perspectives

Social model of dementia

The primary idea behind a social model of dementia is that the condition should be aligned to the status of a disability and contextualized within a social model where the impact of the environment is as important to appreciate as the impact of the condition on the person himself/herself. Thus, how society disables an individual, through poor housing, low income and unemployment, for instance, has a powerful bearing upon how people with dementia are integrated or, more to the point, excluded, from society as a whole (Gilliard *et al.* 2005). While there are many examples we could use to help illustrate this point, a diagnosis of Alzheimer's disease in mid-life causes a biographical disruption to the individual and family system that is not usually seen in later life, such as facing mortgage repayments, university/school fees, loss of (or severely diminished) occupation opportunities and so on (Harris and Keady 2004), and magnifies the need for state recognition and support. However, the lack of adequate financial or work-based compensation for such an adverse life event within current UK social policy legislation, coupled to a patchy (or non-existent) national provision of dedicated services for younger people and their families, succeeds in further marginalizing this group and extenuates their feelings of loss and social exclusion (see also Alzheimer's Society 2005).

The NICE/SCIE clinical practice guideline 42 (NICE/SCIE 2006: 79–80) provides a brief account of the social model of dementia. It suggests that this model has 'important implications' for people with dementia because it highlights that:

- the condition is not the 'fault' of the individual;
- the proper focus is on the skills and capacities the person retains rather than loses;
- the individual can be fully understood (his/her history, likes/dislikes, and so on);
- an enabling or supportive environment can exert an influence;
- appropriate communication is a key value;
- opportunities should be taken for rehabilitation or re-enablement;
- the responsibility to reach out to people with dementia lies with people who do not (yet) have dementia.

Through such a discourse it becomes apparent immediately that the transcending, 'master narrative' (Somers 1994) of experiencing dementia shifts from those of 'illness' and 'burden' to 'retained' and 'recovered' abilities, for instance. This is a direct challenge to the field where, in the past, the language of assessment has been constructed around a 'loss' and 'problem' focus and presented in way that could be seen as inhibitory to positive person work, as the titles of these four scales amply demonstrate:

- The Global Deterioration Scale for Assessment of Primary Degenerative Dementia (Reisberg *et al.* 1982);
- Geriatric Depression Scale (Shiekh and Yesavage 1986);
- The Disruptive Behaviour Rating Scale (Mungas *et al.* 1989);
- The Challenging Behaviour Scale (Moniz-Cook *et al.* 2001).

One way to counter such a negative representation of dementia and ageing is to use the social model of dementia to foster more adaptive and enabling approaches to living and adjusting to its onset and trajectory, for instance through the use of life-story work. To this end, the study by Harris and Durkin (2002) built upon the emerging area of research that examines the coping and adaptation behaviours of people in early stage Alzheimer's disease. This study was based on qualitative interviews conducted with 22 people in early stage Alzheimer's disease and their carers. The analytic framework from which these narratives were examined and organized around common themes of successful coping and adaptation to early stage Alzheimer's disease. Noteworthy from the analysis of these narratives was that the people who adapted successfully used multiple coping strategies and these, together with a brief summary of their associated meaning, are listed below:

- **Acceptance and ownership**: People in early stage Alzheimer's who were coping positively were able to face the reality of their diagnoses and sought no blame for it.
- **Disclosure**: Telling friends, family members, neighbours and, when appropriate, acquaintances that they were diagnosed with probable Alzheimer's disease was a powerful release and coping strategy for many of the people interviewed.
- **Positive attitude and self-acceptance**: Individuals who were coping successfully were able to face Alzheimer's disease from a positive perspective and accept themselves.
- **Role relinquishment and replacement**: Individuals who relinquished the necessary social roles because of dementia, but replaced them with new roles or adapted previous roles, were seen to fair the best.
- **Innovative techniques/use of technology**: Individuals were creative in finding coping techniques to deal with their dementia. Harris and Durkin (2002) give an example of one man in their sample who used travellers' cheques instead of 'normal bank cheques' in his daily transactions because he could no longer write a cheque. With travellers' cheques the person with early Alzheimer's disease just had to sign his name and if he lost the cheque, it could be replaced.
- **Fluidity**: Being able to go with the flow of the disease allowed individuals to manage the daily stresses of dementia.
- **Utilizing pro-active skills**: This action-oriented approach occurred in different ways. For example, some people with dementia utilized 'energy efficiency' in the management of their lives; for instance, one person reported doing chores in the morning rather than the afternoon when he was less fatigued.
- **Connection with past activities**: Using skills developed prior to the diagnosis and finding meaningful uses for them in the 'here and now' was a theme which featured in a number of narratives.
- **Anticipatory adaptation**: Anticipating future needs allowed people to not only become familiar with their next challenge, but also begin to integrate new behaviours. This

anticipation assisted people to adapt to a realistic view of their disease giving them a chance to plan and thus exercise and maintain control.

■ **Altruism**: The ability to still be a productive member of society and give back to their communities was identified as a meaningful coping behaviour by those interviewed.

■ **Holistic practices**: Some people reported enjoying learning new relaxation techniques, such as reiki, tai' chi, meditation, yoga and guided imagery.

■ **Spirituality**: For a number of the individuals, spiritual beliefs were a source of comfort and support, especially on their bad days.

Harris and Durkin (2002) explain that this range of positive coping behaviours assist individuals with early stage Alzheimer's disease to adapt to the challenges of living with dementia by increasing their resilience to the stressors. Moreover, the range of coping behaviours provided people with Alzheimer's disease with some feelings of control over their condition and helped to instil a sense of hope. It is clear that living with the impact of Alzheimer's disease, and other dementias, is not a passive activity and a primary role for the mental health nurse must be to identify and support such positive coping techniques while working to minimize more negative ones.

A diagnosis of Alzheimer's disease, or any other form of dementia, should not be seen as the end of a life journey, but the start of a new chapter of life experience where the opportunity for self-growth and self-discovery have a significant part to play.

Ageism

As our earlier overview of prevalence and demography illustrated, the majority of people with dementia living in the UK (and the rest of the world) are older people. While this may appear an unremarkable observation, it is important to remember that ours is largely an ageist society and despite policy aimed at 'rooting out age discrimination' within the mental health and older person field (DH 2001, 2005a; Welsh Assembly Government 2006), detrimental and negative attitudes remain.

A recent demonstration of this was captured in the Audit Commission's (2000) report *Forget me not: mental health services for older people*. Of all GPs surveyed (n = 1000 + (representing 55 per cent of the study sample)), only around one-half of respondents believed it was important to look actively for early signs of dementia and to make an early diagnosis. As the report went on to explain, many of the GPs saw no point in looking for an 'incurable condition' with a typical GP response being listed as: 'Dementia is untreatable, so why diagnose it?' (Audit Commission 2000: 21).

Challenging such beliefs involves promoting positive person work in dementia care and reconstructing dementia through a rehabilitation, recovery and re-enablement approach. Mental health nurses have a central part to play in this re-orientation of societal values through education, community liaison and health promotion. An encouraging development has been that people with dementia themselves have begun to embrace this agenda, campaigning for change at macro and micro levels of political and health/social care systems (as examples, see the work of the world-wide organization the 'Dementia Advocacy and Support Network International' – www.dasniinternational.org or for national representation, the 'Scottish Dementia Working Group' – www.alzscot.org). Their involvement is typified by the contribution of Gloria Sterin (2002) who wrote with heartfelt passion about her detest of the word 'dementia' and the need to be seen as a person who can cope with the disease, albeit within an altered perception and understanding of time.

It is the voices and experiences of people with dementia that make the social model of dementia so vital and a force for social change.

Family work

The person with dementia does not exist in isolation. Family members and others close to the person are inevitably involved with the journey. Studies have consistently demonstrated that the stressors faced by family carers of people with dementia are among the most burdensome of all chronic illnesses, with carers prone to an increased risk of depression, stress, loneliness and self-injury (Keady 1996). Not only then is there a notable health and social care impact on the carer, but the high potential for a combination effect is apparent with the well-being of the carer and the person with dementia being related.

Recent policy guidance by CSIP maintains that if older persons' mental health services are to be 'fit for purpose' they should provide 'the practical advice and information service users and their carers need as well as developing a consistently high quality, comprehensive package of care and support' (CSIP 2005: 4).

The transactional model of stress and coping has informed the majority of family and care giving studies in dementia and it is important to have a more complete understanding of this literature. The transactional model builds on the work of Lazarus (1966) and, as the name suggests, views stress as resulting from a transaction between an individual and his/her environment. It is based upon a process of assessment, or appraisal, in which, initially, an individual considers the nature of an event and decides whether it poses a threat, harm or challenge. This period of consideration is known as the primary appraisal. If as a result of this appraisal a response is perceived as necessary, the potential response is compared to the individual's available coping resources (secondary appraisal). A coping response is selected and its effect on the original demand is then assessed (reappraisal). Stress is only said to result when there is a perceived mismatch between the nature of the demand and the individual's ability to respond effectively, by reducing the degree of perceived threat, harm or challenge. Using this approach the crucial determinant is not the objective nature of the demand (stressor) itself, but its appraised impact. We will illustrate this further by outlining the four key elements of Pearlin et al.'s (1990) 'Stress Process Model' which is, in our experience, the most robust model for analysing the caregiving process available and it highlights a number of interrelated issues that need to be considered by mental health nurses when undertaking an assessment.

As a way of context, Pearlin et al. argue that in 'some circumstances care giving is transformed from the ordinary exchange of assistance among people standing in close relationship to one another to an extraordinary and unequally distributed burden' (1990: 583). They cite dementia as an example and were critical at the lack of a coordinated approach to the study of such processes at that time. Their aim was to coalesce thinking and improve the level of sophistication of understanding of the processes involved. They articulated a conceptual scheme for the study of caregiver stress derived from their analysis of data from 555 caregivers and promote it as a heuristic device that leads to better understanding of multiple factors impinging on any one caregiving situation. We will now develop the four key elements of Pearlin et al.'s (1990) model a little more.

First, the model highlights that the interplay between the carer and person with dementia's background and the caring context needs to be understood, coupled to the nature and perception of stressors. Potential mediating factors that impinge upon subsequent outcomes for the carer should also be ascertained. This brings to the fore attention on the important impact that age, gender, ethnicity, care giving history, family and network composition, prior relationships, educational and economic attainment and access to social networks have on the experience of caring. Consequently, assessment of the carer's situation needs to consider the role that these factors have on the current situation.

Second, the model highlights those factors related to the person with a dementia diagnosis and distinguishes between 'objective indicators' (e.g. problematic behaviour) and the 'subjective component' (e.g. feeling trapped by the caregiving role).

Third, the model considers what are termed 'secondary stressors' where stress has impinged upon broader aspects of the caregiver's life such as is apparent in family conflict, economic problems and the impact on their social life. As with primary stressors, a subjective component is recognized with potential impact on aspects such as the person's self esteem.

The fourth and final element of the 'Stress Process Model' (Pearlin *et al.* 1990) relates to those factors that are seen to potentially mediate the stress and perceived burden associated with caregiving. This includes formal and informal support mechanisms that might be available. An important consideration is the individual's coping mechanisms.

An interesting consideration is whether any elements of Pearlin *et al.*'s (1990) 'Stress Process Model' are more important than others in understanding the carer's situation. Non-cognitive features of dementia, such as depression and behavioural problems in the care-receiver, have been linked to greater stress and psychological morbidity (Torti *et al.* 2004). The unpredictability of the course of dementia and its manifestations, often referred to as 'progressive losses', cause additional strain (Mittelman *et al.* 2003). On the other hand, the dominance of stress/burden models 'is not without problems' as they have been criticized for their tendency to pathologize caring (Twigg and Atkin 1994); also, the transcending narrative of 'burden', 'stress' and 'strain' hardly denote the application of a social model of dementia, or promote a sense of well-being for the person living with the dementia. Consequently, more attention should be given to promoting a sense of satisfaction and expertise in caregiving as a specific and legitimate target for intervention (for an illustration see Nolan and Keady 2001; Barnes 2006).

The transactional models of stress and coping have been highly influential in the caring literature and help direct interventions. For example, we may aim to reduce 'burden' (objective and subjective) by managing primary stressors through addressing the person with dementia's situation. We can also seek to influence carers' perspectives of the situation through education and support mediating factors by enhancing coping and support mechanisms. However, the question remains as to how 'best' to intervene with the family and person with dementia. The NICE/SCIE clinical guideline 42 (NICE/SCIE 2006) concludes that multi-component interventions, tailored to the individual and family circumstances, have the strongest evidence-base for 'success'. Such interventions might include individual or group psycho-education, peer support groups, support and information through telephone and internet links, training courses about dementia, services and benefits, and dementia-care problem solving.

The crucial element appears to be the necessity to tailor intervention requiring a prerequisite comprehensive assessment. Ideally, planned activity should be seen as meaningful by all major stakeholders and 'goals for treatment should emerge from caregivers themselves' predicated on a model of 'working with' people with dementia and their carers (Nolan and Keady 2001). It is necessary, therefore, to obtain personal accounts about how the condition affects both the person with dementia and those in close contact in order to clarify the family situation and provide a summary of strengths and challenges. As such, assessment material can be organized around key headings such as:

- understanding of the condition;
- positive coping strategies;
- identifying situations that trigger distress;
- strengths of the family unit;
- reconfiguring lifestyle.

Common themes to look out for may include: incorrect beliefs about the aetiology of the condition; beliefs about behaviours being controllable or deliberate; trying to protect the person with dementia from any form of stress; self-sacrificing behaviour and high levels of distress.

Therapeutic effort

Nurses are the largest professional group working in dementia care and are dynamic in the provision of a diverse array of therapeutic services and activities (for a comprehensive examination see Keady *et al.* 2003, 2007). There is often a significant therapeutic overlap between what nurses and other mental health professionals do and this makes it difficult to state accurately what the nurse's role is. As such, we are witnessing a blurring of boundaries and responsibilities between professional groups. However, nurses are present throughout the whole trajectory of the lived experience of dementia, from assessment, through diagnosis into treatment, management and ultimately offering a palliative role at the end of life. It cannot be stated too strongly, or too often, that nurses are in a 'powerful position to influence the care of people with dementia for good or ill' (Clibbens and Lewis 2004: 115). It is the use, application and sharing of that 'power' that will ultimately progress the place of nursing within dementia care.

In the early stages of dementia, nurses are involved primarily in activities related to assessment and historically, under the influence of the biomedical model, this has been aimed at assisting the diagnostic process with nurses gathering information for interpretation by the patient's doctor. Under such a model both nurse and patient have a largely passive role. As the move is made towards a more balanced biopsychosocial model the process of assessment, the way in which it is carried out, is seen to be as important as its purpose and becomes influenced by person-centred principles.

Outlining the practical implications of such influence, Cheston and Bender (2000) suggested that any kind of assessment should be regarded as the first step in a long-term collaborative relationship. They go on to say that assessment only occurs after: informed consent is undertaken (or other safeguards initiated), as outlined in the Mental Capacity Act 2005; is conducted in the person's chosen environment; places the person within the context of their whole life; examines how possible disabilities relate to that person's biography; and significantly, that assessment does not merely give evidence for diagnosis, but has a focus upon that person's specific needs. If Kitwood's (1997) moral philosophy is adopted, then it is clear that assessment is based upon an 'I–Thou' relationship as opposed to an 'I–It' ('I–It' characterizes a very traditional style of assessment which is all about detachment, disempowerment and alienation, while 'I–Thou' characterizes an assessment style which is all about warmth, acceptance and involvement). It is important to have an awareness of the limitations of assessment and to be mindful of the advice from Watkins (2001) that it is simply impossible to know a person in all their 'complexity' from simply having one or two meetings.

As stated in the Introduction to this chapter, mental health nurses have been involved in the provision of treatment to people with dementia for some considerable time, and their involvement in recent years is becoming more significant. While treatment in this context is largely non-medical, there is a growing emphasis upon nurses assuming the role of prescribers and influencing the experience of the prescribing process with movement away from a compliance-oriented model towards one of concordance (for a detailed exposition see Page 2007). The predominant treatments throughout almost the whole of the dementia experience are better termed psychosocial interventions and encompass a wide diversity of therapeutic endeavour that cannot be satisfactorily addressed in this chapter but are available in other parts of this book.

Examples of such interventions may include: post-diagnostic counselling in which we witness the changing role of the nurse moving away from assisting a doctor to make a diagnosis, towards assisting the person to cope with the diagnosis that has been made. Nurses are increasingly active in disclosing the diagnosis of dementia and in offering emotional support thereafter. The aspirations for such support have been outlined by Yale (1995) as being to:

- establish rapport;
- foster interpersonal relationships;
- facilitate grief work;
- assist the person with dementia in 'coming to terms' with their condition.

Such aims promote the notion that people with dementia are able to use strategies that allow them to 'take on their diagnosis' and 'work through it', emphasizing the aspiration of reaching a point, and life, beyond diagnosis. The intention of support would, therefore, appear to be inherently prophylactic, using educational and psychological mechanisms to enhance coping strategies.

Nurses are active in responding to so-called challenging behaviours in the context of dementia, that is any behaviour of people with dementia that is regarded as dangerous to themselves, those around them, either other people with dementia or staff, or is considered antisocial. Current clinical practice guidelines (NICE/SCIE 2006) suggest that all people with dementia who present with a behaviour that challenges should have that behaviour assessed through functional analysis before any treatment or intervention is introduced. As the move away from a first-line biomedical response continues, mental health nurses are ideally placed, whether in community, acute or care home settings, to observe, assess, analyse and advise on changes in behaviour.

Mental health nurses are, of course, significant providers of physical care to people in the more advanced stages of their dementia and increasingly their role in palliative or end of life care is being recognized. Through their website, the WHO (2002) defines palliative care as being:

> 𝄆 an approach that improves the quality of life of the patients and their families facing the problems associated with life-threatening illness, through the prevention and relief of suffering by means of early identification and impeccable assessment and treatment of pain and other problems, physical, psychosocial and spiritual.
>
> (www.who.int/cancer/palliative/definition/en: accessed 29 May 2007) 𝄇

It is, however, debatable at which point in the lived experience dementia care becomes palliative care, and there is a compelling argument that it is essentially an approach to care from diagnosis through to death for anyone with a life-limiting illness and their family, rather than just about care at the end of someone's life. Arguably, we would suggest that the guiding philosophy should be about maximizing health and quality of life from the point of diagnosis, and this value-base fits in well with the nurse adopting a biopsychsocial approach.

Conclusion

This book concerns itself with the 'art and science' of mental health nursing. It is our contention that there is no better exemplar of the appropriateness and necessity of such integration than in the arena of dementia care nursing. The combination of physical and mental co-morbidity, augmented by the complex social and psychological factors associated with ageing and mental ill-health, is arguably at its most complex and challenging in the dementia care field. Consequently, nurses seeking to assist individuals and their families move along the pathway to recovery and/or maintenance of their quality of life will require a depth and sophisticated level of knowledge and skills across a broad range of domains.

Unfortunately, the resources marshalled to address this need appear to fall woefully short. Recently, Pulsford et al. (2007) reported on a UK survey of higher education provision related to dementia care and showed variable, predominantly sparse coverage of dementia within the mental health branch of pre-registration nursing programmes and under-developed provision of post-registration opportunities. Our own experiences as educators, researchers and clinicians, built up over several decades, reinforces the notion that more often than not extra energy is required to adapt negative images and constructions of 'dementia' (often found within our own specialism of mental health nursing) to see the positive within the field. Psychosocial interventions and cognitive behavioural therapy, for instance, are as important for people with dementia and their families as they are in earlier stages of the lifespan.

At present, the transcending narrative and value-base of mental health nursing is located within a 'recovery model' (DH 2006; Scottish Executive 2006). At one level, this is a totally understandable move as recovery as a process is an adaptive state that is imbued with hope and reconfigured abilities. Recovery certainly has a place within dementia care nursing and one of the most pressing challenges ahead is to use, adapt and (potentially) modify this approach for the dementia care field. Moreover, it is important to publish accounts where recovery is seen in dementia care nursing as this literature base is, at present, sparse.

Finally, we would like to highlight the tremendous possibilities and sense of achievement that can come through working with people with dementia and their families at all points in the continua of experience. At its heart, the mental health nursing role in dementia care is built on knowledge (biographical, physiological, practical, social and skills) and the formation of genuine human relationships and partnerships. Simple words, but a life-time of opportunity to test, explore, extend and live their meaning.

Summary of main conclusions

- A long tradition exists of mental health practice with people with dementia and their families.
- The biopsychosocial model of dementia should be used as a foundation for mental health nursing practice and decision-making.
- The recommended implementation of the 'recovery model' is yet to be fully tested and applied to the dementia care field.
- More focused and dedicated training in dementia is necessary on all forms of nursing course curricula.
- Ageist attitudes and stereotypes surrounding the experience of 'dementia' need to be challenged.

Questions for reflection and discussion

1   What would you tell a relative if they asked you what the risk factors for dementia were and what are the implications of these for their lifestyle? What would your answer be if a close relative asked if they were at greater risk of getting dementia?
2   In what ways do you think the perspective adopted on dementia subsequently influences care that is delivered?
3   Does the nature and format of your assessment process promote and maintain dignity and choice for the person with dementia?
4   Consider the extent to which you work in collaboration with the person you assess and what action might you take in future to promote this?

Annotated bibliography

- Kitwood, T. (1997) *Dementia Reconsidered: The Person Comes First.* Buckingham: Open University Press. Groundbreaking book that brings together the body of work that informs personhood, person-centred care and positive person work. The text challenges thinking and attitudes towards the experience of living with dementia, including a belief that a growth experience – or 'rementia' – can occur in people living with dementia if communication styles and the environment are re-tuned to a person-centred philosophy of care. Essential reading.
- Sabat, S.R. (2001) *The Experience of Alzheimer's Disease: Life Through a Tangled Veil.* Oxford: Blackwell Publishing. Written by a respected clinical psychologist in the USA, this book presents new challenges to the dementia care profession by confronting underlying assumptions about what it is to live with dementia. Specifically, Steven Sabat constructs a new way of thinking about 'the self' and its assumed loss in people with

dementia. The book is peppered throughout by case study material and extends the boundaries on the efficacy of therapeutic work with people with dementia.

■ Cantley, C. (ed.) (2001) *A Handbook of Dementia Care.* Buckingham: Open University Press. Comprising of 22 UK-based contributors (including the editor) this comprehensive publication provides readers with an authoritative overview of recent advances in dementia care. The book has a person-centred philosophy to its structure, and the contents address a range of topic areas, e.g. biomedical perspectives, UK policy initiatives, therapeutic advances and service development. The latter topic includes advice on how to include people with dementia and families in developing and evaluating new services. A thoroughly recommended book for students at either undergraduate or postgraduate levels. Existing practitioners will also gain much from a familiarity with the text.

■ Harris, P.B. (ed.) (2002) *The Person with Alzheimer's Disease: Pathways to Understanding the Experience.* Baltimore: Johns Hopkins University Press. Working within dementia care one of the greatest challenge is to 'hear the voice' of people with dementia and to do so in a way which allows us to learn from this voice and apply this new understanding to practice. This publication is a well-selected collection of works from those who have taken the time to 'sit and listen' to people with dementia, and who have presented their work in a way that readers will find both accessible and necessary.

■ Hughes, J., Louw, S.J. and Sabat, S.R. (eds) (2006) *Dementia: Mind, Meaning and Person.* Oxford: Oxford Medical Publications. This collection of works addresses knotty and somewhat complicated philosophical considerations that the notion of personhood raises in the field of dementia care. It attempts to bridge the divide between philosophy and clinical practice moving from theoretical concerns to their application. Within the text, Professor Murna Downs and her colleagues have written a helpful chapter entitled 'Understandings of dementia: explanatory models and their implications for the person with dementia and therapeutic effort' and is particularly useful in outlining how the perspective adopted influences the care that is delivered.

References

Alzheimer, A. (1907) Über eine eigenartige Erkankung der Hirnrinde. *Allgemeine Zeits Psychiatry, Psychisch-Gerichtlich Medicine* **64**: 146–8.

Alzheimer's Society (2005) *Younger People with Dementia: an Approach for the Future.* London: Alzheimer's Society.

Alzheimer's Society (2007) *Dementia UK: A report into the prevalence and cost of dementia prepared by the Personal Social Services Research Unit (PSSRU) at the London School of Economics and the Institute of Psychiatry at King's College London, for the Alzheimer's Society.* London: Alzheimer's Society. Available at: www.alzheimers.org.uk/news_and_campaigns/Campaigning/PDF/Dementia_UK_Full_Report.pdf (accessed 29 May 2007).

Audit Commission (2000) *Forget Me Not: Mental Health Services for Older People.* London: Audit Commission.

Audit Commission (2002) *Forget me not 2002: developing mental health services for older people in England.* London: Audit Commission.

Barber, R., Snowden, J. and Crauford, D. (1995) Frontotemporal dementia and Alzheimer's disease: retrospective differentiation using information from informants. *Journal of Neurology, Neurosurgery and Psychiatry* **59**: 61–70.

Barnes, C. (2006) Working with families and friends as carers, in K. Bryan and J. Maxim (eds) *Communication Disability in the Dementias*. London: Whurr.

Brooker, D. (2004) What is person-centred care in dementia? *Reviews in Clinical Gerontology* **13**: 215–22.

Care Services Improvement Partnership (2005) *Everybody's Business: Integrated mental health services for older adults: a service development guide*. London: Care Services Improvement Partnership.

Cheston, R. and Bender, M. (2000) *Understanding Dementia: the man with the worried eyes*. London: Jessica Kingsley.

Clibbens, R.J. and Lewis, D. (2004) The role of the nurse in the assessment, diagnosis and management of patients with dementia, in S. Curran and J.P. Wattis (eds) *Practical Management of Dementia: a multi-professional approach*. Oxford: Radcliffe Medical Press.

Commission for Health Improvement (2003) *Investigation into Matters Arising from Care on Rowan Ward, Manchester Mental Health and Social Care Trust*. London: HMSO.

Dementia Advocacy and Support Network International: www.dasninternational.org (accessed 25 May 2007).

Department of Health (1989a) *Caring for People: Community Care in the Next Decade and Beyond*. London: HMSO.

Department of Health (1989b) *Working for Patients*. London: HMSO.

Department of Health (1991a) *Care Management and Assessment: Summary of practice guidance*. London: HMSO.

Department of Health (1991b) *Care Management and Assessment: Practitioners' guide*. London: HMSO.

Department of Health (1995a) *Carers (Recognition and Services) Act*. London: HMSO.

Department of Health (1995b) *Building Bridges: A guide to arrangements for inter-agency working for the care and protection of severely mentally ill people*. London: HMSO.

Department of Health (1999) *The Carers National Strategy*. London: HMSO.

Department of Health (2000) *Carers and Disabled Children Act*. London: HMSO.

Department of Health (2001) *National Service Framework for Older People: Modern Standards and Service Models*. London: HMSO.

Department of Health (2004) *Carers Equal Opportunities Act*. London: HMSO.

Department of Health (2005a) *A New Ambition for Old Age: Next Steps in Implementing the National Service Framework for Older People. A Resource Document*. London: HMSO.

Department of Health (2006) *From Values to Action: the Chief Nursing Officer's Review of Mental Health Nursing*. London: HMSO.

Edwards, P. (2004) Is it time for a bit of tough love? *Journal of Dementia Care* **12**(5): 17.

Ferri, C.P., Prince, M., Brayne, C. *et al*. (2005) Global prevalence of dementia: a Delphi consensus study *Lancet* **366**(503): 2112–17.

Folstein, M.F., Folstein, S.E. and McHugh, P.R. (1975) Mini-mental state: a practical guide for grading the cognitive state of patients for the clinician. *Journal of Psychiatric Research* **12**: 189–98.

Gilliard, J., Means, R., Beattie, A. and Daker-White, G. (2005) Dementia care in England and the social model of disability: lessons and issues. *Dementia: the International Journal of Social Research and Practice* **4**(4): 571–86.

Greene, J. (1968) The psychiatric nurse in the community nursing service. *International Journal of Nursing Studies* **5**: 175–84.

Griffiths, R. (1988) *Community Care: an agenda for action*. London: HMSO.

Harris, P. and Durkin, C. (2002) Building resilience through Coping and Adapting, in P. Harris (ed.) *The Person with Alzheimer's Disease: Pathways to Understanding the Experience*. Baltimore: Johns Hopkins University Press.

Harris, P.B. and Keady, J. (2004) Living with early onset dementia: exploring the experience and developing evidence-based guidelines for practice. *Alzheimer's Care Quarterly* **5**(2): 111–22.

Health Advisory Service (1982) *The Rising Tide*. Sutton, Surrey: NHS.

IPA (2007) *Introduction to Behavioral and Psychological Symptoms of Dementia (Revised)*. Available at: http://www.ipa-online.org/ipaonlinev3/ipaprograms/bpsdarchives/bpsdrev/toc.asp (accessed 25 May 2007).

Keady, J. (1996) The experience of dementia: a review of the literature and implications for nursing practice. *Journal of Clinical Nursing* **5**(5): 275–88.

Keady, J., Clarke, C.L. and Adams, T. (2003) *Community Mental Health Nursing and Dementia Care: Practice Perspectives.* Maidenhead: Open University Press.

Keady. J., Clarke, C. and Page, S. (2007) *Partnerships in Community Mental Health Nursing and Dementia Care: Practice Perspectives.* Maidenhead: Open University Press.

King's Fund Centre (1984) *Living well into old age: Applying principles of good practice to services for people with dementia.* Report Number 63. London: King's Fund.

Kitwood, T. (1988) The technical, the personal and the framing of dementia. *Social Behaviour* **3**: 161–80.

Kitwood, T. (1997) *Dementia Reconsidered: the person comes first.* Maidenhead: Open University Press.

Kitwood, T. and Bredin, K. (1992) Towards a theory of dementia care: personhood and well-being. *Ageing and Society* **12**: 269–87.

Lazarus, R.S. (1966) *Psychological Stress and the Coping Process.* New York: McGraw-Hill.

McKeith, I.G., Dickson, D.W., Lowe, J. *et al.* (2005) Diagnosis and management of dementia with Lewy bodies: third report of the DLB consortium. *Neurology* **65**(12): 1863–72.

Ministry of Justice (2007) *The Mental Capacity Act 2005 Code of Practice.* London: Ministry of Justice.

Mittelman, M.S., Epstein, C. and Pierzchala, A. (2003) *Counseling the Alzheimer's Caregiver. A resource for health care professionals.* Chicago: American Medical Association.

Moniz-Cook, E., Woods, R., Gardiner, E., Silver, M. and Agar, S. (2001) The Challenging Behaviour Scale (CBS): development of a scale for staff caring for older people in residential and nursing homes. *British Journal of Clinical Psychology* **40**(3): 309–22.

Morton, I. (1999) *Person Centred Approaches to Dementia Care.* Oxford: Winslow Press.

Mungas, D., Welier, P., Franzi, J. and Henry, R. (1989). Assessment of disruptive behaviour associated with dementia: the Disruptive Behaviour Rating Scales. *Journal of Geriatric Psychiatry and Neurology* **2**(4): 196–202.

National Institute for Health and Clinical Excellence/Social Care Institute for Excellence (2006) *Dementia: supporting people with dementia and their carers in health and social care. NICE clinical practice guideline 42.* London: NICE.

Nolan, M. and Keady, J. (2001) Working with carers, in C. Cantley (ed.) *A Handbook of Dementia Care.* Maidenhead: Open University Press.

Nolan, M.R., Davies, S., Brown, J., Keady, J. and Nolan, J. (2004) Beyond person centred care: a new vision for gerontological nursing. *International Journal of Older People Nursing* 13(3a): 45–53.

Nolan, M., Brown, J., Davies, S., Nolan, J. and Keady, J. (2006) *The Senses Framework: Improving Care for Older People Through a Relationship-Centred Approach. GRIP Report Number 2.* Sheffield: University of Sheffield.

Nolan, P. (2003) Voices from the past: The historical alignment of dementia care to nursing, in J. Keady, C.L. Clarke and T. Adams (eds) *Community Mental Health Nursing and Dementia Care: Practice Perspectives.* Maidenhead: Open University Press.

Packer, T. (2000) Does person centred care exist? *Journal of Dementia Care* **8**: 19–21.

Page, S. (2007) Assuming new responsibilities: nurse prescribing in dementia care, in J. Keady, C.L. Clarke and S. Page (eds) *Partnerships in Community Mental Health Nursing and Dementia Care: Practice Perspectives.* Maidenhead: Open University Press.

Pearlin, L.I., Mullan, J.T., Semple, S.J. and Scaff, M.M. (1990) Caregiving and the stress process: an overview of concepts and their measures. *Gerontologist* **30**(5): 583–94.

Pulsford, D., Hope, K. and Thompson, R. (2007) Higher education provision for professionals working with people with dementia: A scoping exercise. *Nurse Education Today* **27**(1): 5–13.

Reisberg, B., Ferris, S.H., deLeon, M.J. and Crook, T. (1982) The global deterioration scale for assessment of primary degenerative dementia. *American Journal of Psychiatry* **139**: 1136–9.

Rogers, C.R. (1961) *On Becoming a Person.* Boston: Houghton Mifflin.

Royal College of Physicians (1981) *Organic Mental Impairment in the Elderly: A Report of the Royal College of Physicians by the College Committee on Geriatrics.* London: Royal College of Physicians.

Sabat, S. (2001) *The Experience of Alzheimer's Disease: life through a tangled veil.* Oxford: Blackwell.

Sabat, S.R. (2002) Surviving manifestations of selfhood. *Dementia: the International Journal of Social Research and Practice* **1**(1): 25–36.

Scottish Dementia Working Group: www.alzscot.org (accessed 25 May 2007).

Scottish Executive (2006) *Rights, Relationships and Recovery: The Report of the National Review of Mental Health Nursing in Scotland.* Edinburgh: Scottish Executive.

Shiekh, J. and Yesavage, J. (1986) Geriatric Depression Scale; recent findings in the development of a shorter version, in J. Brink (ed.) *Clinical Gerontology: A guide to assessment and intervention.* New York: Howarth Press.

Simmons, S. and Brooker, C. (1986) *Community Psychiatric Nursing: A Social Perspective.* London: William Heinemann.

Somers, M.R. (1994) The narrative constitution of identity: a relational and network approach. *Theory and Society* **23**: 605–49.

Sterin, G. (2002) Essay on a word: A lived experience of Alzheimer's disease. *Dementia: the International Journal of Social Research and Practice* **1**(1): 7–10.

Torti, F.M.J., Gwyther, L.P.M., Reed, S.D.P., Friedman, J.Y.M. and Schulman, K.A.M. (2004) A multinational review of recent trends and reports in dementia caregiver burden. *Alzheimer Disease and Associated Disorders* **18**(2): 99–109.

Twigg, J. and Atkin, K. (1994) *Carers Perceived: Policy and Practice in Informal Care.* Maidenhead: Open University Press.

Walker, L.C. and Rosen, R.F. (2006) Alzheimer therapeutics – what after the cholinesterase inhibitors? *Age and Ageing,* **35**(4): 332–5.

Watkins, P. (2001) *Mental Health Nursing: the art of compassionate care.* Oxford: Butterworth-Heinemann.

Welsh Assembly Government (2006) *NSF for Older People in Wales.* Cardiff: Welsh Assembly Government.

World Health Organization (2002) *Definition of Palliative Care.* Available at: www.who.int/cancer/palliative/definition/en (accessed 29 May 2007).

World Health Organization (2007) *The ICD-10 Classification of Mental and Behavioural Disorders: Clinical Descriptions and Diagnostic Guidelines. 10th Revision.* Geneva: World Health Organization. Available at http://www.who.int/classifications/apps/icd/icd10online/ (accessed 4 June 2007).

Yale, R. (1995) *Developing Support Groups for Individuals with Early-Stage Alzheimer's Disease.* Baltimore: Health Professions Press.

CHAPTER 25

Forensic mental health care

Stephan Kirby and Graham Durcan

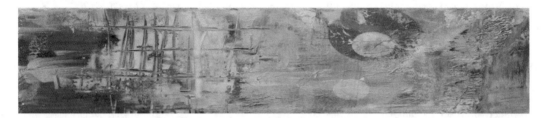

Chapter overview

Since this book's first edition in 2004 there has been considerable change in mental health services across the UK, especially in England. These changes have been to community and hospital services, to forensic provision and most recently to prison services; the latter has considerably expanded the function of forensic mental health services and that of the forensic mental health nurse. Much of this change has resulted from a planned national reform of mental health services described in the *NHS Plan for Mental Health* (DH 2000), but some has been *ad hoc*, resulting from local clinicians, commissioners and other stakeholders identifying a need and a means of meeting it. While not the focus of this chapter, over the same period a small amount of literature has appeared documenting the development of another type of forensic nurse, the 'custody nurse', with a broad caring role for offenders in police custody, but also having a role in supporting the police in their investigations.

Much of what was written by Woods in the first edition of this book still stands and remains recommended reading. However, Woods' focus was on the 'secure' forensic estate, whereas our purpose is to describe the range of services that provide care for patients (generically known as Mentally Disordered Offenders – MDOs) outside of the traditional high and medium secure NHS establishments, and also to describe the growth of services in prisons and the community. Recent changes in forensic mental health services are highlighted and their implications for nursing practice are explored. This chapter covers:

- The forensic estate;
- Prison mental health care;
- Developments in forensic mental health nursing;
- Implications for nursing practice.

The forensic estate

Admission into forensic services can occur in a number of ways and from a variety of routes, the following being the most common:

- Both sentenced and remanded prisoners may transfer to secure services directly from prison and may be returned to prison if treatment ends before the sentence does.

- A court can give a restricted or unrestricted hospital order as an alternative to prison.
- Patients can be transferred to secure services directly from community mental health services.
- Service provision for MDOs is complex and involves many different agencies, professional groupings throughout the public, private and voluntary sectors.
- The boundaries between these groupings and agencies may often be only partially defined and it is the effectiveness of the system as a whole which is important.

Services provided to prisons

Until recently the mental health service provided to prisons was limited, some prisons receiving sessions provided by a small number of forensic psychiatrists (Birmingham 2002). However, *Changing the Outlook* (DH and HM Prison Service 2001), proposed that all prisons would now have access to a community mental health team type service and since then some 360 staff have been recruited (mainly nurses) and some of these were drawn from existing forensic mental health (inpatient) services.

The reform of prison mental health services and the imposition of a minimum standard of transfer to the NHS from prisons of 14 days for transfers (to reduce the often considerable delays in this process) (DH 2005a) has brought about an increase in the proportion of people transferred from prison to forensic inpatient provision (primarily medium secure as very few prisoner transfers go to low or high secure). Although this new standard has been introduced there are still delays in transfer – in one study in London transfers were found to be taking an average of 53 days (Sales and McKenzie 2007). Only about 10 per cent of prison transfers to the forensic estate will return to prison to resume their sentence when their need for hospitalization ends, indeed 41 per cent of all discharges are directly into the community. In addition to an increase in discharges there is also an unfortunate increase in people being recalled into forensic services after being conditionally discharged into the community, even though re-offending rates for those discharged from forensic services are very low (Rutherford and Duggan 2007).

Though there is no substantial research on the profile of forensic inpatients, it is reasonable to assume that the patient group with which forensic nurses work in secure settings in the NHS and independent sector has changed. Other factors that have influenced the changing profile of the forensic inpatient population include increased use of illicit substances and reform and expansion of community mental health provision (Snowden 2007). Illicit substance use rates of between 24 and 37 per cent have been found among general mental health patients with severe mental illness (Graham *et al.* 2001).

A capacity review in 2006, the *Best Practice Guidance: Specification for Adult Medium-Secure Service* (DH 2007a) concluded that the capacity for medium secure care (including specialist groups such as women, learning disabled men, patients with dangerous and severe personality disorder and deaf patients) was gradually rising and as of January 2006 there were 29 NHS medium secure units providing around 1972 beds and a further 1500 beds being provided by the independent sector. The capacity review proposed that by the end of 2010/11 bed numbers will increase. It is projected, for example, that medium secure beds in London will increase from 727 to approximately 906 for male patients and from 94 to 122 for female patients, and in the northern part of the UK from 95 to approximately 159 (for males) and from 11 to 16 for female patients.

There are nearly 4500 secure places (beds) in high and medium secure forensic services (Rutherford and Duggan 2007). The independent sector has, over the years, become a major provider of medium secure beds with around 35–40 per cent of the total capacity and growing (Laing and Buisson 2006). The number of people in adult forensic services has grown steadily year on year and is currently in the region of 4000 (compared to 2650 in 1997) and has increased 7 per cent between 2005 and 2007 (Rutherford and Duggan 2007). Additionally there are low secure facilities which can, in certain instances, be used for voluntary patients as well as for those detained under mental health legislation. These also provide a step down for 'forensic' inpatients, but very seldom a placement for people transferring from prison; between April 2005 and March 2006, only 2 per cent of sentenced prisoners, and 1 per cent of un-sentenced prisoners, were transferred from prison directly to low secure provision (Rutherford and Duggan 2007).

In addition to adult secure provision there are currently five units in England providing medium secure beds for those aged 12–18 years providing a total of just under 70 beds with an additional 20 beds in a sixth unit to be built in the south west of England (currently the English region least well served). A small number of beds are also being commissioned for young people with learning disability (DH 2007b).

While more medium secure services have been built over the past decade during which time the NHS has been working to transfer patients out of high secure accommodation, there is still under provision of medium and low secure units. *Specification for Adult Medium-Secure Services* (DH 2007a) proposed that within medium secure services, there should be two overarching aims of service delivery. First, in common with all other mental health (hospital and community based) services, delivery of high-quality clinical assessments, health care and treatment that is appropriate to the needs of the client group. Second, achieving a balance between the twin goals of treating mental disorder and managing and reducing risk.

This publication recognizes adult medium secure inpatient care as one strand of a pathway of care for MDOs. It acknowledges that patients have individual needs, and that patients with a diagnosis of personality disorder will require differing models of care to those with a learning disability. The principle of access to medium secure services is based on the assessed level of risk and the need of the individual patient receiving care and treatment within a medium secure environment. Patients who do not require a service that provides a medium secure specification should not be admitted (DH 2007a).

It has always been the case and remains so that some forensic patients remain in secure accommodation for many years, but the introduction of new community services and particularly Assertive Outreach and Crisis Resolution Services have increased the capacity of mental health services as a whole to manage 'challenging' patients in the community as well as for 'step-down' from secure inpatient services into the community.

Other forensic services

Community forensic services

Community forensic services are a recent development and their implementation across the UK has been patchy and uneven (Coid *et al.* 2007), as has indeed the development of beds-based forensic services. Community forensic services have developed differently in different localities but the service models can be divided into those which are 'integrated' and those which are 'parallel' (Coid *et al.* 2007). The former is the provision of consultation and advice by a forensic service to a generic community mental health team (CMHT) on the aftercare management of a former forensic inpatient and perhaps direct interventions in conjunction with CMHT practitioners. The latter is an aftercare service (equivalent to the type of care that CMHTs offer to their clients) being offered directly by the specialist community forensic service. The development of integrated models of services may be a product of limited funding and therefore necessity and certainly Coid *et al.* (2007) states that parallel services do not have sufficient resources to provide aftercare for all their discharged patients. As a result, even where they do exist, local CMHTs have to provide care for some discharged patients.

Coid *et al.* (2007) report findings of the only study hitherto of the efficacy of specialist (parallel) community forensic services. This observational study compared outcomes for just over a 1000 people discharged from medium secure service of whom around 40 per cent were cared for post discharge by specialist forensic community services and 60 per cent by CMHTs. Coid *et al.* found that neither type of aftercare was superior and concluded that their study did not support the development of further parallel care. They also describe the benefits of integrated working which can be summarized as:

- combining forensic and generalist services reflects the client's 'natural history of disorder';
- reducing the stigmatization associated with contact with forensic services;
- improving knowledge within general services of forensic clients (Coid *et al.* 2007).

There is also a suggestion that CMHT care may be more cost-effective than specialist forensic care, but this seems to be linked primarily to the tendency of each type of team to readmit their patients to their own facilities rather than to a unit based on need; in the case of CMHTs these would be general psychiatric admission facilities and for specialist teams this would be medium secure or other such forensic facilities, the latter form of care being more expensive to provide.

Court diversion and liaison services

One of the first ventures outside of the secure unit for forensic nurses in the UK was into the courts and in particular the cells beneath them. This was later extended to police custody but the purpose was the same, which was to divert at least a proportion of those with mental health problems away from the criminal justice system and custody in particular and to appropriate mental health care.

Court and Custody Diversion has existed since the 1980s but survey work conducted by NACRO (2005) indicates that there has been a decline in the number of services and where they exist both the quality and extent of provision vary dramatically. Her Majesty's Inspector of Prisons (HMIP) has also addressed the need for more diversion schemes in their thematic report on mental health (HMIP 2007a). It is possible that these scheme have suffered from not being 'must do's' or even mentioned in the NHS Plan for Mental Health, however, diversion is once again becoming a policy priority (DH 2007c).

Diversion for MDOs usually involves moving the person out of the criminal justice system and into the health and social care system (Spurgeon 2005). The reality, however is that many courts have limited or no coverage and also that certain offenders and certain offences (generally those with an element of violence) are unlikely to be diverted to anything other than a medium secure unit. Some judges and magistrates assumed that a custodial disposal within the criminal justice system will guarantee access to mental health care. However, this has largely been untrue until very recently. Another factor to be considered is the reluctance by some mental health services to be a resource for diversion and a failure to see offenders with mental health problems as being a core part of the population they serve. Resourcing (or lack of it) is also a disincentive.

Some critics have argued that diversion and liaison schemes have a negative impact on mental health services, especially on inpatient services, because, they say, people admitted from the criminal justice system are likely to be disruptive because they are prone to violence, drug-taking, non-compliance and criminality. Yet others have demonstrated that such schemes offer significant benefits in other directions because they reduce the need for remands in custody (Exworthy and Parrott 1993), reduce reoffending (James 2000), re-engage people with services (Purchase *et al.* 1996) and reduce or even prevent delays (Joseph and Potter 1993).

Many community forensic teams see their role as being broad, for example offering a multi-agency service for people with a mental health problem who come into contact with the criminal justice system (Spurgeon 2005). Schemes offered by these teams can be (broadly) categorized as:

- *Diversion Schemes*, which aim to increase identification of mental illness and to facilitate and accelerate transfer where appropriate. Options for disposal are wider than just to health services and include the range of social care services whether offered by the statutory or voluntary sector.
- *Diversion Panels* (also known as MDO Panels): These panels formally bring together a range of agencies, most notably police, health, social care and probation, to put forward a coordinated package of care for the courts or the Crown Prosecution Service (CPS) to consider. They will also co-opt other agencies and organizations, including those from the voluntary sector, where relevant to the case – for example a housing or drug team.
- *Assessment Schemes* which are concerned with identifying and assessing people appearing before the courts with a view to assisting magistrates with disposal options. Such schemes significantly reduce the time taken to obtain advice by assessing the defendant at the court rather than on remand in prison.
- *Liaison Schemes:* These schemes work with multiple agencies on behalf of MDOs rather than either just diverting people with mental health problems from prison or providing assessments for the courts. Thus the core function of providing an emergency mental health assessment service to police stations and courts has expanded to include liaising and working with criminal justice and mental health agencies and facilitating appropriate care and supervision of MDOs, both in the community and in prison. Such schemes have become multi-functional; their focal point is now to promote closer multi-agency working.

The reality is, however, that many teams have become eclectic. Rather than being purely a diversion scheme or a liaison scheme a number have elements of both. As well as providing assessments for the courts and arguing for or against diversion depending on the individual case, they will also facilitate assessments, offer advice to a variety of criminal justice agencies and access a range of disposals; that is 'smoothing the way' by helping all agencies to understand the needs of each other and the needs of the client.

While the early schemes were started (and run) by psychiatrists the majority of schemes now are staffed and led by community forensic psychiatric nurses. Ideally, schemes should be multi-disciplinary to allow for a more rounded assessment and to ensure access to a variety of disposal options. However, where that is not practical schemes should ensure that they work with a range of practitioners to ensure input into cases as outlined in the National Offender Pathway (DH 2005b). For schemes to be effective, they must ensure that they are an integral part of the overall strategy for addressing the needs of MDOs, with close links with local services and commissioners, planners and managers. There is no doubt that the interaction between the criminal justice and health and social care services needs to be improved (Spurgeon 2005).

Forensic Child and Adolescent Mental Health Services (CAMHS)

The development of forensic CAMHS has been even less systematic than that of adult services, reflecting the concerns and preferences of local clinicians and commissioners. Forensic CAMHS have developed into two forms. First, those services based around one of the small number of medium secure facilities and which vary in the degree to which they outreach to the community and, second, an even smaller number of entirely community-based forensic services. Forensic CAMHS are a tiny part of the overall forensic mental health service provision. At the time of writing (summer 2008) there are currently five inpatient units providing a total of 68 beds and a small number of community and prison in-reach services. However small there is a strong economic argument for continued growth of this provision as successful intervention during adolescence can potentially reduce of the need for services in adult life.

Several of the forensic CAMHS, both units and community-based, provide in-reach provision to Young Offender Institutes/Juveniles Centres (YOIs), that is young people's prisons, provided by HMPS. These establishments can contain both juveniles, that is young people up to the age of 17 years (services to these are commissioned by the Youth Justice Board), as well as young adults, that is 18 to 21 years old. As a consequence, some forensic CAMHS staff providing an in-reach service to these prisons are encountering a population they would not normally work with in other circumstances.

Clinical experience suggests that a primary function for both adult and younger people's community forensic teams is the provision of consultancy to non-specialist services and therefore the development of liaison skills. The existing evidence also suggests that the integrated approach is more cost efficient. Forensic mental health nurses working in the more traditional secure inpatient environment have in the past worked with a population that has been essentially static and so exposure to other services and the need for liaison skills with these services has been limited, However, for the new fields of forensic mental health nursing practice, the community and also prisons (which we will describe later) liaison skills are vital.

Youth Offending Teams (YOTs)

The Crime and Disorder Act (HMSO 1998) 1998 contained a far-reaching reform of the youth justice system. Section 3 of this Act placed a duty on each local authority with education and social services responsibilities to establish one or more YOTs to coordinate the provision of youth justice services within its area. A YOT, by this understanding is a multi-skilled partnership and (again under Section 39 of the CDA) there is a mandatory requirement that each YOT shall contain at least one probation officer, a local authority social worker, one police officer, a person nominated by the local health authority and another by the chief education officer. This was (and is) a minimum requirement.

All YOTs now have a health practitioner as member; many of these are nurses (though not exclusively) and many of these are mental health nurses. A key role for the health practitioner is to support the young person in accessing mainstream health services. Recent research by the National Association for the Care and Rehabilitation of Offenders reveals that problems in accessing mainstream health care, including mental health care remain, and that often the YOT health-worker attempts to provide this care themselves (NACRO 2007). The Healthcare Commission (2006) state that the NHS has been less than diligent in fulfilling their statutory duties in providing for young offenders. The client group that YOTs work with include many with substance misuse issues and also with poor mental health and often a combination of both. Young people engaged in offending have a variety of health needs and, according to the Healthcare Commission and NACRO, those associated with mental health and substance misuse are predominant. Emerging findings of research on adults with severe personality disorder in the new Dangerous and Severe Personality Disorder (DSPD) Unit, suggests that there are risk factors identifiable in adolescence and in this population of young offenders (Ministry of Justice and Department of Health 2007). This research suggests the possibility of early intervention and it might be that YOTs will in future provide a setting for an early intervention service.

Prison mental health care

Nurses have worked in prisons for decades. Most were, until very recently, direct employees of the prison service rather than the NHS and most were employed as generic nursing practitioners with responsibility for both the general and mental health needs of their charges. A substantial proportion has always held mental health nursing qualifications (e.g. see NHS Executive and HM Prison Service 2000).

There had been no significant provision for prisoners with mental health problems in England until very recently and the poor state of mental health care has consistently been reported by HMIP and others (e.g. HMIP 2007a, b). Concern over prison mental health care is not limited to the UK alone and there is international concern regarding the treatment of prisoners with mental illness (Freshwater 2007).

Prevalence of mental disorder in prison

The most comprehensive study of prevalence of mental ill health in England's prisons was that conducted for the Office of National Census (Singleton *et al.* 1998). Since that study was completed the prison population has grown substantially year on year and despite a recent programme of early release to reduce pressure on prison places the total population is now in excess of 81,000 (NOMS 2007). It is predicted to continue rising to 116,550 by 2013 (Home Office 2006) and it is not known what impact this growth will have had on rates of mental ill health, though doubtless the continued growth in population impacts on the care that can be provided. The Singleton *et al.* (1998) study found that approximately 90 per cent of prisoners have some degree of mental ill health or personality disorder or substance misuse problem; and for young offenders the figure is even higher at 95 per cent (Lader *et al.* 2000). Singleton *et al.* (1998) also revealed that seven out of ten prisoners had a combination of at least two of the above problems and those suffering from a psychosis were likely to have three or four other concurrent problems. See Table 25.1.

	Prevalence among prisoners	Prevalence in general population
Psychosis	6 per cent – 13 per cent	0.4percent
Personality disorder	50 per cent – 78 per cent	3.4 per cent – 5.4 per cent
Neurotic disorder	40 per cent – 76 per cent	16.5percent
Drug dependency	34 per cent – 52 per cent	4.2percent
Alcohol dependency	19 per cent – 30 per cent	8.1percent

Table 25.1 Prevalence of mental health problems in the prison and the general population (After Singleton *et al.* 2001)

Mental health in-reach teams

The responsibility for all health care in English prisons was transferred from the prison service to the NHS, and this process was completed in April 2006. The NHS through primary care trusts now commissions all health care provision in prisons including mental health care. In addition to this shift in responsibility the much neglected state of mental health care in prisons was also addressed. Reforms to prison mental health care were proposed at around the same time as the reforms to the wider community mental health service reforms and the aim was for mental health services within prisons to be 'equivalent' to mental health services in the community (NHS Executive and HM Prison Service 1999). Recent reforms to prison mental health care have involved the introduction of 360 new staff (mainly nurses – see HMIP 2007a) formed into mental health in-reach teams to which most prisons have access. It was proposed that these teams be, in effect, community mental health teams for the prison populations they support (DH and HM Prison Service 2001) and as such that they are focused on those prisoners with severe and enduring mental health problems.

The recent creation of prison mental health in-reach services has meant the development of a new area of mental health nursing practice and many of its practitioners are drawn from forensic mental health services. Indeed the recent national study of prison in-reach teams describes them as part of 'the overall system of forensic mental health care' (Steel *et al.* 2007).

The roles of these teams are yet to emerge, but a sample of staff in London prisons interviewed as part of a research project conducted by SCMH identified the following key elements:

- a service reaching out to the wings of the prisons where prisoners reside;
- a focus on prisoners with severe and enduring mental health problems;
- a community mental health team model of care;
- liaison and support to health care and primary care practitioners in prison;
- liaison and support to wing-based prison officer staff;
- a role in spreading mental health awareness particularly among prison staff;
- evidenced-based interventions (e.g. cognitive behavioural therapy);

■   a multi-disciplinary service such as one might find in a community mental health service (i.e. a mix of nursing, psychiatry, psychology, social work and occupational therapy among others) (Durcan and Knowles 2006).

Other developments in forensic mental health care

In addition to the creation of mental health in-reach teams there has been work to define the offender care pathway and targets have been set to reduce delays in transfers from prisons to secure provision in the NHS (DH 2005a). Coinciding with these changes has been the rollout of a new strategy for dealing with prisoners who attempt suicide or who are deemed to be at risk. Assessment Care in Custody and Teamwork (ACCT) is essentially a form of case management for such prisoners. Though ACCT is led by the prison service, nurses working in prisons are very involved and as part of its rollout many prison staff are receiving training in mental health awareness for the first time (Durcan and Knowles 2006).

In spite of these substantial reforms to prison mental health care to date equivalence with mental health services provided to the wider community has not been achieved. Most mentally disordered prisoners do not suffer from severe and enduring mental illness (though they are often complicated due to co-morbidity with other problems) and most prisoners still receive little or no help with their common mental health problems; and for the significant proportion of prisoners with co-morbid substance misuse and mental health problems, services tend to be disjointed and at best work in a serial fashion (Sainsbury Centre for Mental Health 2007). In short mental health services in prison are far from comprehensive. The reforms have been partial and have not had the sort of evidence base that has underpinned reforms to the wider community's mental health services, nor has there been anything like the policy implementation guidance that has accompanied the wider mental health service reforms. Thus, prison mental health services vary considerably in terms of their make-up and the service they provide across England and are described as 'using limited and idiosyncratic models of care' (Steel et al. 2007).

The great majority of prisoners do not have mental health problems that warrant transfer to external NHS (or private) care and so remain in prison. Many of these will fall below the threshold of the new in-reach teams as these have been primarily targeted to work with prisoners with serious and enduring mental health problems and prison itself may aggravate their mental health problems (HMIP 1996). It has been argued that untreated mental illness contributes to recidivistic behaviour and hampers resettlement in the community after release from prison (Social Exclusion Unit 2002). Hence mentally disordered prisoners are often caught up in a cycle of offending, institutionalization and lack of care in the community.

Burrow (1993) highlighted the 'double barrelled conflict' psychiatric forensic nurses face: caring for mentally ill offenders who are hospitalized for treatment and promoting their interests, while safeguarding the interests of society. Over the years a number of studies have described nurse and patient relationships in practice settings. While these studies give some insight into the experiences of caring, they do not provide insight about caring for inmate patients, within the prison setting.

An objective of *Changing The Outlook* (DH and HMPS 2001) was that, over the next three to five years, there would be a marked reduction of prisoners using prison health care centres for inpatient stays and that the resources and focus of care be redirected to providing day care and more 'localized' care on prisoners' wings. Other objectives were quicker and more efficient transfer of the more seriously ill prisoners to and from the NHS and greater collaboration between NHS and prison health care staff in the management of prisoners who are seriously mentally ill, including those vulnerable to suicide or self-harm.

These objectives entailed major changes for many prisons, but provided an opportunity to take a 'whole systems' perspective on how prisons and the local (mental) health services could work together to improve provision for 'prisoner patients'. Not only the care they received while in custody, but also ensuring, through the development of a number of specialist 'bridging' teams (e.g. mental health in-reach teams) that care was seamless and continued into the community upon prisoners' release.

It has recently been suggested that the introduction of multi-disciplinary mental health in reach teams has led to a much needed emphasis on the care and treatment provided to mentally disordered prisoners located on prison wings so mirroring, as *Changing the Outlook* envisaged, the community scenario (Freshwater 2007). However, recent research and reviews have revealed that the average in-reach team size is four (Durcan 2008b) and largely made up of nurses (HIMP 2007a). The spread of in-reach teams has been slow, by 2005 there were only 101 prisons and Young Offender Institutions covered. Even where in-reach teams are operating, close collaboration is vital with prison and court schemes to provide a seamless service (Spurgeon 2005). Since their introduction there has been surprisingly little debate or analysis as to how a range of prison staff, might contribute to wing-based care and work with in-reach teams to promote the effective care and management of mentally ill prisoners.

The goal of prison officers has always been to ensure safety and custody but their roles are becoming more varied and specialized. Included in their role is identifying, managing and caring for prisoners with mental health problems, but officers are generally not equipped with the skills, knowledge or confidence to do so effectively.

So what has been achieved since the publication of *Changing the Outlook*? The impact of prison in-reach teams is yet to be established, though there is some initial evidence of improvements in prison mental health care offered in some regions (e.g. London and the West Midlands, see Durcan and Knowles 2006; Durcan 2008b). However, there is also evidence of substantial gaps in service and prisoners on release experience poor continuity of care in part because many are not registered with primary care services.

In summary, in the current service delivery climate, 'forensic' is a far from exact term and no longer (if it ever did) defines a particular client group or a specific set of services; certainly the boundaries of the term are fuzzier now than they once were. Forensic nursing or the nursing of forensic patients was in the not too distant past largely carried out in high and medium secure provision mostly within the NHS. Today, though, there has been a general expansion of community services for people with mental health problems which includes some growth in forensic mental health services in the community that provide consultation to generic mental health community services and/or provide direct care via a parallel community service to a small group of their former inpatients. Indeed there has even been the emergence of 'community only' forensic services, to which no beds are attached. Services addressing the mental health needs of young offenders (adolescent offenders) have expanded, which include services specifically designated as forensic mental health and both inpatient and community services.

Implication of service changes for forensic nursing

Forensic nursing is widely regarded as a specialty of mental health nursing. But the types of nurses who work with patients who have an offending (or forensic) profile are almost as varied as the patients themselves. While we have Forensic (Mental Health) Nurses, there are also Forensic (General) Nurses, Forensic (Children's) Nurses, Forensic (Emergency) Practitioner or even Forensic (Elderly) Nurses.

The popular belief that forensic nurses work exclusively with mentally disordered offenders is incorrect. While the term Forensic Mental Health Nursing should be reserved for the forensic branch of mental health nursing, the specialty appears to be defined by the setting in which the nurse works, rather than by specialist qualifications. Traditionally nursing MDO occurs in: prisons; medium or low secure wards of mental hospitals; high secure hospitals and in community settings where the nurse provides care as a member of a mental health team. Forensic Mental Health Nurses work with forensic patients whose problems are invariably linked to some form of criminal or offending/offensive behaviour.

In whatever setting forensic mental health nursing occurs it is important for the nurse to be aware of the legal basis upon which patients are detained, or in the case of patients in the community, the legal basis that is applicable for their supervision and (if necessary) recall. At the same time all patients should be afforded their rights, respected as individuals and worked with closely to empower them to regain and maintain their own mental health.

Custody nursing

Custody nursing is a developing forensic nursing specialty utilized by a number of UK police forces. The Gannon Report (Home Office 2002) found that custody nurses offer a range of skills and services which range from dealing with minor injuries through to emergency care and a range of mental health care skills. Thus the role of the Custody Nurse appears to be varied. There is considerable emphasis on care of the offender with the aim of reducing the incidence of deaths in custody. Since 50 per cent of those who die in police custody have a mental health problem (Joint Committee on Human Rights 2003) there is a strong case for mental health assessment being a core skill of the Custody Nurse. However these nurses may also provide support to the police in evidence collection and may also give evidence in court (West 2004). With regard to the latter aspect of their role the literature focused on the role nurses can play in supporting both the police and victims in rape and sexual assault cases, though this requires specialist training. The range of other 'forensic–judicial' skills required by nurses working in custody nurse roles include taking forensic (blood and bodily fluid) samples, performing intimate searches, assessment of wounds and physical injuries for court reports and giving evidence on a range of matters including fitness to be detained and/or fitness for interview.

Custody Nurses who assist police with rape and sexual assault cases are known as Sexual Assault Nurse Examiners (SANE Nurses) a term which has been derived from similar services in North America. In the UK SANE nurses are still relatively few and restricted opportunities for specialists mean that this is unlikely to change quickly.

There has been considerable debate as to how the NHS could best employ and manage Custody Nurses and in particular how to integrate them into multi-professional teams. Clinical experience suggests that integration of custody nurses into NHS multi-disciplinary teams has not been successfully achieved. One result of this has been the growth of private companies which offer Custody Nurse Services to police services across the UK.

Nursing in the secure environment

There has been much debate and controversy about the development of forensic nursing as a specialty. Advocates argue that the ability to provide therapeutic treatments while maintaining a secure environment is in itself sufficient to ensure specialist status. Opponents maintain there is no empirical evidence to support such a claim and that the dilemma of providing therapy and custody is an issue faced by all mental health nurses. However without a clearly defined role and framework of nationally agreed skills and competencies and with uncertainties over training and educational needs it is difficult to identify a clear career pathway for those nurses wishing to practise within secure environments.

The nurse working in prison has exposure to a wider variety of clients who demand a wider range of nursing skills than the nurse in the secure mental health unit. Additionally the nurse working in prison has virtually no say in the security of those 'clients' whereas 'security' is an integral part of the role of the nurse in the forensic unit; indeed integrating security with therapy or at least trying to reduce the negative impact of depriving a person of their liberty is part of the art of forensic mental health nursing.

The role of nurses working in prison in-reach teams was examined by one of the authors in research by the Sainsbury Centre for Mental Health (Durcan 2008a, b). Nurses in both London and the West Midlands reported that they spent much of their time liaising with mental health, primary care, social care and housing agencies in the community. All of the London teams were working with a number of people who had been remanded to prison and whose length of stay in prison was unpredictable but often short. Many people arrive in prison having fallen out of contact with health care and other agencies (Williamson 2006) and therefore much of this liaison activity was aimed towards re-establishing these connections. The same was true for nurses working in the West Midlands though as more of the population in the five participating prisons were sentenced liaison occurred as part of the resettlement planning for a prisoner. Prisoners interviewed in the West Midlands reported that the involvement of in-reach staff had significantly influenced their resettlement planning; it was occurring earlier than during previous periods of incarceration and was more comprehensive. Prisoners believed that the in-reach teams acted as their advocates.

In virtually all the in-reach patients cases examined in the SCMH research studies probation officers had engaged with the prisoners at a much earlier stage than they had experienced in previous periods of incarceration and there was a difference between these prisoners and those not in touch with in-reach teams. Several prisoners described previous experiences of leaving prison as being poorly planned and some described feeling 'ejected' from prison. Most prisoners in contact with in-reach and who had a release date within a few months of the interview felt more confident than before and noticeably more so than those prisoners with mental health problems not in contact with in-reach teams. The support most prisoners wanted on release was in finding appropriate accommodation and also in having support for what they saw as their problems with substance misuse. Ensuring continuity of care post-release was seen as a huge problem by nurses working in in-reach teams.

The prison setting, unlike other secure settings in which forensic nurses work, is not designed to provide a therapeutic regime, but is primarily concerned with punishment through deprivation of liberty of offenders and ensuring public safety. The great majority of staff working in prisons are primarily concerned with ensuring security and prisoner management, however, given the high prevalence of mental ill health among prisoners, prison staff come into contact daily with mentally ill prisoners. Raising mental health awareness among prison staff is seen by in-reach staff as a key role (Durcan and Knowles 2006) but is also a huge task given the large number of prison staff; around 50,000 (estimated from Her Majesty's Prison Service 2006).

Working with prisoners has meant some considerable challenges for in-reach nursing staff. Nurses working with MDOs have always (as mentioned earlier in relation to adult and younger people's community teams) needed liaison and advocacy skills, however, the move of mental health services into prisons has meant that these skills are more critical as the prison population is socially excluded and often out of contact with health and other services on arrival to prison. An additional challenge to working with this group is unpredictability of the custodial regime. Remanded prisoners can be released at short notice and even sentenced prisoners may be transferred to other establishments again sometimes with little warning.

There are particular challenges in nursing women and black and ethnic minority prisoners, which are discussed briefly below.

Women in secure/forensic settings

In 1998 The Office of National Statistics (Singleton *et al.* 1998) announced that there were 2770 women in prison in England (at the time of writing this has risen to nearly 4500) and of these two-thirds suffered from a neurotic mental disorder. In addition 14 per cent sampled suffered from a functional psychosis (e.g. schizophrenia). A large proportion of women prisoners reported a dependence on drugs (54 per cent of remand and 41 per cent of sentenced prisoners) with heroin dependence reported by 40 per cent of remand and 23 per cent of sentenced prisoners.

Differences between the way men and women in NHS secure establishments are viewed and treated by staff appears as much to do with gender (and gender expectations) as it does with diagnostic or offence category. Some early commentators (e.g. Bland *et al.* 1999) argued that the psychopathic (or borderline personality disorder) label, applied to a large percentage of women in secure settings, was evidence of the medicalization of antisocial behaviour. Had such behaviour occurred in men, it would, they argued, have resulted in them being simply criminalized and so receiving custodial sentences. The relative absence of serious convictions among women in (high) secure care also points to women being considered differently to men.

Women are often admitted to secure services because of damage to property, self-harm or aggression towards hospital staff (Women In Secure Hospitals 1999). For mental health professionals it can be frustrating working with patients who exhibit self-harming behaviour. Such patients are often labelled as having a (borderline) personality disorder or often as being difficult to manage, and are 'relegated' to the 'untreatable' group. Focusing on managing behaviours adds to the sense of hopelessness; instead staff need to focus on patients' interpersonal interactions as the themes of powerlessness, rejection and feeling misunderstood are prevalent in their life histories.

Black and ethnic minority clients

Research since the 1980s has consistently shown that black people are over-represented in UK mental health services, among those detained under the mental health legislation and within secure mental health facilities. Black people are also over-represented in prisons and are more likely to receive custodial sentences than white people (e.g. Healthcare Commission 2007).

Males from black and minority ethnic (BME) communities account for 19 per cent (approximately three times their representation in the population) of those received into prisons nationally, and females from BME communities account for 25 per cent. In London approximately 45 per cent of those discharged from prison are from BME communities (London Resettlement Board 2005).

Thus people from BME communities and particularly those with African and Caribbean heritage are over-represented in the services in which forensic nurses work. Forensic services have been severely criticized in their management of black patients, a recent example being the Bloefeld Inquiry Report into the death of David 'Rocky' Bennett (Norfolk, Suffolk and Cambridgeshire Strategic Health Authority 2003), in which a black patient was mismanaged and died as a result of staff restraint. This report adds to the ample evidence (e.g. Fernando *et al.* 1998) that black people are treated in a more coercive and punitive way within the psychiatric system than white people. Also, that African-Caribbeans are over-represented in locked wards, secure units and Special (High Secure) Hospitals.

In local service evaluations conducted by one of the authors it was noted that people from BME populations were over-represented in assertive outreach teams, for example in one city in the East Midlands less than 6 per cent of the population were of African and Caribbean origin but this group constituted over 25 per cent of the Assertive Outreach Service caseload.

Interestingly, while people from ethnic minority populations are over-represented in prisons, this does not appear to be the case in prison in-reach caseloads (e.g. HMIP 2007a). The explanation for this is unlikely to be that people from these communities are appropriately diverted to secure NHS provision (hence their over-representation there). Prison mental health services, which, though much increased in recent years, are still a limited service and like community services have yet much to do to develop culturally sensitive services. Coid *et al.* (2002) found less mental ill health among African-Caribbean prisoners than among white prisoners, though these findings may be partially explained by a failure to recognize mental illness in African-Caribbean prisoners by health care staff (Rickford and Edgar 2005) and a reluctance to seek help for mental health problems among these prisoners. This reflects the difficult relationship between African-Caribbean communities and mental health services (SCMH 2002).

The proportion of non-English or Welsh nationals has changed rapidly over the past decade by an estimated 152 per cent and they now account for approximately 12 per cent of the overall prison population. The most common reasons for their imprisonment are drugs-related offences (Prison Reform Trust 2004). The mental health needs of this population are not well understood, but some may have experienced considerable trauma prior to their arrival in the UK and many will be very isolated and have no contact with families. Most prisons do not appear to make much use of the translation services that are available. This group accounted for eight out of 94 suicides in prison in 2003 (Prison Reform Trust 2004).

Dangerous and severe personality disorder

The problem of personality disorder is considered in Chapter 26 and so is considered only briefly here and restricted to the problem of psychopathy.

In mainstream psychiatric discourse, psychopaths have come to be regarded as unresponsive to treatment, hence the inclusion under the Mental Health Act (HMSO 1983) 1983 of a treatability clause (cf. Chapter 7). Recently there has been a marked downward trend in the number of inpatients receiving the diagnosis of psychopathic or personality disorder in mainstream services. Yet more than half the residents in high secure hospitals are still classified as suffering from psychopathic personality disorder. This suggests that while mainstream psychiatry is trying to minimize the demands of what are seen as disruptive and undesirable patients, for forensic psychiatry, it remains a large part of their workload.

A new type of high secure service has been launched recently, the Dangerous and Severe Personality Disorder (DSPD) Programme (see http://www.dspdprogramme.gov.uk/home.php), currently consisting of four high secure units, two based in high secure prisons and two based in high secure NHS (High Secure – Special) hospitals. The first unit was opened in 2002 at HMP Whitemoor and the three other units have all been opened since 2004. Community services for those with so-called DSPD are also planned since services in the community for those with personality disorder are few and far between. The programme is seen as a 'pilot' which provides just over 300 places and is aimed at the assessment and treatment of people who have committed a violent and/or sexual crime and who have been detained by the criminal justice system or under mental health legislation.

The impact of the programme is yet to be evaluated as is the contribution of nursing to it. The programme also consists of research into the treatment of personality disorder and the links between personality disorder and offending (Ministry of Justice and DH 2007).

Conclusion

In this chapter we have described the sea change experienced by nurses working with offenders with mental health problems. High and medium secure inpatient settings, though not left unchanged, remain the preserve of forensic mental health nursing, although increasingly the so-called 'forensic' patient can be found in other settings. The role of the forensic nurse working in these settings is quite different, very often liaising and supporting colleagues with less specialist backgrounds in working with a challenging population. Even those nurses working in more traditional 'indoor' settings are working with a changing population, one which matches the characteristics of a prison population, i.e. an extremely socially excluded and transient population.

Just as the secure services have experienced changes in the type of patients they encounter, so too have acute and community mental health services. The demarcation lines that once clearly separated acute, community and forensic services are becoming blurred as more 'generic' services are acquiring a forensic flavour to their clientele. Thus, forensic nursing skills are no longer the preserve of forensic nurses alone, but are increasingly needed to all mental health nurses. The main points of this chapter are as follows:

- Over recent years there has been a substantial increase in medium secure beds, particularly in the independent sector, which in addition to providing general use forensic beds has developed forensic specialist services (e.g. learning difficulty and deaf services).
- There has also been growth in mental health work in prisons through the introduction of mental health in-reach teams. The work of the latter may be leading directly to a further growth in the former, through the identification of those with the most severe mental illness and the facilitation of their transfer to the secure estate.
- This in turn is leading to further changes in forensic services. In-reach teams are learning that they need to comprise a variety of skills, drawn from both the familiar world of forensic mental health (e.g. skills in managing risk), but also general mental health (e.g. skills in facilitating recovery).
- Almost all transfers from prisons go into medium secure units, though it is apparent that were these transfers into the community many would not require this level of security. To some extent patients with more 'routine' psychiatric crises have always been transferred from prison, but the volume of such admission has increased exponentially.
- It is reasonable to assume the proportion of such prisoners in medium secure beds has increased and that possibly the gap between general acute psychiatric care and forensic care has decreased. The skills of forensic inpatient nurses need to reflect this change. Just as acute care nurses need to prepare their patients for life after the ward so do forensic nurses, though they are likely to have much less time to do this than in the past.
- While it is important to meet the health and mental health needs of patients on their release (e.g. connecting them with primary care and local community mental health care) it is important for forensic mental health nurses to have a broad definition of the latter so that basic needs are met; in the case of ex-prisoners this is accommodation, treatment for substance misuse and employment.

Questions for reflection and discussion

1   What is the range of settings in which forensic nursing is currently practised?
2   What are the implications of the current limited provision of diversion and liaison services to both court and custody services?
3   Consider the importance of liaison skills as part of the armoury of the nurse engaged in forensic mental health nursing?
4   Consider some of the potential barriers to reintegrating the 'forensic' patient back into the community and how the forensic nurse practitioner can help address these.

Annotated bibliography

- Chaloner, C. and Coffey, M. (eds) (1999) *Forensic Mental Health Nursing: Current Approaches*. London: Blackwell. This was one of the original texts relating to forensic mental health nursing practice. This multi-authored book demonstrates how forensic mental nursing evolved from its inpatient, secure-services origins to the diverse sub-specialism of mental health nursing that exists today. A range of practice-based issues are addressed, together with an exploration of topics including the skills and knowledge base of this specialism. This book is of interest to forensic mental health nurses; those who may be contemplating a career in this area; and to members of the other professional groups involved in the management and provision of care and treatment within forensic mental health settings, also it serves as a primary resource text for students studying in this area.

■ Dale, C., Thompson, T. and Woods, P. (eds) (2000) *Forensic Mental Health: Issues in Practice.* Oxford: Baillière Tindall. This is a practical text that provides readers with clear guidance on how to tackle care issues in relation to the care and management of this challenging client population. This book draws together a range of expertise from a variety of professionals who draw on available evidence and firmly ground their work in practice. The range of chapters and contributors here reflect the importance of multi-disciplinary teamwork in this area.

■ Kettles, A., Woods, P. and Collins, M. (eds) (2001) *Therapeutic Interventions for Forensic Mental Health Nurses.* London: Jessica Kingsley Publishers. Written by experts in the growing field of forensic mental health care, this text explores interventions in forensic mental health nursing and the care of the mentally disordered offender, with a clear emphasis on clinical practice and clinical competence. It explores the practical issues facing forensic nurses, such as managing the environment and safety issues, as well as the possible emotional trauma of fulfilling such a role. The contributors cover a range of diverse perspectives and examine a range of intervention strategies as well as examining the client group itself and consider new roles for nurses in the light of recent research.

■ Woods, P. (2004) The person who uses forensic mental health services, in I.J. Norman and I. Ryne. *The Art and Science of Mental Health Nursing.* Maidenhead: Open University Press. This chapter in the previous edition of this text provides an excellent summary of the challenges of nursing patients within secure conditions.

References

Birmingham, L. (2002) Commentary. *Advances in Psychiatric Treatment* **8**: 125–7.

Bland, J., Mezey, G. and Dolan, B. (1999) Special women special needs: a descriptive study of female special hospital patients. *Journal of Forensic Psychiatry* **10**: 34–5.

Burrow, S. (1993) An outline of the forensic nursing role. *British Journal of Nursing* **2**(18): 899–904.

Coid, J., Petruckevitch, A., Bebbington, P. *et al.* (2002) Ethnic differences in prisoners I. Criminality and psychiatric morbidity. *British Journal of Psychiatry* **181**: 473–80.

Coid, J., Hickey, N. and Yang, M. (2007) Comparison of outcomes following after-care from forensic and general adult psychiatric services. *British Journal of Psychiatry* **190**: 509–14.

Department of Health (2000) *The NHS Plan.* London: Department of Health.

Department of Health (2005a) *Procedure for the Transfer of Prisoners to and from Hospital under Sections 47 and 48 of the Mental Health Act 1983.* London: Department of Health.

Department of Health (2005b) *Offender Mental Health Care Pathway.* London: Department of Health.

Department of Health (2007a) *Best Practice Guidance: Specification for adult medium-secure services.* London: Department of Health.

Department of Health (2007b) *Secure Forensic Mental Health service for Young People.* London: Department of Health. Available at: http://www.advisorybodies.doh.gov.uk/nscag/services/secure-forensic.htm

Department of Health (2007c) *Improving Health, Supporting Justice: A Consultation Document – A strategy for improving health and social care services for people subject to the criminal justice system.* London: Department of Health.

Department of Health and HM Prison Service (2001) *Changing the Outlook: A Strategy for Developing and Modernising Mental Health Services in Prisons.* London: Department of Health.

Durcan, G. (2008a) Prison Mental Health Nursing In: National Forensic Nurses Research and Development Group (editors) Forensic Mental Health Nursing, Capabilities, Roles and Responsibilities, London: Quay Books.

Durcan, G. (2008b) *From the inside: Experience of prison mental health care.* London: Sainsbury Centre for Mental Health.

Durcan, G. and Knowles, K. (2006) *London's Prison Mental Health Services: a review.* London: SCMH. Available at:
http://www.scmh.org.uk/80256FBD004F3555/vWeb/flKHAL6N3GV4/$file/
policy5_prison_mental_health_services.pdf

Exworthy, T. and Parrott, J. (1993) Evaluation of a diversion from custody scheme at magistrates' court. *Journal of Forensic Psychiatry* **4**(3): 497–505.

Fernando, S., Ndegwa, D. and Wilson, M. (1998) *Forensic Psychiatry, Race and Culture.* Routledge: London.

Freshwater, D. (2007) Editorial. *Journal of Psychiatric and Mental Health Nursing* **14**: 1–3.

Graham, H.L., Maslin, J., Copello, A. *et al.* (2001) Drug and alcohol problems amongst individuals with severe mental health problems in an inner city area of the UK. *Social Psychiatry and Psychiatric Epidemiology* **36**(9): 448–55.

Healthcare Commission (2006) *Let's Talk About It: A review of healthcare in the community for young people who offend.* London: Healthcare Commission.

Healthcare Commission (2007) *Count Me In: Results of the 2006 national census of mental health and learning disability services in England and Wales.* London: Healthcare Commission.

HMIP (1996) *Patient or Prisoner.* London: HMSO.

HMIP (2007a) *The Mental Health of Prisoners: A thematic review of the care and support of prisoners with mental health needs.* London: HMSO.

HMIP (2007b) *Annual Report 2005–2006.* London: HMSO.

Her Majesty's Prison Service (2006) *Annual Staff Ethnicity Review.* London: Her Majesty's Prison Service Available at: http://www.hmprisonservice.gov.uk/assets/documents/10001FEBethnicity_review_2006.pdf

Home Office (2002) *Assessment Report on the Kent Custody Nurse Scheme (Gannon Report).* London: Home Office.

Home Office (2006) *Prison Population Projections 2006–2013. England and Wales 11/06.* London: Home Office.

HMSO (1983) The Mental Health Act 1983. London: HMSO.

HMSO (1998) The Crime and Disorder Act 1988. London: HMSO.

James, D. (2000) Police station diversion schemes: role and efficacy in central London. *Journal of Forensic Psychiatry* **11**(3): 532–55.

Joint Committee on Human Rights (2003) *Deaths in Custody: An analysis of police related deaths in Home Office categories 1, 2 and 3 between April 1998 and March 2003 [written evidence provided by Dr David Best – Police Complaints Authority]. Appendix to Joint Committee On Human Rights – First Report.* Available at:
http://www.publications.parliament.uk/pa/jt200304/jtselect/jtrights/12/12we09.htm

Joseph, P. and Potter, M. (1993) Diversion from custody – 1: Psychiatric assessment at the magistrates' court. *British Journal of Psychiatry* **162**: 325–30.

Lader, D., Singleton, N. and Meltzer, H. (2000) *Psychiatric Morbidity amongst Young Offenders in England and Wales.* London: Office for National Statistics.

Laing and Buisson (2006) *Mental Health and Specialist Care Services UK Market Report 2006.* London: Laing and Buisson.

London Resettlement Board (2005) *London Resettlement Strategy: a commitment to action. Phase One of the London Reducing Re-offending Action Plan* – September 2005. London: Government Office for London.

Ministry of Justice and Department of Health (2007) *Improve knowledge around the Causes of Personality Disorder* (research briefing for Dangerous and Severe Personality Disorder Research and Development Programme). Dangerous and Severe Personality Disorder Programme. Available at: http://www.dspdprogramme.gov.uk/pages/research/research1.php#Improve

NACRO (2005) *Findings of the 2004 Survey of Court Diversion/Criminal Justice Mental Health Liaison Schemes for Mentally Disordered Offenders in England and Wales.* London: NACRO.

NACRO (2007) *The YOT Health Practitioner: Identifying and sharing good mental health practice*. London: NACRO.

NHS Executive and HM Prison Service (1999) *The Future Organization of Prison Health Care*. London: Department of Health.

NHS Executive and HM Prison Service (2000) *Nursing in Prisons: Report by the Working Group considering the development of prison nursing, with particular reference to health care officers*. London: Department of Health.

NOMS (2007) Prison population and accommodation briefing, 28 September 2007. Available at: www.hmprisonservice.gov.uk/resourcecentre/publicationsdocuments/index.asp?cat=85)

Norfolk, Suffolk and Cambridgeshire Strategic Health Authority (2003) *The Independent Inquiry Into The Death Of David Bennett: The Bloefeld Report*. Cambridge: Norfolk, Suffolk and Cambridgeshire Strategic Health Authority.

Prison Reform Trust (2004) *Forgotten Prisoners – The Plight of Foreign National Prisoners in England and Wales*. London: Prison Reform Trust.

Purchase, N., McCallum, A. and Kennedy, H. (1996) Evaluation of psychiatric court liaison schemes in north London. *British Medical Journal* **313**: 531–2.

Rickford, D. and Edgar, K. (2005) *Troubled Inside: Responding to the Mental Health Needs of Men in Prison*. London: Prison Reform Trust.

Rutherford, M. and Duggan, S. (2007) *Forensic Mental Health Services: Facts and figures on current provision*. London: Sainsbury Centre for Mental Health. Available at: http://www.scmh.org.uk/80256FBD004F3555/vWeb/flKHAL796MUF/$file/policypaper7_primary_care_in_prisons.pdf

Sainsbury Centre for Mental Health (2002) *Breaking the Circles of Fear: A review of the relationship between mental health services and African and Caribbean communities. London: SCMH*.

Sainsbury Centre for Mental Health (2007) *Mental Health Care in Prisons*. London: Sainsbury Centre. Available at: http://www.scmh.org.uk/80256FBD004F3555/vWeb/flKHAL74HHH9/$file/briefing32_mh_care_prisons.pdf

Sales, B. and McKenzie, N. (2007). Time to act on behalf of mentally disordered offenders. *British Medical Journal* **334**: 1222.

Singleton, N., Meltzer, H. and Gatward, R. (1998). *Psychiatric Morbidity among Prisoners in England and Wales*. London: Office for National Statistics.

Singleton, N., Bumpstead, R., O'Brien, M., Lee, A. and Meltzer, H. (2001) *Psychiatric Morbidity among Adults Living in Private Households, 2000*. London: Office for National Statistics.

Snowden, P. (2007) Current and potential pressures in the system at *Innovations and Developments for Mentally Disordered Offenders: A one-day conference*. Thursday 6 December 2007 (conference presentation). London: Pavilion.

Social Exclusion Unit (2002) *Reducing Re-offending By Ex Prisoners*. London: Social Exclusion Unit.

Spurgeon, D. (2005) *Diversionary Tactics Safer Society*. London: NACRO.

Steel, J., Thornicroft, G., Birmingham, L. *et al.* (2007) Prison mental health inreach services. *British Journal of Psychiatry* **190**: 373–4.

West, P. (2004) Carry on nurse. *The Superintendent*. Spring (38): 12. Available at: http://www.policesupers.com/TheJournal/issue38.pdf

Williamson, T. (2006) *Improving the Health and Social Outcomes of People Recently Released from Prisons in the UK: A perspective from primary care*. London. SCMH.

Women In Secure Hospitals (WISH) (1999) *Defining Gender Issues Redefining Women's Services, Report From Women In Secure Hospitals*. London: Women in Secure Hospitals.

CHAPTER 26

The person with a personality disorder

Heather Castillo

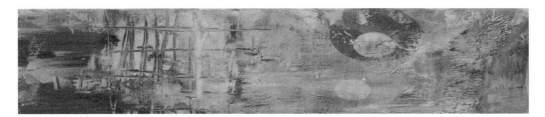

Chapter overview

The diagnosis of personality disorder is often a contested category, and those who attract it can be considered to be difficult patients or untreatable (Lewis and Appleby 1988).

Disrupted attachment experiences in early life can lead to a desperate search, on the part of an individual, to find alternative ways of containing psychological experience. A feeling of relief can sometimes by achieved by cutting, or other forms of self-harm and disruptive behaviour (Fonagy 1997).

Difficult patients create reactions in those who try to care for and treat them and this can result in an emotional retreat on the part of staff (Hinshelwood 1998).

This chapter essentially tells a story of how difficulties around this diagnosis were deconstructed by service users themselves. It outlines a history of the diagnosis and describes service user research about personality disorder and how this preceded service developments locally and nationally. The chapter aims to provide insights into the ways in which service users and professionals can effectively work together to create meaningful progress.

Introduction

'If someone is playing a game, and is playing desperately enough, if I show them I see the game they are playing, they will punish me' (Laing 1971). The mental health system usually becomes trapped in this conundrum along with the person who has attracted a diagnosis of personality disorder. Both suffer. I believe that shedding light on this paradox requires a torch held by those with the diagnosis and may be the best way out of the maze. Although professionals may assume they are pursuing client-oriented goals, decisions about what services are delivered are usually controlled by providers. Roberts and Wolfson (2004) suggest that recovery depends as much on collaboration as on treatment. However, the skills, knowledge and commitment that professionals can bring to the recovery process, while valuing and learning from the client, are stressed. This chapter reflects a ten year journey of collaboration with service users with a personality disorder diagnosis and I hope it will provide some insights into the way in which clients and professionals can effectively work together to create meaningful support, learning and recovery.

Alienation from services

Ten years ago, when I was a mental health advocate working for Mind in Colchester, in north east Essex, and based at the local psychiatric acute inpatient hospital, the advocacy office was a frequent port of call for service users with this diagnosis. The themes they brought were consistent; discharge imminent even though still suicidal; being sectioned and subject to close observation; being transferred to a secure unit; at risk of losing children through child protection procedures; and a whole gamut of desperate outcomes all contributing to a compounding of symptoms and feelings of being fundamentally and irrevocably misunderstood.

In 1998, together with local service users, I formed a research group comprising of 18 people who had attracted the diagnosis. Our aim was to carry out research about personality disorder from service users' perspectives. The group met monthly throughout the year. Attendees were not survivors engaged in a retrospective study but were service users in the midst of their difficulties, struggling for emotional equilibrium while engaged in the research endeavour. Some were inpatients and came to the group meetings from hospital wards each month, others came even though sectioned. In a client group considered inconsistent, undependable and untreatable, the commitment was breathtaking. This determination and dedication was an important clue to future developments.

What is personality disorder?

We began our investigations with a history of the diagnosis of personality disorder, beginning 200 years ago (Table 26.1) when a French psychiatrist (Pinel 1801) spoke of *'manie sans délire'*, mania without delirium. Pritchard formulated the term Moral Insanity, which he defined as 'a morbid perversion of the natural feelings, affections, inclination, temper, habits, moral dispositions and natural impulses' (1835: 126). Negative, judgemental and deeply moralistic language continued throughout the nineteenth century. In 1884 Maudsley wrote 'it is not our business, and it is not in our power, to explain psychologically the origins and nature of these depraved instincts, it is sufficient to establish their existence as facts of observation' (1884: ix). Koch (1891) introduced the term Psychopathic Inferiority and in 1905 Kraepelin was to replace 'inferiority' with 'personality'. He defined the Psychopathic Personality as falling into seven types: excitable, unstable, eccentric, liars, swindlers, anti-social and quarrelsome.

The Mental Deficiency Act 1913 added the term Moral Defective as a legislative control for detention of those considered to fall into this category. Schneider (1923) classified ten sub-categories of personality abnormalities of all types, ranging from those who caused suffering to others to those causing suffering to themselves, including markedly depressive and insecure characters. By 1939, Henderson broadened classifications to include those prone to suicide, drug and alcohol abuse, pathological lying, hypochondria, instability and sensitivity. Borderline personality disorder was a concept which arose in the 1950s to describe people who were considered to be on the borderline between neurosis and psychosis. This concept evolved into a personality disorder classified in the Diagnostic and Statistical Manual of Mental Disorders.

The term psychopathy became included in legislation in the 1959 Mental Health Act, with a clause in the 1983 Act requiring that those detained must be amenable to treatment to justify detention. Problems have arisen regarding the question of treatability and this remains a major consideration in current proposed revisions of the 1983 Mental Health Act. The questions of whether treatability can be considered to be an alleviation of symptoms, or whether treatments need to be meaningfully developed, are encompassed in this debate. In the 1980s the term Severe Personality Disorder began to be used (Kernberg 1984; Tyrer 1988). This started to appear in government documents as Dangerous Severe Personality Disorder (DH 1999) and marked the beginning of action for current revisions of the 1983 Mental Health Act.

	HISTORICAL CONTEXT	
1801	'Manie sans délire' (mania without delirium)	Pinel
1835	Moral insanity	Pritchard
1857	Degenerative deviation (moral imbecility)	Morel
1885	'No capacity for true moral feeling'	Maudsley
1891	The unborn criminal	Lombroso
1891	Psychopathic inferiority	Koch
1905	Psychopathic personality	Kraepelin
1913	Moral defective – Mental Deficiency Act	Mental Deficiency Act
1923	Psychopathy – ten sub-classifications	Schneider
1939	Three groups of psychopaths	Henderson
1941	The mask of sanity	Cleckley
1950s	Borderline personality disorder	DSM I
1959	Psychopathic disorder	The Mental Health Act
1980s	Severe personality disorder	Kernberg & Tyrer
1990s	Ten sub-classifications	DSM IV & ICD 10
1999	Dangerous severe personality disorder	DH & Home Office

Table 26.1 A history of the diagnosis of personality disorder

The modern concept of personality disorder is captured in the ten sub-categories of the European diagnostic manual, ICD-10, and its transatlantic counterpart, DSM-IV (Table 26.2). Categorizing a wide range of personality abnormalities, the clinical definitions range from the most timid, to the most dangerous among us. The diagnosis has been characterized, during its history, by lack of agreement, confusion and contested scientific legitimacy. By the late 1990s, with the appearance of the new concept of DSPD, Dangerous Severe Personality Disorder, where understanding was required fear had emerged. Difficulties in fitting people into distinctly separate clinical syndromes, and the tendency for overlapping symtomatology has, in more recent years, promoted a preference for classification of personality disorder into three clusters (Table 26.3) suggesting that the sub-categories may be unwieldy (Fahy 2003). Classification in the next editions of the psychiatric diagnostic manual may highlight sub-categories or may favour clusters. However, either method describes surface manifestations and fails, fundamentally, to capture the experiences of the sufferer. The defining of deeply ingrained, maladaptive, lifelong behaviour patterns gave the service users in our group little cause for any hope at all.

> 66   It is no wonder that those of us with a Personality Disorder diagnosis feel like second, or more like third class citizens (life's rejects). You only have to look at the definitions given in ICD 10 and DSM IV and read comments such as 'limited capacity to express feelings – disregard for social obligations – callous unconcern for others – deviant social behaviour – inconsiderate of others – incompetence – threatening or untrustworthy'. The list is endless, but one thing that these comments have in common is that they are not helpful in any way.
>
> Service User (Castillo 2003)   99

ICD–10		*DSM–IV*		
Code	*Description*	*Code*	*Description*	*Cluster*
F60.0	***Paranoid*** – excessive sensitivity, suspiciousness and hostile perceptions of others' motives and behaviour, excessive self importance and reference (≥ 3 criteria)	**301.00**	***Paranoid*** – distrust and suspiciousness of others' motives / actions as deliberately demeaning, threatening or untrustworthy (≥ 4 criteria)	A. Odd Eccentric
F60.1	***Schizoid*** – social and affectional withdrawal, preference for fantasy, solitary activities and introspection. Limited capacity to express feelings and experience pleasure (≥ 3 criteria)	**301.20**	***Schizoid*** – detachment from social relationships, restricted range of expression and emotions interpersonally, reduced desire for experience (≥ 4 criteria)	
F21	***Schizotypal*** – (coded under schizophrenia, schizotypal and delusional disorders)	**301.22**	***Schizotypal*** – social and interpersonal deficits, discomfort and reduced capacity for close relationships, cognitive or perceptual distortions and behavioural eccentricities (≥ 5 criteria)	⇨

ICD–10		*DSM–IV*		
Code	*Description*	*Code*	*Description*	*Cluster*
F60.2	***Dissocial*** – disregard for social obligations, callous unconcern for others, low frustration tolerance, tendency to blame others, deviant social behaviour ≥ 3 criteria	**301.70**	***Antisocial*** – disregard for and violation of rights of others since age 15, conduct disorder before age 15 (≥ 3 criteria)	B. Dramatic Emotional
F60.30	***Emotionally unstable, impulsive type*** – emotional instability, poor impulse control, inability to control anger, plan ahead or think before acting, quarrelsome (≥ 3 criteria)		(***Subsumed under Borderline***)	
F60.31	***Emotionally unstable, borderline type*** – disturbed self image aims and preferences, chronic emptiness, intense unstable relationships, self-destructive behaviour (≥ 3 criteria)	**301.83**	***Borderline*** – unstable interpersonal relationships, self-image, affects and impulsivity (≥ 5 criteria)	
F60.4	***Histrionic*** – shallow labile affect, self-dramatization, egocentric, inconsiderate of others, continuous need for appreciation (≥ 3 criteria)	**301.50**	***Histrionic*** – excessive emotionality and attention seeking in various contexts (≥ 5 criteria)	
	Not specifically coded for (***Can be classified under other specific personality disorders [F60.8]***)	**301.81**	***Narcissistic*** – grandiose fantasy or behaviour, need for admiration, lack of empathy (≥ 5 criteria)	⇨

ICD–10		DSM–IV		
Code	Description	Code	Description	Cluster
F60.5	**Anankastic** – doubt, perfectionism, excessive conscientiousness, caution, stubbornness, rigidity, preoccupation with details (≥ 3 criteria)	**301.40**	**Obsessive-compulsive** – pervasive preoccupation with orderliness, perfectionism, mental and interpersonal control at expense of flexibility, openness and efficiency (≥ 5 criteria)	C. Anxious Fearful
F60.6	**Anxious** (**avoidant**) – persistent feelings of tension, insecurity and inferiority. Continuous yearning to be accepted and liked, hypersensitive to rejection, restricted personal attachments, social avoidance due to exaggerated risk (≥ 3 criteria)	**301.82**	**Avoidant** – pervasive social inhibition, feelings of inadequacy, hypersensitivity to negative evaluation (≥ 4 criteria)	
F60.7	**Dependent** – a passive reliance on others for decisions, fear of abandonment, helplessness, incompetence, passive compliance (≥ 3 criteria)	**301.60**	**Dependent** – excessive need to be taken care of, submissive and clinging behaviour, fears of separation (≥ 5 criteria)	
F60.8	Other specific personality disorders – e.g. narcissistic, incompetence, passive compliance (≥ 3 criteria)	**301.9**	Personality disorder not otherwise specified – e.g. passive aggressive personality disorder, depressive personality disorder	
F60.9	Personality disorder unspecified			

Table 26.2 DSM-IV and ICD-10 personality disorders

Cluster A	Personality disorders marked by odd, eccentric behaviour, including *paranoid*, *schizoid* and *schizotypal* personality disorders.
Cluster B	Personality disorders defined by dramatic, emotional behaviour, including *histrionic*, *narcissistic*, *antisocial* and *borderline* personality disorders.
Cluster C	Personality disorders characterized by anxious, fearful behaviour and include *obsessive compulsive*, *avoidant* and *dependent* personality disorders.

Table 26.3 Cluster classification of personality disorders

Psychological perspectives

The group wished to examine aetiology and to explore the inner world of those who had attracted a diagnosis of personality disorder. How did I come to be this way? What have been my experiences in life and in the psychiatric system? What has not worked and what has helped? While members of the group shared lived experiences, I provided the academic papers and books.

Psychological perspectives that resonated with the experiences of group members began with Bowlby's attachment theory and the concept of a secure base (1988). An individual tries to maintain proximity to another clearly identified person who is perceived as being able to cope better with the world and is expected to give care, comfort and security. This encourages us to value and continue relationships. Bowlby recognized that this attachment behaviour is emphasized in childhood but also continues throughout life. A child or adult who has attachment to someone is strongly disposed to stay near and seek contact with that individual, especially in times of threat and emergency. He expanded the theory of separation anxiety by pointing out that both psychoanalysts and psychiatrists had made an unexamined assumption that fear is aroused in mentally healthy individuals only by obviously dangerous or painful situations. He observed that increased risk also carries a signal, for example, threats to abandon a child as a means of control, or parental threat of suicide. He suggested that this might also result in increased arousal, not just in terms of fear, but also intense anger, especially in older children or adolescents.

The dialectical theory of self-development assumes that a sense of self develops through the perception of oneself in another person's mind. An infant builds up a viable sense of self from the repeated internalization of the mother's processed image of the child's thoughts and feelings. This provides containment. Not only does the mother, or close caregiver, interpret the baby's physical expressions, she also gives back to the child a manageable interpretation of what is being communicated. Fonagy (1997) suggests that an absence, or distortion, of this early mirroring experience can lead to a desperate search on the part of the child to find alternative ways of containing psychological experience. This may develop into destructive physical expression, either towards self or others. A child who has not received recognized, but modified, images of behaviour and emotional states may have trouble in differentiating reality from fantasy, and physical from psychic reality. This suggests a tendency, in later life, to cope with thoughts and feelings through physical action. *Do it either to my body or their body.* Not being able to feel oneself from within, that individual is forced to find a sense of self from outside by treating themselves as an object, or by getting others to react to them. This results in experience of self in a more authentic, if very limited, way and the need for re-enactment to augment the incomplete representation of self which has been achieved.

At puberty this factor may become critical because the body changes in shape and function in a way which signifies a far greater change in identity for those whose sense of self has been impaired. This has relevance for the development of existential anxieties and anorexia in adolescents, where the body shape may literally be felt to represent aspects of the personality. A feeling of well-being and relative integrity can sometimes be achieved by cutting or self-starvation. Fonagy suggests this is because the mind is left feeling more contained or bounded, and belonging more to the self, as the body is sacrificed.

Herman and Van der Kolk (1987), in their work with incest victims and Vietnam veterans, discovered that trauma, especially prolonged trauma from caregivers, had a profound effect on personality development and the development of borderline personality disorder. They concurred with Fonagy that behaviour manifestations of self-mutilation, re-victimization, victimizing others, dissociative disorders, substance abuse and eating disorders, are an effort to try to regain internal equilibrium. Van der Kolk (1996: 3) has characterized this condition as 'the black hole of trauma' and has described post-traumatic stress as a failure of time to heal all wounds. For some, there is an inability to integrate the traumatic experience. He pointed out that there is a very complex interrelationship between traumas, neglect, environmental chaos and attachment patterns, and that clinicians fail to pay attention to the effects of early trauma, or to perceive the patterns of reliving, warding-off reminders, or repetitive re-exposure to situations reminiscent of trauma. This inspired the group to begin to seek a systematic way to measure their experiences against such theories.

A new construct

Evans and Fisher (1999) examine power sharing and encourage practitioners to assist users in carrying out research. Our research approach was emancipatory. Described by Freire (1970) as a method which challenges the validity of the privileged effectively analysing the underprivileged, here the research tools would be given to the people. The 'view from above' would be replaced with the 'view from below' or from within. We were fortunate to have two skilled supervisors. Our principal supervisor was Shulamit Ramon, Professor in inter-professional and social studies at Anglia Ruskin University, and our second supervisor was Dr Nicola Morant, senior lecturer from the psychology department and former researcher at the Henderson Hospital. With the help of supervisors we created an interview questionnaire. Four members of the group expressed an interest in being trained as research interviewers and we set out to conduct interviews with 50 people in the area who had a diagnosis of personality disorder. By 20 December 1999 the 50th interview was complete. Capturing the voice of the sample the data collected from the group and the questionnaires yielded a vast quantity of perspectives including 15,000 service user words, together with tables, charts and selected themes.

The study consisted of 20 men and 30 women, aged between 18 and 74 years. The majority of the sample, 86 per cent, fell within age ranges 25 to 54 years.
Eighty-eight per cent were on long-term sickness or other benefits, just one was full-time employed. Sixty-six per cent lived alone and 86 per cent were single, divorced or separated.

Most had secondary, Axis I diagnoses. Eighty-six per cent of the service users involved in the study described their difficulties in terms of depression or anxiety and often combinations of both. So, why should they have attracted a diagnosis of personality disorder? A minority were clearly suffering from some kind of mood disorder. They were not people who had suffered early abuse, but they tended to be outspoken, often articulate, and not slow to express their grievances. It may be that they had attracted the personality disorder label because they were perceived as 'troublemakers'. The question was, could there be a link among the remainder? The findings revealed that 88 per cent of the sample had experienced abuse. For 80 per cent this was childhood abuse, sexual, emotional, violent, and sometimes combinations of all three constituting brutal life experiences.

Twenty per cent made the discovery that they had the diagnosis indirectly from records, reports, or at social services meetings. Others appear to have been told about the diagnosis after many years, yet others were told by professionals only after they asked.

Seventy-two per cent of respondents considered they had received bad treatment because of the label. Confirming that the diagnosis is stigmatizing, they described being treated as a 'service leper', 'let's give her a wide berth', 'you're ignored', 'hostility', 'not mental illness', 'brought on oneself', 'people seem to be scared of the diagnosis', 'it's saying troublemaker'. What service users said during the interviews highlighted the sense of exclusion and hopelessness connected to finding out they had been given this diagnosis, and gave some sense of the impact this information might have on an individual labouring with the desperately hard task of living with the truth of an early abusive history.

An analysis of the diagnoses by gender suggested a bias because over 75 per cent of women had received a borderline categorization and over 75 per cent of men a dissocial diagnosis. A percentage analysis of selected themes showed there was no great variability in self-harming behaviours, regardless of gender or diagnosis. Suicidality showed a remarkably high consistency among men with a borderline diagnosis and women and men with a dissocial diagnosis. It was, however, higher in women with a borderline diagnosis. There was high incidence of childhood trauma across categories although, again, this was highest in women with a borderline diagnosis, including sexual abuse of 70 per cent.

The overall sample showed that 20 per cent of women and 22 per cent of men had been violent to others. Perhaps the most startling variable was that 35 per cent of women with a borderline diagnosis had been violent to others, yet they had retained the borderline categorization. But no men with a borderline diagnosis in our sample had displayed violence. This suggested that men with self-harming behaviours connected to the personality disorder diagnosis may be more likely to receive a dissocial categorization if they display any instance of violence to others. Twenty-six per cent of men in our study had been to prison, compared with 12 per cent of women. This indicated a greater likelihood of a prison disposal on the basis of gender.

The dissocial definition of personality disorder includes 'callous unconcern for the feelings of others' which is not something born out by 50 per cent of our dissocial sample who considered their strengths to be kindness, care or compassion. Rather than the stereotypical notion of the psychopath viewing fellow human beings as 'empty vessels', they characterized themselves as Jekyll and Hyde, an embodiment of both aggression and care. The analysis of selected themes questioned the validity of the classification of personality disorder and the sub-categories within it. For those involved in our study, self states had resulted in suicide attempts of such lethality that survival seemed miraculous. Anger and hate had become dammed up behind a narrow response function. Where early life has been sexually or violently abusive, or simply included an unloving and devastating non-response from care-givers, the blunt limitations of their experience had left some stripped of control and disempowered beyond comprehension.

The study was eventually published as a book (Castillo 2003) and by this time we had linked with the national agenda.

New national guidance

In a climate that emphasized issues of risk and danger, and where personality disorder was considered untreatable in many quarters, part of the purpose in carrying out our study was to engender some kind of compassion and understanding in relation to this diagnosis.

> Isn't it about time professionals started to find out more about the realities of personality disorder and the self-destructive torment, frustration and utmost loneliness sufferers go through. Loneliness? Yes, loneliness because we are so misunderstood, humiliated, desperate and cut-off. Why oh why don't and won't these professionals and health authorities accept that there is such a condition and illness. It is said that personality disorder cannot be treated. I think it can, with the help of different medications, but most of all by just sitting with us and recognizing and trying to understand this condition by listening.

> Can't eat – mind won't let me. Took lactulose – chronic diarrhoea. Wish I could go and talk to –––––––. Daren't though (Paranoid – 'Not HER back here again. Thought we'd seen the last of her for a good few months, or even years'). Just can't slow down – everything I do is done in fast motion. Oh God, help!

> I'm feeling like I'd like to open up my arms but I have no razor blades with me. (My one saving grace – I had the foresight not to pack any.) I'm not sure how I'm feeling. I'm hearing voices but it's not like before. Before the voices were in my head like thoughts that I had no control over. Now I have more control but the voices seem detached, like one step removed from me. It's a really weird feeling and I don't like it. I wish I could tell someone about this but I don't feel that I can. I feel so isolated and alone. I'm scared of practically everything. That might sound like an exaggeration, but the thought of living, paying bills, coping with people, terrifies me. I know what I should be thinking and feeling, but it's not happening at the moment. I am so scared of losing my kids, but I feel that I am losing my grip on reality.

> I do have some insight into the causes of my mental state and I also know I can't simply forget the past. I do not live in this hell for the shear fun of it and, if it was possible to move on I would. My whole adult life, and much of my childhood, has been well and truly blighted by what has happened to me. I am a direct product of abusive influences and it is not possible to just wipe away the last 28 years. I genuinely feel that nothing good will ever happen to me, because I seem to go from one disaster and major trauma to the next, but that doesn't mean I don't want things to change.

> ❝ We make you feel. We also make you suffer. Why? Because in that space after frustration and anger is your desire to wash your hands of us. In a way, we want to make you suffer, because how can there be no answer to this.
>
> Service Users (Castillo 2003) ❞

In 2002 I was contacted by the Department of Health who had formed an expert group to create a National Personality Disorder Strategy. They were interested in our study and how they might meaningfully incorporate the views of service users within the strategy. I was invited to attend a strategy group meeting where renowned national authorities, who had been quoted as references in our study, now sat and listened to my account of the work on personality disorder service users had carried out in north east Essex. The strategy group decided to hold a series of focus groups and it was planned that these groups would involve service users with a personality disorder diagnosis from different parts of the country, including members of our group. Their views were to have a significant impact on national strategy (Haigh 2003). On 23 January 2003, new National Guidance, *Personality Disorder: No Longer a Diagnosis of Exclusion* (DH 2003a) was launched. Proudly, we also believed that our service user research work in north east Essex had a bearing on the development of the national agenda in relation to personality disorder.

Within this meaningful development, concerns about sufficient investment remained. However, by the middle of the year a *Personality Disorder Capabilities Framework, Breaking the Cycle of Rejection* (DH 2003b) had been created with a view to addressing national training needs regarding the diagnosis. At this time the Department of Health began to talk about investment in pilot projects for service delivery and workforce training. Our local research (Castillo 2003) had given clues to better service response, ranging from being listened to, understood and feeling safe, to an out-of-hours helpline, a safe house and a crisis house. But now the local group of service users began to explore, in earnest, what ingredients would comprise a service that could really meet their needs and this is what they had to say.

> ❝ We need more communication – no-one talks to you.
>
> The response is too slow.
>
> We don't want to be told we're not ill.
>
> We need acceptance and staff who understand.
>
> We need a relaxed atmosphere where we are respecting one another and we have peer support.
>
> The day hospital isn't always the right place for us, and nor is the acute ward.
>
> Some of us need substance abuse help and they don't understand it here.
>
> We need help in a crisis.
>
> We need a Crisis House and crisis support.
>
> We need help to prevent suicide attempts.
>
> We can feel very unsupported and need help earlier.

We need mentoring/buddying.

A befriending service.

One to ones.

Groups can be too deep for us.

We need groups when we are ready:
Talking groups
Writing groups
Craft groups
Some service user led groups

We need education:
Positive thinking
Coping strategies
Anger management

We need practical help:
Advocacy
Benefits
Housing
Child protection issues
Legal/Criminal justice support

We like the idea of alternative therapies:
Massage
Acupuncture
Reflexology

Don't forget gay and lesbian support

We need the right kind of therapies to be available:
Cognitive behavioural therapy
Cognitive analytical therapy
Dialectical behaviour therapy
Counselling and psychotherapy

We need all services to be working together:
Medication if we need it
Care Programme Approach
A strong link to statutory services

We need a secure base where:
We are understood
We can help each other
We can get help in a crisis 24/7,
We can get and give ongoing support.   **99**

The national proposals called for eight service pilots throughout England, one for each region of the country. Our next step was to create a multi-agency group which would work to compile a pilot proposal for our area. Members of our local personality disorder group joined with representatives from other local service user groups and Colchester Mind, the Mental Health Trust, local primary care trusts, housing providers, the borough council, the accident and emergency department and Essex Police.

A working name was chosen for the proposal which we called The Haven. Local service users liked the title and the name stuck because it seemed to embody everything we were trying to achieve. The proposal for The Haven Project was planned entirely around the service users' views outlined above. It was a departure in that it did not reflect the models in the new National Guidance (DH 2003a) which were statutory and favoured a hub and spoke approach where therapeutic community day services would be supported by specialist teams providing both service delivery, and expertise and advice to mainstream mental health teams and services. In this context, The Haven was a radical proposal positioned in the voluntary sector, with strong statutory links. It also proposed 24-hour service provision.

Our service users flanked the proposal every step of the way. This began with their presentations at the National Institute of Mental Health Eastern Development Centre, where we made it through the second round of selections. The service user focus groups held at national level were now transformed into a National Personality Disorder Strategy User Reference Group, and some of our local services users joined. This group of 'experts by experience' worked in parallel with the National Expert Personality Disorder Group to select the successful pilot projects. Our local service users had to declare an interest when The Haven came to be considered. In an unprecedented way, the Department of Health continued to involve the Service User Reference Group throughout the three-year pilot period for the national projects and drew on the observations and knowledge of the experts by experience. Eleven service pilots were chosen, each quite distinct in nature with some based on the hub and spoke model in the National Guidance. Details of each pilot are available on the National Personality Disorder website (2009). Of the eleven pilots, one was selected for each region of England apart from London which had three, and Eastern Region where two were selected, one being The Haven. The news came in February 2004 and, being presented with this 'rags to riches' scenario, which represented many years of dreaming and campaigning for service users in our area, we experienced both exhilaration and trepidation, for now we would have to deliver what we had promised.

The Haven

As an advocate, up until then I had been located on the service user side of the divide. Now, I suddenly found myself in the position of being a service provider and the remainder of this chapter reflects not only The Haven's achievements, but also the significant challenges we have encountered, and the lessons we have learned, in working with personality disorder.

From the outset there has been a tremendous sense of goodwill and commitment from the multi-agency group who created the original proposal and who went on to form The Haven Steering Group; from the Board of Directors 50 per cent of whom have used mental health services; from local Commissioners; from the National Personality Disorder Team; from staff who have worked tirelessly; and particularly from the service users themselves because they knew this was their project. Not only had it been created around their views, they would also continue to guide its development. Early abusive experiences represent a violation of boundaries and loss of power. Being party to decisions, and in control of developments, means that someone who has lost power in the past is not subject to and dependent on authority figures in order to progress.

> ❝ I like the Open Notes Policy. That helps me. And I like, again that's about trust, knowing what's written about you. And I also really like the fact that it's client-led, service user-led. I mean it's one of its kind and I think it's setting a lead I think mental health services are going to be following because I think, no I seriously do, I think this is the way forward.
>
> (Client quote from Haven Service Evaluation Group 8/2/05) ❞

> ❝ We're actually involved in all the policies, planning, everything from the start of the centre. They treat you like equals. You're not a second class citizen.
>
> (BBC Essex Radio 7/2/05) ❞

The Haven aspires to be a sanctuary which has a sense of safety, wholeness, caring and home which is a place of refuge and protection (Bloom 1997). It is an old rectory in Colchester with 16 rooms and within its walls the décor is warm and inviting and the artwork is largely painted by clients. Its peaceful atmosphere spreads to the boundaries of its garden. The services offered include a day service programme from Monday to Friday, and a Safe Centre where those in crisis may come for a few hours, at any time of the day or night, on any day of the week. There are also four bedrooms, which constitute a Crisis House, where people may find respite from outside pressures for one night or up to three weeks. People diagnosed with personality disorder often experience high anxiety states born of chronic hyperarousal. Therefore, such a sanctuary should provide a relaxed, de-escalating environment where a range of options are available such as companionship, information, creative and distracting activities and groups, being able to talk to staff about difficulties and safely express emotions at any time of the day or night, skills groups, and more structured therapy. It includes complementary therapies to help sooth the kinds of anxiety symptoms experienced physically as well as mentally. It encourages humour as a form of shared intimacy, promoting laughter and allows playfulness that may recapture a healthy sense of being a child.

> ❝ There's always people around and you can hear them laughing, precious company. ❞

> ❝ I just want to say that I haven't laughed as much in years at the last friendship group I came to here. It was just hilarious. I was crying with laughter, it was just so funny.
>
> (Haven Clients) ❞

Those who have lived too long with untenable emotions often seek to numb unbearable feelings by turning to coping strategies such as self-cutting, alcohol and other substance misuse. Hurting the body can create temporary calm because of endorphin release. To create psychological safety at The Haven these self-destructive behaviours needed to be actively challenged. An approach to bullying, and people's capacity to create negative effects for others, had to be effective. This represented boundary setting and the social and moral limits that needed to be present to create a safe community. Rules and decisions are the concern and responsibility of the whole community and clients and staff alike should be involved in such boundary setting. The Haven Acceptable Behaviour Policy has been constructed, and is administered, by both staff and clients. It requires that community members do not self-harm while on the premises, come to the project while under the influence of alcohol, illegal or non-prescribed drugs, or engage in threatening, upsetting or disruptive behaviour. Not only does this approach help to keep The Haven a safe and peaceful environment, it is also helps clients to acknowledge and gain better control over dysfunctional coping strategies. The success of this policy depends upon The Haven keeping its side of the bargain and ensuring that support is on hand at any time of the day or night, as an alternative to cutting, substance misuse, or other destructive behaviours. On rare occasions when someone is asked to go home because of unacceptable behaviour, they are not abandoned. Staff will telephone later that day and efforts will be made to introduce that person back to the project as soon as possible, usually the next day. If unacceptable behaviour is significantly serious the community may decide that the person concerned should not come to the project for a week or more. Such decisions are made at community discussions where the community comes together with the person, discusses what has happened, and votes to reach a democratic decision. It may be that unwillingness, or inability, to curtail more serious behaviours could mean that a few will effectively bar themselves from the community. The door is left open should that person wish to reapply to the project at a later date.

> I feel safe at The Haven because I know you're not allowed to get away with stuff, are you, like cutting while you're here, which means I don't try. It's like being protected from the negative parts of yourself.

> We have boundaries at The Haven and the boundaries that are applied to one person should be applied the same to everyone. The boundaries help people go forward because they prevent old patterns.

> Since I've been using The Haven, I haven't been admitted once to the acute hospital and that to me is a big breakthrough and I'm sure they're relieved too!

> And stopping overdosing.

> It's helping me to stop self-harming.

> I've stopped cutting. I haven't done anything for eight months now.

> I now pick up the phone before I pick up a drink. I used to drink a lot.

> Before I came to The Haven I used to overdose on a reasonably regular basis. I used to cut myself whenever anything went wrong, and I used to stop eating when anything went wrong.

66 My sobriety is unbelievable, my conscience is clear, I wake up clear. I mean my two things in life that I do now that keep me together is that I eat well and I sleep well.

(Haven Clients) 99

By 2006, an analysis of use of the wider service area, for the first 50 Haven clients who had been with the project for one year, showed a drop in all services measured (Table 26.4). Notably, psychiatric hospital inpatient admissions had dropped for the first 50 clients by 85 per cent. Although continuing to represent a burden for GPs and the A&E department, use had still dropped by 25 per cent and 45 per cent respectively. Calculating the reduction of the use of the wider service area against health and social care figures showed that the project had saved £220,000, over and above the cost of The Haven, on the first 50 clients alone. We had now registered 110 clients and extrapolating savings to this number showed that in excess of £480,000 could be saved, over and above the cost of running the service. The cost per week, per client, for Haven services was around £100, compared to costs ranging from £223 to £1,250 per patient per week, for personality disorder day unit or hospital therapeutic community, in other parts of the country (Chiesa *et al.* 2002).

The Haven had, therefore, fulfilled its original promise to engage the client group in our area and to prove cost savings in the wider service area. However, concerns began to be expressed about whether the project would create a new kind of dependency. Most clients who had registered were still with us and, although many were no longer subject to hospital admission, questions were asked about whether they could move beyond stability achieved at The Haven. These questions also had a bearing on capacity at the project and the need to continue to register new clients. Some clients who were making significant progress in the outside world also began to question the progress of some of their peers.

66 I think, fundamentally, people with PD need a certain amount of love and care and TLC and pampering and I think The Haven's taken that well on board and has supplied that, where other statutory units have failed dismally, but I think there is a danger of overcompensating, and when somebody presents in crisis, this kind of behaviour would tell someone that, if they do it again, they will get the same kind of love and attention. 99

66 I think alcoholism isn't named for what it is. I think that there's too many people that are not using self-management skills and becoming independent, they are going out every night and getting wrecked and coming in here and expecting the staff to get some superglue, rather than learning and using self-management skills. I don't see The Haven as a place to land, it's a place to touch down and spring from 99

66 I think there's an awful lot of people at The Haven that have lived in a world of inner torment for so long, and have lived a psychiatric-based life for so long, that to move away from that and take on something new, is always going to be scary.

(Haven Clients) 99

Service area/ Intervention	Annual average use over two years prior to The Haven	Annual service use since attending The Haven	Percentage reduction in use of service/ intervention
Section 136	42.5	18	−57.64%
Other Sections	11	4	−63.63%
In-patient Admissions	55	8	−85.45%
Use of Day Hospital	32 clients	14 clients	−56.25%
Use of Community MH Team	36 clients	14 clients	−61.11%
Use of NERIL (MH Help-line)	1264 times	317 times	−75.92%
Use of Crisis Team	187 times	42 times	−77.54%
Criminal Justice MH Team	0	0	0
Assertive Outreach	0	0	0
Trust Eating Disorder Service	56 times	14 times	−75.00%
Psychology/Psychotherapy/Counselling	30 clients	21 clients	−30.00%
Annual Use of GP	611 times	459 times	−24.87%
Annual use of A&E	141 times	77 times	−45.39%
General Hospital Admissions	47 times	37 times	−21.27%
Police/Probation/Prison	12.5 times	2 times	−84.00%
Children's Social Services	14 clients	6 clients	−57.14%
Debt Agencies	7 clients	1 client	−85.71%
Housing/Homelessness	11 clients	2 clients	−81.81%
Substance Misuse Voluntary Agency	4 clients	1 client	−75.00%
Eating Disorder Voluntary Agency	5 clients	1 client	−80.00%
Mind Advocate	39 clients	11 clients	−71.79%

Table 26.4 The first 50 Haven clients to complete one year at the project

In a client group beset with attachment difficulties, words such as 'discharge' or 'through-put', and even 'study' and 'work', were likely to produce high anxiety and often instant relapse. Short-termism in personality disorder can result in swift loss of progress as it threatens the fragility of recovery. For many of our clients The Haven is their safe place and for some it is the home they never had as a child. Even if someone has travelled quite far on their journey of recovery, why should they not continue to have a safe space to enable them to come 'home' or phone 'home' when this is needed?

    " The Haven provides for me a replacement role of my parental home, basically I feel safe here, I feel safe. "

    " We don't think we should clip our wings. We just need a nest to come back to.

    (Haven Clients) "

In response to what we felt were the unique needs of people who had attracted a diagnosis of personality disorder, and who often struggle with issues of trust and attachment and abandonment, we decided to create a new category at The Haven called *Transitional Recovery*. This concept separates recovery from cure and it may not be about getting rid of all symptoms, but about learning to understand and manage difficulties better, beginning to take control of one's life, and learning to live well. When someone graduates to the Transitional Recovery category they are likely to be engaged in study or work, or pursuing life in the community that fulfils that person's unique individual goals; however, at this stage, they are able to remain registered at The Haven as a safety net if they wish. A new group was created at the project called *The Transitional Recovery Group* were clients could be supported to move forward, in small steps, to the Transitional Recovery category. Goals range from starting college or work, to getting on a bus or tackling literacy problems. It is about whatever each person wants to do next in order to move forward. The concept of Transitional Recovery was discussed and explained and, once clients understood that progress did not mean they would lose their place at The Haven, an unprecedented 25 per cent of those registered signed up to the group. By Easter 2007, in addition to the four clients who had already begun courses, five more group members started college.

> I started Access Planning Period on 17th April. At first it was quite nerve wracking – sweaty palms – I could hardly hold a pen for the first two weeks. During the first week, after the first two sessions, when I got home I had a panic attack. It's improved now and I'm starting to relax more easily. The academic side is fine. I'm not struggling too badly and came second in the class for English test – not too bad. That was A to C standard GCSE – the best you can get, and I got that for English and Maths. I didn't do too badly at school, so for me it's not so much course content, it's more about confidence and managing anxieties. I feel good about it. I kind of feel proud I suppose, that I've managed to get this far.

> In a way some of us are guinea pigs for Haven clients, we're testing out the study pathways. That is hard because of earlier difficulties and losses at school. I'm getting help at Transitional Recovery Group, with assignments, and I'm hoping for personal tutoring.

> I've been on a hairdressing course for the last few months. To start with it was really difficult and this was the fourth or fifth time I've tried and never got past the second session (second minute!). This time I went with the pain and the panic in a way. It's like a drama in your head, a self-whipped-up drama. I toughed it out this time. It's different when you're not influenced by any intoxicants in your system. I'm now looking to do my next course and I'm just as scared. It's the responsibility and commitment, but I'm going to do it anyway. I feel confident now. I just cut four people's hair this morning. It's not really confidence, it's being absorbed with the skill you've learned, but it comes across as confidence. I used to be like an oak tree with twisted roots.

> Now I'm a sapling beside the old oak tree and sometimes I still live in the shadow of it. But the sapling is growing. I've even planted an oak tree in my garden to symbolize it.
>
> (Haven Clients) **99**

A new Social Inclusion Unit has now been developed at The Haven to address all aspects of becoming part of life, from getting on a bus to starting college, and from accessing good housing or leisure activities to starting voluntary work or employment. It remains vital to us that we encompass the spectrum of support for clients with this diagnosis, from crisis response through containment, to therapeutic work and transitional recovery.

Up close and personal

Because of early traumatic experiences, and overwhelmingly unmet needs in early and later life, people diagnosed with personality disorder often have little sense of boundaries (Mahari 2004). An individual needs to have a sense of their own identity and space, and the space and identity of another, in order to have an awareness of boundaries. Someone with a personality disorder diagnosis may not be aware of where they end and you begin. Demands placed on professionals and others can be experienced as a violation of boundaries and limits and may cause a mental health worker to distance themselves from someone with this diagnosis.

Hinshelwood (1998: 87) suggests that difficult patients create reactions in those who try to care for and treat them which results in an emotional retreat on the part of staff into what he calls the 'scientific attitude'. This retreat causes 'scientific justification' which can blind staff to some aspects of the subjective experience of the patient. 'That blind-spot crucially feeds back directly into the patients' difficulties.' This professional defence causes staff to lose sight of rich information, about the complexity of relating, which is right there in front of them. Rather than the distancing effect of incomprehensible meaning experienced in trying to relate to someone suffering from schizophrenia, the person with a personality disorder may offer 'a relationship too intensely suffused with human feelings – usually very unpleasant ones'. He characterizes such patients as operating 'predominantly in a world of feelings' and they 'directly and deliberately, although unconsciously, interfere with our feelings. We feel intruded upon and manipulated – and indeed, we feel'. Experienced as a kind of abuse of time, help and care, the professional may fail and is in danger of being overwhelmed.

Kerr (2001) speaks about the idea of 'the ailment as ignorance', that is, a lack of understanding may cause others to regard an individual as a difficult patient and this further affects that person's mental health in an adverse way. He explains that behaviour is also a form of communication, and that the way in which a system responds to this behaviour may also be dysfunctional. He urges us to see things in a *systemic* way as a series of dynamics being enacted around that person. Services and people around the client may be reacting in a variety of ways, identifying and sympathizing with them, getting angry with and rejecting them, feeling guilty or burnt out, a variety of responses which fall short of actually understanding how it is for that individual.

Further challenges are represented, first, by the fact that serious trauma can shatter the assumptions on which someone with a personality disorder diagnosis bases their sense of safety, and a way of protecting oneself against ever being hurt or betrayed again is to set up a perfect relationship in which one must never be let down. Clients, therefore, need support to be able to work through the distress generated when mistakes are made and betrayal is experienced because The Haven is not perfect and no longer feels safe. A staff member, who has set out to help someone, may suddenly find themselves cast as an abuser in such a situation, and may need support to ensure they do not take this projection personally. Second, learned helplessness may exist and it has been demonstrated that, when a person has been repeatedly traumatized, or subjected to an environment that is sufficiently out of their control, they will give up trying to make changes (Bloom 1997). Experiences within the mental health system may have compounded such helplessness and the fostering of autonomy for each individual necessarily becomes vitally important. Third, disrupted attachments in early life leave some with this diagnosis unable to currently form healthy attachments (Bowlby 1988). This may manifest in over-use of the project causing dependency and is addressed with good care planning and boundaries which help the client to understand and receive support while encouraging self-reliance. Attachment difficulties can also cause over-attachment to individual staff members and splitting in the staff team, that is, good staff member versus bad staff members. For this reason we do not have a key-worker system at The Haven and encourage clients to attach to The Haven Community as a whole.

Difficulties described above can be experienced as a minefield which presents a significant challenge to any staff team who may be subject to extreme boundary testing. Failure to respond as the client would wish may result in behaviour enacted as a punishment. Manifesting as booby-trapped terms of engagement, this can be dramatized as a deadly game, fraught with risk, in a client group with a mortality rate in relation to suicide and accidents seven times higher than comparable age and sex matched groups (Fahy 2003).

Confronted with a therapeutic community environment, such as The Haven, staff and clients co-existing in a close atmosphere are sometimes exposed to a hazardous excess of emotions. For this reason boundaries must be negotiated, drawn and clearly understood by clients and staff alike. Boundaries must be consistent and allow clients to take stock of thoughts and feelings and learn to take responsibility for how their actions impact on themselves and others.

Not only has it been necessary to create an Acceptable Behaviour Policy for clients at the project, it has also been necessary to create policies for staff which spell out and make boundaries very explicit. However, retaining humanity, while holding firm boundaries, sometimes requires flexibility and can leave grey areas that we believe will always exist with this client group. Opportunities at staff meetings, individual supervision and teambuilding need to be safe enough and to occur often enough for a culture of openness to thrive. If someone is drawn into a compelling situation it can be much easier for colleagues to see what is happening. Our procedure at The Haven is: bring all issues to the staff team, bring them to supervision, write them in client notes, and discuss them openly and in an authentic way with the client. Boundary issues are always up for debate at the project. Where we have run into difficulties in the past is when issues have become hidden. Key learning has included the fact that the degree to which a staff member has unresolved personal difficulties, and un-drawn boundaries, working with this client group can become untenable. Working with personality disorder is not for everyone and requires a truly honest and fairly constant examination of working practices for a staff member, and support systems that allow that person to do so.

Readiness

McGowan (2007) suggests that the therapeutic effectiveness of hospital admissions for people with a personality disorder diagnosis is questionable. In terms of reducing suicidal and self-harming behaviour, Paris (2004) concludes that hospitalization has unproven benefits and may be harmful. However, any area wishing to reduce hospital admissions for those with a personality disorder diagnosis will need to provide alternative support, with sufficient capacity, which affords containment and addresses readiness. Where Haven clients have still been admitted to hospital, reasons for admission are varied. For a few, co-morbid Axis I diagnoses such as bipolar disorder have made this necessary when, for example, a hypermanic episode is experienced. Again, for a small number of clients depressive symptoms have been so intractable, despite admission to a bed at The Haven and a great deal of one-to-one support from staff. Here issues of risk have resulted in hospital admission and may have saved lives. However, a third category has included those who, for a time, have been unwilling or unable to use Haven services effectively. This highlights a spectrum of behaviour and responses that might be characterized as readiness.

Entrenched behaviours and dysfunctional coping strategies, such as self-harm, suicide threats and substance misuse, may be used by a client who is not yet able to ask for help or to explore underlying feelings and experiences. Norton and Dolan (1995) suggest that the damage and violence that can accompany 'acting out' elicits a strong emotional response from others and that services may inadvertently perpetuate behaviour by detaining a client in an institution that has a largely custodial function. In situations where it is difficult to demarcate issues of risk, this scenario is likely to be perpetuated unless multi-agency consultation takes account of information from those who know the client best. Even if such consultation does occur, for some clients hospital admission may be the only way they are currently able to demonstrate their pain and they can use extreme measures to ensure admission.

Determination to gain hospital admission can be viewed at one end of what may be considered a whole spectrum of readiness. For clients attending The Haven this can begin with an inability to phone or come in to ask for help. This receives a proactive response where clients receive short-term care plans with booked support calls for staff to phone the client, or scheduled appointments where the client comes into the project for one-to-one support. They are also encouraged to send texts if they are unable to phone or leave messages. Friendship groups and open, low-key activity groups exist for those who are not yet ready to engage in more formal therapeutic work. Such measures represent the holding aspect of the project where clients are able to take time to build up trust, confidence and a feeling of safety.

In order to achieve effectiveness, psychological treatments, such as CAT – cognitive analytic therapy (Ryle 1997) and DBT – dialectical behaviour therapy (Linehan 1999), also require readiness on the part of the client in the form of trust, confidence, safety and enough stability to attend on a regular basis. Professionals who place hope in referring a client with this diagnosis to a dedicated personality disorder therapy will be sadly disappointed if the time is not right. Formal therapeutic work at The Haven is represented by one-to-one therapy and groups like Life Skills and DBT Skills. However, The Haven environment is a therapeutic community (Campling and Haigh 1999) and can do much to hold an individual until readiness is achieved as clients learn from and support each other. In addition to learning about boundaries and limits, the project has adopted a culture of reward for progress. Crisis beds can mean that someone has to go into crisis to obtain one. Now we plan respite admissions and further admissions are given to those who are progressing. Unacceptable behaviour has consequences and good engagement, constructive behaviour and progress is rewarded with access to formal therapy. We continue to register two people each month and the spectrum of readiness begins again for clients who are new to us.

The Haven represents one service model for the support and treatment of personality disorder, however, we believe it encapsulates key ingredients for successful progress. The project belongs to its clients. It was planned around their wishes and they continue to drive it. It is they who have the control and who are learning to take responsibility for themselves and their community in a journey of recovery from trust, through therapeutic work, to social inclusion.

Questions for reflection and discussion

1   People who have attracted a personality disorder diagnosis are traditionally considered to be difficult patients. Why do they display symptoms and behaviour which constitutes self-harm?
2   Why do people with this diagnosis sometimes provoke extreme reactions in those who try to care for and treat them? Consider this from your own viewpoint and examine your thoughts, feelings and responses.
3   Why are boundaries important in working with this client group? Why is the negotiation of boundaries more effective than their imposition?
4   What do you consider to be some of the key ingredients in achieving readiness for clinical work for someone with a personality disorder diagnosis?

Annotated bibliography

- Castillo, H. (2003) *Personality Disorder – Temperament or Trauma?* London: Jessica Kingsley. This text provides a more comprehensive account of service user research about personality disorder. Although research dates from the late 1990s, it gives a detailed view of personal experiences and the inner world of those with this diagnosis. For anyone wishing to support service users in carrying out research, it also provides a step-by-step description of how this was done.
- Norton, K. and Dolan, B. (1995) Acting out and the institutional response. *Journal of Forensic Psychiatry* **6**(2): 317–32. A seminal paper, this begins to explain why we feel compelled to react in extreme ways to some of the behaviours displayed by people with a personality disorder diagnosis. Kingsley Norton and Brigit Dolan also describe what happens to someone who is contained rather than supported and engaged in an exploration of experiences and feelings and how this reinforces repeating patterns of dysfunctional behaviour which they call 'the scenario of great fidelity'.
- Bloom, S. (1997) *Creating Sanctuary: Towards the evolution of sane societies.* New York: Routledge. This is not a new text but it remains an inspiring account of the creation of a therapeutic environment. Bloom was not specifically concerned with those who have a diagnosis of personality disorder but he devoted his efforts to providing support and

understanding for those suffering unresolved trauma. His story is relevant to anyone seeking alternative and creative ways to provide care and treatment.

References

Bloom, S. (1997) *Creating Sanctuary: Towards the evolution of sane societies.* New York: Routledge.

Bowlby, J. (1988) *A Secure Base.* London: Routledge.

Campling, P. and Haigh, R. (eds) (1999) *Therapeutic Communities: Past, Present and Future.* London: Jessica Kingsley.

Castillo, H. (2003) *Personality Disorder – Temperament or Trauma?* London: Jessica Kingsley.

Chiesa, M., Bateman, A., Wilberg, T. and Friis, S. (2002) Patients' characteristics, outcome and cost-benefit of hospital-based treatment for patients with a personality disorder: A comparison of three different programmes. *Psychology and Psychotherapy: Theory, Research and Practice* **75**: 381–92.

Cleckley, H. (1941) *Traité des Dégéneréscences Physiques, Intellectuelles et Morales de l'Espèce Humaine.* Paris: Baillière.

Cleckley, H. (1982) The Mask of Sanity. St. Louis: CV Mosby Co.

Department of Health (1999) *Managing Dangerous People with Severe Personality Disorder.* London: HMSO.

Department of Health (2003a) *Personality Disorder: No Longer a Diagnosis of Exclusion. Policy Implementation Guidance for the Development of Services for People with Personality Disorder.* London: HMSO.

Department of Health (2003b) *Personality Disorder Capabilities Framework: Breaking the Cycle of Rejection.* London: HMSO.

DSM 1 (1952) *Diagnostic and Statistical Manual of Mental Disorders 1st Edition.* Washington DC: American Psychiatric Association.

DSM IV (1994) *Diagnostic and Statistical Manual of Mental Disorders 4th Edition.* Washington DC: American Psychiatric Association.

Evans, C. and Fisher, M. (1999) Collaborative evaluation with service users: Moving towards user controlled research, in I. Shaw and J. Lishman (eds) *Evaluation and Social Work Practice.* London: Sage.

Fahy, T. (2003) Speech at the Launch Conference for National Guidance: Personality disorder – no longer a diagnosis of exclusion. Harrogate 23 January 2003.

Fonagy, P. (1997) When cure is inconceivable: the aims of psychoanalysis with borderline patients. Paper to New York Freudian Society 4 April 1997.

Freire, P. (1970) *Pedagogy of the Oppressed.* New York: Herder and Herder.

Haigh, R. (2003) *Services for People with Personality Disorder: The Thoughts of Service Users: Personality Disorder: No Longer a Diagnosis of Exclusion. Policy Implementation Guidance for the Development of Services for People with Personality Disorder.* London: HMSO.

Henderson, D. (1939) *Psychopathic States.* New York: W.E. Norton.

Herman, J. and Van der Kolk, B. (1987) *Traumatic Origins of Borderline Personality Disorder in Psychological Trauma.* Washington DC: American Psychiatric Press.

Hinshelwood, R. (1998) The difficult patient: The role of 'scientific psychiatry' in understanding patients with chronic schizophrenia or severe personality disorder. *British Journal of Psychotherapy* November: 187–90.

ICD 10 (1992) *Classification of Mental and Behavioural Disorders.* Geneva: World Health Organization.

Kernberg, O. (1984) *Severe Personality Disorders: Psychotherapeutic Strategies.* London: Yale University Press.

Kerr, I. (2001) Presentation at South London and Maudsley Mental Health NHS Trust Conference on Personality Disorder in H. Castillo (2003) *Personality Disorder – Temperament or Trauma?* London: Jessica Kingsley.

Koch, J.L.A. (1891) *Die Psychopathischen Minderwertigkeit.* Ravensburg, Germany: Otto Maier.

Kraepelin, E. (1905) Personality disorder, in M. Gelder, D. Gath and R. Mayou (eds) *Oxford Text Book of Psychiatry* (2nd edn). Oxford: Oxford Medical Publications.

Laing, R. (1971) *Knots.* London: Penguin.

Lewis, G. and Appleby, L. (1988) Personality disorder: the patients psychiatrists dislike. *British Journal of Psychiatry* **153**: 44–9.

Linehan, M. (1999) *Treating Borderline Personality Disorder.* London, New York: Guilford Press.

Lombroso, C. (1891) Illustrative Studies in Criminal Anthropology. *Monist* **1**: 177–96.

Mahari, A.J. (2004) *BPD from the inside out: Why Boundaries?* Available at: www.borderlinepersonality.ca.borderlinewhyboundaries.htm

Maudsley, H. (1884) cited in H. Kutchins and S.A. Kirk (eds) (1999) *Making us Crazy: DSM The Psychiatric Bible and the Creation of Mental Disorders.* London: Constable.

McGowan, J. (2007) Working with personality disorders in an acute psychiatric ward, in I. Clarke and E. Wilson (eds) *Cognitive Behaviour Therapy for Acute Psychiatric Inpatient Units; working with clients, staff and the milieu.* London: Routledge.

Morel, B.A. (1857) *Traité des Dégéneréscences Physiques, Intellectuelles et Morales de l'Espèce Humaine.* Paris. Baillière.

National Personality Disorder website (2007) www.personalitydisorder.org.uk

Norton, K. and Dolan, B. (1995) Acting out and the institutional response. *Journal of Forensic Psychiatry* **6**(2): 317–32.

Paris, J. (2004) Is hospitalization useful for suicidal patients with borderline personality disorder? *Journal of Personality Disorders* **18**: 240–7.

Pinel, P. (1801) Personality disorder, in M. Gelder, D. Gath and R. Mayou (eds) (Ref. Kauka, 1949, for translation) *Oxford Text Book of Psychiatry* (2nd edn). Oxford: Oxford Medical Publications.

Pritchard, J.C. (1835) Personality disorder, in M. Gelder, D. Gath and R.Mayou (eds) *Oxford Text Book of Psychiatry* (2nd edn). Oxford: Oxford Medical Publications.

Roberts, G. and Wolfson, P. (2004) The rediscovery of recovery: open to all: *Advances in Psychiatric Treatment* **10**: 37–49.

Ryle, A. (1997) *Cognitive Analytic Therapy: The Model and the Method.* Chichester: Wiley.

Schneider, K. (1923) *Psychopathic Personalities.* London: Cassell.

Tyrer, P. (1988) *Personality Disorder, Management and Care.* London: Wright.

Van der Kolk, B. (1996) *Traumatic Stress.* London and New York: Guilford Press.

Part 5

Core procedures

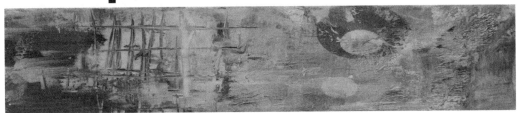

Chapter contents

CHAPTER 27

Engaging clients in their care and treatment

Marc Thurgood

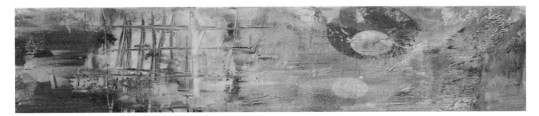

Chapter overview

This chapter defines engagement, outlines its importance for mental health care and identifies the key principles of individual practice and service delivery that best promote it. Criticisms of mental health services that draw upon the experience of service users are described and argued to be the starting point from which services need to change. Barriers and solutions to engagement are expanded upon with reference to key marginalized groups and recommendations for practice illustrated by case-study examples.

Introduction

For more than a decade there has been an increasing policy emphasis upon mental health care for people with severe and enduring mental illness and promoting their 'engagement' with mental health services (DH 1999). This reflects a recognition that many people in this group have often been excluded from effective help and that their negative experience of the mental health system has left them feeling mistrustful and alienated, with some living in conditions of extreme poverty and neglect. The challenge facing mental health services as a whole, and nurses in particular, is to find ways to engage this hard-to-engage group of people.

This chapter focuses on this problem and how nurses might best work to engage their clients. It draws primarily upon literature on the assertive outreach model of community care, which has been defined as an approach that: engages high-risk severe mentally ill clients with complex needs who are resistant to contacting services; proactively reaches out to clients in their own territory in the community; assesses need comprehensively, develops individually tailored care packages and effectively coordinates care across agencies; and optimizes the rehabilitative potential of clients by delivering clinical interventions that enhance client functioning (Ryan 1999: 2).

The assertive outreach model highlights issues that are relevant to engaging service users in all treatment and care settings.

What is 'engagement'?

Engagement can be defined broadly as providing a service that is experienced by service users (including carers) as acceptable, accessible, positive and empowering. If clients perceive a mental health service in this way they are more likely to use it. Creating such a service has implications for both the quality of the relationships that service users have with their individual workers and also for the nature of the services of which these workers are a part.

At a personal level, each client has their own opinion of mental health services that is influenced by factors such as their past experience, ethnicity and culture, needs, difficulties, strengths and aspirations, and the sense that they make of their own experience of mental ill-health, and what helps them. Establishing and maintaining relationships with clients that are experienced as helpful is fundamental to engagement. To do this requires nurses to learn about their clients' unique perspectives and to respect them as valid and meaningful. Respect for the client's viewpoint provides the basis for collaborative working and open negotiation around informed choices for care and treatment.

Service users value mental health nurses as a professional group (Rogers and Pilgrim 1994) and nurses are well placed to improve mental health care practice by virtue of their relatively high contact with clients through their care coordination role and their traditional emphasis on forming long-term therapeutic relationships with clients (cf. Chapter 4). As 'natural allies' (Repper 2000: 585), nurses are able to develop a good understanding of their clients' wider lives and aspirations, and to gain insights into their problematic experiences of services and social deprivation (Campbell and Lindow 1997). These insights are the starting point for engagement.

At an organizational level the engagement agenda has contributed to the implementation of new approaches to service delivery that have taken into account service users' criticisms of traditional mental health services. Examples of these approaches include assertive outreach, home treatment and crisis services in the community, separate community services for black and ethnic minority service users and psychosocial interventions for psychosis (DH 2001). Service users have also created their own 'self-help' services (for example, Clubhouse, the Hearing Voices Network) and are involved increasingly in the design, delivery and appraisal of services. Mental health professionals are now required to share their power with users. Joint-working between statutory mental health, voluntary and social services sectors, particularly with regard to meeting social needs (such as supported housing), is also now recognized as being crucial for effective engagement. The notion of 'recovery' (that people with severe mental illness have the right to and are capable of leading rewarding lives through employment, education and leisure/social opportunities when given access, choice and support) (cf. Chapter 5) supports the development of partnerships between service users and mainstream organizations to promote greater social inclusion (see, for example, NIACE/NIMHE 2003).

If engagement is to be achieved, nurses need to demonstrate their commitment to these organizational and ideological changes. Critical appraisal of one's own work with clients and of the wider service within which individual nurses operate (for example, team and locality service) is essential. Challenging and changing practice in response to the needs and criticisms of service users and involving them in this process needs to be seen as a fundamental part of a service that engages effectively with its clients.

Why some clients do not engage with their care and treatment

Some clients do not engage with their care and treatment because:

- Clients vary in their willingness and ability to engage. Much depends on their previous experience, both of life and of services, and the extent to which their mental ill-health affects their capacity to cooperate with the help offered.
- Services themselves have created significant barriers to engagement in the way that they have been organized and delivered.
- Service users are not always given what they most want.

Service user related factors

Past experience

Many people with mental health problems mistrust statutory services and feel ambivalent or openly hostile towards them, for good reasons. The Sainsbury Centre's review of care for people with severe mental illness who are hard to engage with services (SCMH 1998) points out that many clients' contacts with mental health services may have been characterized by long periods of neglect while in the community and by traumatic experiences of hospitalization at times of crisis (often by detention under the Mental Health Act 1983) with subsequent poor continuity of community support on discharge. An overemphasis on physical treatments (often with bad side effects from medication) at the expense of psychosocial interventions and social support may be experienced by service users as dehumanizing and punitive. Discrimination and insensitivity from mental health service staff (on the grounds of gender, race, culture, sexuality and lifestyle – such as substance use and homelessness) has been a common complaint. Black and ethnic minority clients have been particularly alienated by discriminatory negative experiences, including being subject to more severe and coercive treatments, poorer access to 'talking treatments' and cultural and language barriers in assessments (see also SCMH 2000; DH 2003).

The social disadvantage often associated with mental illness may have also contributed to the traumatic histories of our clients and their experiences of other statutory services could have been as negative as their experience of mental health services. Childhood abuse, local authority care as a child or having their own child taken into care by social services, contact with the criminal justice system in their youth or during a mental health crisis, and difficult dealings with housing and benefits departments are commonplace findings of psychosocial assessments (SCMH 1998). Unstable or inadequate housing is also a common problem and many clients with a history of homelessness relate stories of losing their accommodation through eviction as a consequence of having received insufficient help for their mental health problems (Dean and Craig 1999).

The effects of mental illness

The difficulties associated with serious mental ill-health may also play a major part in an individual's capacity to engage with services. People who have psychotic experiences or significant psychological and emotional instability may find it extremely hard to form trusting and lasting relationships with others. For example, persecutory thinking and the hearing of threatening or derogatory voices can often lead to social withdrawal as a coping strategy and the refusal of even the most basic of survival needs, such as taking up state benefits. Delusional explanations for one's situation, particularly if these relate to services, can be a considerable barrier. Defensive aggression or other anti-social behaviours (for example, begging and petty crime as a survival strategy) can similarly serve to distance someone from help. Cognitive impairments such as difficulties with generating and ordering thoughts, concentration, memory and abstract problem solving will often impede someone's ability to effectively seek out assistance. The use of illicit substances and alcohol as a form of 'self-medication' for chronic distress (or 'symptoms') can serve to exacerbate these problems. Less obvious, but equally disabling, are the 'negative symptoms' of schizophrenia. Loss of volition, motivation and interest ('get-up-and-go') can result in the most extreme self-neglect, whereby the daily tasks of self-care that most of us take for granted can seem insurmountable.

Added to this, the long-term effects of social isolation and loneliness through the progressive loss of meaningful occupation, relationships and income, coupled with the stigmatizing status of being labelled as mentally ill can have a devastating effect on self-esteem and confidence. Many clients experience persecution, exploitation and rejection in their daily lives. This further compromises their ability to assertively communicate their needs and set goals for the future.

Service-related factors

The Sainsbury Centre (SCMH 1998) has identified the main service-related barriers to engagement as:

- difficulties around establishing lead responsibility for care coordination;
- fragmentation of services resulting in poor joint-working between agencies;
- rigid, service-centred practice.

The complexity of need for many people with serious mental illness necessitates coordinated input from a range of agencies. The separation of physical health care, mental health care, substance misuse services, and housing and welfare support typify the traditional rigidity of service boundaries. This can lead to disputes about which agency should take lead responsibility for a client's care with the result that much needed help is denied. The tragic impact of this has been demonstrated by many inquiries into failures of community care (SCMH 1998).

Geographical catchment area boundaries across agencies can serve to exclude people from receiving services, particularly those with no permanent address. The 'no fixed abode' (NFA) hospital admission rota that often dictates which service will take on a homeless client in crisis is inherently discriminatory and commonly prevents continuity of contact with any one service (essential for long-term engagement). It has been argued that this 'lottery' approach' to allocation of homeless people to services ignores the fact that many homeless people have a history of local connection to an area (Timms 1996).

Other service-centred approaches, such as formal appointment systems, do not always meet need and can be positively discouraging. It is unrealistic to always expect someone with a severe mental illness and overwhelming social problems to be sufficiently organized and motivated to attend appointments at a service base or to respond to letters. Non-attendance at appointments will often result in discharge particularly if demand on the service is high (Timms 1993). Some service users therefore tend to delay seeking help until a crisis occurs (via an A&E department, for example). The resulting interventions are too often brief and inadequate, which serves to further alienate the client (Craig and Timms 2000). It is important to note that excellent interventions with clients by individual professionals may often be rendered less effective, or ineffective, by the service framework within which they take place.

A diagnosis of 'personality disorder' (cf. Chapter 26) can lead people to be excluded from receiving help because the disorder is not perceived as a 'severe mental illness' or it may be seen as 'untreatable' and, therefore, beyond the remit of mental health services. Care is also often refused if this label is used in response to anti-social or criminal behaviours. At the same time, other services (such as social care agencies) can paradoxically also refuse help to this group of people on the grounds of a history of high contact with mental health services (SCMH 1998). Many people with a diagnosis of personality disorder are frequent users of mental health services, albeit on the margins, and may experience episodes of 'treatable' mental illness such as psychosis or depression. Mental health policy is now addressing these difficulties through recognition that adequate services need to be provided, some by mental health trusts, and by providing consultation guidelines for best practice and a commitment to funding specialist personality disorder services (NIMHE 2003) (cf. Chapter 6).

Division of responsibility between specialist substance misuse services and mental health teams has meant that clients have often fallen between services. Substance misuse can mean that engagement is even more difficult to achieve due to a worsening of symptoms, increased risk factors (aggression, violence, self-harm and self-neglect), loss of housing and chaotic use of crisis services. Conflicting approaches to the option of coercive treatment for mental illness and the need for motivated voluntary treatment for substance misuse makes this issue difficult to resolve – for example, how does one respond to the intoxicated person with psychosis (SCMH 1998)? Current mental health policy states that mental health services should expect substance misuse in clients with mental illness. The aim is for mental health services to deliver concurrent high quality care and treatment both for the underlying mental illness and the substance misuse via integration with specialists in substance misuse services and by the specialist training of workers within community mental health teams (DH 2002).

Services have often been required to provide managers with evidence of short-term outcomes via brief interventions and 'through-put' to demonstrate their effectiveness and thereby guarantee further funding. This emphasis on through-put data (for example, the numbers of referrals and discharges of clients travelling through a service on their way to a 'cure') has led to criticism of what has been argued to be an overly medical model that is often inappropriate (Craig and Timms 2000). For people with disabling long-term mental illness, short-term improvement is often unrealistic and cure, in the medical sense, is unachievable. Emphasizing short-term outcomes may lead to mental health teams pushing for 'better' results by oppressively imposing interventions on their clients and denying them choice with resulting disengagement from the service. Sustained engagement needs to be an important criterion by which to judge the success of mental health services.

Services neglect what service users want

Repper's (2000) review of studies of service-user views shows that traditional mental health services have not delivered what service users want. In summary service users want:

- practical, socially-oriented support which encompasses help in claiming state benefits and paying bills and in ensuring an adequate income, adequate housing, education, employment, daily living skills, childcare, and satisfying relationships and social networks;
- to be listened to, respected, trusted and demonstrably cared about by friendly, tolerant and non-judgemental workers who are sensitive to and advocate for client preference;
- to be given good quality information and genuine choice around options for care and treatment and help to access appropriate specialist services, including both inpatient units and alternatives to hospital admission when in crisis;
- 'specialist' interventions including help to understand their diagnosis and its potential implications, information and support to achieve an acceptable level of medication, help to cope with symptoms such as worrying beliefs and voices, help to recognize signs of relapse and prevent crises and help in planning ways to cope with crises.

What can be done to engage clients?

Strategies for engaging people with mental health problems have been identified by a number of publications (for example, SCMH 1998; DH 1999, 2003; Repper 2000; Williamson 2003). These are drawn on below, together with my current clinical experience as a worker in an assertive outreach team, to identify principles of engagement, which nurses may wish to consider in their practice. These principles of engagement cover two areas:

- the values and relationship-building interventions of workers;
- the values and organization of the service to support these interventions.

Values and relationship-building interventions of workers

A needs-led, client-centred approach

Allowing the client's priorities to set the agenda wherever possible quickly establishes a working alliance. Socially orientated help, particularly with urgent practical issues (for example, the basic survival needs of housing, income, clothing, food) is often the most effective engagement strategy for people who are most unwilling to engage with mental health services.

Flexibility, responsiveness and creativity

Taking the service to the client on their terms as far as possible will make it more accessible and increase the likelihood of engagement. Negotiation around the timing, venue and what will be done together is needed, and may mean some inconvenience for the worker. The frequency, duration and nature of contact needs to be adapted in response to the client's preference and changing priority of need.

Optimism and hope – viewing clients positively

Instilling hope and building self-esteem are real incentives for clients to remain in contact. Focusing on strengths in the context of an acknowledgement of the disabling long-term effects of illness, discrimination and stigma is important as is recognizing that clients have considerable survival skills and have often coped with far greater difficulties than many other people. Demonstrating a commitment to the possibility of change by not dismissing clients' ambitions but instead seeking realistic ways for them to begin to work towards achieving them creates a positive working climate.

Perseverence, patience and realism

Nurses need to allow for setbacks and to accept a slow or non-existent pace of progress if pessimism is to be avoided. Viewing relapse as part of recovery and taking a long-term view with regard to sustained engagement as a marker of success is a more constructive approach.

Seeing the client as expert and being willing to compromise and negotiate

It is important to avoid a power struggle with clients by trying to impose your own model or explanation on clients. Learning from clients by respecting their perspective on their own experiences as valid and meaningful will inform the process of engagement. This requires an acceptance and tolerance by the nurse of the client's right to reject interventions or to disagree with advice (for example, regarding use of medication) and an openness to explore differences and find acceptable ways forward.

Advocacy and challenging oppressive practice

If they are to genuinely engage with services clients need to be heard and taken seriously. Helping clients to represent their views at care review meetings and including them in Care Programme Approach (CPA) care plans, involving independent advocates where necessary, and highlighting approaches that are overly coercive or paternalistic is essential. Adequate information on individual rights, including the complaints procedures, will also help to create a climate of cooperation.

Positive risk-taking

Allowing clients the freedom to learn and gain from experience where possible (taking into account assessment of risk), even if there is the possibility of failure, promotes engagement by avoiding overly controlling practice. This can be facilitated by a collaborative risk-management approach which involves an open exploration of risk history and honesty about the likely consequences of risk behaviours, coupled with reaching agreement on relapse prevention and coping with crises.

Choice and the sharing of good information

Many clients will have been progressively disempowered by their experiences and regaining a sense of control and self-direction is central to engagement. Active involvement through the promotion of informed choice by providing accessible information about the range of options for care and treatment, including facilitating access to appropriate self-help and non-statutory organizations, will help to restore this. Avoidance of psychiatric jargon is important, because it is a stigmatized and alienating barrier to understanding, but explanations of these terms need to be given as necessary. Finding a meaningful language that is acceptable to the client (for example, 'voice hearing' as opposed to 'auditory hallucinations') should be supported by the provision of educative user-friendly literature and time for discussion.

Cultural sensitivity and anti-discriminatory practice

It is important to recognize that clients' experience of services as discriminatory and oppressive has often been a reason for disengagement. There needs to be active enquiry about cultural beliefs and practices and the respectful consideration of them in care planning. Provision of access to trained interpreters in a preferred language, choice of gender and ethnicity of worker where possible, and the involvement of local religious and cultural organizations will all serve to break down cultural barriers and promote engagement.

Honesty, genuineness, trust and respect

Showing your human side to clients is important. Non-defensive statements about one's limitations, such as 'I don't know but we could find out', is one way of showing this, as is use of humour and having ordinary, problem-free general conversation. Being seen to deliver and do what you say you will do, honesty if you cannot or if there are difficulties or delays, communication of any unforeseen changes to your agreed plan and apologizing for any shortcomings on your part will build trust and respect. Clients can be very forgiving if these features of the relationship are in place.

Values and organization of the service

Some service models are inherently better placed to optimize engagement (for example, assertive outreach and early intervention teams), in that they have the advantage of an explicitly targeted client group with engagement as a stated central goal, and are able to 'gate-keep' referrals and limit workers' caseload size to allow sufficient time for more intensive and comprehensive interventions. The relatively recent integration of mental health and social services in many community teams has helped to address the problems of service fragmentation outlined earlier in this chapter. However, whatever the service model or setting, clinical experience suggests that there are key features of a service which will determine how well (or not) it engages with its clients.

Commitment to engagement

A stated commitment to engagement is needed to underpin all aspects of the team's work and should be central to its operational policy and service specification. Acceptability, accessibility, empowerment, choice and involvement are values that need to be formalized in this way.

Service user involvement

Commitment of a clinical team to engage clients is unlikely to be achieved in full unless there is an effective mechanism for involving clients in team development. Service user-led satisfaction surveys can be a useful way of canvassing opinion but will be perceived as tokenistic if their findings are not then drawn upon to inform changes in practice. The whole team, therefore, needs to be open to criticism and willing to act together positively in response. Service user participation in staff selection can help to ensure that positive attitudes prevail. Being interviewed by a service user prior to joining a team can be an effective way of conveying core service values to a new staff member and establishing their commitment to them.

Effective teamwork

The challenges of engaging a client group that often presents with high risk, complex needs and several concurrent mental health problems means that individual workers may experience a high degree of stress and will be unable to work effectively in isolation. A mutually supportive and respectful team climate is essential if effective teamwork is to be fostered. This can be promoted by good quality clinical debate and team problem solving and care planning that shares responsibility by drawing upon the expertise of all members of the multi-disciplinary team.

Staff support and development

If a team is to engage with its clients it also needs to effectively engage with its staff. Regular clinical supervision by competent and experienced practitioners is needed to facilitate good practice by providing a safe learning environment for workers to recognize achievements, effectively manage their caseload and to feel supported enough to acknowledge their own limitations and gaps in expertise and to ask for advice. This has to be complemented by a commitment to continuing staff training (both external and in-house) and the demonstrable encouragement, valuing, recognition and sharing of good practice and staff innovations within the team.

Leadership

Role-modelling positive and professional attitudes by team managers and senior practitioners is essential to maintain adherence of all workers to the core values and aims of the team. A management style that involves all members in an ongoing critical appraisal of the team's aims, objectives, work and direction is important as it facilitates ownership and commitment to the principles of good practice with regard to engagement.

Joint-working across agencies

Establishing effective working partnerships with relevant allied agencies is essential if the needs of clients are to be fully attended to and their engagement achieved. Central to this is recognition that no one team or service can provide everything, an appreciation of the complementary possibilities of joint-working, and a willingness to work together with other agencies for the best outcomes for clients. The Care Programme Approach (CPA) is the statutory framework intended to facilitate this, and good practice guidelines for its implementation need to be adhered to. Service-level agreements between agencies that commonly work together are an effective way of establishing agreed protocols for joint-working, and should include both statutory and voluntary sectors (for example, primary care, community and inpatient mental health services, voluntary sector housing providers and social services). Collating information on relevant wider community resources (for example, self-help groups, work-skills training and employment agencies, educational, social and leisure opportunities) and making creative use of them in care planning will go some way towards engaging with the priorities of clients.

Resources

Adequate resourcing of services is required if clients are to receive the help that they wish for, and this is an issue that is usually beyond the control of individual workers or their line managers. However, teams should make their views known and need to proactively use the existing mechanisms within their organization to constructively lobby for improvements. Alliances with service users in this respect can be very persuasive. Complementary crisis services with 24-hour access and adequate provision of supported housing projects are just two current areas of shortfall. At a team level, working to achieve a realistic caseload size for individual workers is important for retaining a motivated workforce.

Engagement and cultural difference

Culture is socially determined and shapes many aspects of our identity including our beliefs, values and behaviour. It encompasses many factors including race, ethnicity, religion, gender, sexuality, age, generation, class, life experience and lifestyle. For example, it influences how we perceive 'health' and 'ill health', how we manifest 'illness', decide upon the type of help we prefer, the expectations we have of services and the expectations that the nurse and client have of one another (Luthra and Bhugra 2000). Given that we are likely to differ in some way to each one of our clients, in terms of informing engagement strategies it can be useful to consider every meeting as a cross-cultural encounter. The history and background of both client and nurse are important influences on engagement.

Mental health nurses face the challenge of an increasingly culturally diverse client group and are expected to deliver an equitable service to their clients, irrespective of cultural difference, in the context of mental health services having been criticized for failing to do so (DH 2006, 2007). In the literature this expertise is commonly referred to as 'cultural competence' (DH 2006), although there is a lack of clarity regarding its definition or what it means for the client (Bennett 2006).

Past approaches to promoting cultural competence have been criticized for focusing primarily on providing nurses with information about the cultural differences of particular minority groups (for example, customs, religious beliefs and dietary preferences) to increase 'cultural knowledge'. It is argued that this method can be counter-productive because it can lead to simplified stereotyping of these groups predetermined assumptions about an individual's culture, and a tendency to view differences as problematic, thereby reinforcing negative attitudes towards cultural difference (Narayanasamy 1999).

A broader process of achieving cultural competence has been identified and incorporated into a national policy of training programmes for mental health professionals (DH 2005). This uses the core principles of engagement outlined earlier (arguably the commonalities of needs across cultures) as a basis for maximizing sensitivity and minimizing insensitivity in providing a service to culturally diverse people and communities (Papadopoulos et al. 2004). In their review of the literature on cultural perceptions of nursing and midwifery care, Loveday et al. (2006) support this approach by concluding that there is a universal concept of care, and no substantial difference across cultural groups with regard to what constitutes feeling cared for by nurses.

The successful application of these core principles of engagement is dependent upon the additional dimensions of cultural awareness, attitudes and approach. O'Hagan (2001) page 235 notes:

> 66 The workers need not be, as is often assumed, highly knowledgeable about the cultures of the people they work with, but must approach culturally different people with openness and respect – a willingness to learn. Self awareness is the most important component in the knowledge base of culturally competent practice. 99

While it is recognized that the mental health workforce needs to be ethnically diverse at all levels and thereby representative of the population it serves (DH 2005), it is also important to realize that cultural competency is not about matching the ethnicity of worker and client (although this may be a helpful intervention for some individuals):

> 66   A white mental health worker is no less equipped to provide a culturally responsive service for BME (black and minority ethnic) clients than a Black or Asian staff worker. Competency and commitment will cross all ethnic boundaries.
>
> (DH 2007 page 3)   99

Papadopoulos *et al.* (2004) suggest four core elements of cultural competency training:

■   Cultural awareness: This requires a self-reflective examination of one's own personal value base and beliefs and their origins to become aware that we are not impartial but own a set of culturally – specific attitudes and understandings (some of them professional), and that these may differ from those of our clients. Confronting our own capacity for cultural bias, racism, discrimination and the imposition of inappropriate or unethical care through ethnocentric assessments may feel uncomfortable, but is the foundation for cultural competency.

■   Cultural knowledge: Knowledge about the different cultural groups that we encounter, gained from both training and the experience of meaningful contact with people from different groups, is needed. This allows us to understand the differences and inequalities between groups, particularly with regard to their health beliefs and behaviours (for example, the cultural meanings of mental illness and the differing ways distress is expressed), health inequalities, the influence of societal power relationships (for example, the power of health care professionals), and the origin of common stereotypes and their impact on mental health and access to health care.

■   Cultural sensitivity: This refers to the extent to which nurses demonstrate sensitivity to difference through their interventions with clients and their carers. Enquiring about an individual's cultural identity and needs with an open and respectful acknowledgement of any cultural difference between nurse and client can inform a partnership model based on mutual understanding. Through negotiation the nurse can then become a facilitator and advocate for the client to ensure real choices about treatment and care.

■   Cultural competence in practice: This involves the synthesis and application of previously gained awareness, knowledge and sensitivity. It includes: the practical skills of working with cultural difference, for example, addressing verbal and non-verbal language difference; effective needs assessment, accurate diagnosis; meeting the challenge of care planning with the different family roles, structures and functions in caring that occur across cultures; and involving local minority community agencies as appropriate. These culture-generic competencies can then be applied to culture-specific competencies for individual clients by, for example, working with their culture-specific explanatory models of illness and coping strategies (see Fernando 2002). Recognizing and challenging discrimination and oppressive practice by others should be allied to one's own anti-oppressive practice with clients and their families. At an organizational level, a commitment to engaging and involving local minority communities in service design and delivery is needed to support the work of nurses and their teams (DH 2005).

Two case studies are presented which illustrate some barriers to and strategies for promoting engagement of clients in their care and treatment.

Case study: Terry

Terry is 36 years old with a ten-year history of street homelessness and itinerancy. He often mutters to himself and is suspicious, isolative and aggressive towards others, particularly after binge drinking alcohol. He is often to be seen angrily shouting and gesticulating at passers-by and has been the victim of several assaults. He is extremely thin and wears heavily soiled clothing. He has been excluded from several day centres due to his threatening behaviour.

Barriers to engagement
- hostility towards mental health services due to his exclusion from effective help following a misdiagnosis of his schizophrenia in earlier life and labels of personality disorder and alcohol dependence;
- negative experiences of other services including evictions from hostels, exclusion from day centres and several charges for petty crime;
- persecution and harassment by members of the public;
- long-term isolation and social withdrawal;
- frightening psychotic experiences and threatening behaviour, complicated by alcohol use.

Strategies to promote engagement
- compulsory hospital admission after limited success of non-coercive engagement strategies and in response to increased risk;
- close working between the inpatient team and community team care coordinator, including frequent visits to Terry to provide continuing contact, support, advocacy, and to build trust with an emphasis on engagement around his priorities of maintenance and collection of benefits and wish for clothing and housing;
- facilitation of a carefully planned discharge to voluntary sector high-support special-needs housing with involvement of the housing team in visiting him on the ward prior to the move;
- strengthening the working relationship with Terry by: negotiation and respect for Terry's preference to have relatively brief contacts with mental health staff and his wish to continue to live a largely isolative lifestyle; optimizing benefits entitlement via the securing of disability living allowance; and mutual agreement on the goals of preventing further hospital admissions and a return to homelessness;
- long-term joint-working between the community mental health, housing and home treatment teams to develop acceptable ways to manage risk, build on daily living skills and maintain community tenure;
- gradual, strengths-focused exploration of Terry's past life experiences and illness, pattern of relapse, risk factors and relapse prevention strategies including medication use;
- assistance with working towards his aspirations of renewing contact with his family and returning to his home town.

Case study: Femi

Femi is a 25-year-old single Nigerian man who has experienced a gradual social decline following the death of his mother six years ago with whom he had lived. He now lives in a low-support flat after a period staying in emergency hostels. He has been unemployed for the past four years and has only infrequent contact with his extended family which he experiences as being rather critical of him. He is often distressed by the experience of commanding voices, unpleasant physical sensations and the belief that he is being controlled by persecutory spirits. He feels embarrassed by his involuntary laughter that often occurs when he is in company and, therefore, tends to isolate himself, but has mentioned a wish to find paid employment and thereby regain a social network and a girlfriend. He is extremely sensitive to suggestions that he may be mentally ill and can become very irritable and dismissive of attempts to discuss treatment options, sometimes expressing the belief that services are in conspiracy with the spirits.

Barriers to engagement

- distressing psychotic experiences that impede Femi's ability to trust and feel confident with others;
- negative experience of several dismissals from work and long-term unemployment;
- estrangement from his family with consequent loss of status as the eldest son and disconnection from his own community;
- cultural differences around the explanatory model for his difficulties, complicated by the stigma attached to the mental illness model;
- reluctance to engage with discussion about 'symptoms' and to cooperate with advice regarding medication use.

Strategies to promote engagement

- discussion at the multi-disciplinary clinical review meeting confirms that Femi's need to regain a sense of control over his life should inform all interventions;
- exploring Femi's daily difficulties and aspirations respectfully and empathically from his own cultural perspective and in a way that avoids use of psychiatric jargon. A potential power struggle is avoided through explicit acknowledgement and acceptance of differences of opinion and of the mistrust that he sometimes feels;
- agreement is reached by the mutual identification of the goals of improving his sleep, reducing unpleasant experiences and eventually returning to work;
- exploring the approaches that Femi finds helpful and unhelpful with a view to modifying them through negotiation. For example: respecting Femi's wish to take control at the beginning of visits by deciding whether or not he wishes to discuss 'symptoms' and medication (this can be either 'helpful' or 'unhelpful' depending on how he is feeling); and a flexible approach to medication use whereby Femi is encouraged to try varying doses and assess advantages and disadvantages of this;
- negotiated change of allocation to a Nigerian housing support worker with whom Femi has developed a good rapport. Consequent joint-working gradually involves key family members via formal and informal contacts to build understanding and restore relationships. Input from the family's church pastor to meet Femi's spiritual needs and provide advice;

■ appointments are facilitated with the local disability employment adviser and a referral is made to a supported work-skills training project.

Conclusion

Sustained engagement, often through 'low-level' relationship-building interventions allied to an emphasis on socially oriented practical help (e.g. housing, benefits) is an important criterion by which to judge the success of mental health services. To engage their clients, nurses and other mental health professionals must be willing to relinquish the traditional power relationship of expert–recipient and to use the skills of sensitive compromise. This emphasis requires flexibility and a willingness by mental health workers to put aside their specialist skills in the initial stages of their relationships with clients. 'Psychiatric' interventions (e.g. medication, psychological treatments) may be best introduced later when trust and greater stability has been established (SCMH 1998).

In summary the main points of this chapter are:

■ Engagement in treatment and care of people with serious mental illness is now a national policy and mental health nurses are in a key position to help facilitate this.

■ Many service users have valid reasons to mistrust services, and this must be acknowledged.

■ Engagement requires both individual workers and services to change their traditional practices by responding positively to criticisms by service users and directly involving them in the process of change.

■ There are key principles of engagement that should underpin individual practice and service delivery, whatever the service setting.

■ An individualized and socially oriented approach to care provides a foundation for effective engagement.

Questions for reflection and discussion

1 In what ways have services failed to engage effectively with clients?
2 What principles for practice can help individual workers to engage their clients effectively in care and treatment?
3 Using examples of client work from your own experience, identify possible barriers and solutions to engagement. What needs to change and how might you begin to address these changes?
4 How could your service or team optimize the engagement of its clients?
5 What is your cultural identity? Where do you come from and what makes you the person you are?
6 Consider some of the clients you have recently worked with who differed from you in terms of some of the cultural factors listed earlier. What value judgements or assumptions did you make about them? How knowledgeable were you about their culture? How did this influence your engagement with them?
7 How could you and your service or team become more culturally competent?

Annotated bibliography

- Perkins, R. and Repper, J. (1998) *Dilemmas in Community Mental Health Practice. Choice or Control.* Abingdon: Radcliffe Medical Press. Provides a thorough exploration of the challenges and complexities of practice with regard to empowering and engaging service users.
- Ryan, P. and Morgan, S. (2004) *Assertive Outreach. A Strengths Approach to Policy and Practice.* London: Churchill Livingstone. Although about assertive outreach, this provides an excellent and transferable focus on approaches to engagement for anyone working in mental health.
- Fernando, S. (2002) *Mental Health, Race and Culture.* Basingstoke: Palgrave. Provides a detailed exploration of cultural difference and gives information on culture-specific explanatory models of illness and coping strategies.
- www.refugeecouncil.org.uk. A valuable resource for working with refugees and asylum seekers. Gives information on the cultural norms of key groups and provides links to other sites that provide a wide range of related information and advice.
- Brazier, C. and Hamed, A. (eds) (2007) *The World Guide. An alternative reference to the countries of our planet* (11th edition). Oxford: New Internationalist Publications Ltd. A useful reference book for any service working with clients from diverse home countries. It provides an overview of the key cultural, economic and political features of each country.

References

Bennett, J. (2006) Achieving race equality through training: a review of approaches in the UK. *Journal of Mental Health Workforce Development* **1**(1): 5–11.

Campbell, P. and Lindow, V. (1997) *Changing Practice: Mental Health Nursing and User Empowerment.* London: MIND/Royal College of Nursing.

Craig, T. and Timms, P. (2000) Facing up to social exclusion: services for homeless mentally ill people. *International Review of Psychiatry* **12**: 206–11.

Dean, R. and Craig, T, (1999) *Pressure points: Why people with mental health problems become homeless.* London: Crisis.

Department of Health (DH) (1999) *A National Service Framework for Mental Health. Our Healthier Nation.* London: HMSO.

Department of Health (DH) (2001) *The Mental Health Policy Implementation Guide.* London: Department of Health Publications.

Department of Health (DH) (2002) *Mental Health Policy Implementation Guide. Dual Diagnosis Good Practice Guide.* London: Department of Health Publications.

Department of Health (DH) (2003) *Delivering Race Equality: A Framework for Action. Mental Health Services Consultation Document.* London: Department of Health Publications.

Department of Health (DH) (2005) *Delivering Race Equality in Mental Health Care.* London: Department of Health Publications.

Department of Health (DH) (2006) *From Values to Action: The Chief Nursing Officer's review of mental health nursing.* London: Department of Health Publications.

Department of Health (DH) (2007) *Positive Steps – Supporting race equality in mental healthcare.* London: Department of Health Publications.

Fernando, S. (2002) *Mental Health, Race and Culture.* Basingstoke: Palgrave.

Loveday, H.P., Beake, S. and Rowan, C. (2006) *Caring: Perceptions and context of nursing and midwifery care in London in the 21st century: A preliminary scope of published literature from 1995–2005. London Nursing Network Conference Briefing.* March. London: Network for Nurses and Midwives.

Luthra, A. and Bhugra, D. (2000) Serious mental illness: cross-cultural issues, in C. Gamble and G. Brennan (eds) *Working With Serious Mental Illness. A manual for clinical practice.* London: Baillière Tindall.

Narayanasamy, A. (1999) Transcultural mental health nursing 1: benefits and limitations. *British Journal of Nursing* **8**(10): 664–8.

NIACE/NIMHE (2003) *Access to Adult Education for People Diagnosed with Mental Health Problems.* Report of a national postal survey of colleges of further education, local authority adult education services and workers' educational associations. National Institute of Adult Continuing Education/National Institute for Mental Health (England) Partnership Project. www.nimhe.org.uk

NIMHE (2003) *Personality Disorder: No Longer a Diagnosis of Exclusion.* Policy implementation guidance for the development of services for people with personality disorder. London: National Institute for Mental Health. www.nimhe.org.uk

O'Hagan, K. (2001) *Cultural Competence in the Caring Professions.* London: Jessica Kingsley.

Papadopoulos, P., Tliki, M. and Lees, S. (2004) Promoting cultural competence in healthcare through a research-based intervention in the UK. *Diversity in Health and Social Care* **1**: 107–15.

Repper, J. (2000) Adjusting the focus of mental health nursing: Incorporating service users' experiences of recovery. *Journal of Mental Health* **9**(6): 575–87.

Rogers, A. and Pilgrim, D. (1994) Service users' views of psychiatric nurses. *British Journal of Nursing* **3**: 16–18.

Ryan, P. (1999) *Assertive Outreach in Mental Health*, Nursing Times Clinical Monographs No. 35. London: NT Books/Emap Healthcare.

SCMH (1998) *Keys to Engagement. Review of care for people with severe mental illness who are hard to engage with services.* London: Sainsbury Centre for Mental Health.

SCMH (2000) *Breaking the Circles of Fear. A review of the relationship between mental health services and African and Caribbean communities.* London: Sainsbury Centre for Mental Health.

Timms, P. (1993) Mental health and homelessness, in K. Fisher and J. Collins (eds) *Homelessness, Health Care and Welfare Provision.* London: Routledge.

Timms, P. (1996) Management aspects of care for the homeless mentally ill. *Advances in Psychiatric Treatment* **2**: 158–65.

Williamson, T. (2003) Enough is good enough. *Mental Health Today* April: 24–7.

CHAPTER 28

Problems, goals and care planning

Lina Gega

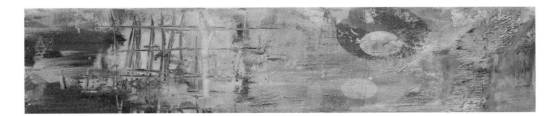

Chapter overview

Care planning in mental health, irrespective of the nature of the problem or the therapeutic approaches used, becomes user-focused when the client and the practitioner develop a shared understanding of what the *problems* are and agree on *goals* to guide their working relationship. Problems and goals are the stepping-stone for an *action plan*, which describes what to be done (*action*) and why or how it may help (*rationale*). Finally, care plan *review* involves the reassessment and evaluation of problems, goals and actions within a specified period of time and with certain methods.

This chapter covers:

- Care planning;
- Defining problems;
- Setting goals and objectives;
- Outlining an action plan;
- Reviewing progress.

Care planning

Care planning is the process by which the nurse arrives at:

1 a shared understanding between nurse and patient of what the problems and needs are and what priority they should take;
2 the desired or expected outcome, which is reflected on the goals and objectives;
3 the interactions/interventions which are the pathway to a certain goal with the ultimate aim to reduce the symptoms, distress and/or disability associated with the problem (action and rationale);
4 the evaluation methods for progress and outcome (care plan review).

Three concepts are pertinent to care planning: problem solving, the nursing process and the Care Programme Approach (DH 2000, 2006). Table 28.1 shows how each part of care planning corresponds to a step in problem solving and a stage of the nursing process.

Care planning	Problem solving	Nursing process
Part 1: Problems and needs	Step 1: Defining and prioritizing problems	Stage 1: Assessment
Part 2: Goals and objectives	Step 2: Setting goals	Stage 2: Planning
Part 3: Action and rationale	Step 3: Identifying all solutions; choose best possible solution; determine tasks to arrive at the solution	Stage 3: Implementation
Part 4: Review	Step 4: Evaluating the effectiveness of the solution	Stage 4: Evaluation

Table 28.1 Relationship between care planning, problem solving and the nursing process

The Care Programme Approach (CPA) is the statutory framework within which bio-psychosocial needs assessment is carried out. CPA forms are set out as care plans for people with mental health problems and complex needs.

Care plans can be either standardized or individualized and uni- or multi-disciplinary. These written records usually have a format which reflects the four components of the care-planning process described above, i.e. problems and needs, goals and objectives, action and rationale, progress review (Figures 28.1 and 28.2). However, the structure and guidelines for care plans vary from one service to another to reflect the needs of specific client groups, or the working methods of a professional team. The patient should be involved in writing their care plan and ideally a copy should be kept by the patient, by the nurse, and be filed in the medical/nursing notes.

The purpose of a care plan can be summarized in six distinct but interlinked areas:

1   As a legal document, it demonstrates that patient care complies with national and local policies.
2   As a means of communication, it forms part of the patient's medical, nursing or multi-disciplinary notes and facilitates information flow and continuity of care among those involved in a patient's care.
3   As a practice guide, it provides a focus for patient needs and planning, implementation and evaluation of care.
4   As a progress record, it demonstrates the patient's journey within a service or across different services.
5   As a teaching tool, it can be used in practice-based learning to develop an understanding of the types of problems and needs that patients may have, and the way nurses may justify and deliver their interventions.
6   As a means of user involvement, it can guide the patient–nurse working relationship and ensure that patients participate and their views are represented in their care.

CARE PLAN for: _____

Problem / area of need / issues to work with: _____
_____
_____

Goals / objectives:

1 _____
_____
_____

2 _____
_____
_____

Action: **Rationale:**

1 _____   1 _____
_____   _____
_____   _____

2 _____   2 _____
_____   _____
_____   _____

3 _____   3 _____
_____   _____
_____   _____

Review: _____
_____
_____

Completed by: _____   _____   _____

Date: _____   _____   _____

Figure 28.1 A care plan format: Example 1

Care plans are, therefore, multi-purpose documents. However, in reality, many of these purposes may not be fulfilled at all times. Care plans can become a 'paper exercise' and their completion can be seen as just an administrative task or a legal requirement. Also, the relationship between care plans and quality of care could be challenged on the basis that time spent writing the care plan can take away time spent with the patient. This line of argument assumes, however, that care plans are done *for* the patient rather than *with* the patient, which is too often the case in busy clinical settings.

Patient/client:		CARE PLAN		
Primary nurse/keyworker:				
Date:				

Problem/ area of need	Goals/objectives	Action	Rationale	Review

Figure 28.2 A care plan format: Example 2

Defining problems

Defining and prioritizing a patient's problems and needs is the first step in care planning. Information gathered during the assessment process through interviewing, observation and measurement is drawn together into succinct problem statements, which are agreed between patient and nurse. Problem statements should reflect a shared understanding of what the problems/needs are, what maintains them and what priority they should take in the care-planning process. Prioritizing problems is not straightforward; we may choose to address the most severe problem first or, alternatively, a problem which could be resolved easily and have an associated effect on other areas of need.

An agreed definition and prioritization of a problem might not be feasible if the patient and the nurse cannot engage in a collaborative working relationship for various reasons. Such difficulties are not a reason to exclude the patient from the care-planning process, however; it is better to draw up preliminary unilateral problem statements and address the lack of a collaborative relationship as a problem in itself. Thereafter the nurse might identify the reasons for lack of collaborative relationship (for example, if the patient is severely distressed or unconscious, the nurse has not spent much time with the patient, etc.), ways to facilitate collaboration (reframing the problem in different terms or with a different focus, involving the family and other members of the team, etc.), and a date by which the problem statements should be reviewed, ideally with involvement of the patient.

If after discussing their understanding of the problem the nurse and patient have still not reached an agreed problem statement, they may have to 'agree to disagree' or 'agree to differ' (Kingdon and Turkington 1994) so to avoid prolonged repetitive discussions. In this case, the patient's understanding should still feature in the care plan; it will just be different to the nurse's. Clinicians tend to describe lack of agreement on problem statements as 'the patient lacking insight' but an alternative way of describing it from our patient's point of view could be, 'Mrs A. does not agree with what the doctors/nurses/family say about what her problem is, and she feels that the only reason for being in hospital is because she has not been behaving as she was expected to.'

Language

A way to reach agreed problem statements is to use language which is user-friendly, non-judgemental and personalized. The nurse may wish to test whether their understanding and phrasing of the patient's problem meets these criteria by asking himself or herself:

- Would this make sense to my patient?
- If this were me, would I mind someone else saying this about me?
- Would I be happy for my patient to read this?
- Does this describe my patient's personal experiences of the problem?

User-friendly language uses direct quotes or paraphrases what a person said, rather than jargon or diagnoses. Some examples of what to avoid and what to say instead are:

- 'The client is depressed' → 'Mrs Smith describes feeling low/unhappy/ sad/miserable/gloomy/down.'
- 'The client exhibits bluntness of affect' → 'Mary describes feeling numb and empty, and not being able to cry even when she wanted to get some relief.'
- 'Self-neglect' → 'John has not looked after himself for several days.'
- 'Lack of motivation' → 'Mrs Smith is finding it very hard to pay the bills and do the shopping. She would like to get back to work but finds it overwhelming and does not know where to start from, so she ends up postponing and "not bothering" to fill in applications.'

Non-judgemental language describes a behaviour and the potential reasons behind it, rather than attributing a characteristic to the person based on the behaviour. The problem statement should also take into account the patient's rather than the practitioner's point of view. Here are some examples:

- 'The patient is acting out and is difficult to manage' → 'John swears and throws things around because he says he is fed up with being in hospital and being treated like an idiot.'
- 'The patient is non-compliant' → 'Mr Smith is unhappy about taking his medication because he is worried about not having any control over it.'

Personalized statements reflect how a person experiences their illness and are specific about what symptoms mean for them. Specificity can also allow for objective evaluation of any change in the problem over time. Examples of general versus personalized statements are:

- 'The patient is lethargic and has low energy levels' → 'Mary feels sluggish and slowed down in the morning, and has a two-hour sleep in the afternoon which she never used to do. She feels exhausted when she does things such as preparing dinner or going out socializing.'
- 'The patient has poor sleep and appetite' → 'Mary sleeps 5 hours as opposed to her 8-hour normal sleep and wakes up 3–4 times during the night. She has stopped enjoying

her food for the past couple of months and she has lost about 10 pounds during this time. Her everyday eating and drinking includes 5–6 cups of coffee and a sandwich.'

Apart from the appropriate language to be used, the format of problem statements depends on the model used to explain how the problem may have developed and is maintained. If the practitioner does not want to tie problem definition to a particular model, the following components can comprise a generic format for a problem statement:

- An *experience or state* (*physical, emotional, mental, behavioural, cognitive, social*), which the patient considers as the primary problem because it causes distress and disability.

Useful questions to ask during assessment include:

- Is anything happening at the moment that upsets you or interferes with your life?
- Is there anything that you are particularly worried about at the moment?
- What does your family think the problem is?
- If there was something that you could change to make your life better or more enjoyable, what would it be?
- What do you fear is the worst thing that might happen?

The *occurrence* of the primary problem: relevant information on what triggers or precipitates it, how often it occurs, when and where it is more likely to occur, how long it has been going on, etc.

Useful questions to ask during assessment:

- When is the problem more likely to happen?
- Is there anything that makes it better/worse?
- When did you start noticing that things were getting out of hand?
- How many times does it happen in a day/week/month?
- Is there anyone who helps or makes things worse?

The patient's *responses* to it and whether they are *helpful or unhelpful*.

Useful questions to ask during assessment:

- How do you make yourself feel better? Does it help? For how long?
- Is there anything that you do more of/less of because of the problem? Is what you do effective? How long does the effect last?
- Is there anything you avoid because of the problem? Is it helpful?
- Are there any disadvantages in avoiding things?
- Do you ever blow up because of what is happening to you/around you? What exactly do you do? Do you do anything to control it?

The primary problem's *impact on self, others and/or life*.

Useful questions to ask during assessment:

- How does it make you feel in yourself?
- How has it been affecting your life?
- Has it affected your relationships with others? In what way?

Problem statement: example 1

John feels unhappy and miserable (*emotional experience as the primary problem*) for most days of the week and for the past month (*occurrence*). Ever since he stopped working, he does not go out much and sits at home (*response*). This makes him feel worthless and even more miserable (*response is unhelpful*), and he worries about being able to go back to work (*impact on life*).

Problem statement: example 2

Mary sleeps less than she would like to and wakes up many times during the night (*physical experience of poor sleep is the primary problem for the patient*). This happens mainly at night when she feels other people's presence in the house (*occurrence and activating event*). She tries to cope with it by telling herself that everything is OK which makes her feel better (*helpful response*) and she occasionally shouts at them (*response*) but she is not sure whether this makes them go away (*unhelpful response*). She feels scared and helpless during the night and tired in the morning (*impact on self*); she is also unable to concentrate on doing everyday things (*impact on life*).

Note that although 'other people's presence in the house' could have been phrased as a problem (e.g. being a symptom of a psychotic illness), Mary chose 'sleep' as the experience that distresses her and interferes with her life more, therefore even if interventions address Mary's psychotic symptoms, this will be done within the context of improving her sleep.

Problem statement: example 3

Mr Smith feels severely anxious (*emotional state*) every time he is about to go out or when he is out (*occurrence*) from fear of doing something stupid and people laughing at him (*cognitive experience*). In *response*, he always goes out very early in the morning and very late at night, and avoids public transport and crowded places (*responses*). Although this prevents anxiety in the short term (*short term helpful response*), he never gets the chance to prove to himself that his fear is unlikely to happen (*response is unhelpful long term*). As a result, he has very little confidence in himself (*impact on self*) and his life has been restricted significantly because he cannot work or socialize (*impact on life*).

Setting goals and objectives

Goals can be long or short term depending on the time and resources available, and the strengths and limitations that the patient is considered to have. Most importantly the nurse needs to identify the objectives to be achieved prior to the patient reaching their goal (i.e. what the person would be able to do and under what circumstances, in order to know that the problem has improved and his/her needs have been met up to a realistic point). It is helpful to include potential or actual obstacles and difficulties in meeting objectives, and to identify, also, what support or resources could assist or smooth the patient's progress. Finally, both problems and goals can be documented and rated in a standard form (Marks 1986) an example of which is given in Figure 28.3.

PROBLEMS AND GOALS

Name: Date:

Problem: _____

_____

_____

_____

_____

_____

_____

_____

_____

How distressing and/or disturbing is the problem?

0---------1---------2---------3---------4---------5---------6---------7---------8
not at all   slightly   moderately   very much   extremely

Goal: _____

_____

_____

_____

_____

_____

_____

_____

_____

If I had to achieve this goal now, how difficult would it be?

0---------1---------2---------3---------4---------5---------6---------7---------8
not at all   slightly   moderately   very much   extremely

Review: _____

_____

Figure 28.3 Problems and goals form

Questions, which may help elicit goals and objectives are:

1   What would you like to be able to do in the near future that you cannot do now because of the problem?
2   What sort of things can people without your problems do?
3   If you woke up tomorrow and the problem was gone, how would you know?

4   How could your family and friends tell if your problem improved?
5   How could people who know you well tell when things start getting difficult for you?
6   If there was one thing that you would like to change in your life/yourself/the world around you, what would it be?
7   What has to change in order for you to be able to …?
8   Some examples of goals and objectives relating to the problem statements of the previous section are:

Example 1

Long-term goal: To be able to go back to work part-time within three months.

■   This could be arranged because my boss is understanding and will not have a problem with an initial trial period of part-time work for me.

Objectives:

■   To be able to get up in the morning at 8.00 a.m., have breakfast and then go out to buy my paper (to do this every day for two weeks and then sleep longer during the weekends).
■   To be able to go out two or three days a week in the evening to see my friends.
■   Potential difficulty could be that my friends may expect too much too soon from me because they do not understand what is wrong with me.

Example 2

Long-term goal: To be able to sleep seven hours without waking up and, if I wake up, not be scared.

   Objectives:

■   To be able to get back to sleep without having to shout at the people in my house and be able to do this every night for a week.
■   To be able to spend one hour, without interruption, doing the housework every day for a week.

Example 3

Long-term goal: To be able to attend an interest group or do voluntary work in a shop within the next six months.

   Objectives:

■   To be able to walk around my local shopping area every day at lunchtime for about 30 minutes or until my anxiety goes down by 50 per cent.
■   To be able to go to the local shop at lunchtime everyday to buy something and make small talk with the shop assistant while making eye contact with him/her.

Outlining an action plan

The action plan includes two elements: (a) the types of interventions or methods of support which will enable the patient to achieve their goals; and (b) the rationale behind these interventions (i.e. why the nurse (and patient) think the intervention may help and how). The focus of interventions/support depends on the ways the nurse understands the problem (i.e. our problem statements) and what the nurse wants the patient to achieve from the interventions (i.e. our goal). Specifically:

- Using diagnostic terms to describe specific signs and symptoms (for example, ICD-10; WHO 1992) forms the basis of pharmacological or other medical interventions whose goal is to reduce these signs and symptoms and restore health or minimize illness.
- Identifying the patient's needs and setting goals based on national policies and guidelines (for example, CPA; DH 2000, 2006) could determine areas of problem-solving priority, such as risk minimization, social inclusion, crisis management, contingency planning and relapse prevention. Apart from the therapeutic purpose of interventions, the objective is to also meet the nurse's ethical, legal and professional obligations, such as ensuring fairness and autonomy for patients, protecting the public, etc.
- Drawing on psychological models to understand the mechanisms by which a problem has developed and is maintained (for example, stress-vulnerability model, Zubin and Spring 1977) could point to effective psychological, social and family interventions. Here, the goal is to remove the distress and disability associated with a problem and to help the person function as closely as possible to how they would wish.

Reviewing progress

Reviewing progress involves evaluating other parts of the care plan, within a specified period of time and with certain methods. Thus, there are three aspects to consider in any care plan review.

What is being evaluated?

Evaluation is usually associated with 'outcome in relation to certain criteria' (that is, whether the problem has improved and goals are met against certain criteria). However, if the scope of the evaluation is broadened to include 'comparisons at different points in time' (a starting point and a review point), then any part of the care plan can be revisited as long as there are changes to be considered. For example, the nurse may choose to review the list of the patient's needs in order to update it, or rephrase the problem statements in order to include the patient's point of view, or perhaps reexamine the patient's priorities in the light of new information. The nurse might want to reconsider their interventions or whether they were successful in problem solving anticipated difficulties. Thus, the care plan review should specify the objective of the evaluation.

How is the evaluation done?

Depending on the objective of the evaluation, the nurse may use idiosyncratic descriptive methods or objective measurement tools to assess actual or required changes in the problems, goals or action plan. *Idiosyncratic descriptive methods* include diaries or verbal accounts of how someone feels or the nurse's own observations regarding the patient's progress. For example, if the objective of the evaluation is the effect of a new medication, the nurse could ask the patient to describe any side effects they experience, or the nurse could note their own observations of any side effects over time. *Objective measurement tools* include rating scales or questionnaires, which can indicate changes from baseline (*relative change*) or changes against certain criteria (*absolute change*). For example, the nurse might choose to take the patient through a standardized questionnaire, which specifies all potential side effects of medication, and rate the severity of each side effect based on the patient's response to each item of the questionnaire. Comparing this rating against a specified cut-off point could tell the nurse whether the medication is well tolerated or not by the patient (*absolute measurement*), and comparing the patient's ratings over time can indicate whether their tolerance of the medication has improved or not (*relative measurement*).

When should the evaluation be done?

Evaluation can be carried out at pre-specified time intervals (for example, weekly), or an arbitrary date can be set. Or evaluation could be triggered by critical events (such as discharge from hospital, change of medication, etc.). Most importantly, the nurse needs to specify whether the evaluation is ongoing or whether there is a cut-off point at which decisions have to be made based on the outcome of the evaluation. For example, the nurse may choose to assess the side effects of medication weekly up to a month at which point a change in medication would be considered. Or the patient's response to cognitive-behavioural therapy might be assessed weekly but an end-point might be specified (for example, the sixth session) at which to evaluate whether continuing treatment is justified.

Conclusion

There is no one definitive way of developing and writing a care plan, but whatever approach is adopted there are core components that must be included: problems and needs, goals and objectives, action and rationale, and progress review. This chapter has addressed these four components of care planning, focusing mainly on defining problems and setting goals.

In summary, the main points of this chapter are:

■ The first step in care planning is to draw the information gathered during assessment into agreed problem statements that reflect a shared understanding of what the patient's problems/needs are, what maintains them and what priority they should take in the care-planning process. A way to reach agreed problem statements is to use language which is user-friendly, non-judgemental and personalized.

■ The goals and objectives in care planning are the desired or expected outcomes that would indicate that the problem has improved and the patient's needs have been met up to a certain level. It is helpful to include potential or actual obstacles and difficulties in meeting objectives, as well as to identify what supports or resources could assist or smooth the patient's progress.

■ An action plan includes the interventions, which will enable the patient to achieve their goals and the rationale behind these interventions (i.e. why the nurse thinks they may help and how). The action plan is shaped by the way the nurse defines the patient's problems and set targets with them (i.e. whether the nurse uses diagnostic criteria, statutory guidelines and/or psychosocial models).

■ Evaluation is an integral part of care planning and need not relate only to outcomes; evaluation can involve a planned reconsideration of problems, goals and actions within a specified period of time. Care-plan review can involve idiosyncratic descriptive methods or objective measurement tools to assess any actual or required changes in the patient's progress and delivery of care.

Questions for reflection and discussion

1 Think about the language you use in your verbal and written communication with or regarding your patients:
  – Have you ever used terms which reflected only the diagnosis rather than the individual person's experiences?
  – Have you ever used statements which were vague and general, and which could not allow you to measure change?
  – Have you ever used value judgements in describing your patient's behaviour?
  – Have you ever written a care plan without your patient being involved?

2 If the answer in any of the above is 'yes', what could you do differently in similar occasions, next time?

3 What framework is prevalent in your everyday practice as a guide for your care planning and delivery? Is it a diagnostic, statutory or psychosocial framework? How do these frameworks complement each other in everyday practice?

Annotated bibliography

■ Johnson, S.L. (2004) *Therapist's Guide to Clinical Intervention: The 1–2–3's of Treatment Planning* (2nd edn). California, USA: Academic Press. A multi-disciplinary resource book which describes the assessment criteria for different types of mental health problems (using DSM-IV rather than ICD-10), and provides useful pointers for appropriate psychosocial interventions for each problem. It is an American book targeted mainly for practitioners working autonomously as therapists but it gives problem-specific goals, objectives and action plans, which makes it pertinent to care planning in mental health care.

References

Department of Health (2000) *Effective Care Co-ordination in Mental Health Services: Modernising the care programme approach – a policy booklet.* http://www.doh.gov.uk/pub/docs/doh/polbook.pdf (last updated 25 January 2000).

Department of Health (2006) *Reviewing the Care Programme Approach 2006: a consultation document.* http://www.DH.gov.uk/en/Consultations/Closedconsultations/DH_063354 (accessed 9 January 2008).

Kingdon, D.G. and Turkington, D. (1994) *Cognitive-Behavioural Therapy for Schizophrenia.* New York: Guilford Press.

Marks, I.M. (1986) *Behavioural Psychotherapy: Maudsley Pocket Book of Clinical Management.* Bristol: Wright.

World Health Organization (1992) *The Tenth Revision of the International Classification of Diseases and Related Health Problems (ICD-10).* Geneva: World Health Organization.

Zubin, J. and Spring, B. (1977) Vulnerability – a new view on schizophrenia. *Journal of Abnormal Psychology* **86**: 260–6.

CHAPTER 29

Self-help

Karina Lovell and Judith Gellatly

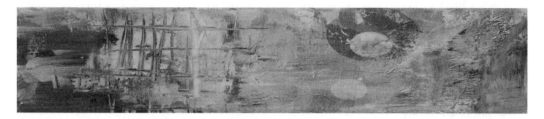

Chapter overview

In this chapter we discuss the rationale for self-help interventions, in particular guided self-help (GSH) interventions within mental health care and emphasize the importance of the nurse within this role. The chapter focuses on GSH for depression and anxiety and identifies key research findings. The application of self-help is illustrated through a detailed case study.

This chapter covers:

- The rationale for self-help;
- What is self-help?
    - Non-guided self-help
    - Guided self-help (GSH);

- Evidence base:
    - Depression
    - Anxiety;

- Application;
- Conclusions.

The need for self-help

Ninety per cent of people identified as having common mental health problems (e.g. anxiety and depression) are managed entirely in a primary care setting (McCulloch 2003) and approximately one third of people who attend a GP's surgery have mental health problems taking up at least a third of the GP's time (ODPM 2004). As it stands there exists a huge disparity between need and provision within current mental health services. There are lengthy waiting lists and waiting times and there is a need for more effective, efficient, accessible and acceptable models of treatment delivery to be considered (Lovell and Richards 2000).

In recent years UK health policies have tended to focus on severe mental health problems (e.g. psychosis and schizophrenia) and little attention has been paid to those people suffering from the more common mental health problems (e.g. depression and anxiety). More recently, partly due to the increasing costs and burden that common mental health problems are placing on health services, it has been recognized that brief and inexpensive interventions such as self-help may be suitable for treating and managing such conditions. Standards two and three of the *National Service Framework (NSF) for Mental Health* (DH 1999) reflect these views and have particular interest in improving identification, assessment, and providing effective, accessible interventions for managing mental health problems.

Concurrently there has been a general move towards involving patients in all aspects of service delivery (DH 1999) empowering them to take more control over their own health and well-being and thus adopting a more proactive approach. Self-help is viewed increasingly as a central part of supporting people (DH 2005) and self-help interventions as a means of overcoming many of the problems that are apparent within mental health settings. Indeed, it has been argued that without the incorporation of self-help our health service will be unable to deliver and achieve the goals they have set (Richards 2004). Many patients have expressed preference for psychological treatments (Tylee 2001; Anderson *et al.* 2005), but due to limited access and lack of therapists delivering such treatments in primary care the vast majority do not receive them (Lovell and Richards 2000; Anderson *et al.* 2005).

With mental health services growing and improving as a result of these policies and initiatives there is an opportunity for the mental health nurse's role to develop. Mental health nurses currently provide a vital valued service to service users in all settings. If, however, mental health services are to focus increasingly on empowering patients, mental health nursing may need a more holistic focus and higher level skills in assessment, health promotion and delivery of evidence-based psychological therapies. Lewis *et al.* (2003) suggest that recruiting non-professional staff and providing them with focused brief training for specific tasks may help solve problems encountered when professionals are in short supply. Rost *et al.* (2001) notes that in practices without onsite mental health professionals, brief training for primary care can have substantial benefits for patients who are commencing episodes of care for depression.

These views on the future of the mental health nurse's role are reflected in a number of policy guidelines. For example, the Care Services Improvement Partnership (CSIP 2006) states that nurses are competent to deliver self-help within primary care mental health because they possess or can be educated to develop core competencies such as engagement, alliance building and responsiveness. Evidence additionally implies that no extra costs are encountered and there are indications that patients are more satisfied by care delivered in this way compared to routine GP care (Richards *et al.* 2003). Furthermore, the UK NHS Plan (DH 2000) encourages GPs, nurses and mental health practitioners to develop their skills and practice-based facilities to enhance mental health services where adequate resources are available.

What is self-help?

Richards (2004) suggests that there are two distinct perspectives on self-help. One emphasizes the importance of utilizing self-help techniques to empower patients whereas the other describes self-help as a solution to the access, demand and professional skill shortages within mental health care. Such interventions differ from self-help groups that provide people with the opportunity to meet and share experiences and coping strategies with others experiencing similar problems. The majority of self-help groups are run for and by users and although they have a therapeutic value they are not the same as self-help interventions. One thing that is apparent however is that with the introduction of self-help, primary care mental health services are moving away from a service which is essentially paternalistic to one that is based upon collaborative relationships between the service users and the health professionals.

As yet there is no agreed definition of what constitutes self-help interventions and how they should be labelled (e.g. self-help, self-care, self-management) and there is also confusion surrounding the differentiation between traditional brief psychological therapies and self-help. In this chapter we incorporate pure self-help and GSH under the umbrella term of brief interventions. We use the term health professional to refer to any professional with a postgraduate mental health qualification (e.g. CBT therapist) or without a postgraduate mental health qualification ('paraprofessionals', e.g. psychology graduate).

Self-help

Whilst no agreed definition exists, there is a general consensus that self-help interventions should guide and encourage the patient to make changes, focusing on methods that can be utilized to sustain change over time. They should do more than provide the patient with information and enable the patient to make choices and decisions and take actions to improve their own health and well-being (Richards *et al.* 2003). Lewis *et al.* (2003) have proposed that a self-help intervention should possess two fundamental features:

1   It requires little or no input from a health professional only involving a small amount of contact beyond initial assessment where the therapeutic rationale is explained.
2   It contains information to encourage the user to develop skills to cope and manage their difficulties through making changes.

The self-help approach fits well with cognitive behavioural therapy (CBT). CBT is a collaborative 'talking therapy' based on a view that the way we act (behaviour) and our thoughts (cognitions) and our physical sensations (feelings) are all interlinked and change what we do. CBT helps to identify the unhelpful and helpful feelings, behaviour and thinking that people have. It can help to change or modify the way people think and act and in doing so reduce the impact that a problem has on people's lives (cf. Chapters 30 and 31 of this volume).

Non-guided self-help
Non-guided interventions require no professional input and thus the patient works through the intervention, usually in the form of a book or computer program alone. In recent years it has been argued that although non-guided interventions could have the biggest impact on access to services, they may be ineffective. For example depressed people who are lacking motivation and confidence are unlikely to benefit from treatments where they receive no professional contact (Mead *et al.* 2005).

Guided self-help
GSH is used to refer to self-help interventions that require minimal therapist contact which may provide the optimal balance between efficiency and effectiveness (Gellatly *et al.* 2007). GSH has been defined by the UK National Institute for Health and Clinical Excellence (NICE) in the Depression clinical guideline as 'a self-administered intervention designed to treat

depression, which makes use of a range of books or a self-help manual that is based on an evidence-based intervention and is designed specifically for the purpose' (NICE 2004).

In practice GSH is:

■ aimed at people suffering from mild to moderate symptoms (although there is no evidence, as yet, to suggest that people suffering from more severe symptoms would not benefit);

■ based on CBT principles;

■ usually mediated through a health technology, e.g. bibliotherapy, computer-administered therapy;

■ intervention is focused on self-management;

■ facilitated by a health professional (or paraprofessional) who monitors and reviews the patient;

■ intervention takes place over six to nine weeks including follow-up;

■ intervention involves no more than three hours of contact with the health professional.

User Focus and Empowerment	*Availability and Accessibility*
■ Reduces stigma associated with formal therapy	■ Easy access to follow-up if relapse occurs
■ Reduces time and costs associated with getting to sessions	■ Reduced waiting lists
■ Patient has control	■ A variety of health professionals can deliver self-help
■ Flexible delivery method and thus minimizes inference with other commitments	■ A wide-range of materials are available
	■ Fewer geographical restrictions on access
	■ Does not have to be delivered face-to-face

Table 29.1 Potential advantages of using a guided self-help approach

Evidence base for guided self-help

There is growing evidence that GSH can be effective for a range of mental health problems managed within primary care (see Table 29.1). The evidence is most substantial for the use of GSH for the treatment of depression and anxieties and these common mental health problems are the focus of the remaining part of this chapter (cf. Chapters 17 and 20 of this volume).

Depression

A recent randomized controlled trial (RCT) by Andersson *et al.* (2005) found that internet-based CBT with minimal therapist contact resulted in a greater reduction of depressive symptoms and increase in quality of life, than a waiting-list control group immediately after treatment and also at six-month follow-up.

A comprehensive systematic review of GSH by Gellatly *et al.* (2007) examined the factors that determine treatment effectiveness; in particular whether variation in benefit was associated with study populations or aspects of study design. Of the 34 studies identified, 24 were guided by either a health professional or paraprofessional. The review examined the nature of guidance (supportive or monitoring), the mode of the guidance (face to face versus other including telephone or computer either CD or internet) and who provided the guidance (paraprofessional or professional worker). A meta-analysis of findings from the 24 studies showed a pooled standardized mean difference of 0.796 (95 per cent CI 1.01–0.58) which gave clear evidence of the effectiveness of GSH interventions compared with pure self-help. Further investigation revealed that the technology used for delivering GSH is not critical, and that a range of delivery methods, professionals and content can be employed successfully.

Anxiety

Van Boeijen *et al.* (2005) conducted an RCT to compare the effectiveness and feasibility of GSH among people suffering from anxiety disorders in primary care. GSH delivered by the GP was found to have significant symptom improvements at 12 weeks and follow up at 52 weeks and was comparable to CBT performed in secondary care by professionals.

Mixed

Several internet interventions have to treat mental health problems were tested in and RCT by Proudfoot *et al.* (2004). This study demonstrated that GSH delivered through an interactive multimedia computerized CBT package ('*Beating the Blues*', *Ultrasis*; http://www.ultrasis.com) over eight therapy sessions is suitable for patients presenting in primary care with mild moderate and severe depression or mixed anxiety and depression. Patients described increased levels of satisfaction with the treatment they were receiving and clinical, work and social functioning symptom improvements remained at six-month follow-up. Furthermore *Beating the Blues* had benefits for patients across the whole range of clinical severity, irrespective of pre-existing illness duration and the programme was as successful in bringing about attributional change, as traditional face-to-face CBT.

A study examined a number of computer-aided self-help programmes for anxiety and depression, highlighted that such programmes not only enabled therapists to treat more patients and reduced treatment costs but patients were satisfied with the treatment, very satisfied with the guidance from the clinicians and there was indication that a large number of the patients achieved improvement in their symptoms (Gega *et al.* 2004).

The results of these and other studies suggest that GSH is an effective treatment for the management of depression and anxiety, that it is more effective than no treatment or waiting list control and that it is more acceptable and cost effective when compared to other psychological treatments. Computerized CBT has been proposed as a key part of Stepped Care models of depression care in both the USA and the UK (National Collaborating Centre for Mental Health 2004).

However, evidence of effectiveness is not uniformly positive. For example, Mead *et al.*'s (2005) RCT of the clinical effectiveness of GSH compared with waiting list control) found no significant benefit of GSH on depression and anxiety symptoms; however there was some evidence of significant benefit to social functioning, albeit difficult to interpret. Although subjects reported high levels of satisfaction with their relationship with assistant psychologists, the treatment manual was evaluated favourably and adherence to the intervention was acceptable.

In a review of self-help books Anderson *et al.* (2005) suggest that, with additional guidance, self-help books based on cognitive behavioural principles are useful for people suffering from mild to moderate depression and that they are a promising treatment in primary care settings. A meta-analysis found that GSH has a greater treatment effect than delayed treatment. Although a positive finding, the authors point out that existing studies have small samples, are poor quality and that a number are biased. Anderson *et al.* conclude that although there is weak evidence to suggest bibliotherapy for depression can be effective it would be wrong to generalize this finding to primary care.

Application of guided self-help in clinical practice

Although the concept of GSH is relatively simple, implementing it into regular clinical practice requires application and practice. To illustrate this, a case study from assessment to completion of GSH is detailed below.

Susan is a 28-year-old woman who lives with her son Sam aged ten. She was referred to a primary care mental health team by her GP for treatment for moderate depression. The mental health worker (MHW) conducted a patient-centred assessment (Mead and Bower 2000) using a semi-structured interview (Newell 2000) (see Box 29.1). Below we summarize Susan's progress over her course of treatment. This case study also serves to illustrate some of the treatment approaches covered in Chapters 28 and 30 of this volume.

Box 29.1   Format of semi-structured assessment

- 4 Ws
    - What is the problem?
    - Where does the problem occur?
    - When does the problem happen?
    - With whom is the problem better or worse?
- ABC
    - **A**utonomic – physical feelings
    - **B**ehavioural – behaviour (e.g. avoidance)
    - **C**ognitive – thoughts
- Current triggers (e.g. is there anything that particularly triggers the problem such as time of day, specific events etc.)
- Impact of the problem on work, home, social, private leisure and family/relationship functioning
- Risk assessment
- Other important information
    - Modifying factors
    - Onset and course of the problem
    - Client expectations and goals
    - Past treatment
    - Drugs and alcohol
    - Any other relevant information the client wishes to discuss
- Problem statement and goals

Session 1 Assessment, goal setting and rationale

Susan described her main problem as feeling depressed, which occurred most of the time, though she felt worse at night and first thing in the morning. She described her physical feelings as poor sleep in that she had difficulty getting off to sleep until the early hours of the morning. She also described increased irritability, poor concentration, frequent crying and a poor appetite.

Because of her low mood Susan had found it increasingly difficult to work and her GP had signed her off sick for a month. She was sleeping a lot in the day and found it difficult to do everyday tasks such as housework, shopping and cooking. She had a number of friends but was avoiding going out or even ringing them. She also felt that she had no energy to do the activities she used to do with her son, such as going to football matches and the cinema.

Susan's main thoughts were: 'I am weak and useless', 'I feel guilty that I am not being a good mother to Sam', 'Everything feels such an effort', 'Why can't I overcome these feelings and just pull my socks up?', 'Much worse things happen to other people in the world and I can't even deal with a relationship ending'.

Susan could not identify specific triggers except that she often felt worse when she saw her son because she felt guilty that she was not doing the things with him that they had done previously.

The problem was having a serious impact in many areas of her life. Due to poor sleep she often did not wake in the morning and Sam was frequently late for school. She thought that her relationship with him had deteriorated as they had little fun and had stopped going out together. Her personal and home life was affected because Susan found it difficult to do her routine household chores. She also thought that she was cooking far more 'junk food' than prior to her depression as this was easier than preparing a 'proper' meal. She thought that the depression had affected her ability to work and she had been off sick from work as a graphic designer for two weeks. Although she wanted to return to work she did not feel well enough to do so. Her social life had been affected. Although Susan had a good network of friends, she had stopped contacting them because she felt ashamed and stigmatized.

The MHW completed a risk assessment and asked Susan directly about risk to self, risk to others, risk from others and risk of vulnerability. Although Susan admitted feeling depressed she had not experienced any thoughts of suicide or of harming herself or others.

Susan described how this episode of depression had begun about a year ago and had gradually worsened. She attributed her depression to a break up of a long-term relationship and work stress. She had suffered from postnatal depression after the birth of Sam which had responded well to antidepressant medication. Susan had been taking Prozac (fluoxetine) 20mg for three months. She felt that the medication had 'taken the edge of her mood' though not improved her depression to the level she had expected.

She rarely drank alcohol and did not take any other medication/drugs.

The MHW asked Susan to complete the Patient Health Questionnaire PHQ-9 (Kroenke *et al.* 2001), a nine item self-rated instrument which enables practitioners and patients to monitor key symptoms of depression/low mood in the previous two weeks. Susan scored 16 which confirmed the MHW's assessment of moderate to severe depression.

The MHW summarized the information that Susan had provided, asked her if it was an accurate reflection of her difficulties and if there was anything else that she thought was particularly relevant to her current difficulties. To ensure that both the MHW and Susan had a shared understanding of the problem, together they devised the following problem formulation.

> 66 Feelings of low mood for one year following the break up of a long-term relationship and work stress resulting in frequent crying, difficulty getting to sleep, a loss of interest in previously enjoyed activities and thoughts of guilt and being a bad mother. The problem impacted on her routine activities, socializing, working and her relationship with her son. 99

The MHW and Susan also identified the following specific goals of treatment, which were to:

- take my son to the cinema once every two weeks;
- meet up with friends once a week;
- return to work.

Delivering a coherent rationale for any intervention is an essential clinical skill which requires giving sufficient information and explanation thereby enabling a client to make an informed choice. The key elements which should be addressed in delivering a rationale for GSH are detailed in Box 29.2.

Box 29.2 Rationale for guided self-help

- **What is guided self-help?**
  - Explain emphasis on self-management
  - Sessions are between 20 and 30 minutes
  - Sessions can be face to face, telephone or email
- **The role of the user**
  - Explain emphasis on self-management
  - They are the expert in their experience of low mood
- **The role of the MHW**
  - To facilitate, support and guide the client with the use of the health technology
  - Use analogy of MHW likened to a personal fitness trainer
  - They are the experts in evidence-based interventions
- **The role of health technology**
  - Explanation of the health technology to be used (e.g. book, CD, DVD, computer program (offer choice and check literacy)
  - Explain the structure of the technology (e.g. contents, how to navigate the structure of the technology)
- **The role of family and friends**
  - Explain how family and friends can help
  - If the user wishes, the facilitator would be happy to discuss any aspects of their care

---

The MHW discussed the rationale of GSH with Susan and gave her a self-help manual and offered the choice of this in the form of a written manual or CD Rom. The self-help manual contained information about depression, GSH, descriptions and application of a range of evidence-based interventions, self-monitoring diaries and 'recovery stories'. The MHW then briefly discussed the evidence-based treatment options for low mood using the ABC model, i.e. interventions could be tailored around the autonomic, behavioural or cognitive components of the model (cf. Chapter 30 of this volume). To help Susan make an informed choice about treatment options, the facilitator indicated she should read or listen to the 'recovery stories'. These illustrated real life accounts of people who had experienced and recovered from low mood/depression using GSH. Each story detailed a specific intervention used – one that described behavioural activation, one describing cognitive restructuring and one describing management of specific symptoms such as sleep disturbance, irritability etc.

Towards the end of the session the MHW sought feedback from Susan on the session, summarized the main points, emphasized the importance of listening or reading the recovery stories and offered Susan the option of the next appointment face-to-face, telephone or email. She opted for a scheduled telephone appointment due to childcare difficulties.

Session 2

In this session a brief review of the week, mood and risk were discussed. Susan had read the 'recovery stories' and opted for behavioural activation as she felt that it was the most practical intervention and one that she felt she could relate to. The MHW discussed the four stages of behavioural activation (see Box 29.3).

Box 29.3   The stages of behavioural activation

- **Stage 1:** Complete a one week behavioural activation diary of current activity.
- **Stage 2:** Decide on the activities that the individual would like to be doing. Some of these things will be routine things. Other things will be pleasurable activities such as going out and meeting people and some things will be important activities that may need to be dealt with quickly.
- **Stage 3:** List these different activities, listing the most difficult things at the top and the easiest activities at the bottom, ensuring that there is a spread of routine and pleasurable activities.
- **Stage 4:** Use the behavioural activation diary to plan the activities, starting with a few easier activities and adding more challenging activities from higher up the list over time.

The MHW explained to Susan how to complete the diary and the first worksheet indicating some of the activities that she would like to be doing. Susan agreed to complete this over the following week and email them to the facilitator the day prior to their next telephone appointment (see Figure 29.1).

Session 3 (Telephone session)

A brief review of the week, mood and risk was discussed. As agreed Susan had emailed the MHW with the completed behavioural activation diary and the list of activities in terms of routine, pleasurable and necessary that she wanted to do (Figure 29.1). Susan said that doing the diary had been useful, but also upsetting as it had highlighted what she needed to do. She also said that the diary had helped to motivate her to change.

		Mon	Tue	Wed	Thur	Fri	Sat	Sun
Morning	What / Where / When / Who	Woke at 9.30 (Sam late for school)	Woke 8.30 called son for school-back to sleep	Woke at 8.00am – called Sam- went back to sleep	Woke at 10.00am (Sam late for school)	Woke at 9.00 (Sam late for school) back to sleep	Slept until 12.00	Slept until 11.00
	What / Where / When / Who	Went back to bed for a couple of hours	Slept	Slept on sofa for an hour	Just sat and did nothing	Did the washing	Slept	Washed and ironed school uniform
Afternoon	What / Where / When / Who	Did a bit of housework	Tried to do some housework but too tired	Did food shopping	Did nothing – just sat staring at TV	Sam's friend came round to play	Promised Sam I would take him cinema but then said I was ill	Watched DVD with Sam but fell asleep
	What / Where / When / Who	Sat and cried	Cooked tea (junk food)	Just sat and did nothing	Went to post office	Cooked tea (more junk)	Went to bed	Slept
Evening	What / Where / When / Who	Friend rang but got Sam to say I was out	sat with Sam and watched TV	Went and got fish and chips for tea	Helped Sam with homework		Cooked tea (mother came over)	Helped Sam with homework
	What / Where / When / Who	Went to bed at about 11.30 did not get to sleep until 4.00am		Could not sleep so watched tv till 3.00am- went to sleep at 3.30am	Went to bed at 2.00 – asleep by 3ish	Went to bed- could not sleep till 4.00am	Went to bed at 1.0pm – fell asleep at 3.00am	Tired –went to bed at 9pm woke at 3.00am

Fig 29.1 Susan's behavioural activation diary

Behavioural Activation Worksheet

Write down your routine activities here: e.g. cleaning, cooking, shopping etc.

Doing some regular housework...
Cooking proper meals and not junk food...........................
..
..
..
..

Write down your pleasurable activities here: e.g. going out/visiting friends or family

Going out with my friends..
Taking my son out (football, cinema etc.).......................
Visiting my parents...
..
..
..
..

Write down your necessary activities here: e.g. paying bills etc.

Going back to work...
Paying bills on time...
Getting my son to school on time....................................
Sort out high school for my son.......................................

Now try to put your lists in order of difficulty
.... Easiest
Doing some regular housework
Taking my son out (football, cinema)
Paying bills on time

....
.... Medium difficulty
Cooking proper meals (not junk food)
Visiting my parents

....
....
....
.... Most difficult
Getting my son to school on time
Sorting out my son's high school
Going back to work...
...

Figure 29.2 Susan's behavioural activation worksheet showing activities in order of difficulty

Susan had received a letter from her son's school asking her to make an appointment to discuss Sam's continued lateness. Using the worksheet the MHW asked Susan to list her activities (Figure 29.1) in order of difficulty (see Figure 29.2). Susan said that one of her most important objectives was to get Sam to school on time even though it was one of the most difficult to achieve. It was agreed that Susan would set an alarm clock, get up at 7.30am every week day morning and get Sam to school. Although difficult Susan also agreed to try not to sleep during the day and to go to bed at a regular time (11.00pm) in order to re-regulate her sleep pattern. She also agreed to do 30 minutes of housework a day and to ring a friend. Susan wrote all these activities onto her diary.

The MHW asked if she foresaw any difficulties with the tasks she had set, summarized the session, asked for any final questions and made a mutually convenient appointment for the following week.

Session 4

This session was a face-to-face session, Susan had managed to get Sam to school everyday on time and had completed 30 minutes housework daily. She had telephoned her friend who had arranged to come to see Susan the following week. She had managed to reduce the time she slept in the day but on two occasions had fallen asleep. Susan was delighted with her progress but said that she was 'stupid as it was so obvious what she needed to do'. The MHW addressed this by commenting on the nature of depression and explaining how it is maintained. Susan and the MHW discussed whether to increase the activities the following week or keep them the same. Susan opted to keep them the same but agreed that if she felt up to it she would make some additions to her diary.

Sessions 5–7

During these telephone sessions, Susan continued to use her daily diary gradually doing the things that she had listed. She had 'bad days' during these weeks but her depression started to improve. Much of the final session focused on how to manage her depression in the future. She was taught by the facilitator to use the PHQ9 once a month to measure her level of depression, and to use her individualized relapse prevention plan. It was agreed that the facilitator would contact Susan in three months for a follow-up session. At the final follow-up session Susan was no longer depressed, was back to work, completing her routine tasks and, most importantly, had re-established her relationship with her son. Her final PHQ9 score was four which indicated that she was not depressed.

Conclusion

In summary, the main points of this chapter are:

- GSH is a valuable part of modern mental health care delivery.
- It plays a key role in increasing access to psychological therapies.
- In spite of this, there remains a mixed evidence base surrounding its effectiveness.
- GSH has, however, been found to be an acceptable and satisfactory intervention for patients and the health professionals delivering it.
- Most of the evidence base surrounding GSH is based on cognitive behavioural therapy principles.
- GSH can be delivered using a number of different delivery modes.
- With 46,000 mental health nurses currently working in the UK there is the opportunity to offer training in brief interventions including guided self-help.

■ Further work is required to determine how the roles of mental health nurses offering brief interventions can be redefined and sustained over time.

Questions for reflection and discussion

1   Think of a client that you have recently seen with mild to moderate depression or anxiety and discuss the following:
    –   The structure of a patient-centred assessment with examples of specific questions you would use to demonstrate collaborative and partnership working;
    –   How you would introduce and deliver a rationale for GSH;
    –   What materials you might suggest (computer programs, books) and why;
    –   How you would support a client using GSH.

Annotated bibliography

■ Lewis, G., Anderson, L. and Araya, R. (2003) *Self-help interventions for mental health problems*. Report to the Department of Health R&D programme. London: Department of Health. Review of self-help interventions commissioned by the Department of Health (England) that demonstrates the increasing interest in the use of self-help for emotional and mental health difficulties. This review identifies weaknesses in previous self-help-based literature in a pragmatic manner in order to summarize key issues that can be drawn from the evidence. The review additionally highlights what recommendations can be made for clinical practice ensuring that practice is evidence based.

■ Richards, D. (2004) Self-help: Empowering service users or aiding cash strapped mental health services. *Journal of Mental Health* **13**(2): 117–23. Richards provides an extremely useful overview of self-help looking at it from the perspective of the user and the health professional. His paper addresses issues surrounding both the clinical and cost effectiveness of its incorporation into the mental health system. Additionally changes that need to be made to incorporate self-help into working practice are stressed and support and training that is required to facilitate self-help is discussed.

References

Anderson, L., Lewis, G., Araya, R. *et al.* (2005) Self-help books for depression: how can practitioners and patients make the right choice? *British Journal of General Practice* **55**: 387–92.

Andersson, G., Bergström, J., Holländare, F., Carlbring, P., Kaldo, K. and Ekselius, L. (2005) Internet-based self-help for depression: a randomised controlled trial. *British Journal of Psychiatry* **187**: 456–61.

Care Services Improvement Partnership (2006) *Designing Primary Care Mental Health Services: Guidebook*. London: DH.

Department of Health (1999) *A National Service Framework for Mental Health*. London: DH.

Department of Health (2000) *The NHS Plan: A plan for investment. A plan for reform*. London: The Stationery Office.

Department of Health (2005) *Self Care – A Real Choice Self Care Support – A Practical Option*. London: COI.

Gega, L., Marks, I. and Mataix-Cols, D. (2004) Computer-aided CBT self help for anxiety and depressive disorders: experience of a London clinic and future directions. *Journal of Clinical Psychology* **60**: 147–57.

Gellatly, J., Bower, P., Hennessy, S., Richards, D., Gilbody, S. and Lovell, K. (2007) What makes self help interventions effective in the management of depressive symptoms? Meta analysis and meta regression. *Psychological Medicine* **37**(9): 1217–28.

Kroenke, K., Spitzer R.L. and Williams, J.B. (2001) The PHQ-9: validity of a brief depression severity measure. *Journal of General Internal Medicine* **16**(9): 606–13.

Lewis, G., Anderson, L. and Araya, R. (2003) *Self-help Interventions for Mental Health Problems.* Report to the Department of Health R&D program. London: Department of Health.

Lovell, K. and Richards, D. (2000) Multiple Access Points and Levels of Entry (MAPLE) ensuring choice, accessibility and equity for CBT services. *Behavioural and Cognitive Psychotherapy* **28**: 379–91.

McCulloch, A. (2003) *Introduction in Primary Solutions: An independent policy review on the development of primary care mental health services.* London: Sainsbury Centre for Mental Health.

Mead, N. and Bower, P. (2000) Patient centredness: a conceptual framework and review of the empirical literature. *Social Science and Medicine* **51**: 1087–110.

Mead, N., MacDonald, W., Bower, P. *et al.* (2005) The clinical effectiveness of guided self-help versus waiting list control in the management of anxiety and depression: a randomised controlled trial. *Psychological Medicine* **35**: 1633–43.

National Collaborating Centre for Mental Health (2004) *Depression: Management of depression in primary and secondary care (National Clinical Practice Guideline 23).* London: NICE.

National Institute for Health and Clinical Excellence (2004) *Depression: management of depression in primary and secondary care.* London: NICE.

Newell, R. (2000) General consultation skills, in R. Newell and K. Gournay (eds) *Mental Health Nursing: an evidence based approach.* Edinburgh: Churchill Livingstone.

Office of the Deputy Prime Minister (2004) *Mental Health and Social Exclusion, Social Exclusion Unit Report.* London: ODPM.

Proudfoot, J., Ryden, C., Everitt, B. *et al.* (2004) Clinical efficacy of computerised cognitive-behavioural therapy for anxiety and depression in primary care: a randomised controlled trial. *British Journal of Psychiatry* **185**: 46–54.

Richards, D. (2004) Self-help: Empowering service users or aiding cash strapped mental health services. *Journal of Mental Health* **13**(2): 117–23.

Richards, A., Barkham, M., Cahill, J., Richards, D., Williams, C. and Heywood, P. (2003) PHASE: a randomised, controlled trial of supervised self-help cognitive behavioural therapy in primary care. *British Journal of General Practice* **53**: 764–70.

Rost, K., Nutting, P., Smith, J., Werner, J. and Duan, N. (2001) Improving depression outcomes in community primary care practice: a randomized trial of the QuEST Intervention. *Journal of General Internal Medicine* **16**(3): 143–9.

Tylee, A. (2001) Major depressive disorder (MDD) from the patient's perspective: overcoming barriers to appropriate care. *International Journal of Psychiatry in Clinical Practice* **5**(suppl.): s37–s42.

van Boeijen, C.A., van Oppen, P., van Balkom, A.J.L.M. *et al.* (2005) Treatment of anxiety disorders in primary care practice: a randomised controlled trial. *British Journal of General Practice* **55**: 763–9.

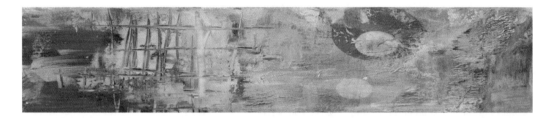

CHAPTER 30

Behavioural techniques

Lina Gega

Chapter overview

Behavioural techniques are focused activities that aim to change behavioural patterns associated with the symptoms, distress and disability of mental health problems. The techniques stem from behaviour therapy, a treatment approach based on learning theories (classical and operant conditioning), that is, that people's behaviours could be sustained or extinct in the presence or absence of strong associations and positive or negative reinforcements.

The clinical application of appropriate behavioural techniques is determined by the problem they aim to treat, and choosing the right technique for the right problem is the cornerstone of evidence-based practice in behaviour therapy. Behavioural techniques have been proven effective for anxiety and stress-related problems (phobias, obsessive compulsive disorder, post-traumatic stress disorder, panic disorder, generalized anxiety disorder), depressive disorders, some medically unexplained symptoms, impulse control problems and habits disorders. Promising results have also been reported for psychotic disorders and bipolar affective disorder.

The delivery of behavioural techniques should be considered as part of the therapeutic process underpinning most types of interventions. This therapeutic process comprises building and maintaining a working relationship, assessing the client and formulating the problem, facilitating and monitoring care, working with families and carers, measuring progress and outcome, and setting up a relapse prevention programme. The structured nature of behavioural techniques allow for flexibility in their delivery according to the client's needs and preferences. For example, professional support could be minimized if the client chooses to carry out the techniques guided by self-help materials.

The first part of this chapter outlines:

- learning theories that explain the maintenance of mental health problems;
- the mechanisms that make behavioural techniques work.

Subsequent sections describe the practical tasks or procedures involved in five fundamental behavioural techniques:

- graded exposure and response prevention;
- controlled worry time;
- symptom management techniques;

- awareness training;
- behavioural activation.

Behavioural explanations of problem maintenance and treatment mechanisms

Mental health problems, or physical problems influenced by mental health factors, are associated with certain experiences both *external* (for example, environmental circumstances, certain objects and situations, etc.) and *internal* (for example, automatic thoughts, bodily sensations, symptoms of an illness, etc.). These experiences trigger various responses which are either a person's way of coping with the experience or simply a reaction to urges and habits. Some of these responses could be helpful for one's problems, such as leaving the room when feeling the urge to 'lash out' and talking to people when feeling low instead of isolating oneself. Others could be unhelpful or even harmful, for example, avoiding going out because of fears and anxieties or using self-injury or substance misuse as a way of relieving tension. Problems are maintained and exacerbated when unhelpful/harmful responses to a trigger are reinforced and helpful/harmless responses are weakened or extinct.

There are three mechanisms which maintain and reinforce unhelpful/harmful responses:

- The trigger-response association becomes automatic and involuntary (*conditioned responses*), therefore, the person has no control over the occurrence and frequency of the response. Examples include habits, tics, certain types of insomnia and some impulsive behaviours.
- The behaviours bring about a temporary relief from unpleasant feelings therefore they become more likely to occur (*negative reinforcement*, Figure 30.1). Negatively reinforced behaviours usually refer to escape, avoidance, reassurance and rituals which a person may use to prevent, reduce or manage distress (for example, in anxiety disorders or psychosis).
- The behaviours result in pleasure and reward therefore they become more likely to occur (*positive reinforcement*, Figure 30.2). Positively reinforced behaviours are usually associated with urges in impulse control problems (such as pathological gambling, kleptomania, paraphilias, etc.).

In addition, a problem may be maintained if helpful/harmless behaviours are weakened or extinct because of:

1 *Lack of practice*: For example, social skills deficits may be the result of social avoidance during which the person has not practised social interactions.
2 *Temporary unpleasant feelings*: For example, people may avoid facing up to their anxieties and problems because this can be stressful and unpleasant.
3 *Lack of response-contingent reinforcement* (reward or pleasure as expected): For example, if a person works hard and there is no reward or problem resolution, then the person may become frustrated or feel hopeless leading to feelings of despair, anger, etc.

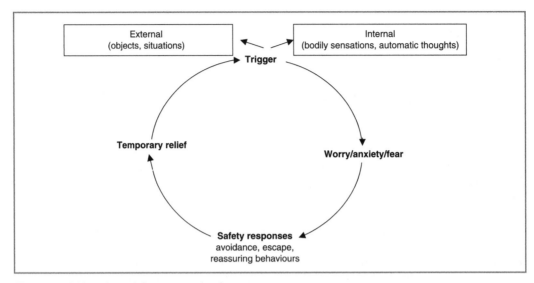

Figure 30.1 Negative reinforcement of safety responses

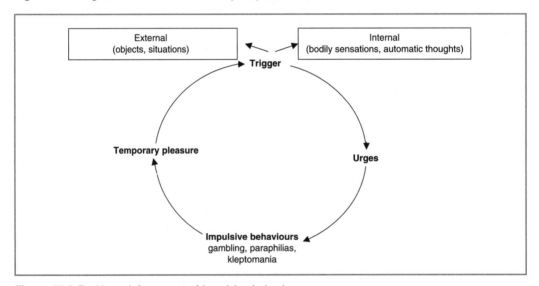

Figure 30.2 Positive reinforcement of impulsive behaviours

Behavioural techniques teach people how to unlearn unhelpful/harmful behaviours and relearn more helpful/harmless responses to external and internal triggers. This is achieved by:

■ breaking the association between trigger and unhelpful/harmful responses and establishing an association between trigger and helpful/ harmless responses;
■ interrupting the cycle of negative or positive reinforcement of unhelpful/harmful responses;
■ reducing the physical symptoms and emotional distress associated with a trigger;
■ introducing a response-contingent reinforcement for helpful responses.

A diagrammatic illustration of how behavioural models explain the maintenance of a problem and the way behavioural techniques work, is given in Figure 30.3.

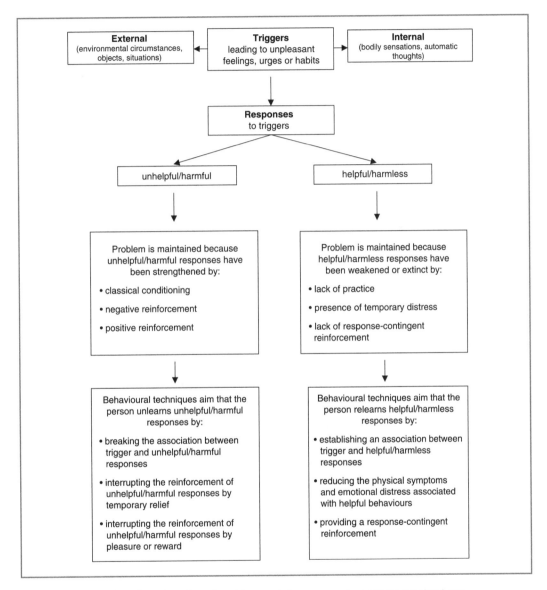

Figure 30.3 Behavioural explanation of problem maintenance and treatment mechanisms

Graded exposure and response prevention

This technique has been extensively studied and proven effective for a range of anxiety and stress-related problems, from phobias and panic to post-traumatic stress and obsessive compulsive disorders. Graded exposure is the process of confronting anxiety and fear-provoking triggers, starting from the least unpleasant and building up to the most dreaded one. The preplanned grading of relevant triggers for exposure is known as 'hierarchy'. Response prevention means that the person refrains from carrying out any behaviours which 'mask' or avoid fear and anxiety (safety behaviours) during and after exposure, for example, seeking reassurance or performing rituals (Marks 1986).

The mechanism which explains how graded exposure and response prevention work is called 'habituation', this is the reduction of anxiety over time when a person encounters an anxiety/fear-provoking trigger without the use of safety behaviours. Consequently, the negative reinforcement of safety behaviours is interrupted, and with repeated exposure and response prevention these behaviours are extinct because they no longer serve the purpose of providing relief from anxiety and fear. An explanation of the mechanism with which graded exposure and response prevention work is given in Figure 30.4.

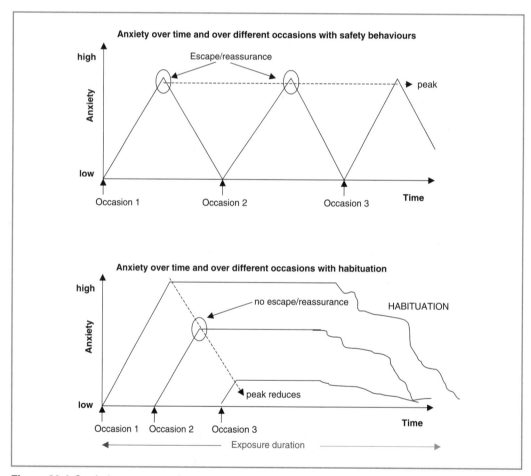

Figure 30.4 Graded exposure and response prevention

Anxiety is the body's natural response to excessive adrenaline production when a person is faced with a situation which is threatening or is perceived as threatening. Adrenaline prepares the body for a flight-or-fight response to an actual or perceived threat. This means that the person experiences physiological changes resulting from increased oxygen flow and blood supply to the muscles, leading to increased heart and breathing rate, increased blood pressure, sweating, blurred vision, etc. Anxiety increases until it reaches a peak when the individual tries to deal with it either by escaping from the situation or by doing certain reassuring or ritualistic things to 'mask' or avoid the anxiety.

With escape and avoidance, the anxiety goes down rapidly but will reappear as soon as the individual comes across the same trigger. If the individual remains exposed to the trigger for a certain period of time without running away or masking the symptoms of anxiety, then the excess adrenaline in the body is gradually depleted and anxiety symptoms eventually subside. Over repeated and prolonged exposure to the same or similar triggers, anxiety peaks at an increasingly lower lever and eventually fades away.

Graded exposure and response prevention involves the following steps:

1   Create a hierarchy of triggers (Figure 30.5). This is a list of all anxiety or fear-provoking experiences with ratings of distress in a 0–8 scale (0 = not at all distressing and 8 = extremely distressing). Triggers could be anything that a person avoids altogether, or situations which the person can cope with only by using safety behaviours. Questions to ask in order to elicit triggers are: 'Is there anything that you avoid because of the problem?' 'What brings your fear/anxiety/worry on?' 'What places, things or people make you feel uncomfortable?'

Set exposure tasks which relate to each trigger (Figure 30.6). These are exercises comprising the following components:

■   behaviours (what to do and in what order);
■   conditions (where, with whom, when, with what response prevention);
■   frequency (how often and how many times);
■   duration (a specified time period or until the anxiety subsides by 50 per cent).

For example, an exposure task for someone who is anxious about going far from home and into public places could be: 'To travel a mile away from home to the nearest shopping centre, everyday for a week, alone without carrying with me my mobile phone or my anxiety pills, and stay there for 1 hour or until my anxiety reduces by 50 per cent.'

In summary, an exposure task should be:

■   *Graded*: i.e. to start from the easiest to achieve and build up towards the most difficult task which could also be the final goal of the exposure programme.
■   *Focused*: i.e. the person should experience the whole range of anxiety without trying to mask it or avoid it with subtle behaviours.
■   *Repeated*: i.e. to carry out the same exposure task as many times as needed until it can be done with relative ease and minimal anxiety.
■   *Prolonged*: i.e. to stay with the anxiety long enough without any safety behaviours to allow habituation to take place.

Practise each exposure task in the list for as many times as needed until the task is performed with relative ease. Keep a record of when the task is carried out, and the anxiety experienced before, during and after exposure (Figure 30.7). Distress and discomfort are part of exposure and although they are unpleasant, they are not harmful. However, if someone finds an exposure task too difficult to achieve then:

■   Grade down the task by choosing a less distressing trigger to confront.

Hierarchy

List and rate all the situations which would trigger anxiety, fear or distress if you had to face them, using this scale:

0---------1----------2-----------3----------4---------5----------6-----------7----------8
not at all   slightly   moderately   very much   extremely

Triggers	*Ratings*
Most dreaded	
1 _____	
2 _____	
3 _____	
4 _____	
5 _____	
6 _____	
7 _____	
8 _____	
9 _____	
10 _____	
11 _____	
Least dreaded	

Figure 30.5 Hierarchy of triggers associated with distressing feelings

- Vary the task by either choosing a trigger with similar fear/anxiety rating or change some of the behaviours, conditions and frequency of the exposure (but not the duration as this would effect habituation).
- Use coping methods, such as controlled breathing, tension release and coping cards (described later on this chapter) which could make the task more tolerable. Such techniques should be dropped at a later stage in exposure because they could become safety behaviours which interfere with habituation.

Exposure tasks

List all the exposure tasks according to your hierarchy of triggers. Practise each task using your daily exposure diary and when you can do your chosen task with relative ease, note the date and move to the next task up the list.

Exposure tasks	*Date achieved*
Most difficult	
1 _____	
2 _____	
3 _____	
4 _____	
5 _____	
6 _____	
7 _____	
8 _____	
9 _____	
10 _____	
11 _____	
Least difficult	

Figure 30.6 List of exposure tasks

■ Use clinician-guided exposure, such as modelling, accompany the patient, etc., to demonstrate how to best carry out the task and as a way of initially managing the discomfort or embarrassment that the person carrying the exposure may feel.

It is important to note that moving too quickly up the hierarchy of triggers and its corresponding exposure tasks may be traumatic, and more harmful than helpful because of the excessive distress it may cause. It can also be disheartening if the person cannot achieve the task and consider themselves to have failed. However, moving too slowly could be

Daily exposure diary

Choose one or more tasks from your list of exposure tasks, note the date and rate the anxiety/distress you felt before, during and after the task using this scale:

0---------1----------2-----------3---------4--------5----------6----------7----------8
not at all   slightly   moderately   very much   extremely

If you used or did anything to make yourself feel better or to be able to carry out the task, make a note under the column 'coping methods'.

Date	Task no.	Anxiety / Distress rating			Coping methods
		Before	During	After	

Figure 30.7 Daily exposure diary

ineffective because the person does not experience the degree of anxiety that would allow habituation to take place. Also, having to practise two or three exposure tasks of slight anxiety could be more unpleasant than having to practise one task of moderate anxiety. In conclusion, the pace of exposure should be negotiated with the person that carries it out and the fine tuning of the tasks is ongoing according to the person's strengths and preferences.

Controlled worry time

The underlying principle of this technique is that worry begins as a coping response to external or internal triggers but becomes uncontrollable and distressing, hence a problem in itself. Controlled worry time (versions of which are described by Borkovec *et al.* 1983 and Wells 1997) aims to reduce worrying thoughts and the distress associated with them by:

■ giving a sense of controllability over the frequency (how often), occurrence (under what circumstances) and duration (for how long) of worrying thoughts;

■ breaking the association between certain external or internal triggers and worry as a coping response to them;

■ change worry from a distressing experience into a problem-solving activity.

This technique has been mainly described and applied for generalized anxiety disorder, however, the relevance of worry control strategies extends to other mental health problems in which worry is a concomitant feature; for example, a schizophrenia sufferer could interpret mental symptoms of worry (muddled thinking, lack of concentration) as a sign of relapse or a depression sufferer could have ruminatory worry about coping with everyday life. The components of controlled worry time are:

1 Identify worrying thoughts. The frequency, occurrence, duration and content of the worrying thoughts depend on the individual's experiences. The person may use a personal or standardized diary to record and monitor their worrying thoughts (Figure 30.8).

2 Establish a 'worry-time' of 30 minutes to take place at the same location every day. There is no ideal place and time; a person may choose a time in the day which allows privacy and solitude or may prefer to have a 'worry-time' when there are other people around who could offer support.

3 If catching yourself worrying at other times, postpone worrying until the designated 'worry-time' and attend to other everyday things. This could be quite difficult at the beginning, but would get easier with practice. Try to transfer your worrying thoughts from your 'head' to a piece of paper (i.e. worry record above) and put this aside until the designated worry-time.

4 Use the worry-time to address your concerns; you may need to carry out a problem-solving plan to deal with factual difficulties or challenge any unrealistic or overestimated fears. Alternatively, you don't have to worry at (and for) the designated time. If you choose not to worry at the designated time, be sure that you do so *not* because you want to avoid it but because you do not feel it is necessary.

Symptom management techniques

Although symptom management techniques may not produce fundamental changes, they facilitate progress by reducing distressing feelings, such as anger, anxiety, fear and worry, and making them manageable to enable other behavioural techniques to take place. Three symptom-management techniques are mentioned here: controlled breathing, tension-release exercises and coping cards.

Worry diary

Under 'situation' note what you were doing, when, where and with whom, every time you feel worried, scared or anxious. Under 'worry' write down what you were worried about, how you felt, what you were thinking, etc.

Day and time	Situation	Worry

Figure 30.8 Example of diary to be used in controlled worry-time

Controlled breathing

The aim of controlled breathing is to restore the oxygen–carbon dioxide balance and acid–alkali balance which can be disrupted because of changes in the breathing rate under conditions of fear or acute stress. The key in controlled breathing is to *breathe in from the abdomen*, keep the chest still, *breathe out slowly and fully* and keep a regular pace between breathing in and out with pauses in-between. A way to know that this is done properly is when the abdomen moves out when you breathe in and moves in when you breathe out. This could be difficult to get used to, because most people breathe in from their chest and their stomach tends to move in as they breathe in. It is better to practise abdominal breathing when calm and comfortable in order to master the technique so that it can be used with the first warning signals of psychological arousal.

Tension-release exercises

Tension-release exercises (Gournay 1995) have been established as part of a comprehensive applied relaxation training programme for anxiety conditions (Ost 1987). Tension-release exercises aim to control physiological arousal symptoms, such as muscle tension, sweating, pounding heart, light-headedness, 'butterflies in the stomach', etc. The person learns to recognize these symptoms early and control them before they reach their peak. This can be achieved by systematically tensing muscle groups in the body for five seconds and then releasing them for about ten seconds. The exercises are first practised for 20–30 minutes in comfortable conditions and then could be done in distress-provoking situations. It is important that:

- the muscles are only tensed until the person feels a sense of 'pulling'; too much pressure may cause injuries or the muscles may not be able to relax after releasing the tension;
- the release of the muscles should be immediate and NOT gradual.

Figure 30.9 describes in detail how to carry out tension-release exercises.

Coping cards

The person uses small index cards or pieces of paper or a certain part of their diary to write a few sentences which are:

- Encouraging: 'I have dealt with worse before, this is just fear and I won't let it get the best of me', 'I'm getting better at this all the time.'
- Challenging: 'Don't jump into conclusions or take it personally', 'There is no need to prove myself, I am good enough as I am.'
- Self-instructions or reminders: 'I must walk away now', 'Time to step back and take a breath', 'I'll make a note of this so I can take it out of my mind now and talk about it with my friend later.'

Awareness training

Awareness training can be used for actions/behaviours which are associated with impulses, urges or habits, such as eating disorders, self-injuries, habits, trichotillomania, kleptomania, anger problems, etc. The purpose of awareness training is to:

1 become aware of the stages before the behaviour occurs, so that the person can break the association between trigger–harmful response and be able to practise an alternative response on time;
2 become familiar with the behaviour itself, so that the person can develop an effective alternative response;
3 become familiar with any unpleasant (potential or actual) consequences of the harmful behaviour, so that any elements of pleasure or relief associated with it are weakened and gradually extinct.

Muscle groups	Tension-release exercise	Time
Hands and forearms	First with right, then with left hand and forearm. • Clench your fist until knuckles are white and the muscles in your forearm feel tense. • Release by letting the hand fall loose.	x2 5 sec. 10 sec.
Arm	First with right, then with left arm. • Clench your fist and bend the arm to 90˚ trying to make your biceps muscle bulge. • Release by letting the hand and arm fall loose.	x2 5 sec. 10 sec.
Head *Forehead and eyebrows*	• Wrinkle the forehead by raising the eyebrows. • Release by letting the eyebrows relax. • Bring the eyebrows close together as in frowning. • Release by letting the eyebrows relax.	5 sec. 10 sec. 5 sec. 10 sec.
Eyes	• Screw up your eyes and hold them tightly shut. • Release by opening your eyes and letting your eyelids relax.	5 sec. 10 sec.
Jaw	• Tense the jaw by biting the teeth together. • Release by letting the jaws relax (they are *NOT* clenched).	5 sec. 10 sec.
Tongue	• Press the tongue flat against the roof of your mouth until you notice tension in your throat. • Release by letting the tongue rest (make sure your jaws are *NOT* clenched together).	5 sec. 10 sec.
Lips	• Press the lips tightly together as in a pout. • Release by letting the lips relax (make sure your jaws are *NOT* clenched together).	5 sec. 10 sec.
Neck	• Let the head fall back (towards the chair) without pushing it back and then let the head fall forward (your chin towards your chest without touching it). • Release by bringing the head in the upright position.	5 sec. 10 sec.
Shoulders	• Hunch the shoulders up towards the ears and then circle the shoulders. • Release by letting the shoulders drop.	5 sec. 10 sec.
Back	• Push your elbows into your side, push your shoulders down, push your head towards your chest and feel your big muscles across your back tense. • Release by letting your elbows relax, your shoulders drop, and your head in the upright position.	5 sec. 10 sec.
Chest	• Push your shoulders back, push your elbows down, tilt your head back and feel the muscles in your chest tighten. • Release by relaxing the shoulders and elbows and bringing the head in the upright position.	5 sec. 10 sec.
Stomach	• Tense the muscles of the stomach and push the stomach inwards. • Release by letting the muscles relax.	5 sec. 10 sec.
Buttocks and thighs	• Squeeze your thighs and buttocks together. • Release by relaxing the muscles.	5 sec. 10 sec.
Calves and shins	• Keeping the leg straight, tense the calves by pushing the feet and toes downwards. • Release by letting the feet fall loose. • Keeping the leg straight, tense the shins by pulling the feet and toes upwards. • Release by letting the feet fall loose.	5 sec. 10 sec. 5 sec. 10 sec.
Feet	• Curl over your toes, trying to make a fist with your toes. • Release by letting the feet fall loose.	5 sec. 10 sec.

Figure 30.9 Tension-release exercises

Awareness training mainly involves self-monitoring using a diary (Figure 30.10) so as to recognize:

1   triggers, cues, warning signals and actions/behaviours associated with the urge;
2   the components of the impulsive action/behaviour itself as a response to the urge;
3   the (potential or actual) consequences of the action/behaviour.

Incident awareness record			
Trigger What were you doing? Who were you with, when and where?	**Urge** How strong was the urge? 0---2----4----6---8---10 not at all extremely	**Response** What did you do as a response to your urge? Describe in as much detail as possible.	**Consequences** What happened afterwards and how did you feel?

Figure 30.10 Self-monitoring diary for awareness training

Awareness training is the first step for the treatment of many problems that involve a certain urge of habit. The technique itself is enough to reduce the occurrence of a certain problem behaviour, but it is also combined with avoiding cues which trigger the urge–response cycle and with rehearsing alternative responses following cue exposure.

Behavioural activation

Behavioural activation has been used to tackle problems associated with low levels of activity and lack of pleasure or satisfaction, as it may happen in depression or negative symptoms of schizophrenia. The aim of behavioural activation is to (a) increase the levels of daily activity which could have a positive effect on energy levels and motivation, (b) introduce pleasant, rewarding and interesting events as a positive reinforcement to daily routine. Behavioural activation comprises the following components: activity monitoring, activity rating, activity scheduling and graded task assignment (Fennell 1989; Greenberger and Padesky 1995).

Activity monitoring

The person needs to use a daily or weekly diary to record the time and type of activities (Figures 30.11 and 30.12). If the sleep pattern of the person is interrupted, then it may be helpful to have a 24-hour diary to monitor their pattern of sleep and what activities take place just before the person goes to bed or just after the person wakes up in the night.

Sometimes a person may write 'doing nothing' if they consider that what they do is not productive or is not what they wanted to do in the first place; things such as sleeping, lying in bed, or watching out of the window are still activities and it is important that they are recorded to demonstrate their link with depressive feelings or negative symptoms.

Activity rating

In the activity monitoring diary, rate each activity using a scale 0–10; 0 meaning 'not at all' and 10 meaning 'extremely'. Intermediate ratings points could be 2 for 'slightly', 4 for 'somewhat', 6 for 'quite a lot' and 8 for 'very much'.

Put a P for PLEASURE with a 0–10 rating next to the activities that may be enjoyable (e.g. watching TV, eating). For example P0 would mean that the person did not enjoy the activity at all, P5 that they moderately enjoyed it and P10 that they very much enjoyed it. The purpose of pleasure ratings is to establish (a) activities that the person used to enjoy but not any more, either because they do not have the motivation or energy to do them or because they do them but do not enjoy them; and (b) activities that the person still enjoys to some extent, and that, therefore, there is scope to build on these activities.

Put an M for MASTERY with the 0–10 rating according to the difficulty of achievement *given how the person felt at the time* (doing the housework, taking children to school). For example M0 would be that the person found the activity quite effortless and did not give them a sense of achievement, M5 that the activity was moderately difficult to achieve but the person managed it, whereas M10 would represent a difficult activity that was an achievement to complete. The purpose of mastery ratings is to demonstrate that (a) a person may achieve more things than they give themselves credit for, because achievement is not what a person *wished they achieved* but what a person *did achieve* considering their circumstances (for example, low energy because of depression, no support, etc.), and (b) if the person does

Week beginning: _____

	Monday		Tuesday		Wednesday		Thursday		Friday		Saturday		Sunday
	a.m.		a.m.		a.m.		a.m.		a.m.		a.m.		a.m.
Time:		Time:		Time:		Time:		Time:		Time:		Time:	
M =	P =	M =	P =	M =	P =	M =	P =	M =	P =	M =	P =	M =	P =
Time:		Time:		Time:		Time:		Time:		Time:		Time:	
M =	P =	M =	P =	M =	P =	M =	P =	M =	P =	M =	P =	M =	P =
Time:		Time:		Time:		Time:		Time:		Time:		Time:	
M =	P =	M =	P =	M =	P =	M =	P =	M =	P =	M =	P =	M =	P =
	p.m.		p.m.		p.m.		p.m.		p.m.		p.m.		p.m.
Time:		Time:		Time:		Time:		Time:		Time:		Time:	
M =	P =	M =	P =	M =	P =	M =	P =	M =	P =	M =	P =	M =	P =
Time:		Time:		Time:		Time:		Time:		Time:		Time:	
M =	P =	M =	P =	M =	P =	M =	P =	M =	P =	M =	P =	M =	P =
Time:		Time:		Time:		Time:		Time:		Time:		Time:	
M =	P =	M =	P =	M =	P =	M =	P =	M =	P =	M =	P =	M =	P =

Figure 30.11 Weekly activity monitoring

Time	Activity What did I do? Where was it? Was anyone there?	Pleasure How interesting and enjoyable was it? 0----2-----4-----6----8----10 not at all very much	Mastery How difficult was it to achieve given my circumstances? 0----2-----4-----6---8----10 not at all very much

Date: _____

Figure 30.12 Daily activity monitoring

things which only require little or no effort, then there is scope to schedule activities with gradually increased effort and consequently increasingly greater sense of achievement.

Activity scheduling

Using a diary similar to the one used for daily activity monitoring, the person plans in advance their hour-by-hour activities (Figure 30.13). There are two types of tasks which need to be scheduled:

■ Tasks which the person *has* to do in balance with tasks that the person *wants* to do. The aim of activity scheduling is not to do as many things as possible in the time we have, but to plan the time we are going to spend on a particular activity in order to complete specific tasks.

■ Sometimes people find it easier to come up with the tasks that *have* to be done rather than activities that could be just pleasurable and interesting. Pleasant/interesting activities rather than chores could crop up from the activity monitoring diary (the ones with high pleasure ratings) or from a detailed history about things that the person used to enjoy in their everyday life but stopped doing because of their depression, or from questions about things that the person always wanted to do but never did.

The person records the planned activity in detail (including what is to be done, with whom and where) and then the actual activity which took place, including whether it was similar, greater or smaller than the planned one. Then, the person records mastery and pleasure ratings as they did in the activity monitoring diary. If the planned activity was too difficult, then the person may have felt disheartened and did not do anything at all, in which case it would be useful to downgrade the task (see Graded task assignment) in order to make the activity manageable.

Graded task assignment

Graded task assignment is helpful for things that the person wants to achieve but are too difficult under their current circumstances and need to be broken down before they are introduced in the activity scheduling diary. Using the Activities list (Figure 30.13) the person could identify all the things they want to achieve during a certain period, always taking into consideration the balance between pleasures (things they *have to* do) and responsibilities (things they *need to* do). For each activity identified, there could be five potential actions:

1   omit, if the activities/tasks exceed the available time;
2   delegate, wherever possible;
3   postpone activities which are of lower priority;
4   seek help and support whenever possible;
5   grade the task: if, for example, the task is 'to get the children ready for school and take them there' but the person cannot do it because he or she feels exhausted or overwhelmed, then a grading could be 'prepare their packed lunch the night before – get up just before they go and just say goodbye – get up in the morning and make them drinks – get up in the morning and prepare drinks and breakfast – get up in the morning, prepare drinks, breakfast and take them to school'.

Date: _____

Time	Planned activity What am I going to do? Where? Will anyone help/be involved?	Actual activity What did I actually do? How did it compare with the planned activity? Was it *similar, greater or smaller* than planned?	Pleasure How interesting and enjoyable was it? 0—2—4—6—8—10 not at all very much	Mastery How difficult was it to achieve given my circumstances? 0—2—4—6—8—10 not at all very much

Figure 30.13 Daily activity scheduling

Conclusion

This chapter described 'what to do' in order to carry out some key behavioural techniques and how these techniques may work based on learning theories. Their application should be based on research evidence about what technique is proven effective for which problems and should be done with guidance by experienced clinicians. Apart from the main activities comprising each behavioural technique, their delivery in practice is more complicated and may yield difficulties because people that nurses care for could have the same problem but vastly different needs, strengths and limitations. Therefore, this chapter aimed to give the main action points and 'conceptual pegs' that practitioners could build upon with further reading, training and supervision.

In summary, the main points of this chapter are:

■   Behavioural models understand mental health problems as a vicious circle of triggers (external, internal), responses (coping behaviours, habits, urges) and consequences (either strong associations, or relief from unpleasant feelings, or ensuing pleasure maintaining a problem-related response).

■   Behavioural techniques are focused activities which aim to manage the symptoms, distress and disability associated with a problem by (a) reducing or removing unhelpful or harmful responses to triggers, and (b) reinforcing more helpful/harmless behaviours.

■   The five fundamental behavioural techniques described were: graded exposure and response prevention, controlled worry, symptom-management techniques (controlled breathing, tension-release exercises and coping cards), awareness training and behavioural activation.

Questions for reflection and discussion

1   Considering that mental health and illness occur in a continuum, what relevance do you think the behavioural techniques described in this chapter may have for your responses to everyday life experiences? Specifically:

(a)   Do you have any fears or anxieties that graded exposure and response prevention may relate to?

(b)   Do you ever worry, so that controlled worry-time may be helpful?

(c)   Do you ever feel miserable, sluggish or overwhelmed by daily tasks, in which case behavioural activation could apply?

(d)   Do you ever act on impulse, which you would like to be more in control of by using awareness training?

(e)   Do you ever get panicky and nervous, in which case symptom management techniques may be useful?

2   Focusing on one of the questions 1(a)–1(e) above, follow the relevant behavioural technique for one week. What difficulties have you experienced in trying to implement this technique and what have you learnt from it which could be useful in its application to your everyday practice?

3   Select one of the behavioural techniques which you find particularly interesting or relevant to your line of work.

(a) Explain to a colleague how the technique works, taking into account learning theories and drawing a trigger–response–consequence diagram.

(b) Find three research papers which study the implementation of this behavioural technique for mental health problems.

(c) How relevant are the papers for the clients/patients you usually care for? The type of service you work in? The expertise you have? The supervision available to you in order to implement the techniques safely and efficiently?

Annotated bibliography

■ Marks, I.M. (2001) *Living with Fear: Understanding and Coping with Anxiety* (2nd edn). London: McGraw-Hill. A best-seller in many countries worldwide, this user-friendly and informative read explains the nature of fear and anxiety in relation to a range of disorders such as phobias, panic, obsessive compulsive disorder and sexual anxieties. The book is enriched throughout with self-help instructions and case examples of people who got help by using various behavioural techniques for their problems.

■ Gamble, C. and Brennan, G. (eds) (2000) *Working with Serious Mental Illness: A Manual for Clinical Practice*. London: Baillière Tindall in association with the Royal College of Nursing. Chapter 9 has very useful applications of the triggers–responses–consequences behavioural paradigm for severe mental illness using the stress-vulnerability model and coping strategy enhancement. Chapter 13 describes behavioural strategies, such as self-monitoring and alternative-response training, in working with people with severe mental illness and anger management problems.

■ Haddock, G. and Slade, P.D. (eds) (1996) *Cognitive-behavioural Interventions with Psychotic Disorders*. London: Routledge. Chapters 2, 3 and 5 provide a theoretical background, evidence base and case examples of behavioural techniques in the management and treatment of psychotic symptoms (mostly in conjunction with cognitive theories and techniques). A comprehensive and stimulating read comprising chapters from nearly all leading specialists in the field of CBT for psychosis in the UK.

References

Borkovec, T.D., Wilkinson, L., Folensbee, R. and Lerman, C. (1983) Stimulus control applications to the treatment of worry. *Behaviour Research and Therapy* 21: 247–51.

Fennell, M.J.V. (1989) Depression, in K. Hawton, P. Salkovskis, J. Kirk and D. Clark (eds) *Cognitive Behaviour Therapy for Psychiatric Problems: A Practical Guide*. Oxford: Oxford University Press, pp. 169–234.

Gournay, K. (1995) *Stress Management: A Guide to Coping with Stress*. Surrey: Asset Books.

Greenberger, D. and Padesky, C.A. (1995) *Mind Over Mood: Change How you Feel by Changing the Way you Think*. London: Guilford Press.

Marks, I.M. (1986) *Behavioural Psychotherapy: Maudsley Pocket Book of Clinical Management*. Bristol: Wright.

Ost, L.G. (1987) Applied relaxation: description of a coping technique and review of controlled studies. *Behaviour Research and Therapy* 25: 397–410.

Wells, A. (1997) *Cognitive Therapy of Anxiety Disorders: A Practice Manual and Conceptual Guide*. Chichester: Wiley and Sons.

CHAPTER 31

Cognitive techniques

Lina Gega

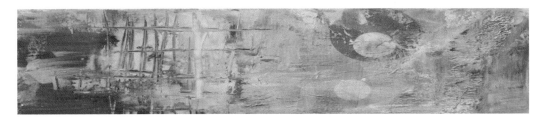

Chapter overview

Cognitive techniques are guided dialogues and focused activities that aim to change inaccurate, distorted or unhelpful beliefs about situations and signs or symptoms that a person may experience. The techniques stem from cognitive therapy, a treatment approach based on information-processing theories, that is, people's emotional, physical and behavioural responses to certain experiences are shaped by how people perceive these experiences and what meaning they attach to them.

This chapter describes the role of perception and thinking in the maintenance of mental health problems and outlines three groups of techniques as part of a process called cognitive restructuring, i.e. identifying misinterpretations and unhelpful ideas, generating alternative interpretations and constructive ideas, and testing and reinforcing the alternatives. This process has been applied successfully for anxiety and stress-related problems, depressive disorders, somatic problems, psychotic disorders and bipolar affective disorder. The chapter concludes by comparing cognitive and behavioural techniques in light of the integrated therapeutic approach known as cognitive behaviour therapy (CBT).

This chapter covers:

- the role of thoughts in mental health;
- techniques to identify misinterpretations and unhelpful ideas;
- techniques to generate alternative interpretations and constructive ideas;
- techniques to test and reinforce alternatives;
- cognitive and behavioural techniques: segregation or integration?

The role of thoughts in mental health

The term 'cognitive' relates to thinking and perception, two processes by which individuals interpret their experiences and form ideas about themselves and the world around them (Beck 1976). Thoughts are formed by words and images, and their content varies according to a person's past and present experiences. Thoughts which contribute to the maintenance of mental health problems share two common characteristics:

- they contain some form of inaccuracy or distortion;

■ they form a significant part of a person's reality and they feed into the symptoms, distress and disability associated with the problem.

The difference between 'normal' thoughts and those associated with mental health problems is not so much in their content as it is in the degree of conviction and significance that a person may attach to them. Such thoughts are considered under four groups below:

■ *Negative automatic thoughts and intrusive thoughts*: They trigger distressing feelings (fear, worry, anxiety or low mood) and the person feels that he or she has no control over their occurrence.

■ *Overvalued ideas and delusions*: They appear to digress from ideas that are acceptable or common within a person's environment and the person has a strong conviction in them.

■ *Catastrophic beliefs and feared consequences*: They are ideas that something awful may happen if a person does not carry out certain behaviours, or does not avoid certain situations.

■ *Assumptions, core beliefs, personal rules and schemas*: These are beliefs which have been developed through life experiences and shape or influence a person's views and actions in response to a critical incident.

Given that thoughts are the result of information processing in relation to past and present experiences, misinterpretations or unhelpful ideas are the result of information processing errors, as outlined below:

■ *Catastrophizing*: expecting the worst to happen and overestimating the probability of it happening.

■ *Emotional reasoning*: using feelings to guide our judgement and confusing how things feel with how things really are.

■ *Dichotomous thinking*: thinking in absolute terms, all-or-nothing, black-or-white, not considering the middle ground.

■ *Arbitrary inference*: jumping to conclusions, making judgements without evidence, believing that we know what others are thinking, predicting the future.

■ *Generalizing*: making sweeping statements based on single incidents, overestimating the importance of isolated events.

■ *Personalizing*: assuming that one has responsibility over everything, blaming ourselves over things that we have little control or influence on.

■ *Selective focus and filtering*: Focusing on the negative and discounting the positive, looking for evidence to back up our ideas and disregarding evidence which challenges them, selecting fragments of evidence without considering the whole picture.

■ *Fixed rules*: using commands rather than wishes and options as the driving force for our behaviours, such as 'I should' and 'I must', rather than 'I would like to' or 'I would prefer it'.

The key aspects of the cognitive model for mental health problems is that our thoughts shape the way we behave and feel (both emotionally and physically) and that in turn our behaviours and feelings may confirm or disconfirm these thoughts, thereby creating a cycle of interlinked thoughts, behaviours and feelings (Figure 31.1). In this chapter, thoughts relevant to mental health problems are referred to as misinterpretations (because of inaccuracies or distortions in them) and unhelpful ideas (because they exacerbate and maintain the problem irrespective of their accuracy, as it may happen with some cultural or religious beliefs).

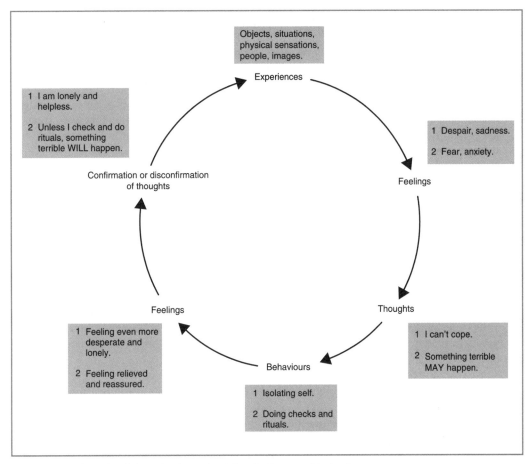

Figure 31.1 The role of thoughts in maintaining feelings and behaviours

Cognitive therapy aims to produce change in a problem through a process called cognitive restructuring or reattribution (that is, reducing a person's belief in their misinterpretations and unhelpful ideas by reinforcing a person's belief in alternative interpretations and more constructive ideas). The description of cognitive techniques in three groups for the purpose of this chapter is to aid clarity, however, in clinical practice cognitive restructuring involves all three groups in a continuous process.

Cognitive restructuring is not simply about positive thinking but about expanding our thinking repertoire so that it includes other options in the way we view ourselves and others, the world around us, our life and future. Furthermore, cognitive restructuring is not so much about challenging inaccurate, distorted or unhelpful beliefs as it is about reinforcing alternatives ones. The reason for this is twofold. Firstly, someone may feel stupid or dejected if a long-held belief which had shaped a person's feelings and behaviours is crashed without an alternative being offered. Secondly, trying to challenge and undermine a person's beliefs may appear threatening and patronizing compared to suggesting and testing alternatives which may be more acceptable and unassuming.

Techniques to identify misinterpretations and unhelpful ideas

The first stage in cognitive restructuring is to identify the content and occurrence of thoughts associated with a problem and rate (a) the person's conviction in them, and (b) the person's feelings and responses to them. This could be achieved in several ways:

■ Keeping thought-monitoring records (Figure 31.2) for a specific period of time, detailing the situation that a thought occurred, what the thought or range of thoughts were, how the person felt and responded at the time, and how much the person believes in that thought. The purpose of thought records is to identify a person's idiosyncratic misinterpretations or unhelpful ideas, establish a pattern of occurrence, demonstrate the link between thoughts and a person's feelings and responses, and finally rate the person's belief in them. An important point to remember while keeping a thought record is to identify which thoughts are the most potent and relevant ones by asking, 'If we could make one or two thoughts go away, which ones would you choose in order to make a real difference in the way you feel?'

■ Going through a recent incident (Figure 31.3) when the person experienced emotions or symptoms associated with the problem. Starting questions could be, 'When was the last time that you felt miserable/angry/anxious/scared?' or 'Looking back during the last week, which was the worst day for you? What was happening at the time that made it so bad?' Then, questions such as, 'What was going through your mind at the time?' and 'Were you saying anything to yourself at the time?' could help elicit thoughts associated with the specific incident.

By using the 'downward arrow technique' (Figure 31.3) it is possible to to elicit the meaning of the individual's thoughts.

The clinician starts by asking the question, 'If this were true …'

– What would be so bad about it?
– What would this tell you about yourself/other people/your future/your life? and carries on by asking the same question to the patient's answer until we arrive at a statement which reflects a core belief or personal assumption. An example is given below:

I am worried I am becoming mentally ill.
↓
If this were true (you became mentally ill) what would be so bad about it?
↓
I would end up in a hospital.
↓
If this were true, what would be so terrible about ending up in a psychiatric hospital?
↓
Everyone would know and also I would never work again.
↓
If this were true, what would be so bad about it?
↓
Everyone would look down on me, feel pity on me and eventually abandon me.

↓

If this were true, what would this tell you about your life?

↓

Life will not be worth living if I end up without a job and friends.

The downward arrow technique, otherwise referred to as *inference chaining*, could yield potent thoughts and powerful emotions which represent the person's ultimate fears. Therefore, this technique should be used only if the practitioner is sure about 'what to do' with the statement that lies at the end of the arrows. Some useful examples of applications of the downward arrow technique are described by Greenberger and Padesky (1995) for anxiety and depression, and Turkington and Siddle (1998) for delusions.

Situation			
· What was I doing	·	·	·
· Who was I with	·	·	·
· When	·	·	·
· Where	·	·	·
	Feelings		
How did I feel?			
How bad was it?			
0----2-----4-----6----8----10			
not at all extremely	**Thoughts**		
What was going through my mind?			
How much did I believe it?			
0%----25%-----50%----- 75%----100%			
not at all completely	**Responses**		
What did I do?			
How did it make me feel?			

Fig 31.2 A record to monitor thoughts

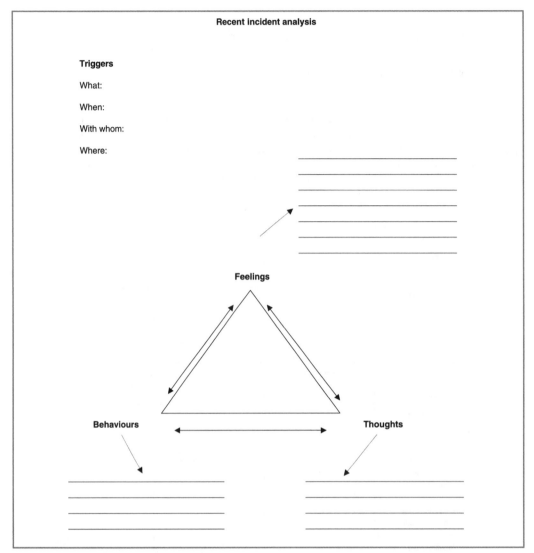

Figure 31.3 Diagram for recent incident analysis

Techniques to generate alternative interpretations and constructive ideas

This is perhaps the most difficult part of cognitive restructuring because the practitioner may be able to see the alternatives, but needs to facilitate the individual client to arrive at these alternatives using one or more of the techniques outlined below (for some examples, see Blackburn and Davidson 1995, Chapter 4). The alternative interpretation or constructive idea is phrased as a *hypothesis*, i.e. a theory or assumption for which we need to come to a conclusion about how accurate it is compared to the initial interpretations and ideas, and/or how helpful it may be in changing the way we feel and behave. At this stage, we may choose not to judge or add value to the alternatives until the next step of cognitive restructuring when we test them for accuracy and helpfulness. Remember, the objective is not to show that we are right and the other person is wrong but to show that there are other options that could be considered.

Prompt sheet

Using a prompt sheet (Figure 31.4), the client could write down their key thoughts (my interpretations and ideas are ...), what made them think this way (these are based on the following observations and experiences ...), and then identify whether there are any information processing errors inherent in these thoughts (In my interpretations and ideas, am I ... e.g. overlooking some facts?). Several alternative interpretations or ideas could derive from rephrasing the initial thoughts so that they do not contain any information processing errors.

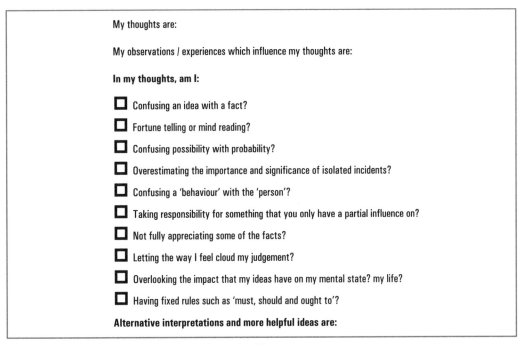

My thoughts are:

My observations / experiences which influence my thoughts are:

In my thoughts, am I:

☐ Confusing an idea with a fact?

☐ Fortune telling or mind reading?

☐ Confusing possibility with probability?

☐ Overestimating the importance and significance of isolated incidents?

☐ Confusing a 'behaviour' with the 'person'?

☐ Taking responsibility for something that you only have a partial influence on?

☐ Not fully appreciating some of the facts?

☐ Letting the way I feel cloud my judgement?

☐ Overlooking the impact that my ideas have on my mental state? my life?

☐ Having fixed rules such as 'must, should and ought to'?

Alternative interpretations and more helpful ideas are:

Figure 31.4 Prompt sheet to generate alternative ideas

Distancing

It is difficult to see different perspectives when we are 'tangled' in a web of our own emotions and thoughts, therefore, creating some distance from our emotional state could be useful in arriving at alternative thoughts and ideas. To this end, we could ask questions such as, 'How would someone else think in your place?' or 'What advice would you give to a friend who experiences the same difficulties as you do?' Alternatively, we could advise our client to write a script of two friends talking, where one is expressing their thoughts and the other is suggesting alternatives ideas.

Role reversal

The therapist will argue in favour of a thought and the patient against it in the place of the therapist. In this way, the therapist could demonstrate an understanding of the patient's point of view and the patient would have the opportunity to identify other perspectives. The patient and therapist could swap chairs, the patient could take notes, or use a flipchart like the therapist may do, and in the end, patient and therapist assume their original positions and discuss the learning outcome of the exercise.

Metaphors

We could use metaphors or everyday examples to demonstrate that our perception of a situation is affected by our emotional state, i.e. anxiety or low mood might cloud our judgement or our ability to appraise a situation objectively. Then we could ask the person to draw parallel links to their specific situations and thoughts.

Advantages and disadvantages

Considering the advantages and disadvantages of holding a certain idea could elicit useful information not about its factual accuracy but about how helpful or unhelpful it is in light of the person's difficulties and needs. This could be very important for engaging a client to consider alternatives when their beliefs are associated with cultural or religious norms. In this case, alternatives are considered not because the beliefs are '.awed' but because they are unhelpful for the specific problem we are addressing. Alternative ideas, which could be more helpful in overcoming the problem, are then considered within the same cultural and religious framework.

Techniques to test and reinforce alternative interpretations and constructive ideas

The aim is to *test* the alternatives interpretations or constructive ideas by either carrying out certain activities or having guided dialogues which highlight the evidence in favour of the alternatives (for some examples, see Wells 1997: 67–85). It is important that before and after testing, the client rates their belief on the alternative thoughts and their feelings in response to these alternatives using the template given (Figure 31.5).

Behavioural experiments

The nature of the experiment depends on the belief it is designed to test and it should aim at reinforcing the alternative belief rather than undermining the old one. The experiments should be negotiated and the therapist should empower the patient to design and implement appropriate behavioural experiments between sessions. A good question to guide us to the appropriate behavioural experiment is, 'If the alternative were true, how would I behave?'

Feelings	Initial thoughts	Alternative ideas	Test	Outcome
How bad is it? 0---2---4---6---8---10 Not at all Extremely	How much do I believe it? 0%---25%---50%---75%---100% Not at all Completely	How much do I believe it? 0%---25%---50%---75%---100% Not at all Completely	- If the alternative idea were true, how would I behave? - How could I find out more about the alternative idea?	What have I learnt? - Re-rate belief in alternative idea - Re-rate belief in initial thought - Re-rate feelings

Figure 31.5 Diary to monitor unhelpful thoughts, test alternative ideas and record emotional changes

Corrective information

This is an exercise which could help gather factual information from various sources, such as asking trusted friends and family, looking at reliable books and journals, talking to professionals. It is important to bear in mind that people would have the tendency to filter information and focus on confirmatory evidence for their initial 'unhelpful ideas'. Therefore, we should highlight that the objective of the exercise is to gather information about the alternative thought because this was likely to be disregarded in the first place.

Rehearsing alternative responses

An observation that people often make after testing alternative thoughts is that although they may believe in them, they do not feel any better. The aim of rehearsing alternative responses is 'not just to think but feel differently', and this is achieved by repeating the same test many times and continuously monitoring one's unhelpful thoughts/ideas and gathering evidence to reinforce alternative ones.

Cognitive and behavioural techniques: segregation or integration?

Although behavioural and cognitive techniques stem from different theoretical backgrounds (behaviour therapy from learning theories and cognitive therapy from information processing theories), in practice they are inextricably bound because any changes in behaviour may influence one's thinking and any changes in thinking are usually reflected in one's behaviour. Let us take, for example, the task of asking someone to confront an anxiety-provoking situation with the aim of controlling and reducing their symptoms of anxiety. This therapeutic activity (i.e. confrontation of an anxiety-provoking situation) which leads to the same outcome (i.e. reduction in anxiety) has a different name and a different working mechanism depending on whether we consider it within a behavioural or a cognitive perspective. A behavioural explanation would use *habituation* as the anxiety-reduction mechanism, would call the anxiety-related thoughts *feared consequences* and would term the treatment activity an *exposure task*. A cognitive explanation would describe anxiety-related thoughts as *catastrophic beliefs*, would consider the *disconfirmation* of catastrophic beliefs as the anxiety-reduction mechanism and would term the treatment task a *behavioural experiment*. In practice, it is virtually impossible to differentiate what brings about the reduction in anxiety; whether it is that people get used to it over time (as in behaviour therapy's habituation) or whether it is that they no longer believe that something terrible may happen (as in cognitive disconfirmation). Therefore, the same activity used as part of a cognitive behavioural treatment may be explained with both a behavioural and a cognitive rationale without substantial differences in its practical delivery and outcome.

Having established the crossover between behavioural and cognitive techniques, it is also important to highlight some of their dissimilarities in the way they are delivered and the emphasis they lay on different aspects of treatment. Behavioural techniques are mainly focused activities which aim to change people's pattern of responses to external and internal stimuli. These responses are the result of acquired strong associations and positive or negative reinforcement. The application of behavioural techniques is symptom-driven and depends on delivering the right technique for the right problem. In contrast, cognitive techniques use both guided dialogues and focused activities in order to change thinking processes and beliefs which are considered the mediating factors between people's experiences and their emotional state or reactions. Cognitive techniques place great emphasis on the process of therapy and their application is guided by an individualized case formulation irrespective of diagnostic classifications relating to the problem.

In summary, behavioural techniques are symptom-driven activities which explain treatment outcome in terms of learned responses, whereas cognitive techniques are process-focused dialogues and activities which explain treatment progress in terms of belief change. In practice, it is usually difficult to distinguish whether it is the behavioural or the cognitive mechanism which produces the reduction in the symptoms, distress and disability associated with a mental health problem. Investigating the differential effect of behavioural and cognitive components of CBT could lead to more efficient treatment models and specific guidelines about which techniques may suit what patients. Whether segregated or integrated, behavioural and cognitive techniques should always be considered within the wider framework of patient care which involved the interpersonal effect of clinician input, the need for risk assessment and management, and the benefits of medical, social, family and psychological interventions other than CBT.

Conclusion

The safe and effective application of cognitive techniques is determined by careful assessment and formulation of an individual's problems and needs. It is difficult to develop an understanding of cognitive techniques without putting them into the context of specific thoughts in case examples, so further reading, training and observation of experienced practitioners is recommended.

In summary, the main points of this chapter are:

- Thoughts shape the way we behave and feel, and in turn our behaviours and feelings confirm or disconfirm these thoughts, thereby creating a cycle of interlinked thoughts, behaviours and feelings.
- Thoughts which contribute to the maintenance of mental health contain some form of inaccuracy or distortion and they are significant but unhelpful for the person.
- Cognitive techniques are guided dialogues and focused activities which aim to manage the symptoms, distress and disability associated with a problem through a process called cognitive restructuring, i.e. reducing a person's belief in their misinterpretations and unhelpful ideas by reinforcing a person's belief in *alternative interpretations* and more *constructive ideas*.
- The main techniques used in cognitive restructuring are described here in three groups: techniques to identify misinterpretations and unhelpful thoughts, techniques to generate alternative interpretations and constructive thoughts, and techniques to test and reinforce the alternatives.
- Cognitive and behavioural techniques co-exist in clinical practice because any changes in behaviour influence one's thinking and any changes in thinking are reflected in one's behaviour. However, they differ in that behavioural techniques are symptom-driven

activities which explain treatment outcome in terms of learned responses, whereas cognitive techniques are process-focused dialogues and activities which explain treatment progress in terms of belief change.

Questions for reflection and discussion

1   Keep a thought record for a week, noting some of your experiences at work, college or home when you felt miserable or angry or anxious. What were the thoughts and beliefs associated with these experiences? Can you identify any information-processing errors within these thoughts? Can you come up with any alternatives? How could you test these alternatives?

2   Consider some of the differences in the care of clients with common mental health problems and with severe/enduring mental illness. What do you think are the implications for the delivery of cognitive techniques for these two client groups, in terms of:
    (a)   pace, intensity and duration of treatment?
    (b)   the professional support required and type of services in which this is usually provided?
    (c)   the comparative benefits of cognitive techniques in relation to other interventions (e.g. medication, family work, counselling)?

3   What is your understanding of the differences between behavioural and cognitive techniques, and how do you think these are integrated for the suitable and effective delivery of CBT in everyday practice?

Annotated bibliography

■   Kingdon, D.G. and Turkington, D. (1994) *Cognitive-Behavioural Therapy for Schizophrenia*. Sussex: Guilford Press. A clear and concise book which outlines the key theoretical frameworks of understanding experiences associated with schizophrenia. It also illustrates the application of specific CBT techniques with case examples, including explanations for psychotic symptoms using a normalizing rationale and stress-vulnerability model, techniques to understand and tackle delusions, and reality testing for hallucinations. Ideal as an introductory book in the field of CBT for psychosis.

■   Hawton, K., Salkovskis, P.M., Kirk, J. and Clark, D.M. (1989) *Cognitive Behaviour Therapy for Psychiatric Problems*. Oxford: Oxford University Press. A classic textbook and comprehensive practical guide for students and practitioners on CBT models and methods for mental health problems. The book covers a historical overview of behavioural and cognitive treatments, and provides detailed guidelines and case examples on CBT assessment strategies, formulation and treatment methods for anxiety disorders (generalized anxiety, panic, phobias, obsessive compulsive disorder), depression, marital problems and physical problems associated with mental health factors (e.g. sleep disorders, medically unexplained symptoms, sexual problems, etc.). In addition, one chapter refers to CBT within the context of caring for patients with high levels of dependence on psychiatric services, and another outlines the delivery and applicability of problem solving.

References

Beck, A.T. (1976) *Cognitive Therapy and the Emotional Disorders*. New York: International Universities Press.

Blackburn, I. and Davidson, K. (1995) *Cognitive Therapy for Depression and Anxiety*. London: Blackwell.

Greenberger, D. and Padesky, C.A. (1995) *Mind Over Mood: Change How you Feel by Changing the Way you Think*. London: Guilford Press.

Turkington, D. and Siddle, R. (1998) Cognitive therapy for the treatment of delusions. *Advances in Psychiatric Treatment* **4**: 235–42.

Wells, A. (1997) *Cognitive Therapy of Anxiety Disorders: A Practice Manual and Conceptual Guide*. Chichester: John Wiley.

CHAPTER 32

Medication management to concordance

Sue Gurney

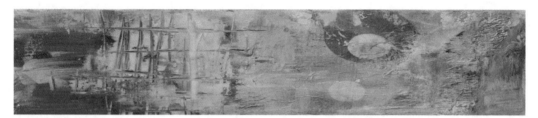

Chapter overview

Since the mid-twentieth century, compelling evidence has evolved on the efficacy of a range of psychotropic medications in reducing and managing the symptoms of an array of mental health problems. This chapter gives an overview of medication concordance and implications for nursing practice. This chapter covers:

- Introduction and overview of the concept of medication concordance;
- Exploring the language of medication management;
- Factors affecting adherence;
- The rationale for interventions;
- Reviewing the evidence;
- Implications for mental health nursing practice.

Introduction

As discussed in Chapter 16 the three main classes of psychotropic preparations in use for symptom relief are: antidepressants for treating depression, anxiolytics for anxiety and anti-psychotics for treating symptoms of psychosis (WHO 2001). The developments of new generations of psychotropic preparations, although not necessarily possessing improved symptom reduction-relief efficacy, generally do cause fewer side effects (NICE 2003).

Psychotropic medications often need to be taken continuously over a sustained period of time in order to reduce symptoms and potential relapse. Conformity to prescribed medications is often referred to as adherence or compliance. Ceasing or partial conformity to the prescription is referred to as non or partial adherence/compliance. These are value-laden terms (Marland and Sharkey 1999) and the literature and best practice refers to the concept of concordance in promoting an equal partnership between the prescriber and the user (RPS 1997). Mental health nurses (MHNs) are not only routinely involved in dispensing and administering medication but are now actively embracing non-medical prescribing roles, hence medication concordance is central to MHN practice. However, there are reports that

MHNs are often ill-prepared for this aspect of practice (Gray *et al.* 2001), and that they have poor professional responsibility in prescribing psychotropic medication. There is little research into medication errors in mental health (Maidment 2006).

The terms concordance, adherence and compliance are used interchangeably throughout this chapter. The phrase 'people who use our services' is used to encompass the terms: service user, client and patient. The chapter refers primarily to the literature on compliance to anti-psychotic medication. However, many of the issues and concepts discussed here are transferable to other forms of psychotropic and generic medication management-concordance practice.

Exploring the language of medication concordance

The use and understanding of the language in this area has significant meaning and impact for professional practice (Repper and Perkins 1998). The literature reveals a development in terminology reflected in a shift in the balance of power of the relationship/alliance of the prescriber and health care worker with the person using mental health services. Overall, this describes a change in value, from the individual as a passive recipient of health care to an informed partner in health care decision-making. Kemp *et al.* (1997) identified successful collaboration between professionals and the individual as the most valuable approach in improving compliance, assuming that compliance is appropriate. The concept of collaboration has since shifted to one of concordance. This implies that an equal partnership needs to exist between health care workers and the individual, before compliance is achieved, assuming the latter is appropriate (RPS 1997). Permeating into the literature and into current health policy is a further shift along the language continuum with the concept of choice (Hogman and Sandamas 2000; Jones and Jones 2007).

What is adherence/compliance?

Agreement on defining compliance is diverse. Dodds *et al.* (2000) define compliance as the extent to which a person's behaviour regarding taking medication coincides with medical or health advice. Marland and Sharkey (1999) discuss the value-laden term of 'compliance' and that interpretation varies with each individual professional. They also propose two further dimensions to the concept. The first as being process defined, influenced by the degree of conformity to the prescription. The second as being outcome defined, being determined by the maintenance of wellness. Interestingly, this latter dimension implies that wellness may not correspond with compliance.

There is a clear relationship between compliance with prescribed medication and best practice in medication management. However, it is imperative that compliance is not the main target. In fact non-compliance for someone suffering from severe adverse reactions might be life-saving in cases of inappropriate prescription. Hence, a crucial element of best practice in medication management-concordance is about health professionals and the individual recognizing that a problem may be medication related.

Measuring compliance

There are challenges in measuring compliance. Measures may include methods of observation, self-reporting, pill counts and biological assays such as urine and blood specimens; and these only determine current compliance (Gray *et al.* 2006). In clinical practice, individual and carers' reports, clinical assessment and observation are the commonly employed (subjective) measures of compliance.

Compliance rates

Interpreting the literature is difficult as there are no agreed definitions of non-compliance. Non-compliance/adherence with all types of medication is common. Studies report rates of compliance with anti-psychotic medication ranging from 10 to 80 per cent (Kemp *et al.* 1997). Cramer and Rosenheck (1998) suggest an average compliance rate of 42 per cent. This is similar to compliance rates for people with physical disorders (Carter *et al.* 2005). More recent work suggests non-compliance with antipsychotic medication (including the newer anti-psychotic preparations) is as high as 74 per cent (Lieberman *et al.* 2005).

Factors which influence adherence with medication

Little work has been undertaken on the relationship of medication adherence with theoretical models of health behaviour change, which might provide explanation, understanding and potential for therapeutic development (Gray *et al.* 2002). However, compliance is clearly linked to a complex, dynamic decision-making process (Marland and Cash 2005). The literature identifies a wide range of factors that appear to influence adherence to prescribed medications. These can be categorized into the following three themes, as illustrated below with some examples (Kemp *et al.* 1997).

1　**The person:** Culture, values, beliefs, prejudices, experience, support networks, family and carers' involvement, personality, awareness and understanding of the problem, use of non-prescribed substances, e.g. cannabis or alcohol.
2　**The illness:** Cognitive impairment, thought disorder, depression, features of hallucinations.
3　**The treatment:** Value of alliance with clinicians, complexity of the treatment, the form of treatment, the treatment setting, the experience of side effects, stigma, effectiveness of the medication, polypharmacy, ease of accessing medications.

In summary compliance with medication is a multi-faceted issue. Decisions on whether to comply with a prescribed medication regime can be influenced by a wide range of factors, the reduction/relief of symptoms being just one.

The rationale for interventions

Although the literature exploring the benefits of improved medication compliance is limited (NPA 1998), there is a strong rationale for addressing this area for the following reasons. The first is a moral-ethical one, related to symptom reduction/relief and improving and maintaining the perceived quality/quality of life of the person; taking into account the holistic needs of the individual, a cost-benefit analysis of the prescribed medication and an awareness that improvement of health may not always be a motivating factor. The second is related to the impact of adverse reactions to medication. General studies have identified that a high proportion of all hospital admissions, general practitioner and outpatient consultations are a result of the impact of non-adherence and/or adverse drug reactions (NPA 1998). The third is related to costs of health and social care. The direct cost of schizophrenia in England and Wales is estimated to be in excess of £1 billion, with drug costs accounting for 5 per cent of this sum (NICE 2003). In 2002 overall prescription costs rose to £6.1 billion, one-tenth of all NHS spending, with £230 million of medicines returned to pharmacies and an uncalculated cost/amount being privately disposed of (Crouch 2003). There are also indirect costs: the costs of caring, loss of employment and the loss of active citizenship. In 1990/1 the indirect costs of schizophrenia in the UK were estimated to be at least £1.7 billion (NICE 2003). From the evidence there is obviously a clear rationale for careful, individual tailored prescribing and support in improving the quality of life for people receiving prescribed medication treatments. There is also the added potential of a positive effect in reducing direct and indirect costs.

Reviewing the evidence base of medication management/concordance

Interventions to improve adherence

A detailed systematic review of the literature on interventions to improve the taking of all types of prescribed medication can be found in the Cochrane Library (Haynes *et al.* 2002). The review analysed 39 randomized controlled trials for short- and long-term interventions and concluded that methods for improving compliance are generally complex and require development.

A meta-analysis of clinical interventions for treatment of non-adherence in psychosis reviewed 24 studies. Clinical interventions were grouped into educational strategies, psychotherapy, prompts, specific service policies and family interventions. The study concluded that interventions were positive and recommended improvements in research design (Nose *et al.* 2003). Two recent studies (Gray *et al.* 2006; McIntosh *et al.* 2006) have found no clear evidence to suggest that compliance therapy, as a discrete intervention, is beneficial for people with schizophrenia.

Similarly no approaches that clearly increased adherence in people experiencing depression have been identified, but findings have suggested that mental health professionals need to be better equipped in enquiring about adherence, providing appropriate information and managing side effects (Pampallona *et al.* 2002). Delivering information/education are important areas in facilitating informed choice and mastery (Bollini *et al.* 2004). If people are not adequately informed then informed consent has not been obtained (Harris *et al.* 2002).

The views of people using our services

Medication issues are a frequent source of tension between mental health professionals and people using services, with some people requiring section under the Mental Health Act to enforce compliance (Langan and Lindow 2004).

There is also a growing body of work that identifies a range of strategies that those suffering mental distress find useful with a recognition of a place and value of medication among a number of strategies (Faulkner and Layzell 2000) (see Box 32.1).

In a qualitative analysis of the views of inpatient mental health services Goodwin *et al.* (1999) found comments around medication centred around two common themes: informed consent and the effects of medication. The majority of people thought they had not received any/sufficient information on side effects, and of those who thought themselves adequately informed nearly all had viewed themselves as having to request the information. A community survey of people taking antipsychotic medication found that the majority of people experienced side effects, had not received written information, had not been offered alternative approaches and took the medication as a professional had told them to do so (Gray *et al.* 2005). A study of people's views of 'as needed medication' has highlighted the process associated with its use as stigmatizing and confusing. These findings raise issues of power and control and the need to provide adequate information is a key priority (Baker *et al.* 2006). Boyle and Chambers (2000) also highlight the neglected area of informing and working with carers.

Nursing

It has already been mentioned that mental health nurses are often ill-prepared for this area of practice (Gray *et al.* 2001). In particular the literature identifies areas for improvement in: objective assessment, pharmacology, management of side effects and the ability to facilitate physical health care interventions in reducing physical problems (Jones and Jones 2005). Specific medication management training for mental health nurses to address these issues has resulted in improved clinical outcomes and adherence rates for people with schizophrenia (Gray *et al.* 2004).

Box 32.1 'Most helpful' strategies and supports

Relationships with others	Medication
■ Friends	
■ Other service users/people with similar problems	Physical exercise
■ Mental health professionals	
■ Counsellors/therapists	Religious and spiritual beliefs
■ People encountered in day centres, drop-ins, voluntary sector projects	
	Money
Personal strategies	Other activities
■ Peace of mind	■ Hobbies and interests
■ Thinking positively, taking control	■ Information
	■ Home
	■ Creative expression

Overall picture of different strategies and supports in living and coping with mental distress. Many people found a number of strategies useful.

Implications for MHN practice

Medication concordance is a crucial area of nursing practice and is increasingly so with the advent of non-medical prescribing (Jones and Jones 2005).

From the literature the key areas for practice implications are:

1 *Foundation skills*: reliant on interpersonal skills, partnership working, person centred-person led approach (Kemp *et al.* 1997);

2 *Assessment*: baseline and systematic assessments of general health, lifestyle, quality of life, syndrome, symptom and side effects of medication (NICE 2003, 2004);

3 *Pharmacology*: tailoring medication to individual needs with reference to best practice prescribing (NICE 2003), systematic assessment of side effects utilizing valid and reliable measures, e.g. Day *et al.* (1995), and in-depth knowledge of the prescribed medication in the following areas:

   ■ pharmacokinetics: how the medication biologically functions in the body through the process of absorption, distribution, metabolism and elimination

   ■ pharmacodynamics: where, how and why the medication acts

   ■ pharmacogenetics: awareness of the variation of ethnic and racial responses to medication;

4 *Exploring the person's illness story*: experience, attitudes, beliefs, awareness and understanding; utilizing interpersonal skills, information exchange, in normalizing and health-promotion opportunities. It is also essential to maintain awareness that there can be negative connotations to improved adherence and that it is imperative to understand the reasons for non-compliance;

5 *Exploring ambivalence towards treatment*: utilizing interpersonal, problem solving, CBT and motivational interviewing approaches, skills and techniques;

6 *Providing information*: in a number of formats on medication: how it works, side effects and the condition. Consent to treatment is the precursor to involvement in the treatment process, information giving is seen as a starting point in enabling people to adhere to prescribed medication;

7 *Maintaining wellness*: exploring strategies, skills and techniques for managing health;

8 *Involvement of carers:* providing information, as in number 6;

9 *Service protocols, designs, strategies:* enhancing ways to provide support, e.g. discharge protocols, telephone support.

Case study

Preda (56) lives with her partner Joe (64). They are both retired. Preda has a diagnosis of schizophrenia; she acknowledges this but is very opposed to medication and is now refusing to take it. Jo contacts the CMHT stating that she is deteriorating. The crisis resolution team undertakes an assessment and is convinced that she needs inpatient assessment. Preda is sectioned and admitted under the Mental Health Act. Mental health professionals now face many challenges in terms of Preda's care and support. The care coordinator starts to regularly explore Preda's views of her situation, using a range of strategies from medication concordance best practice the care coordinator works with Preda and her partner and the team in implementing a range of approaches in facilitating Preda's improved well-being, one of which is medication. Preda's medication adherence is regularly monitored and reviewed. Clinical judgement is informed by measures such as the:

■ Beliefs about medication questionnaire (Horne *et al.* 1999);
■ Drug attitude inventory (Hogan *et al.* 1983);
■ LUNSERS (Day *et al.* 1995).

Conclusion

This chapter has provided an overview of medication concordance. The concept of medication concordance is that of an equal partnership with the individual, a move along the continuum from a paternalistic model towards a person-centred approach. There is increasing emphasis on the role of the health worker in exploring issues and exchanging information, so that people can make informed choices. This is a shift from an illness to a health focus model.

In summary the main points from this chapter are:

■ The concept of medication concordance is that of an equal partnership with the client, a move along the continuum from a paternalistic model towards a person-centred approach and to one of choice.
■ Compliance rates to psychotropic medication appear similar, or slightly higher, to those of generic medication prescribing.
■ Findings from the literature indicate that interventions to improve compliance and outcomes are generally complex and require innovation.
■ The literature indicates mental health professionals have much work to do in facilitating concordance/choice; this has important implications for MHN practice.
■ The current preferred concordance approach is in a composite strategy of education, psychological, behavioural and socio-economic interventions.
■ Medication concordance is a complex activity and is fundamentally about health behaviour change.

Questions for reflection and discussion

1 Consider the rationale for the use of psychotropic medication and what negative effects there might be from improving compliance.

2 Put yourself in the position of a person taking medication which dulls your emotions, lessens your energy and increases your weight. What changes would you like to make? How would you do this? What help might you need? How could you tell if things had improved?

3 Medications have side effects; there is a cost–benefit to usage. Think of a person you have known or nursed who has received a medication treatment. Make two lists, one of the costs and the other of the benefits of the treatment. What is your conclusion? Now give each element in the list a weighting, say from 1 (not important) to 8 (very important) then total the figures. Are your findings the same? Has this highlighted any other issues?

Annotated bibliography

- Taylor, D., Paton, C. and Kerwin, R. (2007) *The Maudsley Prescribing Guidelines* (9th edn). London: Informa Healthcare. An essential text that provides information and guidance on issues of psychotropic medication prescribing.
- Stahl, S. (2000) *The Essential Psychopharmacology: Neuroscientific basis and practical applications* (2nd edn). Cambridge: Cambridge University Press. Another essential and creatively illustrated text which explores the complexity of the nervous system and the effects of medications.
- Svedberg, P., Jormfeldt, H. and Arvidsson, B. (2003) Patients' conceptions of how health processes are promoted in mental health nursing. A qualitative study. *Journal of Psychiatric and Mental Health Nursing* **10**: 448–56. This paper explores the current barriers and opportunities related to the health promoting behaviour of MHNs.
- Usher, K., Foster, K. and Park, T. (2006) The metabolic syndrome and schizophrenia: the latest evidence and nursing guidelines for management. *Journal of Psychiatric and Mental Health Nursing* **13**: 730–4. This review article discusses the issues related to poor physical health for people with severe mental illness and metabolic conditions associated with schizophrenia with focus on second generation antipsychotics.

References

Baker, J., Lovell, K., Easton, K. and Harris, N. (2006) Service users' experiences of 'as needed' psychotropic medications in acute mental healthcare settings. *Journal of Advanced Nursing* **56**(4): 354–62.

Bollini, P., Tibaldi, G., Testa, C. and Munizza, C. (2004) Understanding treatment adherence in affective disorders: a qualitative study. *Journal of Psychiatric and Mental Health Nursing* **11**: 668–74.

Boyle, E. and Chambers, M. (2000) Medication compliance in older individuals with depression: gaining the views of family carers. *Journal of Psychiatric and Mental Health Nursing* **7**: 515–22.

Carter, S., Taylor, D. and Levenson, R. (2005) A question of choice-compliance in medicine taking: A preliminary review (3rd edn). Available from www.medicines-partnership.org/research-evidence/major-reviews/aquestion-of-choice

Cramer, J.A. and Rosenheck, R. (1998) Compliance with medication regimens for mental and physical disorders. *Psychiatric Services* **49**: 196–201.

Crouch, D. (2003) Sharing medication agreements with patients. *Nursing Times* **99**(38): 34–6.

Day, J.C., Wood, G., Dewey, M. and Bentall, P. (1995) A self rating scale for measuring neuroleptic side effects. *British Journal of Psychiatry* **166**: 650–3.

Dodds, F., Rebair-Brown, A. and Parsons, S. (2000) A systematic review of randomized controlled trials that attempt to identify interventions that improve patient compliance with prescribed antipsychotic medication. *Clinical Effectiveness in Nursing* **4**: 47–53.

Faulkner, A. and Layzell, S. (2000) *Strategies for Living: A Report of User-led Research into People's Strategies for Living with Mental Distress.* London: Mental Health Foundation.

Goodwin, I., Holmes, G., Newnes, C. and Waltho, D. (1999) A qualitative analysis of the views of in-patient mental health service users. *Journal of Mental Health* **8**(1): 43–5.

Gray, R., Wykes, T., Parr, A-M. and Hails, E. (2001) The use of outcome measures to evaluate the efficacy and tolerability of antipsychotic medication: a comparison of Thorn graduate and CPN practice. *Journal of Psychiatric and Mental Health Nursing* **8**: 191–6.

Gray, R., Wykes, T., and Gournay, K. (2002) From compliance to concordance: a review of the literature on interventions to enhance compliance with antipsychotic medication. *Journal of Psychiatric and Mental Health Nursing* **9**: 277–84.

Gray, R., Wykes, T., Edmonds, M., Leese, M. and Gournay, K. (2004) Effect of medication training on clinical outcomes for patients with schizophrenia. *British Journal of Psychiatry* **185**: 157–62.

Gray, R., Rofail, D., Allen, J. and Newey, T. (2005) A survey of patient satisfaction with and subjective experiences of treatment with antipsychotic medication. *Journal of Advanced Nursing* **52**(1): 31–7.

Gray, R., Leese, M., Bindman, J. *et al.* (2006) Adherence therapy for schizophrenia: European multicentre randomized control trail. *British Journal of Psychiatry* **189**: 508–14.

Haynes, R.B., McDonald, H., Garg, A.X. and Montague, P. (2002) *Interventions for Helping Patients Follow Prescription for Medications* (*Cochrane Review*), in *The Cochrane Library*, Issue 4, 2003. Chichester: John Wiley and Sons.

Harris, N., Lovell, K. and Day, J. (2002) Consent and long-term neuropletic medication. *Journal of Psychiatric and Mental Health Nursing* **9**: 475–82.

Hogman, G. and Sandamas, G. (2000) *A Question of Choice*. London: Rethink.

Hogan, T.P., Awad, A.G. and Eastwood, R. (1983) A self-report scale predictive of drug compliance in schizophrenics: reliability and discriminative validity. *Psychological Medicine* **13**: 177–83.

Horne, R., Weinman, J. and Hankins, M. (1999) The Beliefs about Medicines Questionnaire: the development and evaluation of a new method for assessing the cognitive representation of medication. *Psychological Health* **14**: 1–24.

Jones, A. and Jones, M. (2005) Mental health nurse prescribing: issues for the UK. *Journal of Psychiatric and Mental Health Nursing* **12**: 527–35.

Jones, M. and Jones, A. (2007) Delivering the choice agenda as a framework to manage adverse effects: a mental health nurse perspective on prescribing psychiatric medication. *Journal of Psychiatric and Mental Health Nursing* **14**: 418–23.

Kemp, R., Hayward, P. and David, A. (1997) *Compliance Therapy Manual*. London: The Maudsley Hospital.

Langan, J. and Lindow, V. (2004) *Living with Risk: Mental health service user involvement in risk assessment and management*. York: Joseph Roundtree Foundation.

Lieberman, J., Stroup, S., McEvoy, J. *et al.* (2005) Effectiveness of antipsychotic drugs in patients with chronic schizophrenia. *New England Journal of Medicine* **353**(12): 1209–23.

Maidment, I. (2006) Medication errors in mental healthcare: a systematic review. *Quality and Safety in Health Care* **15**(6): 409–13.

Marland, G. and Sharkey, V. (1999) Depot neuroleptics, schizophrenia and the role of the nurse: is practice evidence based? A review of the literature. *Journal of Advanced Nursing* **30**: 1255–62.

Marland, G. and Cash, K. (2005) Medicine taking decisions: schizophrenia in comparison to asthma and epilepsy. *Journal of Psychiatric and Mental Health Nursing* **12**: 163–72.

McIntosh, A., Conlon, S. and Stanfield, A. (2006) Compliance therapy for schizophrenia. *Cochrane Database of Systematic Reviews*. Issue 2. Art No: CD003442.DOI: 10.1002/14651858.CD003442.pub2.

National Pharmacy Association (1998) *Medication Management: Strategies to Meet the Needs of Vulnerable People*. St. Albans: NPA.

NICE (2003) *Schizophrenia: full national clinical guideline on core interventions in primary and secondary care*. Available from: www.nice.org.uk

NICE (2004) *Clinical Guideline 23. Depression: management of depression in primary and secondary care*. Available from: www.nice.org.uk.

Nose, M., Barbui, C., Gray, R. and Tansella, M. (2003) Clinical interventions for treatment non-adherence in psychosis: meta-analysis. *British Journal of Psychiatry* **183**: 197–206.

Pampallona, S., Bollini, P., Kupelnick, B. and Munizza, C. (2002) Patient adherence in the treatment of depression. *British Journal of Psychiatry* **180**: 104–9.

Repper, J. and Perkins, R. (1998) Different but normal, language, labels and professional mental health practice. *Mental Health Care* **2**: 90–3.

RPS of Great Britain and Merck Sharp Dohme (1997) *From Compliance to Concordance: achieving goals in medicine taking*. London: Royal Pharmaceutical Society of Great Britain.

WHO (2001) *The World Health Report. Mental Health: New Understanding, New Hope*. France: World Health Organization.

CHAPTER 33

Therapeutic management of aggression and violence

Susan Sookoo

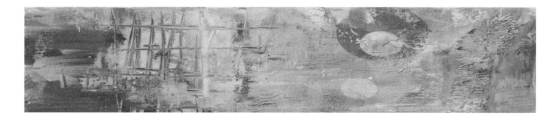

Chapter overview

The therapeutic management of violence and aggression is not separate to, but rather an integral part of routine care. Aggressive incidents are not isolated events, but take place within a clinical, psychological, environmental and social context. Consequently a broad range of interventions is required in order to manage violence and aggression and prevention is always more desirable than intervention. This chapter is largely concerned with methods used to safely manage anger, aggression and violence when they occur or are imminent. As such, the techniques described can be seen as 'as required' interventions aimed at short-term management. The focus is on methods used in ward environments. Although non-physical interventions may also be applicable to community settings, safe management of aggression in the community is built on effective risk assessment processes, multi-disciplinary team working and attention to local policies on safety when visiting clients.

However, methods for dealing with imminent aggression alone do not constitute complete management of violence and aggression: an understanding of the underlying factors that influence such behaviour and reduce the need for short-term intervention is also necessary. In addition, this chapter should be read in conjunction with Chapter 27 on engaging with clients, Chapter 12 on the creation of a therapeutic milieu and Chapter 11 on assessing and managing risk as these are key preventative measures. In summary, this chapter covers:

- The factors which influence the incidence of violence and aggression in inpatient mental health services;
- Mechanisms underlying anger and aggression;
- Observation and de-escalation techniques;
- Physical interventions.

As a starting point, some definition of commonly used terms is needed:

- Anger – a subjective emotional state involving physiological arousal and associated cognitions. This can be adaptive, but frequency, intensity and duration of anger can make it dysfunctional (Novaco 1983).
- Aggression – a disposition to inflict harm. This may be verbally expressed in threats to harm people or objects, or result in actual harm (Wright *et al.* 2002).
- Hostility – a personality trait, which reflects a style of appraisal in which the actions of others are seen as harmful. This can result in anger or detachment (Novaco 1983).
- Violence – acts in which there is use of force to attempt to inflict physical harm (Wright *et al.* 2002).

Background

There is a public perception of the psychiatric patient as dangerous to the community at large (Vinestock 1996), as well as increasing concern about the level of violence and aggression occurring within health care settings. Violence against staff in the UK National Health Service (NHS) as a whole rose at least 13 per cent in the period 2002–3 (National Audit Office 2003) with 95,000 reported incidents during this period. The level of incidents within mental health and learning disability Trusts has been reported to be three times higher than the average in all other Trusts (NHS Executive 1998/9, in Gournay 2000). A survey of care in acute psychiatric wards (Sainsbury Centre for Mental Health 1998) found that nearly a third of patients were involved in incidents of non-physical aggression, 9 per cent carried out assaults on staff or other patients without causing injury and 5 per cent carried out assault causing minor injury. Reported rates are likely to be far less than real incidence (Gournay 2000).

It is not the purpose of this chapter to explore the nature of the relationship between mental disorder and violence, as, in any case, the exact nature of the relationship is not straightforward (see for example, Monaghan 1993). Nor should the above figures suggest that a relationship between mental illness and violence is inevitable. It is worth noting that mentally ill people living in the community are twice as likely to be the victim of violent abuse as the general population (NMC press release 2003). The reasons for an apparent increase in the level of violent incidents within health services are not clear but may include a higher level of violence within society in general (Wright *et al.* 2002), the reduced number of hospital beds resulting in only the most disturbed patients being admitted to inpatient units, or the effect of non-therapeutic hospital environments (Sainsbury Centre for Mental Health 1998).

The evidence base

Violence is a complex phenomenon and it is not possible to state a theory in terms of 'violent behaviour is caused by *x, y* and *z*'. As Mason and Chandley (1999) state, there are probably as many theories of violence as there are aggressive incidents. Neither is there definitive evidence on the effectiveness of methods to manage violence and aggression, as acknowledged by the National Institute for Health and Clinical Excellence (NICE 2005). Most of the evidence considered by the group developing the current NICE guideline on short-term management of violence is graded Level 4, that is 'expert opinion or formal consensus'. However, it is still worth examining practice and experience to discuss factors which might contribute to violence and ways to manage it. Indeed, over recent years, professional bodies have produced guidance and summarized the evidence base for managing violence and aggression. The Royal College of Nursing (RCN) published a position statement on dealing with violence and aggression in 1997. In 2002, Wright *et al.* produced a report for the then UKCC (now the Nursing and Midwifery Council) providing a detailed exploration of the literature around both causes of violence and aggression and the various methods of managing them. The Royal College of Psychiatrists (RCP) Research Unit also produced a detailed report: *Management of Imminent Violence: Clinical practice guidelines to support mental health services* (1998). This report reviewed the evidence base and made practice recommendations as a result. In 2005 NICE produced a guideline *Violence: the short-term management of disturbed/violent behaviour in in-patient psychiatric settings and emergency departments* (NICE 2005). This guideline is based upon and both updates and replaces the RCP guideline. This chapter considers findings from all of these reports, but it must be emphasized that all staff working in mental health settings or emergency departments should be familiar with and follow the recommendations of the NICE guideline as this is the current guide to best practice and has a legal standing: 'Failure to act in accordance with the guideline may not only be a failure to act in accordance with best practice, but in some circumstances may have legal consequences' (NICE 2005: 10).

Factors which influence violence and aggression

Prevention of violence requires understanding of the factors which may contribute to levels of violence and aggression and is an important part of management. Some factors are considered here, although these should always be interpreted within the context of an individual, collaborative risk assessment.

Demographic or personal factors

The NICE guidance (2005) cautiously lists several demographic or personal variables which may be risk factors for aggression (Box 33.1).

Clinical factors

Wright *et al.* (2002) report an increased relative risk of violence in patients with psychotic illnesses, although, once again, there is not a clear relationship between specific symptoms and violence, and the relationship does not seem to be consistent. For example, one study (Lowenstein *et al.* 1990) found manic patients to have higher levels of inpatient violence than any other diagnostic group. Non-compliance with treatment and use of drugs or alcohol also complicate the picture. NICE guidelines (2005) suggest clinical factors that range across diagnoses, listed in Box 33.2.

Wright *et al.* (2002) conclude that although symptoms may have some role in influencing violence and aggression, it is more likely that it is the effect of symptoms in reducing ability to deal with external demands and interpersonal conflict that is implicated in violent and aggressive behaviour.

> ### Box 33.1   Demographic or personal risk factors for aggression
>
> ■   a history of violence or disturbed behaviour
> ■   history of substance misuse
> ■   carers' reports of previous violence or anger
> ■   previous expression of intent to harm
> ■   previous use of weapons
> ■   previous dangerous impulsive acts
> ■   denial of previous (proven) dangerous acts
> ■   severity of previous acts
> ■   known personal trigger factors
> ■   verbal threat of violence
> ■   evidence of recent severe stress, particularly loss or threat of loss
> ■   one or more of the above plus any of the following:
>   –   cruelty to animals
>   –   reckless driving
>   –   history of bed wetting
>   –   loss of a parent before age 8

> ### Box 33.2   Clinical factors associated with increased risk of aggression
>
> ■   substance abuse
> ■   agitation or excitement
> ■   hostility or suspiciousness
> ■   a preoccupation with violence
> ■   poor collaboration with treatment
>
> ■   delusions or hallucinations focused on a particular person
> ■   delusions of control with a violent theme
> ■   impulsive personality traits
> ■   poor collaboration with treatment
> ■   organic dysfunction

Environmental factors

The Royal College of Psychiatrists Research Unit (1998) acknowledged that hospital wards are unnatural environments, which nevertheless should aim to create a safe, homely atmosphere which allows for safety and for privacy. The supporting social environment is equally important. Patients in a US maximum security facility reported that they often did not understand the reasons for ward rules and expectations (Caplan 1993), while patients in the Sainsbury Centre for Mental Health survey of acute wards (1998) reported disliking the constant refrain from staff of 'the policy is …'. Boredom and lack of structured activity may also be contributory to violence and aggression. Katz and Kirkland (1990) examined levels of violence on psychiatric wards in the USA and concluded that 'violence was more frequent and extreme in wards in which staff functions were unclear, and in which events such as activities, meetings or staff-patient encounters were unpredictable' (1990: 262). Shah (1993) summarized research suggesting that levels of violence increase at times when patients congregate with little structured activity, e.g. medication and meal times. (See Box 33.3.)

Staffing factors

Patients surveyed by the Royal College of Psychiatrists Research Unit (1998) emphasized that talking and listening are key interventions not to be undervalued. They focused on boredom, staff attitudes and staffing levels as factors affecting levels of violence. Patients in the Sainsbury Centre for Mental Health (1998) survey indicated that they wanted more access to staff; however, organizational and resource factors may militate against this. Shah (1993) summarized possible staff factors associated with higher levels of violence including: use of temporary staff, under-involvement of medical staff, poor communication among staff, demoralization and incompetence among staff and high staff turnover. It may be that these factors create a 'high expressed emotion' environment. Establishing an ideal number of nursing staff is complex. Owen *et al.* (1998) found an association between higher numbers of nursing staff and higher levels of violence, which may reflect increased numbers of staff as a response to violence. On the other hand, Morrison and Lehane (1995) found that over a two-year period in one psychiatric hospital, as staffing levels increased, use of seclusion fell. This study also reported that fewer seclusions took place when experienced nurses were on duty, while Owen *et al.* (1998) reported that increased violence is associated with lower levels of experience and lack of staff training in control of aggression techniques.

The Royal College of Psychiatrists Research Unit (1998), in reviewing the evidence on the influence of the physical and social environment concluded that the quantitative evidence is too weak to draw firm conclusions about relationships between these and incidence of aggression. However, they also argue that addressing these issues makes intuitive sense. The NICE guidance (2005) concords with this and also makes recommendations about the environment in mental health wards. Box 33.3 summarizes some of the evidence on physical and social environmental factors which may influence levels of violence and aggression.

Box 33.3   Aspects of the physical and social environment affecting levels of aggression

Physical environment should:
- be clean
- allow for daylight and fresh air
- avoid overcrowding
- have controlled noise levels (for example, a separate TV room)
- allow for control of temperature and ventilation
- provide designated smoking and non-smoking areas
- allow for privacy in bedrooms, bathrooms and toilets
- provide sightlines allowing people to see what is happening in different parts of the ward.

Social environment should have:
- rationale offered for ward expectations
- open communication processes between patients, ward staff and management
- patient involvement in decision-making
- planned, predictable activity
- opportunity for social and recreational activity
- clear staff functions
- adequate and consistent staffing
- effective multi-disciplinary working
- commitment to staff training and support.

Although these points may seem self-evident, findings of a national audit of psychiatric wards for the period 1999–2000 indicated that many aspects of the physical and social environment and staff training and communication fell short of the recommendations above (Royal College of Psychiatrists Research Unit 2000). The RCP have also devised audit criteria based on all the recommendations in the NICE guideline which will be used to monitor clinical environments on behalf of the Healthcare Commission.

Practice model

Improving services and practice in light of the factors above is likely to have a long-term and lasting impact in levels of violence. However, in the best planned environments, anger, aggression and violence will still occur, and in this case an understanding of the appropriate level of intervention matched to the phase of aggression is needed.

One model which lends itself to a range of interventions is that proposed by Novaco (1983) in his development of an anger management treatment programme. In this model, anger is seen as a state of physiological arousal leading to tension and irritability which lead to cognitions producing antagonistic thought patterns. As exposure continues, antagonistic thought patterns lead to faulty appraisal of others' behaviour or situations. Inappropriate coping mechanisms in response to increasing stress can then cause aggression. Goleman (1995) in his book on *Emotional Intelligence* describes a similar cascade of events in which a sense of threat or danger evokes the fight or flight mechanism, invoking a train of angry thoughts which in turn contribute to increased physiological arousal, rendering the person more susceptible to external triggers, each wave becoming more intense and increasing the level of physiological arousal. These models suggest that anger and aggression can often be observed to escalate, and physical harm can be prevented if the escalating situation is observed and early intervention made.

Observation and engagement

The 2005 NICE guidelines include observation and engagement as methods for predicting and preventing escalation of anger into violence. Observation is defined in the same way as when used in the management of self-harm, i.e. on four levels from general observation through intermittent observation to 'within eyesight' and 'within arms length'. The minimum level of observation necessary should be used and engagement with the service user is a key aim of the intervention.

It could be argued that intrusive levels of observation are both provocative to patients at risk of harm to others and place observing staff at risk. Risk assessment should be rigorous and recorded in both medical and nursing notes and consideration should be given to having more than one staff member observing the service user. All staff involved in observation should be familiar with the ward environment and methods of summoning help. In accordance with the NICE guidance, observation should be considered a short-term (72 hour) intervention. More specific methods of prediction and prevention are incorporated into de-escalation techniques.

De-escalation

The Sainsbury Centre for Mental Health (2001) includes understanding of de-escalation skills as a core capability for mental health nurses working in acute settings. The term 'de-escalation' refers to the 'processes by which a patient's expressed anger or aggression is defused, so that a calmer state ensues' (RCN 1997). In this position statement, the RCN (1997) described these short-term interventions as utilizing a combination of immediate risk assessment together with verbal and non-verbal communication skills. Application is divided into several phases, as follows:

Understanding reasons for anger or aggression

As well as the clinical and social factors underlying aggression, the individual's specific situation has to be considered. The person may have experienced (or perceive that they have experienced) personal criticism, restriction or control, unfair treatment, frustration of intentions or the irritating behaviour of others. Nurses therefore need to be aware of what is happening both on the ward in general and for the patient in particular, and may be contributing to their anger. Stressors might also include staff behaviours. Wright *et al.* (2002) report that research shows violent incidents to be more likely when there is aversive stimulation from staff in terms of imposing limits or frustrating requests.

Assessing immediate risk

The NICE guideline (2005) emphasizes that staff should be aware of both general and personal factors which can provoke an individual service user. This includes an awareness of the effect of staff behaviour, both verbal and non-verbal. Staff should also encourage service users to be able to recognize and monitor their own triggers and record this in care plans. These individual factors are important to recognize as similar behaviours may mean different things when displayed by different people. A study by Whittington and Patterson (1996) matched aggressive and non-aggressive patients and found that the groups were distinguished by levels of verbal abuse, threatening gestures and either very high or very low activity. Verbal abuse was the most common behaviour and preceded two-thirds of physical attacks. However, the caveat is that in many cases key behaviours were exhibited for long periods without being followed by violence. Despite this, possible antecedents to aggression derived from the Royal College of Nursing (RCN 1997) and RCP Research Unit (1998) are indicated when the person (see Box 33.4).

Box 33.4   Possible indicators of anger and aggression

- focuses attention on what is causing anger and continues to dwell on this
- perceives threat from others or is suspicious
- reacts in an exaggerated manner to problems
- shows increased physical arousal – restlessness, pacing, erratic movements

- refuses to communicate or withdraws
- makes verbal threats or gestures
- reports angry or violent feelings
- shows increased volume of speech
- has a tense facial expression – fixed stare, clenched jaw, makes constant eye contact

---

Monitoring safety

Having identified an increased risk of violence, maintaining safety is also necessary. Practice points drawn from the RCN (1997) and RCP Research Unit (1998) guidelines are listed in Box 33.5.

Box 33.5   Practice points for monitoring safety

- Don't isolate yourself – check that colleagues know your whereabouts.
- Check that you are familiar with mechanisms for calling for help and that you have access to these.
- Check escape routes – avoid corners.
- If isolated when a violent incident occurs, the priority is to get away from the situation and summon help. Do not tackle a violent person alone, whatever your or the patient's gender or size.

- Make a visual check of the immediate area for potential weapons. For example there may be chairs, cups or glasses in the day area or dining room; if in a kitchen there may be knives or boiling water; in a bathroom razors or aerosols may be present. If identified, the priority is to maintain distance and offer the option to person to leave the area and continue discussion elsewhere.

Once a risk assessment and safety check indicate that it is possible to approach the person safely, de-escalation techniques can be used. NICE guidelines (2005) provide specific descriptions of the techniques which should be used and recommend that one person should approach the service user and assume control of the situation (rather than several staff surrounding one service user, which can clearly be seen as threatening). Some key non-verbal and verbal interventions (derived from NICE and the RCN) are:

Non-verbal communciation
- Maintain an adequate distance – this is more than usual when dealing with an angry person as closeness may be interpreted as a threat or increase tension.

- Stand at an angle to the patient to avoid appearing confrontational. Do not point and do not touch the person.
- Maintain normal eye contact – staring can be threatening, avoiding can seem dismissive.
- Appear calm and speak slowly using clear and short sentences. However, avoid being patronizing (avoid telling patient to calm down!). Be courteous, and use the person's name.
- Be aware of your own reactions, which may be fear or anger, and try to consider the patient's point of view – they might be anxious as well as angry. Do not feel that you have to win any argument or that you have to deal with this situation alone and effectively in order to be a 'good nurse'. Try to show concern and attentiveness.

Verbal communication

The aim here is to continue communication and move on to problem-solving. Some key techniques are:

- Engage in conversation and most importantly acknowledge concerns, allowing the person time to express their worries or complaints. Ask the person to sit down with you or go to a quieter area (as long as other staff know where you are and your initial risk assessment indicates this is safe). Ask the person for the facts of the problem as they see them.
- Use reflective listening to acknowledge concerns. This is more skilled than it appears and is not simply stating the obvious or parroting what the person says. Be specific – 'I can see you're disappointed and upset that you won't be able to go home this weekend.'
- Convey that you want to help the person find a solution, e.g. 'give me half-an-hour to try to find out what has happened'. Be realistic and do not make promises that cannot be kept. Allow the person to start generating options for dealing with the problem. Do not lecture or challenge.
- Attempt to establish rapport and emphasize cooperation.
- Negotiate realistic options and avoid using threats.
- Ask open questions.
- Listen carefully and show empathy.

Physical intervention

NICE guidance (2005) clearly states that de-escalation techniques should be seen as part of an ongoing response to escalation of anger and aggression. They should always be attempted before other interventions are employed. However, verbal interventions work up to a certain point of moderate anger but may fail to calm a situation. Goleman (1995) argues that after a certain stage, they have no effect as people are unable to process information. Further, the relationship between anger and aggression is not straightforward. Absence of overt anger does not mean that aggression will not occur. Where aggression leads to gain – material, social or psychological – anger is not necessary to precipitate it. If, at this stage, aggression or violence occurs, physical intervention may be needed to maintain safety.

Restraint

The aim here is not to describe techniques for physical restraint. These should be taught on an approved course and involve an assessment of competence to use physical techniques. However, they should be used judiciously with an understanding of the legal, professional and ethical context. The Mental Health Act Code of Practice (DH 1999) makes clear that providers of inpatient psychiatric care should have policies on the use of physical restraint.

However, restraint is a 'last resort' intervention. NICE guidelines place restraint, rapid tranquillization and seclusion at the end of a care pathway where prediction and prevention have failed. However, the RCN (1997) acknowledged that use of restraint should not necessarily be seen as a failure, as people in an extreme state of anger or provocation might not be able to respond to verbal interventions.

Physical intervention techniques developed from Control and Restraint (CandR) training used by the Prison Service (Wright *et al.* 2002). The term C&R should not however be used within psychiatric services as techniques have been adapted for this setting. Specific techniques have also evolved and changed in the face of deaths and injuries sustained using physical intervention in mental health settings. The NICE guidance, for example, takes account of some of the findings of the 2003 inquiry into the death of David Bennett during restraint. Staff should attend regular updates to ensure that they are familiar with changes. In a survey of acute wards in London (Gournay *et al.* 1998) only one trust out of 11 did not routinely train ward staff in use of physical restraint. One of the most important recommendations of the NICE guidance is the development of standardized and accredited training in both physical and non-physical management of violence and aggression. In October 2005, NHS Security Management Services published *Promoting Safer and Therapeutic Services: Implementing the national syllabus in mental health and learning disability services.* This provides learning outcomes for all non-physical aspects of training and should form the basis for physical skills training being developed by the National Institute for Mental Health in England (NIMHE) and the National Patient Safety Agency. All relevant staff in mental health settings should be trained in accordance with the Promoting Safer and Therapeutic Services (PSTS) curriculum by 2008. The NICE guidance makes several recommendations about the principles of use of physical restraint including:

- Staff should continue to use de-escalation techniques during physical intervention.
- Physical restraint should be avoided if possible and should not be used for prolonged periods because of risks to physical health. Rapid tranquillization or seclusion should be considered as an alternative.
- The level of force used must be justifiable and appropriate to the situation.
- The application of pain has no therapeutic value and could only be justified for the immediate rescue of others.
- Pressure should never be applied to the neck, thorax, abdomen or pelvic area. The patient's airway and breathing should be monitored throughout.

Both the RCP Research Unit (1998) and the Nursing and Midwifery Council (Wright *et al.* 2002) reviews found that studies of the effectiveness of restraint in reducing levels of violence and aggression tend to be poorly designed and descriptive in nature. Many studies are from countries other than the UK and 'restraint' may have different meanings across countries. Wright *et al.* (2002) also argue that there are significant ethical and methodological issues in conducting research in this area. There are likely to be many other intervening factors apart from restraint training which influence the incidence of violence and it is arguably unethical to withhold training from some staff in order to maintain a control group. The RCP Research Unit (1998) concluded that evidence suggests that injury during restraint can be reduced as a result of training although the frequency of violence may not reduce. Wright *et al.* (2002) conclude that 'it is reasonable to believe that the evidence base is sufficient to indicate what is likely to constitute good practice that is clinically, logically, ethically and medico-logically defensible' (2002: 41). What does seem clear is that the use of restraint is emotive for both patients and staff. However, patients and carers consulted by the RCP acknowledged that restraint was sometimes necessary to prevent harm to others, what was important was the judicious and rational use of physical intervention.

Seclusion

Many wards manage violence without the use of seclusion; however, its use is still widespread and remains controversial with both staff and patients expressing negative attitudes. Soliday (1985) found that patients expressed more negative feelings about seclusion than did nurses, who saw seclusion as necessary at times. As with restraint, research into the therapeutic use of seclusion lacks controlled studies. Wright *et al.* (2002) state that outcome studies are problematic because 'improvements' may be perceived as a result of a change in the patient's behaviour rather than mental state.

The Mental Health Act Code of Practice (DH 1999) defines seclusion as: 'the supervised confinement of a patient in a room which may be locked to protect others from significant harm. Its sole aim is to contain severely disturbed behaviour which is likely to cause harm to others' (para. 18.16). In addition, it should be used as a last resort and for the shortest possible time. It should not be used as a punishment or threat, as part of a treatment programme (it should not be confused with the use of 'time out' which is a specific behavioural intervention) because of shortage of staff or where there is any risk of suicide or self-harm. The decision to seclude should not be an automatic one following restraint. The Mental Health Act Code of Practice (DH 1999) states that the decision to seclude can be made by a doctor or the nurse in charge (para. 18.18). If seclusion is initiated, the NICE guidelines recommend that:

- Seclusion should be recorded in accordance with the Mental Health Act Code of Practice.
- An observation schedule should be established and the patient observed constantly by a trained person.
- Seclusion must be reviewed at least every two hours and should be for the shortest time possible.
- The patient should not be deprived of clothing or personal items such as jewellery as long as there is no risk to self or others.
- If rapid tranquillization has been used, seclusion should terminate once medication has taken effect.

In addition, the seclusion room should be kept clean and free of anything that could be used as a weapon. The patient should also be checked for weapons before seclusion is initiated.

Use of seclusion is controversial and emotive. The RCP Research Unit (1998) argued that service users should be involved in the development of local protocols and that patients who are secluded should always be given an explanation at the time, which is repeated later.

Wright *et al.* (2002) also suggest that debriefing is offered afterwards to patients and that use of seclusion in principle should be discussed at ward or patient meetings.

Rapid tranquillization

Again, the decision to use medication should not be an automatic one. The aim of rapid tranquillization is to calm a situation and may or may not involve the use of anti-psychotic medication depending on the service user. The patients in the RCP Research Unit (1998) consultation exercise expressed concern about the use of medication in people they felt were not mentally ill, but felt that informed use of medication was preferable to physical restraint. However, it is worth noting that the Mental Health Act Code of Practice (1999) warns that prolonged use of medication can become a form of constraint if used solely to control aggressive behaviour.

Staff should also be aware of the legal context for medication administration before incidents (this is covered by Part IV of the Mental Health Act 1983. Sections 57 and 58 cover treatment requiring consent or a second opinion; Section 60 relates to withdrawal of consent; and Section 62 covers urgent treatment). The Mental Health Act Commission also provides guidance to nurses on the administration of medication (2001). Decisions should be multi-disciplinary and a rationale always recorded.

The NICE violence guideline (2005) reiterates the rapid tranquillization protocol for patients with schizophrenia (NICE 2002). Their treatment algorithm emphasizes the need for staff training in tranquillization protocols, in the properties of benzodiazepines, antipsychotics, flumenazil (a benzodiazepine antagonist), and in cardiopulmonary resuscitation. Use should be balanced against the risks of over-sedation causing loss of alertness or consciousness and damage to the nurse–patient relationship. If the patient is secluded and rapid tranquillization used, extra vigilance is needed. Oral medication should be offered first – lorazepam, olanzepine and haloperidol are suggested (use of the latter may also require the administration of an anticholinergic). If intramuscular (IM) administration is necessary, single use of one of the above drugs is advocated, again with the proviso that where typical antipsychotics are used, an anticholinergic should also be given. The NICE guidelines (2005) state that in urgent cases IM haloperidol and lorazepam can be given together if psychosis is indicated. There is no evidence that combining several medications of the same group or using doses above BNF limits has any better effect.

Again, the decision should be a multi-disciplinary one and a rationale clearly documented. Vital signs also need to be monitored following medication. The 2005 NICE guideline states that staff who are involved in rapid tranquillization should be trained to the level of Immediate Life Support and should be trained in the use of a pulse oximeter. As soon as possible, the patient should be given an opportunity to discuss the use of medication and receive an explanation for its use.

Dealing with serious incidents

Advice on dealing with situations which involve weapons has unfortunately been unclear and contradictory. RCP Research Unit (1998) guidance calls for staff to ask for a weapon to be put down rather than handed over, while the RCN (1997) advised that the area should be cleared and the police called. The NICE guideline (2005) recommends that the patient is asked to put down any weapon in a neutral space. Wright *et al.* (2000) state that all trusts should have policies on when to involve the police. The Mental Health Act Commission (2003) argue that clear guidance is needed as police may be resentful of being involved in minor incidents, but that nursing staff need reassurance that the necessity to prevent crime (and harm) also applies to mental health settings.

Post-incident management

Many nurses will be uncomfortable about using physical interventions as it is difficult to see them as 'therapeutic'. The Mental Health Act Commission, in their Tenth Biennial Report (2003) argue that restraint and seclusion are justifiable to maintain safety, but that the power to use these interventions should not be abused and they should not become punitive measures. Gunn and Rodgers (2002) argue that use of restraint and seclusion cannot be justified on treatment grounds, but that the most appropriate ethical basis is in 'common law justification', i.e. the requirement to use the least force necessary to prevent harm. The difficulty for nurses is that they may have to use these interventions while building and maintaining therapeutic relationships. It would be naive to assume that physical intervention does not affect staff–patient relationships. However, the legal, professional and ethical context which frames their use can serve to provide safety and reassurance for both patients and staff, and good post-incident management may help to reduce the longer-term effects. NICE guidance recommends both incident reporting and post-incident review following any instances of aggression or violence.

The emotional impact of coping with aggression, even if managed effectively, should not be overlooked. Wykes and Whittington (1994) found that staff reactions to assault included fear, anxiety, guilt, self-blame, anger and hatred. Crichton *et al.* (1998) suggested that staff response to aggression involves an element of moral censure of the patient related to level of perceived threat and assessment of moral responsibility. Coping with these strong feelings has an effect on relationships with patients, possibly leading to hostility, avoidance and controlling behaviour, which feeds back to levels of violence among patients (Whittington and Wykes 1994). Post-incident review is therefore vital to allow expression of difficult emotions and enable learning from the incident (critical incident analysis is one such mechanism). Patients who have been involved in or observed aggressive incidents also need support. Neither should the impact of verbal abuse be underestimated. Community staff may be particularly affected by this given that they often see clients alone and are often called on to make day-to-day practice decisions in isolation (ENB 1998).

Conclusion

There is no 'cookbook' approach to managing anger, violence and aggression. Interventions need to be adapted to the needs of the patient. The current NICE guideline emphasizes the recognition of the individual needs of service users including all aspects of diversity such as social, physical and spiritual needs. On a positive note, research suggests that nurses do actually use a creative mixture of techniques when dealing with violence and aggression (Haber *et al.* 1997, in Wright *et al.* 2000) adopting an approach which tailors interventions to seriousness of situation. However, there is overwhelming consensus that the interventions discussed above are no substitute for competent and confident staff working as a team in a safe and therapeutic environment. To summarize:

- The quality of the physical and social environment on mental health wards is likely to have an impact on the level of violence and aggression.
- Talking and listening to patients are fundamental interventions in preventing violence and aggression.
- Intervention should be matched to the level of anger or aggression; there is a hierarchy of methods from verbal to physical techniques. NICE (2005) guidance emphasizes that any staff response should be proportionate to the level of risk.
- Physical intervention occurs within a legal, professional and ethical framework. Staff should make sure they understand these considerations before any incident.
- Patients and staff need to be offered support after an incident of aggression.

Questions for reflection and discussion

1   Think about wards you have worked on. Did the physical and social environment impact on levels of aggression? Were there any improvements which could have been made? (Consider the points in Box 33.3.)
2   You arrive at work for an early shift and receive a handover about Richard. He was brought to the ward during the night by the police after throwing a brick through a neighbour's window. He felt they were secretly filming him and was trying to break the recording equipment in their house. He smelt of alcohol when admitted and looked disoriented and scared. He has only slept for a few hours. After the night staff leave, Richard comes into the day area. He looks agitated; pacing the day area and talking to himself. What do you consider before approaching him? (See Box 33.4.)
3   What beliefs do you have about angry and aggressive people? What nursing skills do you think are most important when dealing with potentially aggressive situations? (See de-escalation techniques.)
4   Richard agrees to sit down and talk to you. He doesn't understand why he is in hospital and the thinks the police may have fitted him up. He would like to go home and at least get some money and clothes. He still sounds angry when talking about his situation. What verbal interventions could you use?

Annotated bibliography

- Wright, S., Gray, R., Parkes, J. and Gournay, K. (2002) The recognition, prevention and therapeutic management of violence in acute in-patient psychiatry: a literature review and evidence-based recommendations for good practice. London: UKCC. This report, prepared for the NMC, provides a comprehensive review of the research on violence and aggression in mental health settings and discusses the evidence base for factors which influence violence as well as the effectiveness of management interventions.
- Royal College of Psychiatrists College Research Unit (1998) Management of imminent violence: clinical practice guidelines to support mental health services. Occasional Paper

OP41. London: RCP. This report provided practical guidance based on a review of research evidence and consultation with users and carers. It has been replaced by: Violence: the short-term management of disturbed/violent behaviour in in-patient psychiatric settings and emergency departments (National Institute for Health and Clinical Excellence, clinical guideline 25, February 2005). This is the current definitive guide to practice in the management of violence or aggression. The full guideline also provides a review of the most recent evidence in the area. The guideline was developed in conjunction with service users.

■ Mason, T. and Chandley, M. (1999) Managing Violence and Aggression: a manual for nurses and healthcare workers. Edinburgh: Churchill Livingstone. This provides a practice based discussion of interventions used during different phases of aggression. The sections on longer-term, structured intervention such as behavioural programmes give another perspective on management of aggression.

■ Vaughan, P.J. and Badger, D. (1995) Working with the Mentally Disordered Offender in the Community. London: Chapman Hall. For guidance on managing aggression in the community, Chapter 4 contains practical advice on maintaining safety in community mental health centres and when visiting clients.

References

Caplan, C.A. (1993) Nursing staff and patient perceptions of ward atmosphere in a maximum security forensic hospital. *Archives of Psychiatric Nursing* **3**(1): 23–9.
Crichton, J., Callanan, T.S., Beauchamp, L., Glasson, M. and Tardiff, H. (1998) Staff response to psychiatric inpatient violence: an international comparison. *Psychiatric Care* **5**(2): 50–6.
Department of Health (1999) *Mental Health Act 1983 Code of Practice*. London: HMSO.
ENB (1998) *Research Highlight 34: risk assessment and management in multi-agency, multi-professional health care: education and practice*. London: ENB.
Goleman, D. (1995) *Emotional Intelligence*. London: Bloomsbury.
Gournay, K. (2000) *The Recognition, Prevention and Therapeutic Management of Violence in Mental Health Care: a consultation document;* London: UKCC.
Gournay, K., Ward, M., Thornicroft, G. and Wright, S. (1998) *Crisis in the Capital: in-patient care in inner London Mental Health Practice* **1**(5): 10–18.
Gunn, M. and Rodgers, M. (2002) Mental health nursing, in J. Tingle and A. Cribb (eds) *Nursing Law and Ethics* (2nd edn). Oxford: Blackwell Science.
Haber, L.C., Fagan-Pryor, E.C. and Allen, M. (1997) Comparison of registered nurses' and nursing assistants' choices of interventions for aggressive behaviours. *Issues in Mental Health Nursing* **18**: 325–8.
Independent Inquiry into the Death of David Bennett (2003). An independent inquiry set up under HSG(94) 27.
Katz, P. and Kirkland, F.R. (1990) Violence and social structure on mental hospital wards. *Psychiatry* **53**: 262–77.
Lowenstein, M., Binder, R.L. and McNiel, D.E. (1990) The relationship between admission symptoms and hospital assaults. *Hospital and Community Psychiatry* **41**(3): 311–13.
Mason, T. and Chandley, M. (1999) *Managing Violence and Aggression: a manual for nurses and healthcare workers*. Edinburgh: Churchill Livingstone.
Mental Health Act Commission (2001) *Guidance note: nurses, the administration of medicine for mental disorder and the Mental Health Act 1983*, Commission ref: GN 2/2001. Trent: MHAC.
Mental Health Act Commission (2003) *Tenth Biennial Report 2001–2003: Placed Amongst Strangers*. Trent: MHAC.
Monaghan, J. (1993) Mental disorder and violence: another look, in S. Hodgins (ed.) *Mental Disorder and Crime*. London: Sage.

Morrison, P. and Lehane, M. (1995) Staffing levels and seclusion use. *Journal of Advanced Nursing* **22**: 1192–202.

National Audit Office (2003) *A Safer Place to Work: Improving the management of health and safety risks to staff in NHS trusts.* London: HMSO.

National Institute for Clinical Excellence (2002) *Schizophrenia: core interventions in the treatment and management of schizophrenia in primary and secondary care.* London: NICE.

National Institute for Health and Clinical Excellence (2005) *Violence: the short-term management of disturbed/violent behaviour in in-patient psychiatric settings and emergency departments* (clinical guideline 25). London. NICE.

Nursing and Midwifery Council (2003) Press release, 3 February 2003.

Novaco, R.W. (1983) *Stress Inoculation therapy for Anger Control: a manual for therapists.* Irvine: University of California.

Owen, C., Tarantello, C., Jones, M. and Tennant, C. (1998) Violence and aggression in psychiatric units. *Psychiatric Services* **49**(11): 1452–7.

Royal College of Nursing (1997) *The Management of Aggression and Violence in Places of Care: an RCN position statement.* London: RCN.

Royal College of Psychiatrists Research Unit (1998) *Management of Imminent Violence: clinical practice guidelines to support mental health services.* Occasional Paper OP41. London: RCP.

Royal College of Psychiatrists Research Unit (2000) *National Audit of the Management of Violence in Mental Health Settings 1999–2000.* London: RCP.

Sainsbury Centre for Mental Health (1998) *Acute Problems: a survey of the quality of care in acute psychiatric wards.* London: Sainsbury Centre for Mental Health.

Sainsbury Centre for Mental Health (2001) *The Capable Practitioner: a framework and list of the practitioner capabilities required to implement The National Service Framework for Mental Health.* London: Sainsbury Centre for Mental Health.

Shah, A.K. (1993) An increase in violence among psychiatric in-patients: real or imagined? *Medical Science Law* **33**(3): 227–9.

Soliday, S.M. (1985) A comparison of patients and staff attitudes toward seclusion. *Journal of Nervous and Mental Disease* **173**(5): 282–6.

Vinestock, M. (1996) Risk assessment: 'a word to the wise'. *Advances in Psychiatric Treatment* **2**: 3–10.

Whittington, R. and Patterson, P. (1996) Verbal and non-verbal behaviour immediately prior to aggression by mentally disordered people: enhancing the assessment of risk. *Journal of Psychiatric and Mental Health Nursing* **3**: 47–54.

Whittington, R. and Wykes, T. (1994) An observational study of associations between nurse behaviour and violence in psychiatric hospitals. *Journal of Psychiatric and Mental Health Nursing* **1**: 85–92.

Wright, S., Lee, S., Sayer, J., Parr, A. and Gournay, K. (2000) A review of the content of management of violence policies in in-patient mental health units. *Mental Health Care* **3**(11): 373–6.

Wright, S., Gray, R., Parkes, J. and Gournay, K. (2002) *The Recognition, Prevention and Therapeutic Management of Violence in Acute In-patient Psychiatry: a literature review and evidence based recommendations for good practice.* London: UKCC.

Wykes, T. and Whittington, R. (1994) Reactions to assault, in T. Wykes (ed.) *Violence and Healthcare Professionals.* London: Chapman and Hall.

CHAPTER 34

Nursing people who self-harm or are suicidal

Ian Noonan

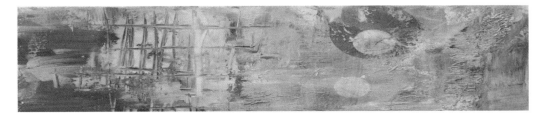

Chapter overview

Working with people who harm themselves or feel and act upon suicidal thoughts can pose a dilemma: how do you help someone who is trying to hurt himself/herself or attempt to end his/her life? In health care we often assume that the person we are working with will negotiate, want and be a partner in the care that is being provided for them, or that, at some level, we are able to find a goal that is shared in the work that we undertake.

When someone is self-harming, the behaviour itself can seem like the opposite of what we are trying to achieve, but for the client the need to cut, for example, might be so great that they fear what would happen without it. Equally, for a client who feels suicidal, they may not be able to see a future and find it very difficult to imagine a way of resolving how they feel.

For the nurse, there is a risk that we might end up resenting or feeling angry with the person who has self-harmed, as it can be perceived as deliberately undoing the work you have done.

This chapter aims to explore the range of self-harm behaviour and suicidal thoughts, feelings and actions, and show that, although the two phenomena are different, there is an overlap between self-harm and suicide. Ways of thinking about people who self-harm or are suicidal will be suggested, to help nurses understand this client group. Different treatment options will be explored using case study examples to help identify ways of nursing this client group that are positive and hopeful. Further details on assessment of risk in people who self-harm or are suicidal, can be found in Chapter 11.

This chapter covers:

■ definition and types of self-harm behaviour;
■ the relationship between self-harm and suicide;
■ nursing someone who self-harms:
  – understanding – mechanism and meaning,
  – therapeutic assessment,
  – motivation,
  – harm reduction,

- – solution-focused interventions for self-harm;
- ▪ what people who self-harm want;
- ▪ nursing someone who is suicidal;
- ▪ therapeutic engagement through the process of observation;
- ▪ special groups:
  - – young people,
  - – older adults,
  - – people with psychosis;
- ▪ being safe.

Defining self-harm

The language used to describe how and why people harm themselves can reflect the judgements that are often made about this client group: 'self-abuse' and 'self-mutilation' assume emotive aspects such as guilt or self-loathing, whereas purely descriptive terms such as 'cutting' or 'blood letting' convey neither the choice that the client has made nor the fact that the act is harmful.

Weber (2002) cites several terms that have been used to describe such behaviour: self-injury, self-abuse, indirect self-destructive behaviour, para-suicide, self-inflicted injury, self-injurious behaviour, self-mutilation, as well as deliberate self-harm. The terms used often reflect the theoretical standpoint of the clinician using them rather than the client who harms himself or herself. Self-abuse, self-destructive behaviour or self-mutilation suggest a psychodynamic understanding of the motivation for the behaviour, whereas self-injury or deliberate self-harm convey some sense that the person has chosen to act in this way and that it is a behaviour rather than an illness per se.

House *et al.* define deliberate self-harm as 'intentional self poisoning or self injury (such as cutting), irrespective of the apparent purpose of the act' (1999: 137). Weber, however, goes on to exclude suicidal intent as a possible purpose or meaning of the act: 'I used the term self-destruction as the broad encompassing category of behaviours that are self-inflicted, of which self-abuse, or the deliberate harm to one's own body without suicidal intent, is one type' (2002: 118). Gallop and Tully expand further on the meaning of the behaviour in their definition, 'Self-injury is often an attempt to communicate distress, relieve pain and maintain connection to oneself and others. Suicide attempts, on the other hand are directed at discontinuing all connections and ending consciousness' (2004: 236). See Table 34.1.

The NICE guidelines for the short-term management of self-harm (NICE 2004) have chosen to remove the term deliberate in acknowledgement of the fact that some people may self-harm in a dissociative state and that intent varies from individual to individual and on each occasion that someone harms themselves. Their broad scoping definition 'self-poisoning or self-injury irrespective of the apparent purpose of the act' (NICE 2004: 16) aims to ensure that people presenting with a wide range of self-harm will be offered access to a psychosocial assessment and appropriate support and follow-up.

1 *Self-harm which breaks the skin or causes bleeding*

Cutting with knives, razor blades, broken glass

Excessive scratching by removing the top layer of skin to cause a sore

Excessive nail biting to the point of bleeding and ripping cuticles

Burning skin by chemical means using caustic liquids

Burning by physical means using heat

Friction burns to skin using abrasive materials

Gnawing at flesh

Blood letting

2 *Self-harm by more violent methods*

Pinching hard enough to cause bruises

Head banging against the floor or walls

Hitting the head with fist or hard objects

Punching windows or walls

Bone breaking

Jumping from heights without suicidal ideation

Tying ligatures around the neck, arms or legs to restrict the flow of blood

Hair pulling from head, eyelashes, eyebrows or armpits (trichotillomania)

3 *Self-harm with internal/medical effects*

Medication abuse (overdoses) without the intention to die

Poisoning by ingesting small amounts of toxic substances to cause discomfort or damage

Deliberately ingesting food to cause a known allergic reaction

Wound interference to prevent wounds from healing or to deliberately infect them

Insertion of foreign objects

Binge-eating or starvation

Alcohol misuse

Illicit drug use

Table 34.1 Self-harm: mechanisms of injury

Self-harm therefore can include a wide range of behaviours that damage an individual's body, either externally or internally, with a meaning or purpose that can vary for any one client on each occasion that they self-harm, and from person to person. The act might be impulsive or planned, with immediate or long-term effect. The term only describes the behaviour and is not an illness. This does not mean that the person who self-harms will not benefit from treatment, rather that there are likely to be coexisting mental health needs which will also need to be addressed in order to help that person change their self-harming behaviour.

The relationship between self-harm and suicide

According to the Office of National Statistics (2008), just over 11,000 people committed suicide in the United Kingdom in 2006, and suicide is the most common cause of death in men under 35 (DH 2003). Although self-harm and suicide are different phenomena, there is a statistical relationship between the two. Of the population who self-harm 1–2 in 100 will be dead by suicide within one year, 3–4 in 100 will be dead by suicide within four years and more than 10 will be dead by suicide eventually. For example in the London Borough of Southwark 15 of the 52 people who committed suicide in 2002–3 had attended an accident and emergency department within the year preceding their death (Hodgkiss 2007). In Leeds, 39 per cent of the people who committed suicide had attended an accident and emergency department in the 12 months before their death: 40 per cent of these had attended with self-harm (Gairin et al. 2003). One of the key relationships between self-harm and suicide is therefore the necessity to assess everyone who self-harms to try to identify those who might be at risk of suicide and care for them accordingly.

It is important to remember that the death of an individual impacts on his community, family and society in general. One of the target groups that the government has identified for reducing suicide rates is the high-risk group of clients who commit suicide in the year following an incident of self-harm. If this group is combined with people who are currently, or have recently been, in contact with mental health services, it represents almost half of the number of people who kill themselves each year.

Bongar (2002) suggests that the 'murky' discriminations between self-harm, attempted suicide by a non-lethal method, survived and completed suicide attempts, are of more use to the researcher than the clinician. He argues that any act where someone self-harms or states their intention to do so should be treated as a communication of psychological pain, which should be thoroughly assessed. Bongar (2002) views suicide as a complex bio-psychosocial phenomenon which includes the death of those who intended to kill themselves and individuals with patterns of self-harm who accidentally die as a result of their injuries. The relationship between suicide and self-harm also depends on the client's understanding of the risk to his or her own life. Stengel defined attempted suicide as follows:

> 66 A suicidal attempt is any act inflicted with self destructive intention, however vague and ambiguous. For the clinician, it is safer still to regard all cases of potentially dangerous self-poisoning or self-inflicted injury as suicidal attempts, whatever the victim's explanation, unless there is clear evidence to the contrary. Potentially dangerous means in this context: believed by the attempter possibly to endanger life.
>
> (Stengel 1965: 64) 99

Although there is some value in Stengel's definition in terms of immediate assessment, it has the potential to devalue the client's own knowledge, experience and reasons for self-harming. Without question, it is important to find out from the client what their intentions were and are, and in fact this could provide the 'clear evidence to the contrary' which Stengel seeks.

There are grounds for distinguishing between self-harm and suicidal thoughts, feelings and actions, as many people who self-harm are not suicidal. Someone who feels suicidal may not act in any way to self-harm. However, the meaning or purpose of self-harm will vary from person to person, and it may be more useful to view self-harm on a continuum with suicide.

Table 34.2 shows that self-inflicted damage to the body may be deliberate but without the intent to harm oneself – for example with tattoos, body piercing, plastic surgery or tribal marking/cutting the face. The self-harm can be deliberate and immediate, such as cutting or taking overdoses, or prolonged, such as starvation or poisoning. In turn, the intent of the person who self-harms may or may not be to end their life. Someone may feel suicidal, have suicidal thoughts but not actually make any attempt to kill himself or herself. Often referred to as attempted or para-suicide, the final group that we can nurse are clients who feel suicidal and make an attempt to end their life, but do survive.

Any client might have suicidal thoughts, feelings or plans, whether or not they actually self-harm
MEANING
Behaviours that may be socially acceptable, but cause harm and could result in accidental or premature death
Self-harm as a coping mechanism for psychological distress
Behaviours with varying risk of completed suicide. Remember to consider the client's view of whether an act might be lethal
SELF-HARM
Tattoos, body piercing, tribal cuts or scaring
Risk taking: driving too fast, unsafe sex
Smoking or drinking to excess
Illicit drug use or excessive use of prescribed drugs
Binge- eating or starvation
Cutting or overdosing without suicidal ideation
Non-lethal cutting or overdosing with the intent to kill oneself
Overdoses, hanging, cutting or immersion with suicidal intent
Attempted suicide with lethal method resulting in death
COMPLETED SUICIDE
MOOD
Boredom, thrill seeking, frustration, experimentation, socialization, self-expression
Feeling 'out of control', angry, guilty, low self-esteem, need to punish or purge oneself
Depressed, hopeless, unable to see a future, guilty, angry, resolved to die or apathetic about living

Table 34.2 Self-harm – suicide continuum

When considering clients who self-harm or attempt suicide it is clear that each group has different but overlapping qualities. In defining self-harm and suicide, a relationship between the two phenomena becomes evident. Displayed on a continuum, in Table 34.2, it shows that although the two acts can be separated in terms of the client's intent, there are many similarities in feelings and actions. Population studies provide the demographic data for identifying whether or not an individual falls into a high-risk group. This does not however inform the clinician of that individual's risk. Only by assessing the mechanism and the meaning of an act when somebody self-harms or attempts to commit suicide, can a plan of nursing care be made to address the behaviour.

Nursing someone who self-harms

'Listen, believe, imagine, stay, find hope'

The core mental health nursing skills required to work with someone who has self-harmed are no different from those required in any other clinical setting. Joshua, a 19-year-old bank clerk who regularly attends accident and emergency having cut himself, suggests that the following key qualities are essential in a nurse looking after him: the ability to *listen* to what has happened, to *believe* what the person is telling you, to *imagine* what that must be like, and to *stay/be with him* even if you don't like what you have imagined or thought. There is a crucial further stage – that of *finding hope* which will be discussed further in the section below on nursing someone who is suicidal.

Mechanism, meaning and motivation – a model for assessing self-harm

Understanding – mechanism

It is important to assess the mechanism of someone's self-harm – this will provide you with important information to plan the emergency aspects of their care. Someone who has self-harmed does feel physical pain in the same way as anyone else and will need the same first aid and pain relief. They are likely to be psychological distressed as well. The NICE guidelines clearly recommend that this psychological distress be taken into account when prioritizing their care (NICE 2004). Assessing the mechanism of injury will also help inform the risk assessment. Consider the difference in risk between someone who impulsively breaks a glass and cuts themselves in the context of an argument, and someone who has been saving up their medication for weeks in order to take an overdose. Providing first aid, helping to relieve someone's pain or administering prescribed treatments can be an opportunity to engage with the client and to prevent any further deterioration in their physical health.

Understanding – meaning

The next stage in nursing someone who has self-harmed is to understand what meaning the act has for them. In order to do this we have to ask about and explore with the client what happened and how they felt, before, during and after they self-harmed. This requires us to have an attitude, and use language, that is non-judgemental. Showing that we are interested in the client as an individual and that we do not blame them for self-harming will help to establish a therapeutic relationship through which we can help the client to identify what they would like to change and how they can change their behaviour. Above all we need to be interested in the person, what has happened to them and what they would like to happen – aiming to fulfil Joshua's criteria to be listened to and believed. These two stages together form the basis of a therapeutic assessment.

Therapeutic assessment

Case study: Jenny

Jenny is a 21-year-old music student training as a classical violinist. She attended the emergency department in the early hours of the morning having made ten 4 cm cuts in a row along the length of her forearm. She had played in an end-of-term concert that evening and been for a drink with her fellow students, consuming approximately 12 units of alcohol. Upon her return home she had felt an overwhelming desire to release a feeling of tension, which she described as being located in her arm. Having cut herself she felt an immediate release of tension, but very quickly felt her anxiety levels rise again as she began to fear lest she had damaged her arm, worry about what her friends, teachers and family would think, and was angry that the tension seemed to be returning. She told one of her flatmates what she had done, and was persuaded to attend the emergency department.

Although this was the first time that Jenny had cut herself, she had taken an overdose one year ago and from the age of 13 had starved herself when feeling stressed. When she was 7 years old her father, who was also a professional musician and her first teacher, left her mother. Jenny excelled at school and gained a place at the university of her choice, but always felt that she was somehow 'scraping by'. Since arriving at university she had struggled, and although passing her course, felt she was near the bottom of the class. She described in her own words a 'love–hate' relationship with her peers. Performing at university motivated her, but she resented doing it. As the end of her course approached she feared what would happen and was angry that she had failed to get onto a postgraduate course. Jenny seemed able only to see things as poles apart: she would either become a professional musician or she would be a failure; her teachers loved or hated her.

During her assessment with a psychiatric liaison nurse, Jenny was able to identify that when things went wrong she 'blamed' and 'hated' herself. She had a belief that she wasn't good enough for her father, her school or her university, and only felt better if she 'punished' herself by starving, taking an overdose or cutting herself. Jenny agreed that she wanted to do something to change this pattern of behaviour. She identified that drinking alcohol when she was feeling distressed made it more likely that she would do something to harm herself, or starve herself the following day because she felt guilty at having had too many calories in the alcohol. She also felt that she was 'testing' her body, and to some extent that she wanted 'it' (her body) to fail her so that she would be able to justify not becoming a professional violinist.

The nursing intervention as a result of this assessment was essentially pragmatic. Jenny was educated about the risks of binge drinking, and given some written information to back this up. Jenny identified that it would be helpful to speak to the careers adviser at her university to see if she could identify a realistic option that fell between her ideal career and her view of failure. A 'crisis plan' was devised including what Jenny would do if she felt like harming herself again. This included trying to think of a middle-ground between her extreme beliefs and feelings, asking a friend to come round rather than going to the pub, calling a student helpline, and how to access emergency mental health services.

Jenny was offered a referral for psychotherapy. However, she felt it would be 'too much to deal with' at that time, but would consider it as an option for the future.

Jenny gave permission for her case to be used as an example. Her name and other details have been changed to protect her anonymity.

The case study of Jenny illustrates the importance of this first stage. During the assessment of her self-harm, Jenny was able to formulate her own ideas about how she had come to a point where she used cutting as a coping mechanism. Even if this is your only contact with someone who has self-harmed there are treatment options available: psycho-education, solution-orientated interventions, distraction or harm-reduction techniques can all be employed in the context of a therapeutic assessment.

Anyone who self-harms and has capacity has the right to refuse treatment. In Jenny's case she did not feel able to cope with psychotherapy at that time, and so chose not to take up the offer of referral. The nurse's role includes ensuring that treatments remain accessible to their clients and acknowledging that people change their minds over time. If Jenny repeatedly attended the emergency department, the nurse could suggest to her that she needed more support to change her behaviour and re-offer the referral to psychotherapy.

Understanding – motivation

To nurse someone who self-harms we need to make an assessment of their motivation to change their self-harming behaviour. An interesting analogy can be made between models of change used in addictions nursing and nursing someone who self-harms. Prochaska *et al.* (1993) demonstrate how a transtheoretical model of a cycle of change can be used to promote behavioural change in people with addictive behaviours. The six stages of change: pre-contemplation, contemplation, preparation, action, maintenance and termination, can equally well be applied when assessing and nursing someone who self-harms. At any stage during the cycle, an individual may relapse. Prochaska and Velicer (1997) demonstrate that when interventions are matched to the client's assessed stage of change, there is a dramatic improvement in recruitment, retention and progress in treatment programmes. Table 34.3 maps the characteristics and suggests techniques for someone who self-harms, at each stage of change.

Stage of change	Client characteristics	Nursing techniques
Pre-contemplation	Not considering change.	Acknowledge and accept the client's lack of readiness.
	Does not consider that self-harm is a problem.	Respect the client's choice and that it is their decision.
	Denying that the behaviour exists and not seeking help.	Encourage thinking about the meaning of self-harm rather than action.
		Explain and personalize the risk of self-harm.
Contemplation	Ambivalent about changing self-harm behaviour.	Acknowledge and accept the client is not ready to change.
	Thinking about the role of self-harm in their life.	Respect the client's choice and that it remains their decision.
	No plans for change in the immediate future.	Encourage evaluation of the benefits and risks of self-harming.
	Sitting on the fence, but interested in treatment options.	What would it be like if you didn't self-harm?
		Identify possible positive outcomes of reducing or stopping self-harm behaviours. ⇨

Stage of change	Client characteristics	Nursing techniques
Preparation	Some experience with trying to stop self-harming – testing the waters. Feels ready to change and wants to stop self-harming. May have been finding out about self-help groups or been in touch with other people who self-harm. Enquiring about different treatment options.	Help to identify any barriers to change. Use solution-orientated techniques to diminish or remove barriers. Help to identify sources of support – self-help groups, friends and social support. Identify the client's strengths, skills and abilities to change. Set small, SMART goals.
Action	Living without self-harm. Using other coping mechanisms. Engaging with treatment. Risk of replacing self-harm with other destructive or addictive behaviours.	Acknowledge this achievement and highlight the positive outcomes of not self-harming. Identify feelings of loss and anxiety. Ask about other behaviours, drug/alcohol use, gambling, etc.
Maintenance	No self-harm for over six months. Continued commitment to living without self-harm. Conscious awareness of healthy management of stress and anxiety.	Plan long-term follow up. Reinforce success and internal benefits of not self-harming. Discuss techniques for coping with relapse, and that relapse does not equal failure.
Relapse (can occur at any stage of change)	Self-harming or unable to cope with the thoughts of self-harm. Feeling guilty, angry or hopeless.	Identify triggers for relapse. Explain that relapse is a part of change. Reassess motivation. Review coping strategies. Screen for depression or suicidal thoughts.
Termination	No self-harm. Reduced anxiety about not self-harming. Strong social support and interpersonal relationships.	The end of a therapeutic relationship needs to be planned. Treatment no longer required.

Table 34.3 Nursing interventions for different stages of change in clients who self-harm (After Prochaska *et al*. 1993)

In Jenny's case, she could be described as moving between the contemplation and preparation stages of changing her self-harm behaviour. She wants to change, and has been trying albeit unsuccessfully, to change her behaviour. Although she does not feel ready for psychotherapy – she has not ruled it out for the future. She is willing to try to drink less and see a careers adviser. Achieving small steps towards her goal will support her changing behaviour whereas viewing any further self-harm as a failure would reinforce Jenny's beliefs about herself. Preparing a crisis plan acknowledges that relapse is possible, moreover likely, during the process of change.

Harm minimization

In the fields of health promotion and addictions nursing the concept of harm minimization is well established. For example, in addictions, by acknowledging that someone is going to continue to use if they are in the pre-contemplative, contemplative or preparation stages of change, the risk of infection, accidental overdose, not knowing what they are ingesting, can be reduced by needle-exchange programmes, health education and methadone maintenance programmes. The client engages with services while still using so that the therapeutic relationships and hopefully the client's confidence in a service is established at the time they do want to change their behaviour.

It may be particularly challenging to engage with someone who is self-harming as it is possible that your client may have had previous negative experiences of health care. If you make nursing care conditional on not self-harming, you will communicate to your client that you blame them. Service users report that signing 'no self-harm' contracts is unhelpful and that short-term tolerance of risk leads to increased honesty about self-harm (South London and Maudsley 2001). While ensuring that the responsibility for self-harm remains with the client, nurses should accept that the behaviour will continue into treatment.

Specific harm-minimization techniques such as distraction are widely used. Some people have suppressed the need to cut by snapping elastic bands against their wrist, holding ice in their hands, or punching pillows. In the short term these may reduce the risk involved in self-harm. However, they perpetuate the client's need to experience an immediate physical response to psychological distress. Positive distraction techniques that engage the client in creative rather than destructive behaviours, such as exercise, listening to music, watching television, drawing/painting, etc. are more likely to change their behavioural response to self-harm.

In Jenny's case, examining the role alcohol may have to play as an antecedent to her self-harm could be considered a harm-reduction strategy. Educating Jenny about the risks of binge drinking and finding an alternative to going to the pub may help to reduce the potential frequency and severity of her self-harm.

Solution-focused interventions

Systematic reviews of research evidence for treating self-harm have found that problem-solving therapies result in decreased repeat self-harm rates (Centre for Review and Dissemination 1998; Hawton *et al.* 2003). The lack of longitudinal studies and small numbers involved in the studies mean that these results are not statistically significant. However, they identify a clinically significant trend of reduced repetition rates, which would support the use of solution-focused techniques when working with people who self-harm. In Chapter 28 Gega explores the art of problem solving with clients.

If we apply these principles to Jenny's case, the nurse's perspective of Jenny's problem might focus on her self-harm. Jenny, however, viewed the risk to her career as her current, most important problem. Jenny's thinking about her violin playing was catastrophic; she thought that she was a failure and that she should give up if she 'couldn't make it' as a professional violinist. The nurse's role is to help Jenny to find a solution to this dilemma. If the solution is one that Jenny can come up with, she is more likely to believe that it is achievable and, therefore, possible.

However, when someone like Jenny is distressed, her thinking can become very fixed and she might believe that there is no possible solution. Rather than just suggesting a solution that you think fits, questioning Jenny regarding her beliefs and feelings about her career can help her to see her situation from another perspective and to develop a solution. Once Jenny has a solution in mind, you can help her to set goals towards achieving it. Table 34.4 gives some examples of questions you might ask in order to help Jenny find her own solution.

Purpose	Examples
Defining the problem	What do you think is the main problem?
	What would you like help with?
	What would you like to achieve?
	What would it feel like to pass your course?
	How do you feel you are doing?
	How do others think you are doing?
	What options are there available to you?
Challenging negative thinking errors/seeking the exception	Are you actually failing?
	What have you passed before that you had to work hard for?
	Could you use those skills/techniques in this situation?
	How do your tutors think you are doing?
	What careers are your peers thinking of?
	What else would you view as being successful?
	What is the worst thing that could happen if you did fail?
Identifying possible solutions	What would your colleagues do in your shoes?
	Is there a middle ground?
	What would be 'good enough' for you?
	Can you think of alternatives?
	What do you think of these alternatives?
Refining solution choice	What do you think is most likely to work?
	Which would you like to try?
	What steps do you need to take to achieve this?
	What help would you like to achieve this?
	How would you feel when you achieve this?

Table 34.4 Purpose and examples of questions for Jenny

Although in this case, Jenny's anxieties about her career may seem secondary to her self-harm behaviour, this is the problem she identifies as most significant. Jenny plans to go and see the careers adviser at her university. Although her friends had already suggested this solution, she had not before thought that she would actually go. It is not implied that this one small shift would fundamentally change Jenny's beliefs about herself, but it is achievable and very strongly linked to her own understanding of why she self-harms. It moves Jenny's focus from what she considers to be her past failures, towards what she can achieve in the future. Stevenson *et al.* (2003) suggest that nurses are required to undergo a change in their philosophy in order to work with the priorities that the client brings, and to have a solution-orientated, prospective approach rather that a retrospective 'fixing' of the underlying causes of any crisis.

Clinical practice recommendations

In 2004 the National Institute for Health and Clinical Excellence issued the following clinical practice recommendations. While these are based on the best available evidence there are limitations with the research into treatments for self-harm. Many of the studies have a small number of participants and the follow-up period is quite short. There are also issues around the highly heterogeneous nature of some of the groups studied which makes generalization difficult. Nonetheless these guiding principles offer a framework within which nursing care could be tailored to the individual:

- Following psychosocial assessment for people who have self-harmed, the decision about referral for further treatment and help should be based upon a comprehensive psychiatric, psychological and social assessment, including an assessment of risk, and should not be determined solely on the basis of having self-harmed.
- Clinicians should ensure that service users who have self-harmed are fully informed about all the service and treatment options available, including the likely benefits and disadvantages, in a spirit of collaboration, before treatments are offered. The provision of relevant written material with time to talk over preferences should also be included for all service users.
- The mental health professional making the assessment should inform both mental health services (if they are already involved) and the service user's GP, in writing, of the treatment plan.
- For people who have self-harmed and are deemed to be at risk of repetition, consideration may be given to offering an intensive therapeutic intervention combined with outreach. The intensive intervention should allow frequent access to a therapist when needed, home treatment when necessary and telephone contact; and outreach should include following up the service user actively when an appointment has been missed to ensure that the service user is not lost from the service. The therapeutic intervention plus outreach should continue for at least three months.
- For people who self-harm and have a diagnosis of borderline personality disorder, consideration may be given to the use of dialectical behaviour therapy. However, this should preclude other psychological treatments.

(NICE 2004: 178)

What people who self-harm want

The main principles in this section should apply to all the clients whom we nurse. In the past, people who self-harm have experienced judgemental and sometimes painful treatment at the hands of health care professionals. This has been the case not only in emergency departments, but also in mental health services. Reasons for this may be that carers do not understand self-harm and therefore feel angry or frustrated with a client who may repeatedly self-harm. In general, people who self-harm want to be treated with respect and non-judgementally. This means treating injuries and assessing people in private, respecting confidentiality within the clinical team, thinking about the timing of psychosocial assessments and allowing appropriate time to recover from any injury. It is a myth that people who self-harm either enjoy, or do not feel pain.

The NICE guidelines give advice for health care professionals working in any setting which are based on service-user evaluations and reports of their experience receiving treatment for their self-harm. These include:

- Always treat people with care and respect.
- Ensure privacy for the service user.
- Take full account of the likely distress associated with self-harm.
- Offer the choice of male or female staff for assessment and treatment.
- Involve the service user in clinical decision-making and provide information about treatment options.
- Include family or friends if the service user wants their support during assessment and treatment.
- Offer emotional support to relatives and carers.
- Assume mental capacity, unless there is evidence to the contrary (NICE 2004: 6–7).

Conflict may arise as some people who self-harm do not wish to discuss this with a mental health professional. Both the Royal College of Psychiatrists (1994) and NICE (2004) advise that everyone who self-harms should have a psychosocial assessment by a trained professional before they leave the emergency department. Furthermore, the *National Suicide Prevention Strategy for England* (DH 2003) states that anyone who has self-harmed within the previous three-month period should receive follow-up within seven days of discharge from hospital. As nurses we have to balance these policy requirements with the right that any capable adult has to refuse treatment. Where conflict arises, discuss with the client why they wish to refuse treatment, ensure they understand what is being offered, and whenever possible discuss the case with other members of the multi-disciplinary team.

Nursing someone who is suicidal

Many of the principles outlined above in nursing someone who self-harms apply to nursing someone who is suicidal. Someone who is suicidal has basic needs: to be listened to, in relationship with others, cared for, understood and valued. Anything less risks reinforcing the hopelessness they may already feel.

The UK government's focus on the reduction in suicide as the key target in mental health (DH 1990, 2001, 2003) has contributed to a culture of risk assessment and management in mental health care. There is a growing body of evidence regarding how to assess risk of suicide, but little that supports nurses in working with clients who are suicidal. The most recent National Confidential Inquiries into Suicide and Homicide by People with Mental Illness (DH 2006) identified that there were 6367 cases of suicide by current or recent mental health patients representing 27 per cent of all suicides in the period April 2000 to December 2004. Having examined the circumstances in detail 1108 cases were identified where the suicide was considered to be 'most preventable' and were clearly related to service failure. The inquiry made recommendations for practice that fall into the following nine broad categories:

- Reduce absconding

- – Understanding triggers
- – Technology
- ■ Manage transition from ward to community
    - – Regular assessment of risk during trial leave
    - – Plans to address stressors
    - – Crisis contacts during leave
    - – Early follow-up by phone immediately and in person within a week
    - – Support for people who self-discharge
- ■ Use of CPA
    - – Closer alignment of CPA and risk management
    - – Always use enhanced CPA for high risk groups
    - – Joint review of high risk groups with other clinical teams
- ■ Responding when care breaks down
    - – Robust use of CPA
    - – Assertive outreach teams
    - – Modern pharmaco-therapy as first-line treatment
- ■ Attitudes to prevention
    - – Culture of 'inevitable deaths' needs to be challenged
    - – Previous recommendations have resulted in fewer deaths
- ■ Ward environment
    - – Improvements in ward environment have lead to a reduction in deaths by hanging
    - – Removal of ligature points and non-collapsible curtain rails/hooks/handles etc.
- ■ Observation
    - – Intermittent observations not suitable for high risk people
    - – No gaps in one-to-one observation – these must be strictly carried out
- ■ Dual diagnosis
    - – Staff training in substance misuse management
    - – Joint working with drug and alcohol teams
    - – Local clinical leadership
    - – Use of enhanced CPA for severe mental illness and substance misuse patients
- ■ Older adults
    - – Better clinical care for physical illness
    - – Higher risk after recent bereavement

Reid and Long (1993), Cleary *et al.* (1999) and Bowers *et al.* (2000) all agree that if a client is placed under continuous observation, it provides an opportunity for the nurse working with the suicidal client to form a therapeutic relationship. However, clients' experiences of being continuously observed are often reported as being restrictive, punishing, humiliating and clearly far from therapeutic (Fletcher 1999; Jones *et al.* 2000). Numerous problems exist with continuous close observations:

- ■ There is a lack of, and inconsistent application of policy, with observations often being carried out by junior or agency staff (Bowers *et al.* 2000).
- ■ People still kill themselves while on inpatient acute admissions wards (DH 2001, 2006).

- It is stressful for the nurses doing the observation (Cutcliffe and Barker 2002).
- It may put the nurse at risk if the client's impulsive behaviour becomes directed towards them (Cleary *et al.* 1999).

So the question remains, how can we nurse someone safely who is suicidal? One example of how this can be addressed has been proposed by South London and Maudsley NHS Foundation Trust. Their Engagement and Formal Observation Policy for inpatients emphasizes the importance of 'empathy, listening skills, initiating conversation which is meaningful, use of silence, discussing the patient's feelings and thoughts which have led to their behaviours, giving clear information back to the patient about those feelings and thoughts, *naming them for the patient*, and helping them discover ways of making those feelings and thoughts less distressing' (SLAM 2001: 5). Enhanced observations form part of this enhanced engagement and include the levels:

- within arms length;
- within eyesight.

The standard level of engagement, general observations applies to all inpatients, and the interim measure of intermittent observations should only ever be used as a step-down from enhanced observations and not started with a new patient when the risk of self-harm or suicide has been identified.

An example of when and how this type of intervention might be used and reviewed is given in the case study of Serena.

Case study: Serena

Serena is a 35-year-old woman who was diagnosed with bipolar affective disorder in her early twenties. She has tried to kill herself on four occasions, each shortly after a depressive episode. Her suicidal behaviour has been impulsive and high risk: trying to hang herself, running out in front of oncoming traffic, and jumping from a high building. Over the past fortnight, her community nurse has been increasingly concerned about Serena. She had been depressed, and although her mood was still low, she was becoming increasingly irritable and angry. In the days before her admission, she started telephoning staff at the hospital stating she was going to 'be with God' as 'He wanted her back at his right side' and that she was 'ready to die'. Her community nurse arranged a Mental Health Act assessment at Serena's home, and they found that Serena had tied a noose with her dressing gown cord, which was hanging from the banisters on her landing. She did not want to come into hospital, was assessed as being at risk of harm to herself and was admitted to an acute psychiatric admissions ward under Section 3 of the Mental Health Act 1983.

Serena gave permission for her case to be used as an example. Her name and some other details have been changed to protect her anonymity.

In such an emergency situation as Serena's, the assessment of risk should be multi-disciplinary, and the purpose, level and duration of the observation made explicit. Where possible, the client should be involved in the decision about whether observation will be helpful and reduce the identified risk, and should always be informed about why and how they will be observed. The nursing staff doing the observation must be appropriately trained, know the local observation policy and should not be expected to continuously observe a client for more than two hours at a time. When it is decided that someone should be continuously observed, the team should also agree when this will be reviewed, and what changes in the client's thoughts, feelings and behaviours will result in the observation level being reduced.

The aim of continuous, close observation should be to engage with the client, to try to form a relationship with them, so that they can express their suicidal thoughts and feelings and be prompted to identify what else would be helpful. This can be achieved by listening to, and talking with, the person you are observing. However, constant focus on being 'nursed' can be exhausting – so negotiating activities, and doing them with the client, will help to form the therapeutic relationship as well as provide a break for both the client and the nurse.

For observation to be of any value, the nurse's observations of their client must be documented and discussed with the multi-disciplinary team responsible for his or her treatment. An example of how this might be done in Serena's case is given in Box 34.1.

Box 34.1   An example of an observation care plan and monitoring form

Care need

Serena has a history of violent suicide attempts and today was found at home with a noose tied to her banister. Serena is also known to act impulsively. She is expressing a desire to die in order to 'be with God' and appears irritable in mood.

Plan

Serena will be closely observed at all times by registered nursing staff. The purpose of this observation is to maintain her safety by preventing her from impulsively harming herself and de-escalating any conflict that arises with other clients. The nurse in charge and duty psychiatrist will review this level of observation in six hours' time, once an initial risk assessment has been undertaken. During this period of observation, the nurse observing her will explain the purpose of her observation, show her around the ward, introduce her to the other staff and clients, explain emergency procedures, and document Serena's mood, suicidal thoughts, behaviour and any other concerns she may raise.

Observations

Time	Observations
14:00– 16:00	Serena appears frustrated at being back on the ward. She feels angry that we won't leave her alone, and has been slamming her room door and asking me to sit outside. I have explained that we will try to keep this period of observation as short as possible and that our aim is to make sure she is safe on the ward. Serena says that there are times when she wishes she were dead. She says she tied the noose to her stairs to 'wind up' her CPN and denies any suicidal plans at present. In the coffee room she was laughing when telling other clients she was 'on special'. ⇨

Observations	
16:00–18:00	Spent half an hour in the quiet room telling me that she feels angry with herself for coming back into hospital. On reflection, Serena thinks she knew she was becoming unwell again and that she did think about killing herself because she feels stuck in a cycle of 'hospital, depression, hospital, depression'. She finds it hard to look forward to anything, because although she is beginning to feel 'happy' and 'powerful', she knows it won't last. From 16:30 until 18:00 Serena was with the duty psychiatrist and her named nurse, doing her admission assessment.
18:00–20:00	Serena felt tired after her assessment and wanted to eat her supper in her room. She spent time in the day room, watching TV and talking to other clients in the smoking room. Her mood seemed irritable when another client asked her for a cigarette, and she knocked the ashtray over before running out of the room. Serena did not want to talk about this. In the garden, she mentioned that she enjoyed gardening and asked if the OT still worked with people in the garden.

Evaluation

The duty psychiatrist, named nurse and charge nurse met to discuss Serena's observation. Assessment reveals she is thinking about suicide and displaying impulsive behaviour such as slamming her door and knocking over the ashtray – however, these have been in response to the frustration of being observed and being asked for a cigarette. She has made no attempt to harm herself or leave. She has no specific plan at present, and her own belief is that she will not harm herself on the ward. She has been prescribed 7.5 mg zopiclone at night.

The process of observation may be exacerbating Serena's irritable mood. However, a moderate risk of an impulsive suicide attempt still exists. If the zopiclone is effective, and Serena sleeps well tonight, the observation level can be reduced to general observation, and then reviewed when she awakens in the morning.

If she has slept well, and her impulsive behaviours have not increased, it is agreed that the team will consider reducing the observation level.

Finding hope

Cutcliffe and Barker (2002) suggest that there are two approaches to the care of suicidal clients: 'observation' and 'engagement and inspiring hope'. They argue that the observation approach limits the role of the nurse to that of a custodian, and has little therapeutic value. Using the interpersonal processes of engagement and inspiring hope may help to address the problem of how to nurse someone who is feeling suicidal.

They describe the engagement process as forming a relationship, conveying acceptance and tolerance, and hearing and understanding. If the client is valued by their nurse, this sense of worth can be conveyed to the client who may be experiencing feelings of hopelessness and worthlessness. In the absence of a relationship with a client, the mental health nurse is inhibited from doing anything else, and in itself the relationship is valuable.

As with self-harm, acknowledging, accepting and tolerating the client, without conditions supports the process of engagement. Thurgood discusses engaging clients in detail in Chapter 27.

Engaging with someone who is suicidal can itself inspire hope. There is a sense of expectation created in the relationship – you expect your client to live, to recover. Imagine the contrast with continuous close observation, where you are expecting your client to do something harmful. In their study of what relatives of suicidal people found hope-inspiring, Talseth *et al.* (2001) identified six themes:

■ being seen as a human being;
■ participating in an 'I–You' relationship;
■ trusting staff, treatment and care;
■ feeling trusted by staff;
■ being consoled;
■ entering into hope.

These themes were fundamental for the relatives to feel that they had 'been met' during the crisis of their relatives being suicidal. Being met, Talseth *et al.* (2001) propose, is a passageway to hope. This could equally be applied to the client as the relative or carer. Table 34.5 shows what Collins and Cutcliffe (2003) describe as the key elements of hope and hopelessness.

Hope	Hopelessness
Multi-dimensional	Multi-dimensional
Dynamic	Dynamic
Empowering	Disempowering
Central to life	A threat to the quality and longevity of life
Related to external help	Related to the absences of caring, or uncaring practitioners
Related to caring	
Orientated towards the future	Orientated towards the past
Highly personalized towards each individual	Highly personalized towards each individual

Table 34.5 Key elements of hope and hopelessness
(Source: Collins and Cutcliffe 2003)

Cutcliffe and Barker (2002) suggest that the same processes involved in engaging with a client, demonstrating unconditional acceptance, tolerance and understanding, inspire hope because of the relationship between caring and hope. In their wide-ranging literature review Cutcliffe and Stevenson (2008) conclude that caring for someone who is suicidal is an interpersonal endeavour at the centre of which are talking and listening. The caring response must include self-awareness, confidentiality, unconditional positive regard, congruence and empathy (McLaughlin 2007), if we are to engage clients and help them to identify reasons to live.

For Serena, her main emotions appear to be anger and frustration at being readmitted to hospital and a fear of being depressed again when she is eventually discharged. It will be important for staff to listen to, accept and tolerate her anger, frustration and help her to explore these feelings. Although Serena fears for her future, she does envisage it. She has also demonstrated a positive interest in her sharing a joke with another client, and enquiring about the occupational therapy gardening group. Promoting or facilitating these interpersonal relationships and experiences will help to create purpose, and therefore diminish hopelessness in Serena's life.

Although there is a gradual shift in focus in the care of people who are suicidal, the majority of NHS trusts have policies and an expectation that people at high risk of attempting suicide are closely observed. As Bowers *et al.* (2000) have shown, where these policies exist they differ greatly across the country. As you will be expected to closely observe clients, it is important that you consult the local policy in your clinical area. Ideally, continuous, close observation should only be used as an emergency provision, but where it is required, you must be clear of what is expected of you, and wherever possible use it as an opportunity to engage with, form a relationship, accept, tolerate, listen to and understand the person with whom you are working.

Special groups

When working with people who self-harm or are suicidal, there are groups of the population who need special consideration: young people, older adults, and people with psychosis who are self-harming in response to psychotic experiences.

Young people

The Royal College of Psychiatrists (1998) have made specific recommendations for the management of self-harm in young people. In summary, they recommend that all young people under the age of 16 who self-harm should be admitted to an appropriate paediatric or medical ward so that a comprehensive assessment of risk and the young person's mental health can be undertaken. This assessment will involve the young person, their family, mental health, social and education services, and, therefore, will take some time. Ideally an agreed local protocol should exist in order to manage these cases. NICE (2004) recommend that for young people who repeatedly self-harm, group psychotherapy with other young people who self-harm may have a clinically significant impact on reduction of repetition. Following the National Inquiry into self-harm in 2006 and based on what young people who self-harm had said they found useful Richardson (2006) produced an extremely useful booklet for young people and their families and carers – *The Truth about Self-harm*. This booklet suggests useful ways for young people to think about, talk about and get help for their self-harm, as well as providing support for people who are worried that someone they know might be self-harming.

Older adults

Older adults are less likely to self-harm, but those that do are at an increased risk of suicide (Marriott *et al.* 2003) and are identified as one of the target groups for the promotion of mental health in the National Suicide Prevention Strategy (DH 2003). Marriott *et al.* (2003) found that people over the age of 55 who had self-harmed were more likely than those under 55 to be admitted to a mental health unit for further assessment and treatment. When working with an older adult who is either suicidal or who has self-harmed, it is important to consider this increased risk.

People with psychosis

There is a markedly increased risk of suicide for clients with psychotic illnesses (Harris and Barraclough 1997) and this risk is further elevated in those who have a co-morbid psychosis and personality disorder (Moran *et al.* 2003). There is the potential for a further exacerbation of risk if an individual's experience of psychosis includes command auditory hallucinations (instructing them to self-harm or commit suicide) or beliefs that they should harm or kill themselves. While the risk is high, nurses can help clients to identify the strengths and strategies the client has used to resist these instructions or beliefs. If the client is in such distress that they are compelled to act on the instructions they hear or believe, emergency measures such as continuous close observation in an inpatient setting may be necessary to try to protect the individual's physical safety.

Being safe

Rather than addressing risk-assessment issues, this section is concerned with maintaining the physical and psychological safety of nurses who work with people who self-harm or are suicidal. Any mental health work can be stressful, but the added pressure of working with someone with potentially life-threatening behaviour, means that extra support is required. Furthermore, this chapter has emphasized the importance of the relationship between client and nurse as the key to any therapeutic intervention. Relationships are not risk free. People who self-harm have often had traumatic relationships in their past, and the ways in which they form and break relationships may mirror the impulsivity displayed in their self-harming behaviour. Not only do suicide attempts often follow the loss of an interpersonal relationship (Hall and Platt 1999), but people who self-harm may have had previous negative experiences of their relationships with health care workers (Smith 2002).

There is also a risk when trying to de-escalate someone who is in the process of self-harming. If someone is using a knife, razor blade or glass to cut themselves, there is a risk that this could be used against a nurse trying to intervene. It is not suggested that someone who self-harms is likely to be violent to others, rather that at the point of self-harming, they might be emotionally charged and acting impulsively. This combination can put health care professionals at risk of being injured.

The following key points may help nurses to maintain their physical and psychological safety:

- The responsibility for self-harming behaviour always remains with the client.
- Supervision is essential, both as an individual nurse working with clients who self-harm, and as a team.
- Risk assessments should be made by the multi-disciplinary team, and risk-management plans agreed.
- Continuous close observation should only be used as an emergency provision.

■ Ask clients to hand in any sharp objects they may have and do not attempt to remove any sharps by force.

If someone self-harms, it is neither a failure on the nurse's part, and nor should the client be blamed. Incident reporting may help to highlight other contributory factors that have influenced the client's distress as well as monitoring the rates and type of self-harm in any clinical area. Also, if there is an incident where someone self-harms or attempts suicide, part of the purpose of incident reporting is to ensure that the health care professionals involved receive appropriate support from their manager or supervisor.

Conclusion

This chapter has given an overview of the different types of self-harm behaviour and explored the relationship between self-harm and suicide. In summary, the main points are:

■ Self-harm is a behaviour not an illness. However, there is a strong association between self-harm and suicide and nurses have a health-promoting role to try and help reduce the psychological distress that underlies the behaviour.

■ In all cases, the therapeutic relationship is the key to working with these client groups.

■ Models of care from addictions nursing have scope for application to working with people who self-harm: assessing motivation, considering where someone is in a cycle of change and harm-minimization techniques have been suggested as ways of engaging clients who self-harm.

■ The science, or research evidence, suggests that techniques such as problem solving are likely to reduce the frequency of further self-harm, though there are insufficient, large-scale, longitudinal studies to advocate one particular treatment (Hawton *et al.* 2003).

■ The art is to use interpersonal skills of engagement (forming a relationship, conveying acceptance and tolerance, and hearing and understanding), and inspiring hope to help clients who may be suicidal shift their position from one of hopelessness to possibility (Cutcliffe and Barker 2002; McLaughlin 2007).

■ People who self-harm want to be treated with respect, and conveying acceptance and tolerance is a key to understanding how and why they are using self-harm as a coping mechanism.

■ Continuous observation should be used for people who are at high risk of harm to themselves, but is only effective when the focus is on enhanced engagement with the client.

■ Anyone who works with people who self-harm or are suicidal must have clinical supervision in order to manage the anxiety, frustration and anger that may arise from being in a therapeutic relationship with clients for whom relationships are difficult.

Questions for reflection and discussion

1   What are your beliefs about and attitudes towards people who self-harm?

2   Consider Jenny's case, outlined in the case study. If you were nursing Jenny, how might you encourage her to engage with treatment?

3   Serena still feels suicidal. Reflecting on the brief details given in the case study and Table 34.5, think about how you could 'inspire hope' with Serena.

4   What do you think about continuous close observation? Try to imagine having someone with you 24 hours a day and list the different feelings you might have.

Annotated bibliography

- Barker, P. and Cutcliffe, J.R. (2000) Creating a hopeline for suicidal people: a new model for acute sector mental health nursing. *Mental Health Care* **3**(6): 190–3. Barker and Cutcliffe outline a new model of care for suicidal people. They propose a combination of restoring hope through individual, in-depth assessment and developing a personalized 'security plan'. The model can be applied to other aspects of acute psychiatric care.

- Hawton, K., Townsend, E., Arensman, E. *et al.* (2003) Psychological and pharmacological treatments for deliberate self-harm. *The Cochrane Library*, Issue 2. Oxford: Update Software. A systematic review of randomized control trials relating to the treatment of self-harm. Raises issues of the lack of longitudinal follow-up and large-scale studies in self-harm research. This text provides summaries of the effectiveness of problem-solving interventions, short- and long-term therapy, intense intervention plus outreach, emergency card provision, dialectical behaviour therapy, general hospital admission and treatment with antidepressants.

- McLaughlin, C. (2007) *Suicide Related Behaviour. Understanding, Caring and Therapeutic Responses.* Chichester: John Wiley and Sons. Uses case and interaction examples to work through establishing and using a therapeutic relationship to care for someone who is suicidal. Uses cognitive behavioural and solution-focused approaches in addition to reviewing standard medical and psychological treatments.

- National Self-Harm Network (2008) The National Self-Harm Network website: http://www.nshn.co.uk provides an invaluable resource in terms of service user experience and opinion, links to self-help groups and other support agencies, information for health care professionals, people who self-harm and their carers. It is regularly updated and has links to other online resources and organizations.

References

Bongar, B. (2002) *The Suicidal Patient. Clinical and Legal Standards of Care* (2nd edn). Washington DC: American Psychological Association.

Bowers, L., Gournay, K. and Duffy, D. (2000) Suicide and self-harm in inpatient psychiatric units: a national survey of observation policies. *Journal of Advanced Nursing* **32**: 437–44.

Centre for Review and Dissemination (1998) Deliberate self-harm. *Effective Health Care* **4**(6). NHS Centre for Review and Dissemination: University of York http://www.york.ac.uk/inst/crd/ehc46.htm

Cleary, M., Jordan, R., Horsfall, J., Mazondier, P. and Delaney, J. (1999) Suicidal patients and special observation. *Journal of Psychiatric and Mental Health Nursing* **6**: 461–7.

Collins, S. and Cutcliffe, J.R. (2003) Addressing hopelessness in people with suicidal ideation: building upon the therapeutic relationship utilizing a cognitive behavioural approach. *Journal of Psychiatric and Mental Health Nursing* **10**: 175–85.

Cutcliffe, J.R. and Barker, P. (2002) Considering the care of the suicidal client and the case for 'engagement and inspiring hope' or 'observation'. *Journal of Psychiatric and Mental Health Nursing* **9**: 611–21.

Cutcliffe, J.R. and Stevenson, C. (2008) Feeling our way in the dark: the psychiatric nursing care of suicidal people – a literature review. *International Journal of Nursing Studies* **45**: 942–53.

Department of Health (1990) *Health of the Nation*. London: HMSO.

Department of Health (2001) *Safety First – Five Year Report of the National Confidential Inquiry into Suicides and Homicides by People with Mental Health Problems*. London: HMSO.

Department of Health (2003) *National Suicide Prevention Strategy for England*. London: DH. http://www.doh.gov.uk/mentalhealth/suicideprevention.htm

Department of Health (2006) *Safety First – Five Year Report of the National Confidential Inquiry into Suicides and Homicides by People with Mental Health Problems*. London: HMSO.

Fletcher, R.F. (1999) The process of constant observation: perspectives of staff and suicidal patients. *Journal of Psychiatric and Mental Health Nursing* **6**: 9–14.

Gairin, I., House, A. and Owens, D. (2003) Attendance at the accident and emergency department in the year before suicide: a retrospective study. *British Journal of Psychiatry* **183**(1): 28–33.

Gallop, R. and Tully, T. (2004) The person who self-harms, in P. Barker (ed.) *Psychiatric and Mental Health Nursing: The Craft of Caring*. London: Arnold.

Hall, R.C.W. and Platt, D.E. (1999) Suicide risk assessment: a review of risk factors for suicide in 100 patients who made severe suicide attempts: evaluation of suicide risk in a time of managed care, *Psychosomatics* **40**(1): 18–24.

Harris, E.C. and Barraclough, B. (1997) Suicide as an outcome for mental disorders. A meta analysis. *British Journal of Psychiatry* **170**: 205–28.

Hawton, K., Townsend, E., Arensman, E. *et al.* (2003) Psychological and pharmacological treatments for deliberate self-harm. *The Cochrane Library*, Issue 2. Oxford: Update Software.

Hodgkiss, A. (2007) The emergency department. Chapter 32 in G.G. Lloyd and E. Guthrie (eds) *Handbook of Liaison Psychiatry*. Cambridge: Cambridge University Press.

House, A., Owens, D. and Patchett, L. (1999) Deliberate self-harm. *Quality in Health Care* **8**: 137–43.

Jones, J., Ward, M., Wellman, N., Hall, J. and Lowe, T. (2000) Psychiatric inpatients' experiences of nursing observation. A United Kingdom perspective. *Journal of Psychosocial Nursing* **38**(12): 10–19.

Marriott, R., Horrocks, J., House, A. and Owens, D. (2003) Assessment and management of self-harm in older adults attending accident and emergency: a comparative cross-sectional study. *International Journal of Geriatric Psychiatry* **18**: 645–52.

McLaughlin, C. (2007) *Suicide-Related Behaviour. Understanding, Caring and Therapeutic Responses*. Chichester: John Wiley and Sons.

Moran, P., Walsh, E., Tyrer, P. *et al.* (2003) Does co-morbid personality disorder increase the risk of suicidal behaviour in psychosis? *Acta Psychiatrica Scandinavica* **107**: 441–8.

NICE (2004) *Self-Harm. The Short-Term Physical and Psychological Management and Secondary Prevention of Self-Harm in Primary and Secondary Care*. Clinical Guideline 16. London: National Institute for Clinical Excellence and National Collaborating Centre for Mental Health http://www.nice.org.uk/guidance/CG16

Office for National Statistics (2008) *Suicide Rates in the UK 1991–2006*. http://www.statistics.gov.uk/downloads/theme_health/suicide_uk_1991to2006_table.xls

Prochaska, J.O. and Velicer, W.F. (1997) The trans-theoretical model of health behaviour change. *American Journal of Health Promotion* **12**(1): 38–48.

Prochaska, J.O., DiClemente, C.C. and Norcross, J.C. (1993) In search of how people change: applications to addictive behaviours. *Addiction Nursing Network* **5**(1): 2–16.

Reid, W. and Long, A. (1993) The role of the nurse providing therapeutic care for the suicidal patient. *Journal of Advanced Nursing* **18**: 1369–76.

Richardson, C. (2006) *The Truth about Self-Harm for Young People and their Friends and Families*. London: Camelot Foundation and Mental Health Foundation.

Royal College of Psychiatrists (1994) *The General Hospital Management of Adult Deliberate Self-harm: A Consensus Statement on Standards for Service Provision* (*Council Report CR 32*). London: Royal College of Psychiatrists.

Royal College of Psychiatrists (1998) *Managing Deliberate Self-harm in Young People* (*Council Report CR 64*). London: Royal College of Psychiatrists.

Smith, S.E. (2002) Perceptions of service provision for clients who self-injure in the absence of expressed suicidal intent. *Journal of Psychiatric and Mental Health Nursing* **9**: 595–601.

South London and Maudsley (SLAM) (2001) *Crisis Recovery Service: A Service for Individuals who Self-Harm. Philosophy and Protocols for the Management of Self-Harm.* London: South London and Maudsley NHS Foundation Trust.

Stengel, E. (1965) *Suicide and Attempted Suicide.* Bristol: MacGibbon and Kee.

Stevenson, C., Jackson, S. and Barker, P. (2003) Finding solutions through empowerment: a preliminary study of solution-orientated approach to nursing in acute psychiatric settings. *Journal of Psychiatric and Mental Health Nursing* **10**: 688–96.

Talseth, A., Gilje, F. and Norberg, A. (2001) Being met – a passageway to hope for relatives of patients at risk of committing suicide: a phenomenological hermeneutic study. *Archives of Psychiatric Nursing* **15**(6): 249–56.

Weber, M.T. (2002) Triggers for self-abuse: a qualitative study. *Archives of Psychiatric Nursing* **16**(3): 118–24.

Future directions

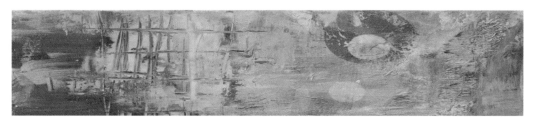

Chapter contents

CHAPTER 35

Future directions: taking recovery into society

Ian Norman and Iain Ryrie

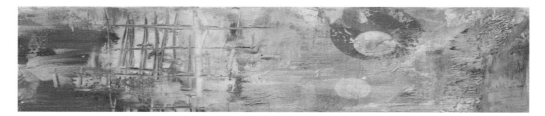

Chapter overview

The main message of the final chapter of the first edition of this book was for mental health nurses to develop recovery oriented practice. Five years on we are pleased to see that this has been endorsed strongly by international reviews of mental health nursing – in Scotland (CNO Scotland 2006) and in England (CNOE 2006) which highlight the importance of: nurses working to maintain the rights of service users and ensure that they have every opportunity to exercise choice; the central importance of positive relationships as a starting point for all interventions with service users and carers; a commitment to evidence-based practice; and recovery as the underpinning principle and focus of all interventions. Mental health policy internationally has become recovery oriented and the widespread acceptance of recovery as a principle for practice has paved the way for reconciliation between the artists and scientists within mental health nursing (see Chapter 4). Today mental health nursing involves delivering evidence-based interventions in a recovery oriented way through the medium of the relationship between the nurse and service users and their carers.

The traditional focus of attention for mental health nursing has been the individual person with mental health problems, albeit it within the context of her/his family and friends. Individualized care has become the ideal, reinforced by the adherence of professional nursing to the adapted problem solving cycle known as the nursing process. Individualized care will continue to be a major goal for nurses to counter the tendency towards batch treatment which can so easily occur within inpatient wards, but also in community settings too, including patients' own homes. However, emerging evidence from the public health field presented by Friedli in Chapter 3 suggests that population-based interventions have the potential to shift the mean mental health of the population in a positive direction, and that this could lead to a substantial decrease in the number of people in the population suffering from mental disorder.

While mental health nurses will continue to work primarily with people with high levels of need in terms of severity, acuity or complexity (i.e. individuals with mental illness and additional needs, such as substance misuse, physical ill health or learning difficulties) our argument in this chapter is that nurses need to extend their remit to incorporate a new public health role. They need, as the title of this chapter indicates, to take recovery oriented practice into society if they are to increase their positive impact on the lives of those with mental health problems and their families.

The first part of this chapter sets out what has been achieved over the recent past with particular reference to mental health care reform in the UK. We refer in particular to progress subsequent to the National Service Framework for Mental Health (DH 1999) and also to the 2006 Chief Nursing Officer for England's (CNOE 2006) review of mental health nursing, which endorsed the recovery, social inclusion agenda discussed in detail in Chapter 5.

The second part of the chapter sets out the case for improving the mental health of all citizens. We examine the potential benefits of shifting the mean happiness of the population in a positive direction for people with mental disorder and the potential contribution of mental health nurses to this endeavour through interventions which improve the environmental conditions of people's lives and change their attitudes and behaviour.

In summary this chapter covers:

- Developments in mental health services in the UK subsequent to the National Service Framework for Mental Health (DH 1999);
- Recovery oriented mental health nursing as endorsed by the Chief Nursing Officer for England's review of mental health nursing (CNOE 2006);
- The contribution of environmental factors to mental disorder;
- The potential benefits for mental health service users of promoting positive mental health of the population as a whole;
- The contribution of mental health nurses to individual and population level positive mental health strategies.

Recent achievements

We focus in this section on developments in England, to illustrate broader trends within the UK more generally. As described by McCulloch and Ford in Chapter 6, the NSF for Mental Health (NSF-MH) (DH 1999), published in September 1999, provided an evidence-based template for the development of mental health services and set out a ten-year reform programme for mental health services in England. It covered the following care standards: mental health promotion, access to services, effective service models in primary and secondary care, support of carers and suicide prevention. The NSF-MH, was the first step in transforming mental health care. The second was the NHS Plan (DH 2000), which identified mental health as a key priority, sought to strengthen community care and so relieve pressure on hospital services and set targets for mental health services nationally. And the third was the creation of the National Institute for Mental Health for England (NIMHE) which had the job of supporting the redesign of local services. These policy initiatives were followed by substantial additional investment in health and social services, although mental health spending as a proportion of all NHS spending has remained stable at around 8–9 per cent (Appleby 2007).

There have been two reports on the implementation and achievements of the NSF-MH, both by Louis Appleby, the National Director of Mental Health for England (Appleby 2004, 2007). These reports chart substantial achievements in a number of areas of care and treatment which are the focus of chapters in this volume. These achievements include:

- A major increase in the number of specialized crisis resolution (home treatment) teams offering an alternative to inpatient admission, assertive outreach teams offering intensive support to services users with complex needs, and early intervention teams providing rapid assessment and treatment to young people who have developed severe mental illness for the first time;

- An expansion in the mental health workforce (including an increase of 24 per cent in the number of mental health nurses, which was estimated at 48,400 in April 2007), new ways of working (including nurse prescribing and nurse consultants) and new ways of delivering therapies, with an emphasis on self-help (cf. Chapter 29);

- An increase in the use of more modern treatments, underpinned by clinical guidelines produced by the National Institute for Health and Clinical Excellence (NICE) including: an increase in the numbers of staff, including nursing staff, who can deliver psychological therapies; and a 20-fold increase in the prescription of 'atypical' anti-psychotic drugs as first-line treatment for schizophrenia and decrease in the use of older drugs with more severe side effects (cf. Chapters 16 and 32);

- Substantial investment to replace or refurbish acute inpatient wards which by the late 1990s had become neglected places both physically and therapeutically (cf. Chapter 12) and investment to improve psychiatric intensive care units for patients who need intensive nursing or observation, places of safety for people detained by the police and also women patients. Single sex day areas and washing facilities have now been adopted by most Trusts within the British NHS;

- A reduction in the suicide rate of the population of around 7.4 per cent since 1997 to around 350 deaths per year, which means, however, that there is still a long way to go to meet the target of a 20 per cent reduction in 2010. Encouragingly, there has been a reduction in suicide of mental health inpatients of around 29 per cent (over 60 deaths per year), which suggests general improvement in ward safety as well as a specific government initiative to remove ligature points (cf. Chapter 34);

- The 2006 national patient survey conducted by the Healthcare Commission report generally positive views of services, with 77 per cent describing their care as good (22 per cent), very good (30 per cent) or excellent (25 per cent). Encouragingly 90 per cent of patients reported that they are listened to and treated with dignity and respect, which is a tribute to the good work of nurses who are often the first point of contact with mental health services.

There is no doubt that there have been very substantial improvements in the standards of mental health services and care over the past ten years, and that mental health nurses have contributed to these. Appleby (2007) reports that Matt Muijen, WHO European Regional Advisor for Mental Health (who contributed the Foreword to this volume) has commented publically that England now has the best mental health service in Europe and that this is widely acknowledged by other countries; however, there is what Muijen has described as a 'culture of criticism' in England, which prevents it being acknowledged here.

While there have been many positive developments it is also true that most progress so far has been in specialist mental health services and, as Appleby (2007) acknowledges 'less has been achieved on mental health promotion and social exclusion' than on some of the other NSF-MH standards (Appleby 2004: 80). As he points out in his 2007 report (Appleby 2007) the focus now must turn from reforming specialist mental health services to improve the mental health of the community as a whole. This is a goal which we endorse and which is the main focus of this chapter.

The Chief Nursing Officer for England's review of mental health nursing

Some of the achievements of the past ten years, particularly in service users' more positive views of services, reflect the widespread adoption by mental health nurses of recovery oriented practice, which is discussed by Perkins and Repper in Chapter 5. The clearest statement of recovery oriented practice with regard to mental health nursing is the Chief Nursing Officer for England's review of mental health nursing (CNOE 2006), which sought to answer the question: How can mental health nursing best contribute to the care of service users in the future? The main recommendations of the review are summarized in Figure 35.1.

The CNOE's review has had a mixed, although predominantly positive, reaction from mental health nurses. Some commentators, for example Brooker (2007), have been critical of the review for being high on aspiration but 'desperately thin on detail on implementation' (2007: 329), and for failing to acknowledge the challenges that implementing values such as recovery, equity and inclusion present in practice. Brooker is also critical of the review for making no specific recommendations about research, saying little about the role of education and training and for consigning findings from the extensive literature review commissioned to inform the review (on the efficacy of MHN interventions, service users' and carers' views of mental health nursing; and work stress and recruitment and retention of mental health nurses) to an appendix.

In our view, Brooker's criticisms are overstated. We are inclined to agree with Brimblecombe and Tingle (2007) who, in a response to Brooker, point out that challenges of implementation, such as how nurses can fulfil their professional responsibilities while offering service users increased choice, are best managed by individual nurses themselves in consultation with their clinical managers and are probably not best the subject of national recommendations.

Although containing little that is new the review's recommendations, summarized in Figure 35.1, describe an approach to contemporary mental health nursing practice based upon broad mental health policies which promote user centred goals, a recovery approach and evidence-based health care. The review appears to have raised the profile of mental health nursing within mental health services, and in its emphasis on nurses delivering evidence-based interventions in a recovery oriented way through the medium of their relationship with service users and their carers, it has helped to draw together a practice discipline, which had been in danger of fragmentation. It is too early to judge the impact, if any, of the CNOE's review on mental health nursing or patient care more generally. However, a self-assessment toolkit has been produced to support the implementation of the recommendations and a research team led by Professor Patrick Callaghan is due to report on a preliminary evaluation of the review's impact shortly.

Theme 1: Putting values into practice
- Ensure that all social groups receive an equitable mental health service from a nursing workforce that reflects the local population.
- Adopt a recovery oriented principles into their work which involves:
  - working to goals that are meaningful for service users;
  - being positive about users' ability to change; and
  - working wherever possible with service users and carers to promote their social inclusion. Social inclusion (as discussed in Chapter X – Repper) is important not only because service users want this, but because, as discussed later, there is much evidence that socially included people have better mental health outcomes (OPDM 2004).
- Providing evidenced based care

Theme 2: Improving outcomes for service users
- Work with people with high levels of need and support other workers to meet less complex needs, so utilising their skills to best effect.
- Develop and sustain positive relationships with service users and carer, as a starting point for all interventions with service users and carers.
- Adopt an holistic approach which takes account of service users' physical, psychological, social and spiritual need and for nurses to gain appropriate competencies, within pre-registration training, to be able to identify and assess these meet these needs and respond to them. Skills mentioned specifically by the review include those required for assessment, delivery of evidenced based psychological therapies and health promotion activities.
- Support the physical well-being of service users since people with severe mental health problems are more likely to have higher levels of morbidity than other people and also be overweight, smoke and be physically inactive.
- Improve the quality of inpatient care by spending more time in direct clinical contact with patients and less on administrative tasks, review the roles of support workers and ensure that patients are treated with dignity and respect.
- Assess and manage risk appropriately (c.f. Chapter 11), and work in partnership with others to develop realistic care plans.

Theme 3: A positive and modern profession
- Develop new roles and ways of working to meet local needs. For example, nurse prescribing, shared roles between in-patient and crisis-home treatment staff; review the roles of non-professionally qualified workers and how they can be deployed and supported in their care to optimal effect; review senior clinical roles (including those of nurse consultants) to take account of service users needs, legislative developments and skill and professional shortages.
- Strengthen relationships between service providers and higher education institutions and ensure that pre-registration training courses ensure that essential competencies are met by the point of qualification.
- Develop initiatives to improve recruitment and retention of nurses through presenting positive messages about mental health in the media and fostering links with schools and colleges. The report highlights the need for MH nursing to be a self-confident professional group whose members can function in an assertive and professional manner as members of in multi-disciplinary teams.
- Support continuing professional development and access for nurses to support, supervision and professional advice.

Figure 35.1 Main recommendations of the Chief Nursing Officer for England's review of mental health nursing

Broadening the focus of mental health nursing

Recovery oriented mental health nursing is widely endorsed but the focus of nurses' work remains very much focused upon the individual suffering from mental health problems within the context of their family. The remainder of this chapter makes the case for broadening this focus to improve the mental health of the population as a whole. In this regard there is much for nurses to learn from the positive psychology literature, which focuses on what it is that helps individuals and communities to thrive and what makes normal life fulfilling. In this focus positive psychology provides a timely corrective to the overwhelming focus of psychology over the past 60 years on curing or alleviating mental illness (see Seligman 2002). So what is positive mental health and how is it achieved and maintained?

What is positive mental health?

Positive mental health and well-being has been defined from two main perspectives: the hedononic perspective emphasizes subjective life satisfaction, presence of positive mood and absence of negative mood; whereas the eudaimonic perspective emphasizes a sense of fulfilment and expression of true nature (eudaimon). These perspectives are reflected in the main three areas for positive psychology research identified by Seligman (2002): the pleasant life (i.e. how people experience the positive emotions associated with things like relationships, hobbies and entertainment, which are all parts of normal healthy living; the good life (i.e. the benefits from engagement or absorption in the activities of life); and the meaningful life (i.e. the experience of affiliation, the sense of belonging and purpose the individual experiences as part of something (e.g. belief systems, nature, social groups) which is larger and more enduring than themselves). A term used widely by positive psychologists is 'happiness' which refers to a combination of positive emotion, engagement and meaning in life.

Research studies show that within modern affluent societies the wealthiest people are happier than the poorest, which supports the fundamental economic position that wealth creation is a good thing. But there is also a sound body of evidence which demonstrates that once basic needs are satisfied increases in an individual's income produce diminishing levels of return in terms of happiness, and that at a certain threshold, wealth and possessions make very little difference to life satisfaction and happiness – some psychologists suggest that they explain only 10 per cent of the variation in happiness between individuals overall (Lyubomirsky *et al.* 2005). Much more important is what is referred to as 'intentional activities', that is those aspects of their lives over which individuals have more control – such as having meaningful and challenging work, socializing, the way that they behave towards others, the goals they pursue. Moreover, it is sometimes argued that the more materialistic people are the more likely they are to suffer from stress, 'time poverty' and impaired social relationships, which may decrease their well-being.

The importance of intentional activities is reflected in the six feelings which foster psychological well-being, identified by Keyes (2002): self-acceptance; positive relations with others; autonomy (or ability to think for yourself); environmental mastery (the sense that you can change your circumstances for the better); life purpose (having goals and not feeling helpful); and personal growth (being able to learn from the stresses and challenges in life). Experiencing these positive feelings may be relevant markers for mental health services users on their own journeys of recovery.

Positive psychology is beginning to exert a major influence on public policy. Layard's (2005) book on economics and happiness laid the foundation for the *Depression Report* (CEP *et al.* 2006) which argued that because one in six of us suffers from depression the greatest contribution the UK government could make to promoting well-being is to improve mental health care. At the time of writing the UK government has acted on the report by funding the training and deployment of 10,000 new cognitive behaviour therapists, who will be deployed in psychological treatment centres. There are calls too from Seligman and others for governments to create national well-being accounts to supplement mainly economic data and in the UK Government's Securing the Future (UK Government 2005) endorses for the first time that the promotion of well-being is a legitimate aim of public policy, since it is seen as at the heart of sustainable development.

What sets the set point for happiness?

Research confirms our personal experience that people with an underlying positive temperament tend to feel more positive and happy than those with an underlying negative temperament. Psychologists of personality refer to this underlying disposition as a trait, as distinct to variation in people's reaction to changing events and circumstances, which is referred to as a state. The trait concept is closely linked to the concept of what is referred to as a set point for happiness (Huppert 2005), which suggests that each individual has a basal level of happiness or general well-being, to which they will return even if they experience major positive or negative fluctuations.

So how is this set point for happiness determined? This question raises the age old nature or nurture debate, that is how far our sense of happiness or well-being is influenced by our genes or by our environment. It has been widely assumed that the set point for each individual is genetically determined and so unalterable, but in recent years this assumption has been challenged and it is becoming clear that the influence of the environment on a person's set point for happiness is much greater than previously assumed.

Of these environmental influences those which occur in early life would appear to be the most influential. From classic studies by Bowlby (1951) and later researchers we know that children who experience warm and loving relationships with parental figures grow up feeling secure and trusting of others and perceive the world as benevolent. In contrast children who experience inconsistent parenting, or who experience neglect or abuse grow up feeling insecure, cannot trust others and perceive the world as a hostile place, which in turn impacts negatively on their sense of well-being, their mental health and their ability to form and sustain positive relationships. However, these studies do not necessarily demonstrate the influence of environmental factors on mental health and adjustment. As Huppert (2005) points out, it could be that nurturing itself is under genetic control. Thus, children who grow up into well-adjusted adults do not do so because of the nurturing they themselves receive, but because of the genes that influence nurturing and their later adjustment.

However, evidence in support of the influence of environmental influences on well-being comes also from studies of non-human mammals in which it is possible to experiment to test the role of early nurturing on later adjustment. One such study by Meaney (2001) demonstrated the impact of early experiences by rearing the offspring of anxious, emotionally reactive female rats with calm, stress-resistant mothers who provide high levels of licking and grooming; in these studies the temperaments of these rats resembled those of their adoptive, rather than their biological mothers, so providing evidence for the potential powerful influence of early environmental factors on adult mental health.

There are also studies which demonstrate the short-term benefits of positive emotions on performance and on physiological responses. For example, Levy *et al.* (2000) demonstrated that older subjects perform well on cognitive tasks following exposure to subliminal positive images of ageing but that their performance is substantial impaired following exposure to negative images. This study raises the question of how far age-related problems are a consequence of negative social attitudes towards the elderly and ageing. As with Meaney's study, it also points to the possibility of reversing the negative effects of adverse influences through changing a person's attitudes.

Happiness and positive functioning

Positive mental health or well-being may be a goal worth pursuing for its own sake. But there is evidence that well-being is related also to positive functioning, although the causal direction between these is difficult to unravel. For example, it might be that happiness leads to positive thoughts, which in turn leads to more happiness; or it might be that both happiness and positive thoughts are influenced by a third factor, such as temperament. Huppert's (2005) assessment of experimental studies on induced mood states is that happiness or other positive emotions influences appraisal of situations and social relationships. Support for this comes from Fredrickson's 'broaden and build' theory of positive emotions, which proposes that the frequent experience of positive emotions can: broaden people's attention and thinking; promote psychological resilience; enhance personal coping resources; promote feelings of greater well-being into the future; and undo the negative consequences of negative emotional arousal (see Fredrickson 2005). Overall, the evidence suggests that the causal pathway between hedonic and eudaimonic well-being runs in both directions; positive feelings can produce positive functioning and vice versa.

Environmental determinants of mental disorder

The debate about the relative influence of genes and environmental factors is relevant too to those whose set points for happiness are at the bottom of the scale, often within the range which may be considered mental disorder. While, as discussed above, having more money has an increasingly negligible impact on happiness after a certain income has been reached it also true that those in poverty and who experience social deprivation are at much higher risk of mental disorder than the rest of us, and so relative poverty does appear to be a major risk factor; so the risk of mental disorder falls disproportionately on some social groups than others.

As Friedli points out in Chapter 3, mental disorder is more common in areas of deprivation and poor mental health is closely associated with unemployment, less education, low income and low material standards of life, and it is also associated with poor physical health and adverse life events. Ramon (2007) summarizes the evidence on the relationship between social structural aspects of inequality on mental ill health as follows:

■ Poor people, however defined, are much more at risk of psychotic and neurotic disorders (now referred to as common mental health problems) than those who are not poor.

■ Having less education and being unemployed or economically inactive greatly increases the risk of both psychosis and common mental health problems.

- People who have a physical illness are six times more likely to suffer from mental illness than people who are physically well.
- People who have had two or more recent adverse life events are three times more likely to suffer from mental illness than people without life events.
- Being a lone parent or perceiving lack of social support are risk factors, but not as high as those of physical illness or adverse events. Significantly more women experience common mental health problems than men, while rates of psychosis and gender vary with age; younger men and older women are more at risk than their gender counterparts; and people above 65, and particularly above 80, experience more depression and dementia than younger people.
- A number of previous studies have found that members of ethnic minority groups have a higher rate of mental illness and under-utilize mental health services. More recent studies show that minority ethnic groups suffer a similar rate of common mental disorders to the general population, but that there are variations; for example, compared to the indigenous white British population, depression is higher in African-Caribbeans and Africans, anxiety is higher in Irish and non-British white groups, and phobias are more prevalent among Asian and Oriental people. Thus, rates of mental illness do not divide along colour or racial lines – rather poverty appears to be the key factor, poor people in the ethic minorities are more likely to experience mental illness than those who are not poor.
- Rogers and Pilgrim (2003) point to the greatly increased risk of mentally ill people being victims of violence and contrasts this with the relatively few in which they perpetuate violence. While misuse of drugs and alcohol can lead to violent behaviour, such violence is often misattributed to mental disorder.

Social causation or social selection?

The relationships between mental illness and the markers of inequality mentioned above suggest that poor mental health is both a cause and a consequence of inequality. This reflects two dominant explanations of this inequality in mental health; social selection explanations, which assume that people who are mentally ill become poor because they are unable to function, and social causation explanations which hold that people become mentally ill because they are poor. Social selection explanations highlight the role of genetic and biomedical factors in mental disorder, whereas social causation explanations highlight the role of the early experiences and social context. Whichever type of explanation is preferred is important because it is reflected in mental health policies, treatment approaches and the messages received by people who are mentally ill and their families. For example, the current emphasis on the importance of social inclusion initiatives, discussed by Perkins and Repper in Chapter 5, is a variant of a version of social causation developed by Durkheim (1897) in his classic study to explain differences in suicide rates across European countries. Specifically that abnormally low (or high) levels of social integration may increase the suicide rate; low social integration results in a disorganized society in which people commit suicide either because they do not have sufficiently close ties to others (egoistic suicide) or because are unable to identify with the norms of their society and commit suicide as a form of escape (anomic suicide).

Whilst social selection explanations continue to be important, there is increasing evidence in favour of social causation explanations. Sociologists such as Rogers and Pilgrim (2003) have highlighted a particular form of social causation, in which mental health inequalities are in fact caused by mental health services themselves as a result of the imbalance in power between professionals and service users. Possible mechanisms include: rejection of lay knowledge which may arise from claims to professional expertise; selective diagnosis through which some groups are at greater risk of receiving a stigmatizing label than others, which can exert a major influence on likely future functioning and the chances of recovery; differential access to interventions, for example to psychological therapies by money (available privately to avoid long waiting lists) and decisions on suitability influenced by ethnicity and being judged articulate or otherwise; differential utilization of services affected by views of the trustworthiness of the services provided. A final factor is pessimistic assumptions about the chances of recovery from schizophrenia, which until 1987 was widely considered in Anglo-Saxon countries as between 25 and 33 per cent; this was only revised following publication of Harding *et al.*'s (1987) longitudinal study and reports of other European studies, which indicated a recovery rate of above 50 per cent. This rate is now widely accepted and this is perhaps the major reason for the adoption of recovery policies across European countries (Ramon 2007).

In sum, while both social selection and social causation place a key role in explaining mental disorder, it is now clear that the role of social factors, those aspects of the person's environment, in causing mental disorder has been under-rated.

What are the benefits for people suffering from mental disorder of raising the mean set point for happiness?

The Chief Nursing Officer for England's (CNOE 2006) review of mental health nursing reaffirms that the focus of work will continue to be those with the highest level of need that is those suffering from serious mental illness. This raises the question, then, of why nurses ought to concern themselves with raising the mental health of the population as a whole. Why will this benefit those suffering from mental disorder?

The answer to this question lies in our understanding of mental health (as discussed by us in Chapter 1 and by Friedli in Chapter 3) as having a continuous distribution in the population, rather than being mistakenly regarded as a dichotomous variable, in which most of us have it and some of us (those with a mental illness) do not. This is illustrated in Figure 35.2 which shows the mental health spectrum ranging from those who are flourishing through to those who have moderate mental health, languishing and who suffer from mental disorder. According to Keyes (2002) those who are flourishing are enthusiastic for life, are active and productively engaged with others and with social institutions. In contrast those who are languishing, which may have a high prevalence among young people, have a greatly increased risk of depression, suicide and physical illness.

The epidemiologist Rose (1992) proposed a population-based approach to reducing the number of people in a population with a disorder, based on his finding that the prevalence of many common diseases in a population is directly related to the population mean of the underlying risk factors. The implication is that by changing the mean, the prevalence of the disorder would also change. Huppert (2005), drawing on Rose's work, proposes that that since mental health is continuously distributed it is a suitable target for a population level intervention to shift the whole population in a positive direction. This is illustrated by Figure 35.2, which shows that a small shift in the mean of symptoms or risk factors will lift a

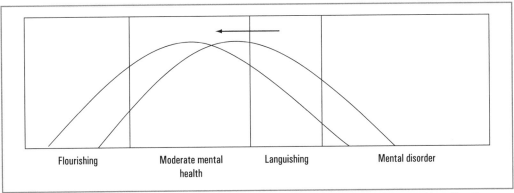

Figure 35.2 The effect of shifting the mean of the mental health spectrum in a positive direction (from Huppert 2005)

proportion of people out of the languishing and mental disorder tail of the distribution and, by reducing the mean number of symptoms in the population, a greater proportion of people will cross the threshold for flourishing.

As Friedli points out in Chapter 3, Keyes' (2002) model of the mental health continuum has been criticized for implying that people suffering from mental disorder cannot also be flourishing, and points out that Keyes has found that some individuals who meet clinical criteria for mental disorder may also lack mental health, have moderate mental health or be flourishing. This suggests that the categories along the mental health spectrum are not independent and that the model needs refinement. However, it raises also the potential for applying public health models to combat mental disorder.

How stable is the set point for happiness?

Many chapters in this volume detail treatments and care practices which are effective in improving the set point of happiness for individuals who suffer from mental disorder. But how far is it possible to increase the mean of happiness in the population and so move people who are languishing towards the group who are flourishing?

The previous sections of this chapter have challenged the traditional view that an individual's set point for happiness is almost wholly determined by genetic factors. It has highlighted the hitherto under recognized influence of a person's environment, which is particularly striking in the case of people whose set points fall into the spectrum of mental disorder. But how stable is a person's set point? A frequently cited study which illustrates how we adapt to changes in circumstances and return to a basal level of happiness is Brickman *et al.*'s (1978) study which showed that while the well-being of lottery winners soared initially and that of accident victims who were rendered paraplegic plummeted, within a relatively short period the well-being of both groups had returned to its original level. This phenomenon, known as hedonic adaptation, implies that any gains in well-being are followed inevitably by adaptation back to baseline; thus the potential of social policies for increasing the happiness of the population are limited.

Yet, as Huppert (2005) reminds us, certain events can have a far-reaching and sustained influence on our lives for some people; for example, loss of a spouse or job has been shown to produce a sustained lowering of well-being, and so for some can establish a new set point for happiness. Nevertheless, studies of the impact of life events also suggest that the magnitude of changes to the set point for happiness is relatively modest, if they change at all, which raises the important question of whether happiness of the population can be increased in a sustainable way.

Strategies for promoting mental health

The evidence points to the relative stability of the set point for happiness, but most of this comes from studies of how people adapt to the events and circumstances that they encounter during the course of their lives and adapt to in a rather passive way. We know also that most people want to be happier than they are and will actively pursue things that make them happy. These considerations suggest active strategies for promoting mental health at the level of individuals and populations, which nurses should be aware of in their work.

Individual level strategies

We have previously mentioned the potential of intentional activities in promoting subjective well-being. Sheldon and Lyubomirsky (2004) suggest that these are of three types: overt behaviours, such as taking regular exercise; positive cognitions, e.g. interpreting events in a positive way, appreciating the moment; and motivations towards activities and goals which are perceived as worthwhile. These goals should also be achievable and involve action rather than avoidance (e.g. pursing the goal of becoming healthy, rather than the goal of giving up fatty foods or smoking) and motivations to participate in social activities and with one's community is also associated with increased life satisfaction. The effectiveness of some of these intentional activities in enhancing well-being is beginning to be demonstrated in controlled trials and replication studies, some of which reported in the positive psychology research literature (see Seligman 2002).

Engaging in intentional activities have the potential of solving the hedonic adaptation problem, mentioned earlier, because they are under our control and so can be changed; for example, while a person might no longer derive pleasure from routine attendance at the same social event, enjoyment can return by making small changes to the sequence, content or location of intentional activities. Moreover, the categories of intentional activities outlined by Sheldon and Lyubomirsky do not pursue pleasure and happiness (hedonic well-being) but fulfilment (eudaimonic well-being). As Huppert (2005) points out these activities produce subjective well-being not because feeling happy is their aim, but because happiness is a by-product of being fully engaged and functioning.

An increasing variety of interventions have been tested in trials for their contribution to happiness and well-being. Examples given by Huppert (2005) include:

- cognitive behaviour therapy, which has been shown to reduce the impact of negative emotions (see also Layard 2005);
- pleasant activity training helps us to identify the activities that make us happy and through practising them enhances our stock of positive emotions;
- mindfulness meditation, which involves helping people to focus on what is taking place at the moment in their internal and external environment has been shown to enhance subjective well-being and to reframe their problems positively.

And Seligman *et al.* (2005) highlights the positive impact on well-being of interventions that include:

- listing three good things that happen every day for a period of weeks;
- making gratitude visits to people who have helped you in life but who you have never properly thanked;
- practising one's signature strengths as a way of enhancing meaning in life.

Population level interventions

There are many programmes for preventing mental disorder in 'at risk' groups but these run the risk of stigmatizing the individuals targeted and miss the opportunity of improving mental health for all. Population level interventions are those that are regarded as desirable for everyone. Compulsory wearing of seat belts, fluoridation of drinking water and avoiding smoking are examples of such interventions to prevent physical illness. School-based interventions which teach children life skills, identify positive life goals, value the process of goal attainment rather than the outcome alone, and to find or create social support are the equivalent of these in preventing mental disorder. Huppert (2004) cites the *Going for Goal* programme for school children in Virginia as an example of a universal programme which incorporates many of these interventions (Danish 1996), and Greenberg *et al.* (1999) review universal school-based interventions for the prevention of mental disorders.

Huppert (2004) comments that most current population level interventions are for children and that few are reported for adults. An exception is positive parenting programmes, such as the Triple P (Positive Parent Program) programme for parents of pre-school children in Western Australia which Huppert writing in 2004 reports being taken up by over 4000 parents. Programme evaluation documents an increase in positive parenting and a reduction in punitive strategies, a decrease in the intensity and frequency of child problem behaviours, a reduction in parental anxiety stress and depression and an increase in relationship satisfaction. It has been estimated that if carried out at a universal level and all families took up the opportunity, Triple P would reduce the total proportion of children with substantial behaviour problems by a staggering 40 per cent (Lewis 1996). This level of success is unlikely to be achieved in practice because such programmes are likely to be taken up by a proportion of the pre-school parent population only, and probably by those who have a more positive approach to parenting than the average and so are unrepresentative of the population. For this reason Huppert (2004, 2005) concludes that interventions via the mass media, such as television and the Internet, potentially provide the best vehicle for delivering population-based interventions for the general adult population, possibly using principles of 'social marketing' through which product marketing principles are adopted to sell ideas, attitudes and behaviours which have social benefits (Box 35.1).

> ### Box 35.1   Population based intervention
>
> The Mental Health Foundation's 'Feeding Minds' campaign was designed as a population-based intervention using television, newspapers, magazines and the internet to raise public awareness of the relationship between food and mental health, and to equip people with strategies, ideas and recipes to support their mental health. It was undertaken in partnership with Sustain: the alliance for better food and farming. The key products for this campaign were a report on the relationship between food and mental health (MHF 2005), and web pages for the public that included mentally healthy recipes, top tips, personal stories, a nutrition table and web guide http://www.mentalhealth.org.uk/campaigns/food-and-mental-health/
>
> The Foundation's Director of Research, a mental health nurse, was at the forefront of this campaign in partnership with the Foundation's Chief Executive and their Director of Communications. The project's dissemination strategy used traditional media channels, which on the day of the report's launch included:
>
> - a broadsheet front page story (*Guardian* 16 January 2006)
> - 13 national television items featuring campaign staff
> - 16 national radio items featuring campaign staff
> - the website to support healthy eating.
>
> Subsequent to its launch the story was reported a further 19 times in national newspapers and 49 times in consumer and trade magazines. The report was downloaded from the Foundation's website 135,000 times in the three months following publication. Following this work the Big Lottery Fund (BLF) sought advice from the Foundation regarding a funding round. A total of £180 million was subsequently allocated by BLF to be spent on projects that addressed mental health, diet and exercise.

Huppert argues too that mental health promotion strategies should adopt a life-course approach, which ensures that parents of pre-school children are targeted, the children themselves, employers to create positive work environments which provide high levels of engagement, opportunities for autonomy, challenge, demonstrating competence and positive relationships and which combat negative stereotypes (e.g. of women, older people, ethnic minorities, people suffering from mental disorder) which damage well-being of people in these groups and limit their opportunities to thrive and demonstrate their potential.

Creating environments that promote flourishing

The focus of this section hitherto has been on interventions which involve individuals stepping forward to take the initiative to change their behaviour and attitudes and on delivering universal interventions to populations. A third approach to promoting mental health is to identify societal factors that influence our well-being and through public policy make changes to these to create environments in which more people can flourish. Dedicated programmes to tackle the stigma and discrimination surrounding mental health in England (*Shift*) and Scotland (*See Me*) are examples. The programme of work in England has included:

- a speakers' bureau to train and support people affected by mental health problems who can then contribute to training initiatives and talk to the media;
- a media alert system for people to give positive and negative feedback to journalists and their regulatory bodies;
- a partnership with Ofcom to monitor complaints about the portrayal of people with mental health problems in the media.

This chapter has demonstrated the close relationship between social structural aspects of inequality and mental ill health and, within this, the central role played by poverty in reinforcing vulnerability and diminishing resilience. Thus, in addition to helping people change their attitudes and behaviour it is crucial that nurses adopt a public mental health promotion role to address social structural inequalities; this is the focus of Chapter 3 by Friedli, and we would refer readers also to the National Institute for Mental Health's (2005) good practice guide to support the development and delivery of action to improve mental health and well-being in England.

Implications for mental health nursing

Most mental health nurses are working currently in recovery-oriented ways with individuals suffering from severe and enduring mental disorders and their families, and with service users with complex needs. This population is likely to continue to be the focus of nurses' work into the future, which raises the question of whether they ought to become involved in improving the mental health and well-being of the population as a whole, or should they leave this to others?

While working with mentally disordered individuals with complex needs will remain fundamental to the nurse's role, our argument in this chapter is that nurses of the future need to expand their professional horizons. There is good evidence that a shift in the positive mental health of the whole population will effectively reduce the number of people suffering from mental disorder and also, as Friedli reminds us in Chapter 3, mental health nurses' traditional focus on delivering individualized care could lead to nurses endorsing and reinforcing an inadequate 'disembodied psychology' which separates what goes on inside our clients' heads from their social and economic circumstances. Implications for nurses include:

- recovery-oriented work with mental health service users and their families;
- increased engagement in initiatives to:
    - reduce and eradicate poverty, which includes active commitment to promoting social inclusion (cf. Perkins and Repper, Chapter 5)
    - promote mental health for all, through interventions delivered to individuals and populations to change individual attitudes and behaviour.

Conclusion

This chapter has outlined the potential benefits for people suffering from mental disorder of increasing the positive mental health of the population as a whole and it has provided some pointers for mental health nurses who wish to move beyond working with individual mental health service users and their families, to promoting the mental health of the population as a whole through interventions to change attitudes and behaviour and to create environments under which people's mental health can flourish.

In summary, the main points are:

- There has been substantial improvement in mental health services across the UK over the past decade, subsequent to the National Service Framework for Mental Health (DH 1999) standards but there has been less progress on mental health promotion than in other standards.

- Mental health care has become recovery oriented, as reflected in recent reviews of mental health nursing, and many nurses are delivering evidence-based interventions in a recovery oriented way in their work with individual mental health service users and their families.

- Nursing remains very focused on the delivery of individualized care, in spite of evidence that improving the mental health of the population as a whole will reduce the proportion suffering from mental disorder.

- Positive psychology alerts us to the benefits of positive emotions for health and well-being, and for helping to explain why people thrive and flourish or show resilience in spite of negative events and adversity.

- But emotions are inevitably influenced by the circumstances of people's lives and so nurses need to work both at the level of the individual and of communities and society to address the key risk factors of mental illness – debt, poor housing, poverty and negative childhood experiences.

Questions for reflection and discussion

1 With reference to the evidence and/or logical argument discuss the following critiques of positive psychology:
    (a) The current preoccupation with 'happiness' is a self-indulgent concern of prosperous and comfortable people living in wealthy countries, and positive psychology is a movement for selling self-help to the 'worried well' (see White 2007);
    (b) Personality is not as flexible as positive psychologists suggest and they are naive if they think that a positive attitude can solve complex human problems (see Held 2005);
    (c) Measurement of subjective well-being and happiness is problematic, because happiness can involve self-deception, excessive optimism and an overestimation of control over life (see O'Neil 2006).

2 Reflect on the community in which you live and:
    (a) Make a note of any attitudes, behaviours or structural factors that promote a positive sense of mental health;
    (b) Make a note of any attitudes, behaviours or structural factors that threaten the mental health of the community;
    (c) What practical steps can you take in your own life to improve the mental health of people who you come across?
    (d) Identify public policies for your community that would create environments in which more people can flourish.

Annotated bibliography

- Huppert, F.A., Baylis, N. and Keverne, B. (eds) *The Science of Well-being*. Oxford: Oxford University Press. This landmark text draws together contributions from scholars of physiology, neuroscience, psychology, sociology and economics to provide a comprehensive summary of the scientific study of 'well-being', and so what we know currently about life characterized by health, vitality and fulfilment and the social relations and civic institutions required to foster and support these positive experiences.
- National Institute for Mental Health in England (NIMHE) (2005) *Making it Possible: Improving mental health and well-being in England*. Leeds: IMH/CSIP. Written for NIMH by Lynne Friedli, a contributor to this volume (see Chapter 3), this report documents good practice to improve mental health and well-being. It sets out a framework for action to: raise public awareness about how to safeguard our own and others' mental health; and mobilize communities and organizations to promote and protect mental well-being. There are plenty of practical examples here which nurses can draw on to develop their public health role.
- Positive Psychology Center website, University of Pennsylvania, USA http://www.ppc.sas.upenn.edu/. Professor Martin Seligman's positive psychology centre website provides an excellent resource for all interested in the therapeutic benefits offered by positive psychology, and also an opportunity to participate in his on-line research programme.

References

Appleby, L. (2004) *The National Service Framework for Mental Health – five years on.* London: Department of Health.

Appleby, L. (2007) *Mental Health Ten Years On: progress on mental health care reform.* London: Department of Health.

Bowlby, J. (1951) *Maternal Care and Mental Health.* Geneva: World Health Organization.

Brickman, P., Coates, D. and Janoff-Bulman, R. (1978) Lottery winners and accident victims: is happiness relative? *Journal of Personal and Social Psychology* **36**(8): 917–27.

Brimblecombe, N. and Tingle, A. (2007) National reviews of nursing: challenges, corrections and cynicism. Response to Brooker (2007) The Chief Nursing Officer's review of mental health nursing in England: an ode to 'motherhood and apple pie'? *International Journal of Nursing Studies* **44**: 857–8.

Brooker, C. (2007) Guest Editorial: The Chief Nursing Officer's review of mental health nursing in England: an ode to 'motherhood and apple pie'? *International Journal of Nursing Studies* **44**: 327–30.

Centre for Economic Performance's Mental Health Policy Group (2006) *The Depression Report: a new deal for depression and anxiety disorders.* London: London School of Economics and Political Science. http://cep.lse.ac.uk/textonly/research/mentalhealth/DEPRESSION_REPORT_LAYARD.pdf

Chief Nursing Officer (England) (2006) *Review of Mental Health Nursing: from values to action.* London: DH.

Chief Nursing Officer (Scotland) (2006) *Rights, Relationships and Recovery.* Edinburgh: Scottish Government Publications. http://www.scotland.gov.uk/Publications/2006/04/18164814/0

Danish, S.J. (1996) Going for goal: a life-skills program for adolescents, in G.W. Albee and T.P. Gullotta (eds) *Primary Prevention Works.* Newbury Park, CA: Sage Publications, pp. 291–312.

Department of Health (DH) (1999) *A National Service Framework for Mental Health.* London: DH.

Department of Health (DH) (2000) *NHS Plan.* London: DH.

Durkheim, E. (1897) *Le suicide.* Paris: Alcan.

Fredrickson, B.L. (2005) The broaden and build theory of positive emotions, in F. Huppert, N. Baylis and B. Keverne (eds) *The Science of Wellbeing.* Oxford: Oxford University Press, pp. 217–40.

Greenberg, M.T., Domitrovich, C. and Bumbarger, B. (1999) *Preventing Mental Disorders in School Age Children: a review of the effectiveness of prevention programmes.* Report for Center for Mental Health Services, US Department of Health and Human Services.

Harding, C.M., Brooks, G.W., Ashikaga, T., Strauss T.S. and Breier, A. (1987) The Vermont longitudinal study of persons with severe mental illness: long term outcome of subjects who retrospectively met DSM III criteria for schizophrenia. *American Journal of Psychiatry* **144**: 727–35.

Held, B.S. (2005) The 'virtues' of positive psychology. *Journal of Theoretical and Philosophical Psychology* **25**: 1–34.

Huppert, F.A. (2004) A population approach to positive psychology: the potential for population interventions to promote well-being and prevent disorder, in P.A. Linley and S. Joseph (eds) *Positive Psychology in Practice.* New York: John Wiley and Sons.

Huppert, F.A. (2005) Positive mental health in individuals and populations, in F.A. Huppert, N. Baylis and B. Keverne (eds) *The Science of Wellbeing.* Oxford: Oxford University Press, pp. 307–40.

Keyes, C.L.M. (2002) The mental health continuum: from languishing to flourishing in life. *Journal of Health and Social Research* **43**: 207–22.

Layard, R. (2005) *Happiness: lessons from a new science.* London: Allen Lane.

Levy, B., Hausdorff, J., Hencke, R. and Wie, J. (2000) Reducing cardiovascular stress with positive self-stereotypes of aging. *Journal of Gerontological Psychology* **55**: 205–13.

Lewis, J. (1996) *Triple-P Positive Parenting Programme: evidence based action in child health promotion.* Report of the Eastern Perth Public and Community Health Unit, Western Australia.

Lyubomirsky, S., King, L. and Diener, E. (2005) The benefits of frequent positive affect: does happiness lead to success? *Psychological Bulletin* **131**(6): 803–55. http://www.apa.org/journals/releases/bul1316803.pdf

Meaney, M.J. (2001) Maternal care, gene expression and the transmission of individual differences in stress reactivity across generations. *Annual Review of Neuroscience* **21**: 1161–92.

Mental Health Foundation (2005) *Feeding Minds: The impact of food on mental health.* London: MHF.

National Institute for Mental Health in England (2005) *Making it Possible: improving mental health and well-being in England.* NIMH, London.

O'Neil, J. (2006) Feature review. *New Political Economy* **11**: 447–50.

Ramon, S. (2007) Inequality in mental health: the relevance of current research and understanding to potentially effective social work responses. *Radical Psychology* **6**(1). http://www.radpsynet.org/journal/vol6-1/ramon.htm

Rogers, A. and Pilgrim, D. (2003) *Mental Health and Inequalities.* Basingstoke: Palgrave Macmillan.

Rose, G. (1992) *The Strategy of Preventive Medicine.* Oxford: Oxford University Press.

Seligman, M. (2002) *Authentic Happiness.* New York: Free Press.

Seligman, M.E.P., Steen, A., Park, N. and Peterson, C. (2005) Positive psychology progress: empirical validation of interventions. *American Psychologist* **60**: 410–21.

Sheldon, K.M. and Lyubomirsky, S. (2004) Achieving sustainable new happiness: prospects, practices and prescriptions, in P.A. Linley and S. Joseph (eds) *Positive Psychology in Practice.* New York: John Wiley and Sons.

UK Government (2005) *UK Government Strategy for Sustainable Development: Securing the future:* London: The Stationery Office.

White, A. (2007) A global projection of well-being: a challenge to positive psychology? *Psychtalk* **56**: 17–20.

Index

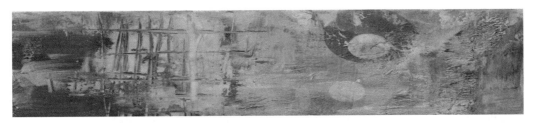

Mental Health and Well Being in Later Life

Mima Cattan

"This book's main contribution ... is to say to us all there is no single solution, no magic bullet, no instant cure, for the discomforts and illnesses of older age, and that not all ageing is comfortable. But it also tells us that it is in our control to do something about much of this, that older people's mental well-being could be vastly improved, and that public policy, and private attitudes, need to change. I hope that it is as influential as it deserves to be."

Taken from the foreword by Baroness Julia Neuberger, Former Chief Executive of the King's Fund and author of 'Not Dead Yet'

Mental health issues amongst older adults are becoming ever more prevalent. This fascinating book looks broadly at the mental health and well being issues that affect adults in later life. Taking a holistic approach to mental health and mental health promotion, the book explores the debates around what is meant by mental health and mental illness and the wider social determinants of mental health.

All chapters have a common thread running through them – each of which was identified as being a key theme for mental health and well-being by adults in later life. Among them are issues relating to:

- Gender
- Ethnicity
- Societal diversity
- Poverty
- Class
- Cultural differences

A range of examples from the UK and other countries, along with insights gained from older people's own perspectives, are used to emphasise the evidence base for effective interventions to promote mental health. Case studies, vignettes and quotes demonstrate how social theory and principles of health promotion can be effectively applied to improve practice.

Mental Health and Well Being in Later Life is key reading for those working or intending to work in public health, health promotion and health and social care professions, especially those who work with older people.

Contents: Introduction – What is mental health and mental well-being – Theoretical perspectives of ageing and health promotion – The application of policy and practice in the promotion of mental health and well-being in later life – Work, retirement and money – Relationships – Keeping active [physically and mentally] – Maintaining capability – Retaining independence and control

2009 184pp

ISBN-13: 978-0-335-22892-8   (ISBN-10: 0335-2-2892-5) Paperback
ISBN-13: 978-0-335-22891-1   (ISBN-10: 0335-2-2891-7) Hardback

Physical Health and Well-Being in Mental Health Nursing

Michael Nash

With recent evidence showing very high prevalence of ill-health amongst groups of mental health service users, this new text is extremely timely and will be valuable for all those working and studying in mental health.

The first book of its kind, this book considers the risk factors and assessment priorities amongst different mental health client groups and provides the necessary clinical insights into how best to work with service users to ensure their health is assessed and improved. It explores the impact of physical illness on people with severe mental illness, the current barriers and practice issues to good physical health and the core concepts of mental and physical health that should underpin practice – with the emphasis on providing the tools and insights to improve your own practice.

All of the chapters include case studies, examples, diagrams and exercises for self-testing and reflection. This is a must-have text for students and practitioners working in mental health nursing.

Contents: An introduction to physical health in mental illness – An introduction to key concepts in health and illness – A public health context to physical health in mental illness – General principles and approaches to physical assessment – Physical assessment – Medication side effects and physical health – Physical health emergencies in mental health settings – Practical steps in improving the physical health of people with severe mental illness

2009 232pp

ISBN-13: 978-0-335-23399-1   (ISBN-10: 033-5-23399-6) Paperback
ISBN-13: 978-0-335-23398-4   (ISBN-10: 033-5-23398-8) Hardback

Introduction to Mental Health Nursing

Nick Wrycraf

Full of insights into what it's like to be a mental health nursing student, including direct quotes from current students!

This engaging new textbook provides a student focused introduction to the main issues and themes in mental health nursing. The book requires no previous knowledge and the content has been carefully chosen to reflect the most significant aspects of this important and rewarding area of nursing.

The book includes specific chapters on:

- Social inclusion and the Ten Essential Shared Capabilities.
- Mental health promotion
- Mental health at different stages of the life course
- Physical health issues in mental health settings
- Mental health law
- Therapeutic interventions, specifically Cognitive Behavioural Therapy (CBT) and psychoanalytic/psychodynamic approaches
- The concept of recovery

Scenarios and exercises are used to demonstrate integration of theory and practice. These can be easily linked to your placement experience and overall learning and development. Readers are encouraged to develop an analytical and investigative approach to their studies.

Other important areas covered in the book include the National Service Framework (NSF) for Mental Health, the Care Programme Approach (CPA) and the Tidal Model of mental health nursing.

Introduction to Mental Health Nursing is the perfect introduction for all nursing students with an interest in a career in mental health nursing.

Contributors: *Geoffrey Amoateng, Amanda Blackhall, Alyson Buck, David A. Hingley, David Dean Holyoake, Richard Khoo, Mark McGrath, Mary Northrop, Tim Schafer, Julie Teatheredge, James Trueman, Henck Van- Bilsen, Steve Wood.*

Contents: Background to mental health nurse training – Learning on practice placements – Mental health and recognition of mental illness – Risk assessment: Practicing accountably and responsibly – Mental Health Nursing and the Law – Mental health promotion – Section 2 – Children and adolescent mental health – Adult mental health services in the community – Secure inpatient and forensic mental health care for adults – The mental health of older adults – Section 3 – Physical health issues in mental health practice – CBTN – Psychodynamic and psychoanalytic therapeutic interventions in mental health – Recovery – Social inclusion – Conclusion

2009 368pp

ISBN-13: 978-0-335-23358-8   (ISBN-10: 033-5-23358-9) Paperback
ISBN-13: 978-0-335-23357-1   (ISBN-10: 033-5-23357-0) Hardback

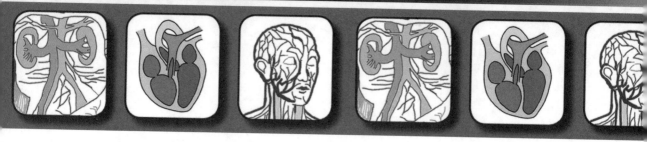
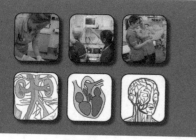
        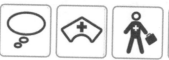